VOLUME NINETY THREE

ADVANCES IN PHARMACOLOGY

Behavioral Pharmacology of Drug Abuse: Current Status

VOLUME NINETY THREE

ADVANCES IN PHARMACOLOGY

Behavioral Pharmacology of Drug Abuse: Current Status

Edited by

JUN-XU LI
Jacobs School of Medicine & Biomedical Sciences, University at Buffalo, The State University of New York, NY, United States

ELSEVIER

ACADEMIC PRESS
An imprint of Elsevier

Academic Press is an imprint of Elsevier
50 Hampshire Street, 5th Floor, Cambridge, MA 02139, United States
525 B Street, Suite 1650, San Diego, CA 92101, United States
The Boulevard, Langford Lane, Kidlington, Oxford OX5 1GB, United Kingdom
125 London Wall, London, EC2Y 5AS, United Kingdom

First edition 2022

Notices

Knowledge and best practice in this field are constantly changing. As new research and experience broaden our understanding, changes in research methods, professional practices, or medical treatment may become necessary.

Practitioners and researchers must always rely on their own experience and knowledge in evaluating and using any information, methods, compounds, or experiments described herein. In using such information or methods they should be mindful of their own safety and the safety of others, including parties for whom they have a professional responsibility.

To the fullest extent of the law, neither the Publisher nor the authors, contributors, or editors, assume any liability for any injury and/or damage to persons or property as a matter of products liability, negligence or otherwise, or from any use or operation of any methods, products, instructions, or ideas contained in the material herein.

ISBN: 978-0-323-91526-7
ISSN: 1054-3589

For information on all Academic Press publications
visit our website at https://www.elsevier.com/books-and-journals

Publisher: Zoe Kruze
Developmental Editor: Jhon Michael Peñano
Production Project Manager: Vijayaraj Purushothaman
Cover Designer: Miles Hitchen

Typeset by STRAIVE, India

Contents

Contributors *ix*
Preface *xiii*

1. Interactions between opioids and stimulants: Behavioral pharmacology of abuse-related effects **1**

David R. Maguire and Vanessa Minervini

1. Introduction 2
2. Abuse-related effects of opioid/stimulant combinations 4
3. Conclusion 21

Acknowledgements 23
Conflict of interest 23
References 24

2. In vitro and in vivo pharmacology of kratom **35**

Takato Hiranita, Samuel Obeng, Abhisheak Sharma, Jenny L. Wilkerson, Christopher R. McCurdy, and Lance R. McMahon

1. Introduction 36
2. Pharmacodynamics of kratom alkaloids in vitro 38
3. Pharmacokinetics of kratom alkaloids 41
4. Behavioral effects of kratom alkaloids 50
5. Conclusion 65

Acknowledgments 66
Conflicts of interests or disclaimers 66
References 66

3. Human behavioral pharmacology of stimulant drugs: An update and narrative review **77**

Ashley Strzelecki, Jessica Weafer, and William W. Stoops

1. Introduction 78
2. Human behavioral pharmacology of cocaine 80
3. Human behavioral pharmacology of amphetamine 87
4. Conclusion 94

Conflict of interest 96
References 96

4. Human behavioral pharmacology of psychedelics **105**

Justin C. Strickland and Matthew W. Johnson

1. Introduction 106
2. Classic psychedelics 107
3. Special considerations 108
4. Psilocybin 113
5. LSD 119
6. DMT 123
7. Conclusion 125

Funding 126
Conflicts of interest 126
References 126

5. Stimulus functions of nicotine **133**

Mark G. LeSage

1. Introduction 134
2. Stimulus functions of nicotine 137
3. Role of stimulus functions in tobacco use theory 157
4. Conclusion 159

Acknowledgments 161
Conflict of interest statement 161
References 161

6. The incentive amplifying effects of nicotine: Roles in alcohol seeking and consumption **171**

Christopher P. King and Paul J. Meyer

1. Introduction 172
2. Appetitive effects of nicotine 174
3. Consummatory effects of nicotine 183
4. Neurobiological underpinnings of nicotine's reinforcing and incentive amplifying effects 188
5. Conclusion 197

Acknowledgments 200
Conflict of interest 200
References 200

7. Environmental influence on the preclinical evaluation of substance use disorder therapeutics **219**

Matthew L. Banks

1. Introduction 220
2. Drug dependence and withdrawal on candidate medication effectiveness 223

3. Schedule-related variables on candidate medication effectiveness 225
4. Subject housing variables on candidate medication effectiveness 230
5. Subject variables on candidate medication effectiveness 231
6. Conclusion 232
Acknowledgments 233
Conflicts of interest 233
References 234

8. Examining the effects of psychoactive drugs on complex behavioral processes in laboratory animals **243**

Brian D. Kangas

1. Introduction 244
2. Cognitive tasks in pharmacology 245
3. Caveats and considerations 262
4. On terms coda 263
5. Conclusion 264
Acknowledgments 265
Conflict of interest statement 265
References 265

9. Receptor mechanisms underlying the CNS effects of cannabinoids: CB_1 receptor and beyond **275**

Briana Hempel and Zheng-Xiong Xi

1. Introduction 276
2. Cannabinoid receptors 277
3. Cannabinoid tetrad effects 288
4. Cannabinoid subjective effects 299
5. Cannabinoid effects on anxiety 304
6. Cannabinoid cognitive effects 309
7. Conclusion 314
Acknowledgments 314
Conflict of interest 315
References 315

10. Potential therapeutic targets for the treatment of opioid abuse and pain **335**

Norikazu Kiguchi and Mei-Chuan Ko

1. Introduction 337
2. Opioid abuse 338
3. Pain 346
4. Treatment of pain by spinal and supraspinal actions 353

5. Conclusions 357
Acknowledgments 358
Conflict of interest 358
References 358

11. Trace amine-associated receptor 1 and drug abuse 373
Ruyan Wu, Jianfeng Liu, and Jun-Xu Li

1. Introduction 375
2. The implication of TAAR1 in the brain 376
3. Neural mechanisms of TAAR1 in drug addiction 378
4. TAAR1 and psychostimulants 386
5. TAAR1 and opioids 390
6. TAAR1 and alcohol 392
7. Current challenges 392
8. Conclusion 394

Acknowledgments 395
Conflict of interest 395
References 395

12. Substance abuse and neurotransmission 403
Sarah Davis and Jun Zhu

1. Introduction 404
2. Cocaine 406
3. Methamphetamine 409
4. Amphetamine 411
5. Opioids 412
6. Alcohol 417
7. Nicotine 419
8. Drugs of abuse and HIV-1 421
9. Considerations regarding COVID-19 423
10. Conclusion 423

Acknowledgments 424
Conflict of interest 424
References 424

Contributors

Matthew L. Banks
Department of Pharmacology and Toxicology, Virginia Commonwealth University School of Medicine, Richmond, VA, United States

Sarah Davis
Department of Drug Discovery and Biomedical Sciences, College of Pharmacy, University of South Carolina, Columbia, SC, United States

Briana Hempel
Addiction Biology Unit, Molecular Targets and Medications Discovery Branch, Intramural Research Program, National Institute on Drug Abuse, Baltimore, MD, United States

Takato Hiranita
Department of Pharmacodynamics, College of Pharmacy, University of Florida, Gainesville, FL, United States

Matthew W. Johnson
Department of Psychiatry and Behavioral Sciences, Johns Hopkins University School of Medicine, Baltimore, MD, United States

Brian D. Kangas
Behavioral Biology Program, McLean Hospital, Belmont; Department of Psychiatry, Harvard Medical School, Boston, MA, United States

Norikazu Kiguchi
Department of Physiological Sciences, School of Pharmaceutical Sciences, Wakayama Medical University, Wakayama, Japan

Christopher P. King
Department of Psychology; Clinical and Research Institute on Addictions, State University of New York at Buffalo, Buffalo, NY, United States

Mei-Chuan Ko
Department of Physiology and Pharmacology, Wake Forest University School of Medicine, Winston-Salem, NC, United States

Mark G. LeSage
Hennepin Healthcare Research Institute; Departments of Medicine, Pharmacology, and Psychology, University of Minnesota, Minneapolis, MN, United States

Jun-Xu Li
Department of Pharmacology and Toxicology, University at Buffalo, Buffalo, NY, United States

Jianfeng Liu
Department of Psychological and Brain Sciences, College of Liberal Arts, Texas A&M University, College Station, TX, United States

David R. Maguire
Department of Pharmacology; Addiction Research Treatment and Training Center of Excellence, University of Texas Health Science Center at San Antonio, San Antonio, TX, United States

Christopher R. McCurdy
Department of Medicinal Chemistry; Department of Pharmaceutics; Translational Drug Development Core, Clinical and Translational Sciences Institute, College of Pharmacy, University of Florida, Gainesville, FL, United States

Lance R. McMahon
Department of Pharmacodynamics, College of Pharmacy, University of Florida, Gainesville, FL, United States

Paul J. Meyer
Department of Psychology, State University of New York at Buffalo, Buffalo, NY, United States

Vanessa Minervini
Department of Psychological Science, Creighton University, Omaha, NE, United States

Samuel Obeng
Department of Pharmacodynamics; Department of Medicinal Chemistry, College of Pharmacy, University of Florida, Gainesville, FL, United States

Abhisheak Sharma
Department of Pharmaceutics; Translational Drug Development Core, Clinical and Translational Sciences Institute, College of Pharmacy, University of Florida, Gainesville, FL, United States

William W. Stoops
University of Kentucky, Department of Psychology; University of Kentucky, Department of Behavioral Science; University of Kentucky, Department of Psychiatry; University of Kentucky, Center on Drug and Alcohol Research, Lexington, KY, United States

Justin C. Strickland
Department of Psychiatry and Behavioral Sciences, Johns Hopkins University School of Medicine, Baltimore, MD, United States

Ashley Strzelecki
University of Kentucky, Department of Psychology, Lexington, KY, United States

Jessica Weafer
University of Kentucky, Department of Psychology, Lexington, KY, United States

Jenny L. Wilkerson
Department of Pharmacodynamics, College of Pharmacy, University of Florida, Gainesville, FL, United States

Ruyan Wu
Medical College of Yangzhou University, Yangzhou, China; Department of Pharmacology and Toxicology, University at Buffalo, Buffalo, NY, United States

Zheng-Xiong Xi
Addiction Biology Unit, Molecular Targets and Medications Discovery Branch, Intramural Research Program, National Institute on Drug Abuse, Baltimore, MD, United States

Jun Zhu
Department of Drug Discovery and Biomedical Sciences, College of Pharmacy, University of South Carolina, Columbia, SC, United States

Preface

Behavioral pharmacology as a unique and identifiable discipline is more than 65 years old. It is commonly recognized that the 1955 paper by Peter Dews entitled "Differential sensitivity to pentobarbital of pecking performance in pigeons depending upon the schedule of reward (*J Pharmacol Exp Ther*, 113(4): 393–401)" represents an important landmark as the birth of behavioral pharmacology. In that study, Dews showed for the first time that the sensitivity of pigeons to pentobarbital was determined by the level of operant performance (rate of pecking), which was controlled by different schedules of reinforcement. This was truly a groundbreaking discovery as never before had an environmental variable been found as a deciding factor to control an individual's sensitivity to a drug. In the past six decades, numerous behavioral scientists and pharmacologists have contributed tremendous amounts of work to foster the growth of behavioral pharmacology as an independent entity, which now has its own societies, scientific journals, and textbooks, and plays an indisputable role in the understanding of various brain disorders and the development of behavioral and pharmacological treatments.

One of the most extensively studied topics engaging behavioral pharmacologists has been drug abuse. Indeed, over the years, one clear observation I have made after examining the annual behavioral pharmacology society meeting agendas is that studies focusing on drug abuse claim the lion's share of the presentations. This probably is not surprising given the fact that drug abuse is in essence a behavioral disorder, and federal funding agencies have for decades been providing generous funding support toward the study of the mechanisms and treatment developments of drug abuse and dependence.

Behavioral pharmacology generally includes two types of research: the study of how drugs affect behavior and the behavioral analysis of drug actions. During its early era, many experimental psychologists were crucial players who were most interested in understanding the behavioral mechanisms of drug action. However, over the past several decades, pharmacologists interested in understanding the pharmacological mechanisms of psychoactive drugs (notably, drugs of abuse) have been dominating the field. In this regard, several prominent scientific questions attract the majority of scientific endeavors. For example, many scientists have spent decades to understand the pharmacological mechanisms of how drugs of abuse control behavior, the environmental influence on pharmacological actions of drugs of abuse, and the pharmacotherapy developments to treat drug dependence.

Quite a few books and monographs were published from the late 1960s to the late 1980s surveying the new developments of behavioral pharmacology. The popular series of *Advances in Behavioral Pharmacology,* of which all four volumes were coedited by Travis Thompson and Peter Dews, along with William McKim on Volume 3 and James Barrett on Volume 4, were published between 1977 and 1984. However, I know of no other published book that focuses on the behavioral pharmacology of drug abuse in the past 15 years. This volume of *Advances in Pharmacology* attempts to fill this void by providing an update on the current status of behavioral pharmacological research of drugs of abuse. The goal of the volume is not to offer a complete and comprehensive review of the discipline, which would require a much heavier volume. Instead, the volume provides a collection of expert reviews on select topics that we believe are the most relevant to modern behavioral pharmacology research. These selections include the application of quantitative pharmacological approaches in drug abuse research, the behavioral pharmacological evaluation of emerging drugs of abuse, the new developments in human behavioral pharmacology, the roles and contributions of environmental factors in drug abuse, drug target-based medication developments, and the incorporation of neurochemical mechanisms in the interpretation of drug effects on behavior. The topics covered in this volume are not limited to the traditional comfort zone of behavioral pharmacology because modern behavioral pharmacology research has evolved into much broader outreaches and applications; so, the volume intends to reflect that reality.

I am sincerely grateful to all the friends and colleagues who contributed to this volume, which I trust will be a useful reference source and, hopefully, an inspiration to scientists, be they novices in the field or seasoned experts.

Jun-Xu Li
Jacobs School of Medicine and Biomedical Sciences,
University at Buffalo, The State University of New York

CHAPTER ONE

Interactions between opioids and stimulants: Behavioral pharmacology of abuse-related effects

David R. Maguire[a,b,*] and Vanessa Minervini[c]

[a]Department of Pharmacology, University of Texas Health Science Center at San Antonio, San Antonio, TX, United States

[b]Addiction Research Treatment and Training Center of Excellence, University of Texas Health Science Center at San Antonio, San Antonio, TX, United States

[c]Department of Psychological Science, Creighton University, Omaha, NE, United States

*Corresponding author: e-mail address: maguired@uthscsa.edu

Contents

1. Introduction 2
2. Abuse-related effects of opioid/stimulant combinations 4
   2.1 Drug self-administration 4
   2.2 Reinstatement 10
   2.3 Drug discrimination 13
   2.4 Place conditioning 17
   2.5 Intracranial self-stimulation (ICSS) 20
3. Conclusion 21
Acknowledgements 23
Conflict of interest 23
References 24

Abstract

Opioid abuse continues to be a significant public health challenge, with rates of opioid-related overdose deaths increasing continuously over the last two decades. There also has been a sharp increase in overdose deaths involving stimulant drugs, primarily cocaine and methamphetamine. Recent estimates indicate a high prevalence of co-use of opioids and stimulants, which is a particularly complex problem. Behavioral pharmacology research over the last few decades has characterized interactions between opioids and stimulants as well as evaluated potential treatments. This chapter describes interactions between opioids and stimulants, with a focus on pre-clinical studies of abuse-related behavioral effects using self-administration, reinstatement, drug discrimination, place conditioning, and intracranial self-stimulation paradigms in laboratory animals. In general, the literature provides substantial evidence

Advances in Pharmacology, Volume 93
ISSN 1054-3589
https://doi.org/10.1016/bs.apha.2021.10.002

of mutual enhancement between opioids and stimulants for abuse-related effects, although such results are not ubiquitous. Enhanced abuse-related effects could manifest in many ways including engaging in drug seeking and taking behaviors with greater persistence, effort, and motivation and/or increased likelihood of relapse. Moreover, studies on opioid/stimulant combinations set the stage for evaluating potential treatments for polysubstance use. Behavioral pharmacology research has proven invaluable for elucidating these relationships using rigorous experimental designs and quantitative analyses of pharmacological and behavioral data.

Abbreviations

CTAP D-Phe-Cys-Tyr-D-Trp-Arg-Thr-Pen-Thr-NH2;
CTOP D-Phe-Cys-Tyr-D-Trp-Orn-Thr-Pen-Thr-NH2
ICSS intracranial self-stimulation
OUD opioid use disorder
NOP nociceptin/orphanin FQ peptide

1. Introduction

Nearly 300 million people worldwide use controlled substances for non-medical purposes, with 35 million people globally and close to 20 million in the United States likely meeting the criteria for a substance use disorder (SAMHSA, 2020; UNODC, 2019). Although drug misuse and abuse have long been significant public health challenges, opioids have become the primary focal point over the last two decades as rates of drug overdose deaths have increased dramatically (i.e., the opioid epidemic). In the United States, deaths involving opioids increased more than fivefold from 1999 to 2019, and, over the last several years, increased 60% from approximately 40,000 in 2016 to over 65,000 in 2020 (e.g., Ahmad, Rossen, & Sutton, 2021; Hedegaard, Miniño, & Warner, 2020). The severity of the opioid crisis has prompted official declarations of public health emergencies, resulting in deployment of substantial resources for treatment and prevention which include expanding access to medications for opioid use disorder (OUD) and opioid overdose, revising opioid prescribing guidelines, improving public health surveillance and data collection, increasing access to harm reduction programs such as safe injection sites, and increasing investments in research, treatment, and training.

Despite these heroic efforts, rates of drug overdose deaths continue to climb, in part, because the epidemic is not restricted to opioids. Although availability of highly potent and efficacious opioids such as fentanyl and related synthetic compounds continue to be key drivers (e.g., Mattson et al., 2021), other factors contribute to high rates of overdose deaths, particularly polysubstance use. In recent years, a majority of opioid overdose related deaths involved synthetic opioids such as fentanyl, 80% of which also involved other drugs or alcohol (e.g., Jones, Einstein, & Compton, 2018). Undoubtedly, many deaths involving synthetic opioids were the result of unintentional ingestion through a contaminated drug supply. Nevertheless, polysubstance use is highly prevalent, which significantly increases the risk of dangerous drug-drug interactions and complicates treatment. A majority of people meeting criteria for OUD often engage in co-occurring substance use and likely meet criteria for multiple substance use disorders (e.g., Crummy, O'Neal, Baskin, & Ferguson, 2020; Hassan & Le Foll, 2019; Jones & McCance-Katz, 2019; Mahoney et al., 2021; Zhu & Wu, 2020). In addition to increased overdose and mortality risk compared to single substance use, polysubstance use is associated with greater unmet health care needs, increased risky behavior, and higher rates of involvement in the criminal justice system; for individuals in treatment, polysubstance use is associated with poorer treatment outcomes, including lower treatment retention and higher rates of relapse.

Co-use of opioids and stimulants in particular has been an enduring problem. For example, in the United States, from the 1960s heroin was often used along with cocaine or amphetamine, commonly referred to as "speedballing." Cocaine and amphetamine use among heroin users not in treatment ranged from 30% to 80%, with approximately 50% of patients seeking treatment for OUD reporting co-use of a stimulant (reviewed in Leri, Bruneau, & Stewart, 2003). Combining heroin and cocaine or amphetamine is especially problematic because both drugs are often taken by intravenous injection which significantly increases risk of infectious diseases, poisoning, and cardiovascular disease. Concerns regarding use of opioids and stimulants have intensified over the past decade. In fact, use of opioids with other drugs, especially stimulants such as methamphetamine and cocaine, has contributed to the so-called fourth wave of the drug overdose epidemic (e.g., Ciccarone, 2021). Methamphetamine use has doubled in individuals with OUD that are seeking treatment, and the percentage of heroin users reporting recent use of methamphetamine has increased nearly fivefold (e.g., Ellis, Kasper, & Cicero, 2018; Strickland, Havens, & Stoops, 2019; Strickland, Stoops, Dunn, Smith, & Havens, 2021). While overdose deaths involving cocaine increased fourfold from 2009 to 2019, overdose deaths involving other psychostimulants (primarily methamphetamine) increased 10 fold, and nearly 50% of psychostimulant-related deaths involved an opioid (Jones, Underwood, & Compton, 2020; Kariisa, Scholl, Wilson, Seth, & Hoots, 2019).

Although the high prevalence of polysubstance use is not a new phenomenon (e.g., Peppin, Raffa, & Schatman, 2020), recent trends underscore the need for more effective treatment and prevention measures. Mitigation strategies targeting opioids alone likely are not sufficient to stem the tide of drug overdose deaths. Understanding factors that contribute to co-use of opioids and stimulants is critical for developing effective treatment and prevention strategies. Some effects, such as ratings of "drug liking" and "high," are often greater when mu opioid receptor agonists are administered in combination with stimulants than when either drug is given alone, yet other (e.g., physiological) effects of opioid/stimulant combinations can be mutually antagonistic (e.g., Foltin, Christiansen, Levin, & Fischman, 1995; Foltin & Fischman, 1992; Jasinski & Preston, 1986; Preston, Sullivan, Strain, & Bigelow, 1996; Walsh, Sullivan, Preston, Garner, & Bigelow, 1996). Behavioral pharmacology research has proven invaluable for characterizing the complex and dynamic interactions between opioids and stimulants as well as evaluating potential treatments. This chapter highlights contributions of behavioral pharmacology research to understanding interactions between opioids and stimulants with regard to abuse-related effects focusing on commonly used pre-clinical procedures, including drug self-administration, reinstatement, drug discrimination, conditioned place preference, and intracranial self-stimulation.

2. Abuse-related effects of opioid/stimulant combinations

2.1 Drug self-administration

Drug self-administration is considered the gold standard for assessing the abuse potential of drugs. In a typical arrangement, drug delivery is contingent on a response such that the subject determines if and when drug is delivered. Generally, drugs that are abused by humans also maintain reliable self-administration in laboratory animals (e.g., Johanson & Balster, 1978; O'Connor, Chapman, Butler, & Mead, 2011). Drug self-administration procedures are thought to have high predictive validity and have been used extensively to examine interactions between opioids and stimulants. In early studies, morphine maintained responding in monkeys trained to self-administer cocaine (e.g., Hoffmeister & Goldberg, 1973), demonstrating that an individual animal would self-administer both drugs. Monkeys with a history of codeine self-administration tended to have higher intake of a variety of drugs than those with a cocaine history, suggesting the reinforcing properties of some drugs might depend upon self-administration history (Hoffmeister & Schlichting, 1972; see also Leri, Flores, Rajabi, & Stewart, 2003; Ward, Läck, Morgan, & Roberts, 2006).

Studies also have examined interactions by giving one drug as a pretreatment before sessions in which another drug was available for self-administration. For example, morphine given as pre-session treatments decreased responding in monkeys working for cocaine but did so at doses of morphine that also decreased other overt behaviors (grooming, exploratory activity, locomotor activity and orienting responses), suggesting that some interactions might be the result of general (non-selective) suppression of behavior (Wilson & Schuster, 1973). In a later study (Winger, Skjoldager, & Woods, 1992), acute pre-session treatment with buprenorphine decreased self-administration of alfentanil and cocaine; however, much larger doses of buprenorphine were required to decrease responding for cocaine compared to responding for alfentanil. This study provided a demonstration of how different pharmacological activities of one drug could decrease self-administration of another. Buprenorphine, having high affinity for but relatively low efficacy at mu opioid receptors, likely blocked the reinforcing effects of alfentanil through competitive binding at mu opioid receptors, whereas effects of buprenorphine on cocaine self-administration might have been mediated by other mechanisms associated with larger doses. In contrast to buprenorphine, heroin also decreased self-administration of alfentanil and cocaine, but did so at equivalent doses, likely the result of the same (e.g., rate-suppressant) effects in each case. In rats, pretreatment with indirect-acting dopamine receptor agonists such as amphetamine enhanced responding for heroin, shifting the self-administration dose-effect curve leftwards, possibly indicating enhanced reinforcing effects; however, this effect was not specific to opioid self-administration which could be interpreted as a generalized rate-increasing effect (Hiranita et al., 2014). Chronic opioid treatment and opioid withdrawal have also been shown to alter cocaine self-administration. For example, daily treatment with fentanyl, morphine, nalbuphine, or buprenorphine attenuated cocaine self-administration in some studies (Gerak, Galici, & France, 2009; Lukas, Mello, Drieze, & Mendelson, 1995; Negus & Mello, 2002) but had little effect in others (Gerak, Galici, & France, 2008; Winger & Woods, 2001). Likewise, opioid withdrawal appeared to enhance the positive reinforcing effects of cocaine in monkeys (Gerak et al., 2009; Wade-Galuska, Galuska, & Winger, 2011) but not in rats (Cooper, Shi, & Woods, 2010; see also Seaman Jr & Collins, 2021).

Given the propensity of users to take opioids and stimulants in close temporal proximity, a significant amount of effort has gone toward understanding the nature of interactions when drugs are available for self-administration as mixtures. The strategy for selecting dose combinations varies across studies. In some cases, a fixed dose of one drug is paired with a range of doses of another drug whereas in other studies, the ratio of doses (e.g., 3:1, 1:1, 3:1, etc.) is fixed. Although the approach varies, it is clear that studying several dose pairings is optimal for characterizing interactions. One of the first published studies investigating self-administration of opioid/stimulant mixtures was conducted in monkeys (Mello et al., 1995). Heroin, cocaine, and heroin/cocaine mixtures maintained responding in a dose-related manner. Effects appeared to be additive in so far as combining relatively small unit doses of heroin and cocaine maintained higher levels of intake than that same unit dose of either drug alone; however, the maximal level of drug intake was not significantly greater than either drug alone. This study demonstrated that mixtures had positive reinforcing effects in nonhuman subjects and was among the first in a series of investigations across multiple laboratories attempting to characterize interactions. For example, in rats responding under a fixed-ratio schedule, addition of a fixed unit dose of heroin dose-dependently shifted the descending limb of the cocaine dose-effect curve downward suggesting that heroin increased the potency of cocaine to maintain responding (Hemby, Smith, & Dworkin, 1996; see also Smith, Co, Coller, Hemby, & Martin, 2006). Interestingly, although interactions for self-administration did not appear to be greater than additive, intake of heroin/cocaine mixtures doubled extracellular dopamine levels in the nucleus accumbens, compared to intake of cocaine alone, in a manner suggesting that effects of mixtures on dopamine signalling were synergistic (Hemby, Co, Dworkin, & Smith, 1999; Smith et al., 2006).

Various types of schedules have been employed to evaluate reinforcing effectiveness of opioid/stimulant mixtures. For example, under progressive ratio schedules, the number of responses required to obtain a reinforcer increases with successive reinforcer deliveries. Eventually the requirement grows so large that the individual fails to obtain a reinforcer; in that case, the last ratio completed (breakpoint) is taken as an index of reinforcing effectiveness. Generally, more effective reinforcers maintain higher breakpoints.

In a series of studies with rhesus monkeys responding under progressive ratio schedules, heroin/cocaine mixtures resulted in reciprocal increases in potency to maintain responding relative to either drug alone; that is, combining heroin with small doses of cocaine shifted the heroin dose-effect curve leftward and vice versa. However, combining heroin and cocaine did not maintain higher breakpoints than either drug alone, suggesting that although mixtures were more potent, they did not appear to be more effective reinforcers (Rowlett, Platt, Yao, & Spealman, 2007; Rowlett, Rodefer, & Spealman, 2005; Rowlett, Wilcox, & Woolverton, 1998; Rowlett & Woolverton, 1997). This interaction generalized to other mu opioid receptor agonists, alfentanil, etonitazene, and nalbuphine, varying in intrinsic efficacy at mu opioid receptors as well as to some direct- and indirect-acting dopamine receptor agonists (Achat-Mendes, Valdez, Platt, Rowlett, & Spealman, 2009; Rowlett et al., 2005; Rowlett et al., 2007). In rhesus monkeys responding for cocaine or the ultra-short acting mu opioid receptor agonist remifentanil, isobolographic analysis indicated that interactions between cocaine and remifentanil with regard to potency were either additive or supra-addictive depending on the ratio of remifentanil to cocaine; however, consistent with other studies, maximum breakpoints maintained by mixtures were not greater than those maintained by either drug alone (Woolverton, Wang, Vasterling, & Tallarida, 2008). Results in monkeys generalized to rats where the dose-effect curve for the heroin/cocaine mixtures were shifted leftward in a parallel manner compared to heroin or cocaine alone, consistent with an additive interaction, and the mixture did not maintain higher breakpoints than either drug alone (Duvauchelle, Sapoznik, & Kornetsky, 1998). Although many studies employing progressive-ratio schedules showed enhanced potency of reinforcing effects, others demonstrated what appeared to be enhanced reinforcing effectiveness as indicated by higher breakpoints. For example, in rats, mixtures of heroin with either cocaine or methamphetamine maintained higher breakpoints compared to cocaine or methamphetamine alone across a range unit doses, reflecting an upward shift in the dose-effect curve (Lacy, Strickland, Brophy, Witte, & Smith, 2014; Ranaldi & Munn, 1998; Ranaldi & Wise, 2000).

Another method used to investigate reinforcing effectiveness of opioid/stimulant mixtures is demand analysis based on principles of behavioral economics. Generally, consumption of a commodity decreases as its price increases, and the slope of the function relating consumption to price reflects demand elasticity, with shallower slopes, indicating less elasticity and, in the case of a self-administered drug, likely greater abuse potential (Hursh, Galuska, Winger, & Woods, 2005). Demand analyses have been utilized to evaluate reinforcing effectiveness of drugs of abuse, including combinations of opioids and stimulants. For example, in rhesus monkeys responding for cocaine or remifentanil, consumption of each drug decreased as the response requirement ("price") increased. When given a choice between cocaine and remifentanil, consumption of one drug offered at a fixed price increased as the response requirement for the other drug increased, indicating that these drugs served as economic substitutes (Wade-Galuska, Winger, & Woods, 2007). In rhesus monkeys responding for smoked heroin and/or cocaine, the demand function for a heroin/cocaine mixture was shifted upwards compared to the demand curve for either drug alone, indicating increased intensity of demand (i.e., higher drug intake at the lowest price); however, the slope of the demand function was not different. The parallel upward shift in the demand function was interpreted as an increase in reinforcing effects (Mattox, Thompson, & Carroll, 1997). On the other hand, another study showed that demand for remifentanil/cocaine mixtures delivered iv was not more inelastic than demand for either remifentanil or cocaine alone, suggesting that mixtures were not more effective reinforcers (Winger, Galuska, Hursh, & Woods, 2006; but see Rowlett et al., 2005). In a recent study (Crummy, Donckels, Baskin, Bentzley, & Ferguson, 2020), separate groups of rats were trained to self-administer cocaine only, heroin only, or cocaine and heroin on alternating days; demand for cocaine was higher than for heroin in rats that self-administered either cocaine or heroin but not for rats with a history of self-administering both.

Choice procedures also have been used to investigate interactions between opioids and stimulants. Under choice procedures, subjects choose between two or more alternatives with the primary measure of reinforcing effects being based on allocation of behavior among the alternatives rather than overall response output (i.e., response rate). In rhesus monkeys responding under concurrent fixed-ratio schedules, choosing between iv infusions and food, heroin, cocaine, and heroin/cocaine mixtures dose-dependently increased choice over food, and dose-effect curves for heroin/cocaine mixtures generally were shifted left of curves for either drug alone, again suggesting increased potency with drug mixtures. According to dose-addition analyses, interactions for choice were sub-additive or additive, depending on the ratio of heroin to cocaine, but not synergistic (Negus, 2005). Interestingly, the nature of the interactions differed across endpoints with effects of some mixtures being sub-additive for choice but additive for response rate measures. Rhesus monkeys responding under a concurrent schedule for iv infusions preferred remifentanil/cocaine mixtures to a dose of cocaine alone that was predicted to be equally reinforcing based on dose addition, suggesting that mixtures are more effective reinforcers (Freeman & Woolverton, 2011; see also Gerak, Weed, Maguire, & France, 2019). In rhesus monkeys responding under single alternative fixed-ratio schedules for oral drug solutions, response rates maintained by cocaine or methadone/cocaine mixtures were similar when compared across sessions; however, when responding under concurrent fixed-ratio schedules for oral drug solutions, monkeys often (>80% of comparisons) preferred methadone/cocaine mixtures over either of the constituent drugs alone, suggesting that the mixture had greater reinforcing effects (Wang, Brown, Grabowski, & Meisch, 2001). Likewise, in rats responding under a progressive ratio schedule for iv infusions, breakpoints maintained by heroin/cocaine mixtures were not different from breakpoints for cocaine alone; however, in rats responding under a concurrent schedule for iv infusions, heroin/cocaine mixtures were preferred over a larger dose of cocaine available alone (Ward, Morgan, & Roberts, 2005).

Establishing self-administration of opioid/stimulant mixtures set the stage for exploring underlying pharmacological mechanisms as well as evaluating potential treatments. Mu opioid receptor antagonists such as naloxone, naltrexone, and quadazocine attenuate self-administration of heroin but not cocaine (e.g., Maguire et al., 2019; Winger et al., 1992), whereas dopamine receptor antagonists such as flupenthixol attenuate reinforcing effects of cocaine but not heroin (e.g., Ettenberg, Pettit, Bloom, & Koob, 1982). In addition to establishing pharmacological selectivity, these studies also demonstrated that antagonists acting at either mu opioid or dopamine receptors alone are unlikely to serve as pharmacological treatments across drug classes (e.g., using a mu opioid receptor antagonist to treat stimulant use disorder), and, therefore, might not be effective for treating polysubstance abuse. This is consistent with studies examining effects of selective antagonists on responding maintained by drug mixtures. For example, opioid receptor antagonists such as naltrexone blocked responding for opioids when available alone and in a mixture with cocaine at doses that did not alter responding for cocaine alone. Generally, opioid receptor antagonists shifted the heroin/cocaine mixture dose-effect curve back to a pattern resembling cocaine alone, and the dopamine receptor antagonist eticlopride selectively attenuated effects of cocaine in a mixture (e.g., Hemby et al., 1996; Martin, Coller, Co, & Smith, 2008).

In rats responding under a progressive ratio schedule for a heroin/cocaine mixture, injection of a combination of the dopamine D1 receptor antagonist SCH 23390 and the mu opioid receptor antagonist CTOP into the nucleus accumbens reduced breakpoints without affecting locomotor activity, presumably because a small dose of the mu opioid receptor antagonist and a small dose of the dopamine receptor antagonist sufficiently blocked reinforcing effects of the heroin and the cocaine, respectively (Cornish, Lontos, Clemens, & McGregor, 2005). In rhesus monkeys, a combination of the dopamine receptor antagonist flupentixol and the opioid receptor antagonist quadazocine selectively decreased self-administration of heroin/cocaine mixtures, shifting the mixture dose-effect curve rightward without altering food-maintained responding (Mello & Negus, 1999; see also Mello & Negus, 1998). In these studies, combination treatments comprised doses of the constituent drugs which were ineffective when administered alone, suggesting that relatively small doses of potential medications could be combined to produce sufficient therapeutic effects while avoiding adverse effects associated with larger doses of either drug.

Taken together, studies on self-administration of opioid/stimulant mixtures often indicate mutual enhancement of reinforcing effects. In a majority of cases, combining opioids and stimulants increased potency to produce reinforcing effects in so far as combinations of small doses of each drug maintained levels of responding equivalent to levels maintained by larger doses of each constituent drug alone. However, there are some examples of enhanced reinforcing effectiveness indicated by higher breakpoints under progressive ratio schedules and choice of drug mixtures over larger doses of either constituent drug alone. Importantly, studies with drug mixtures have also established conditions for evaluating potential pharmacological treatments for co-abuse of opioids and stimulants.

2.2 Reinstatement

Although understanding factors that maintain ongoing drug taking is critical, resumption of drug taking following a period of abstinence (relapse) remains a key hurdle for successful treatment of substance use disorders. Reinstatement procedures emerged as an efficient method for studying relapse-related processes. After self-administration of a drug (or drug mixture) is established, access to the drug is discontinued for a period of time and conditions are presented that prompt resumption of drug-taking behavior. Reinstatement procedures are thought to be relevant to relapse because stimuli such as non-contingent drug administration (priming), presentation of drug-paired cues and contexts, and stress tend to reinstate responding previously maintained by drug delivery. These types of stimuli appear similar to factors that influence relapse in individuals with substance use disorders, so the model is considered to have reasonable face validity (e.g., Epstein, Preston, Stewart, & Shaham, 2006). Reinstatement procedures have been used extensively, including to characterize the interactions between opioids and stimulants.

Initial studies using reinstatement procedures in subjects with a history of drug self-administration suggested that reinstatement was pharmacologically selective. For example, cocaine and amphetamine dose-dependently reinstated responding in rats trained to self-administer cocaine (de Wit & Stewart, 1981), and heroin and morphine dose-dependently reinstated responding in rats trained to self-administer heroin (de Wit & Stewart, 1983). However, findings of "cross-reinstatement" between opioids and stimulants have been reported, likely owing to common neurobiological mechanisms involved (e.g., Stewart, 2000). Indeed, amphetamine and cocaine reinstated responding in animals trained to self-administer an opioid (de Vries, Schoffelmeer, Binnekade, Mulder, & Vanderschuren, 1998; de Wit & Stewart, 1983; Stewart & Vezina, 1988) and morphine reinstated responding in rats that self-administered cocaine (Stewart, 1984). However, although cross-reinstatement can occur, it is not always consistent (e.g., reviewed by Shalev, Grimm, & Shaham, 2002). For example, amphetamine produced some, albeit very modest, reinstatement in rats that self-administered heroin, while cocaine was without effect (de Wit & Stewart, 1983). Likewise, morphine produced weak reinstatement of cocaine-maintained responding while heroin was ineffective (de Wit & Stewart, 1981). Later studies also demonstrated that several opioids such as morphine, buprenorphine, and butorphanol failed to reinstate responding previously maintained by cocaine (e.g., Comer, Lac, Curtis, & Carroll, 1993; de Vries et al., 1998; Lynch, Heaser, & Carroll, 1998; Schenk & Partridge, 1999). Whether cross-reinstatement occurs depends on a number of factors including the time since the last self-administration session (e.g., de Vries, Schoffelmeer, Binnekade, Raasø, & Vanderschuren, 2002; de Vries, Schoffelmeer, Binnekade, & Vanderschuren, 1999; Lu & Dempsey, 2004) and drug history. For example, drugs that reinstate responding often produce locomotor sensitization and vice versa, suggesting an important relationship between drug-induced reinstatement and sensitization (de Vries et al., 1999; Vanderschuren, Schoffelmeer, Mulder, & de Vries, 1999).

There are also reports of drugs from one pharmacological class preventing reinstatement of responding previously maintained by a drug from another. For example, buprenorphine, butorphanol, and methadone attenuated cocaine-primed reinstatement of responding previously maintained by cocaine (Comer et al., 1993; Leri, Tremblay, Sorge, & Stewart, 2004; Lynch et al., 1998; Sorge, Rajabi, & Stewart, 2005). However, some opioids are not as effective. For example, although the high efficacy mu opioid receptor agonist etonitazene partially attenuated cocaine-primed reinstatement, it did so only at very large doses (Comer et al., 1993). Morphine decreased ongoing self-administration of cocaine in rats but failed to alter cocaine-primed reinstatement (Lynch et al., 1998).

Relatively few studies have examined reinstatement in animals with a history of self-administering opioids and stimulants either sequentially or as mixtures, although a series of studies demonstrated distinct patterns of reinstatement could be established within the individual subjects. For example, in rats trained to self-administer heroin and cocaine in separate sessions, heroin selectively reinstated responding directed toward the lever and conditioned stimuli previously associated with heroin, whereas cocaine selectively reinstated responding directed toward the lever and conditioned stimuli associated with cocaine, demonstrating a high degree of stimulus control within subject (Leri et al., 2004; Leri & Stewart, 2001; Sorge et al., 2005). The propensity of heroin and cocaine to reinstate responding appears to be differentially modulated by context in so far as cocaine reinstated responding more effectively in rats that self-administered cocaine in an environment that was distinct from the home cage, whereas heroin reinstated responding more effectively in rats that self-administered heroin in their home cage (Montanari et al., 2015). Although effects of drug-primed reinstatement varied, cue-induced reinstatement did not differ between rats that self-administered a single drug (cocaine or heroin) and rats that self-administered cocaine and heroin across alternating sessions (Crummy, Donckels, et al., 2020), and re-exposure to the drug self-administration context resulted in renewal of responding that did not differ between rats with a history of self-administering a heroin/cocaine mixture compared to rats that self-administered cocaine only (Crombag, Grimm, & Shaham, 2002; Crombag & Shaham, 2002). One study examined the potential therapeutic effects of the α2A adrenergic receptor agonist lofexidine, which was approved to treat opioid withdrawal, on reinstatement of responding in rats trained to self-administer a mixture of heroin and cocaine (Highfield, Yap, Grimm, Shalev, & Shaham, 2001);

although lofexidine did not alter ongoing self-administration of the combination or extinction of responding, it decreased footshock- but not cue-induced reinstatement of responding.

Results from studies with reinstatement indicate that opioids and stimulants can produce some degree of cross-reinstatement; however, the relationship appears to be asymmetrical in so far as stimulants are more likely to reinstate opioid-maintained responding than vice versa (Shalev et al., 2002). Other studies have shown that drugs from one pharmacological class can attenuate reinstatement produced by drugs from another class; however, interactions are not always consistent across studies. Cross-reinstatement has significant implications for risk of relapse to drug taking. For example, an abstinent individual with a history of OUD might be at a high risk of relapse following ingestion of a stimulant.

2.3 Drug discrimination

Drug discrimination is an operant conditioning procedure often used alongside self-administration procedures to characterize abuse-related effects of drugs (see Swedberg, 2016; Bolin et al., 2018 for recent reviews). In a typical experiment, subjects are trained to discriminate the injection of a particular dose of drug ("training drug") from the injection of the drug vehicle using differential reinforcement. After stimulus control is established (i.e., the subject reliably emits an injection-appropriate response), tests occur during which different doses of the training drug, other drugs, or drug combinations are administered. The distribution of responses during test conditions reflects similarity of the test injection to the training stimulus. Drug discrimination performance is pharmacologically selective in so far as drugs with pharmacological properties similar to those of the training drug will occasion drug-appropriate responding whereas drugs that are not pharmacologically similar will occasion responding on the other alternative. Although having discriminative stimulus effects per se is not indicative of abuse potential, drugs that share discriminative stimulus effects with commonly abused drugs are also likely to have abuse potential. In general, there have been two types of studies examining interactions between opioids and stimulants with regard to discriminative stimulus effects. The first includes substitution tests that determine whether a drug from one pharmacological class produces discriminative stimulus effects similar to those of drugs from another class, that is, whether opioids and stimulants share discriminative stimulus effects. The second examined discriminative stimulus effects of drugs given in combination to determine whether addition of one drug modifies the discriminative stimulus effects of another, that is, whether opioids modify the discriminative stimulus effects of stimulants and vice versa.

In many studies, stimulants fail to substitute in subjects trained to discriminate an opioid, and opioids fail to substitute in subjects trained to discriminate a stimulant, reflecting a high degree of pharmacological selectivity. However, full cross-substitution at the group level has been reported albeit rarely (e.g., Shannon & Holtzman, 1979). Interestingly, full cross-substitution between opioids and stimulants is not uncommon when examining the response of individual subjects. Cocaine and amphetamine have been reported to occasion significant drug-appropriate responding in subjects trained to discriminate an opioid and vice versa (e.g., Colpaert, Niemegeers, & Janssen, 1980; Cook & Picker, 1998; Platt, Rowlett, & Spealman, 2010; Spealman & Bergman, 1992; Zhang, Walker, Sutherland 2nd, & Young, 2000). However, when averaged for the group, results tend to show partial substitution, which is typically defined as 20%–80% drug-appropriate responding. Although not robust, there is clear evidence of overlap between the discriminative stimulus effects of opioids and stimulants, with at least one third of studies reporting full cross-substitution in a subset of subjects. This sort of partial substitution at the group level occurs in most species tested (rats, pigeons, squirrel monkeys, rhesus monkeys, and cats [Kilbey & Ellinwood, 1979]) and in both opioid- and stimulant-trained subjects. For example, cocaine substituted in two of six rats trained to discriminate heroin (Lamas, Negus, Gatch, & Mello, 1998), and cocaine, amphetamine, and GBR12909 increased drug-lever responding in three of five squirrel monkeys trained to discriminate morphine (Platt, Grech, Rowlett, & Spealman, 1999). Likewise, morphine increased drug-appropriate responding in approximately half of rats discriminating amphetamine or cocaine (Colpaert, Niemegeers, & Janssen, 1979; Hernandez, Holohean, & Appel, 1978), and opioids increased drug-appropriate responding in 25-50% of non-human primates (squirrel and rhesus monkeys) trained to discriminate cocaine (e.g., Mello et al., 1995; Rowlett & Spealman, 1998).

It remains unclear why cross-substitution occurs in some individuals; however, training dose appears to be an important determinant. For example, amphetamine produced greater than 90% drug-lever responding, on average, in rats trained to discriminate a relatively small dose of morphine (1.75 mg/kg) but little more than 10% drug-lever responding in rats trained to discriminate a larger dose (5.6 mg/kg) (Shannon & Holtzman, 1979). Likewise, in groups of rats trained to discriminate different doses of fentanyl (0.005–0.04 mg/kg), amphetamine produced a maximum of 30% drug-lever responding in any group, and the maximum level of responding averaged for the group was inversely related to fentanyl training dose (Colpaert et al., 1980).

A majority of studies examining discriminative stimulus effects of opioid/stimulant mixtures did so by testing drug combinations in subjects trained to discriminate either an opioid or a stimulant. Results are mixed with regards to the nature of the interaction; however, more than half of the studies demonstrate mutual enhancement of discriminative stimulus effects. For example, amphetamine and cocaine potentiated the discriminative stimulus effects of morphine in rats, pigeons, and squirrels monkeys trained to discriminate morphine (e.g., Gaiardi, Bartoletti, Gubellini, Bacchi, & Babbini, 1998; Gauvin & Young, 1989; Platt et al., 1999), and several studies have shown that opioids can enhance the discriminative stimulus effects of cocaine and amphetamine (e.g., Dykstra, Doty, Johnson, & Picker, 1992; Kamien & Spealman, 1991; Negus, Gatch, & Mello, 1998a; Platt et al., 2010; Spealman & Bergman, 1992; Suzuki et al., 1997). However, there are studies showing no apparent interaction (Cook & Picker, 1998; Lamas et al., 1998; Wood & Emmett-Oglesby, 1986) or even attenuation of discriminative stimulus effects (e.g., Gauvin & Young, 1989; Platt et al., 2010; Young, Masaki, & Geula, 1992).

In one study (Negus, Gatch, & Mello, 1998b), three rhesus monkeys were trained to discriminate a 10:1 mixture of cocaine (0.4 mg/kg) to heroin (0.04 mg/kg) from the vehicle. In substitution tests, cocaine alone, heroin alone, as well as cocaine/heroin mixtures (ratios ranging from 3:1 to 30:1 cocaine:heroin) increased drug-lever responding above 80%, though heroin alone only did so at doses that produced very low rates of responding. Amphetamine, alfentanil, and fentanyl alone as well as a 10:1 mixture of amphetamine and morphine also increased drug-lever responding. Effects of the cocaine/heroin mixture were blocked by pretreatment comprising a combination of the dopamine receptor agonist flupenthixol and the opioid receptor antagonist quadazocine at doses that alone were ineffective. Taken together, these findings suggest that a combination of cocaine and heroin produces a discriminative stimulus complex that includes aspects of both constituent drugs.

Interestingly, many of the same patterns that emerged for substitution tests also applied to drug-combination tests. For example, when combinations showed altered (enhanced or attenuated) discriminative stimulus effects compared to drugs alone, the magnitude and direction of the change was related to the dose of the training drug. Across groups of pigeons discriminating different doses of morphine, relatively small doses of amphetamine potentiated whereas larger doses attenuated the discriminative stimulus effects of morphine, and the magnitude of change in either direction was inversely related to training dose (Gauvin & Young, 1989). In rats trained to discriminate either a low (3.2 mg/kg) or a higher (5.6 mg/kg) dose of morphine, amphetamine attenuated the discriminative stimulus effects of the training dose of morphine in the low- but not high-training dose group (Young et al., 1992), and in rats trained to discriminate either a low (3 mg/kg) or a high (10 mg/kg) dose of cocaine, morphine enhanced effects of cocaine in the low but not high training-dose group (Kantak, Riberdy, & Spealman, 1999).

Whether a stimulant enhanced the discriminative stimulus effects of an opioid in an opioid-trained individual was related to the substitution profile of stimulants in that individual. For example, in squirrel monkeys trained to discriminate morphine, cocaine and amphetamine enhanced the discriminative stimulus effects of morphine, but only in the three monkeys for which cocaine and amphetamine increased drug-appropriate responding when tested alone; amphetamine and cocaine attenuated effects of morphine in the remaining two monkeys for which they did not substitute (Platt et al., 1999). In squirrel monkeys discriminating cocaine, heroin shifted the dose-response curves for cocaine and the dopamine transporter blocker GBR 12909 leftward in the three monkeys for which heroin engendered cocaine-lever responding but not in the other two monkeys (Rowlett, Spealman, & Platt, 2001). Similarly, in rhesus monkeys discriminating cocaine, morphine, fentanyl, and nalbuphine enhanced the discriminative stimulus effects of cocaine, and in some cases, amphetamine (Negus et al., 1998a; Negus & Mello, 2002).

Studies examining interactions using drug discrimination procedures demonstrate many cases of cross-substitution and mutual enhancement of the discriminative stimulus effects of opioids and stimulants. Especially interesting are patterns of inter-subject variability whereby some individuals clearly show cross-substitution (and often enhancement of discriminative stimulus effects) whereas others do not. As with reinstatement of drug taking behavior, cross substitution of discriminative stimulus effects produced by one drug class might prompt behavior associated with another drug class. Enhanced discriminative stimulus effects might contribute to increased co-use of opioids and stimulants. Whether these patterns of interaction extend to other classes of drugs is unclear but worthy of additional consideration.

2.4 Place conditioning

Place conditioning procedures have been used extensively to evaluate abuse-related effects of drugs as well as interactions between opioids and stimulants. Place conditioning is a Pavlovian discrimination procedure wherein the subject is exposed to one context paired with presentation of an unconditioned stimulus (e.g., drug) and exposed to another distinct context in its absence (e.g., vehicle). After several pairings, test sessions occur in the absence of the unconditioned stimulus during which subjects have unrestricted access to both contexts, and time spent in the context paired with the unconditioned stimulus relative to the other reflects the "hedonic value" of the stimulus. If the unconditioned stimulus has rewarding properties, subjects spend more time in the drug-paired context (i.e., "preference"), whereas if the unconditioned stimulus has aversive properties, subjects spend less time in the drug-paired context (i.e., "aversion"). There is high correspondence between drugs that induce a place preference and those that maintain self-administration (e.g., Bardo & Bevins, 2000). Interactions between opioids and stimulants also have been studied using place conditioning procedures in which subjects are exposed to one drug prior to conditioning with another as well as co-administration of drugs during conditioning.

Administration of amphetamine or cocaine in the days prior to conditioning enhanced morphine place preference and vice versa (Lett, 1989; Shippenberg & Heidbreder, 1995; Shippenberg, Heidbreder, & Lefevour, 1996; Shippenberg, LeFevour, & Thompson, 1998). The treatment regimens employed in those studies also produced behavioral sensitization (e.g., enhanced locomotor effects) which might contribute to enhanced place conditioning. In contrast, repeated drug treatment regimens that result in tolerance did not produce the same interaction. For example, chronic morphine treatment before conditioning, which was sufficient to produce tolerance to morphine and fentanyl place conditioning, failed to alter amphetamine place preference (Shippenberg, Emmett-Oglesby, Ayesta, & Herz, 1988), further supporting the notion that cross-sensitization might play an important role in opioid/stimulant interactions. Interestingly, daily treatment with buprenorphine or continuous infusion of methadone via osmotic mini-pumps prior to or after conditioning attenuated cocaine place preference, suggesting that these opioids, which are mainstays of treatment for OUD, block acquisition and/or expression of stimulant place conditioning when given under the right conditions (Kosten, Marby, & Nestler, 1991; Leri, Zhou, Goddard, Cummins, & Kreek, 2006). The facilitatory effects of amphetamine also depend critically on timing of injections. In rats, amphetamine administered immediately, but not 6 h, after conditioning sessions enhanced morphine place preference; the authors reasoned that effects of amphetamine might depend on enhanced memory consolidation (Blaiss & Janak, 2006).

Other studies demonstrated that drug treatments occurring during critical developmental periods can have long-lasting effects. For example, prenatal exposure to buprenorphine (but not morphine or methadone) enhanced methamphetamine place conditioning in rats trained during adulthood (Chiang, Hung, & Ho, 2014). Rats treated daily with methylphenidate during the preweanling period (post-natal days 10–20; Crawford et al., 2007) or treated daily with mephedrone during adolescence (post-natal days 30–36; Joanna et al., 2017) before conditioning exhibited enhanced morphine place preference. On the other hand, although rats exposed prenatally to morphine showed normal levels of methamphetamine place preference, the place preference was more resistant to extinction and showed more robust reinstatement when primed with methamphetamine (Shen et al., 2016).

Combining an opioid receptor agonist with stimulants such as cocaine, amphetamine, or methamphetamine during conditioning generally results in enhanced place preference indicated by greater potency and/or maximal effect (Bilsky, Montegut, Delong, & Reid, 1992; Brown, Finlay, Wong, Damsma, & Fibiger, 1991; Lan, Chang, Liu, Ho, & Lin-Shiau, 2009; Masukawa, Suzuki, & Misawa, 1993). Buprenorphine also potentiated cocaine-induced increases in extracellular dopamine concentration in a greater-than-additive manner supporting the notion that increased dopamine transmission contributes to enhanced place conditioning (Brown et al., 1991). Interestingly, a buprenorphine analog with a similar pharmacological profile to buprenorphine, BU08028, administered during conditioning did not alter cocaine place conditioning (Khroyan et al., 2011). Just as opioids and stimulants have been shown to produce mutual enhancement of conditioned place preferences, effects of opioid or dopamine receptor antagonists demonstrate involvement of opioid receptors in stimulant place conditioning and vice versa. Dopamine receptor antagonists such as haloperidol as well as the D1 receptor antagonist SCH23390 (but not the dopamine D2 receptor antagonists sulpiride or spiperone) have frequently been shown to attenuate morphine and heroin place conditioning (Leone & Di Chiara, 1987; Schwartz & Marchok, 1974; Shippenberg & Herz, 1987; Shippenberg & Herz, 1988; Spyraki, Fibiger, & Phillips, 1983). Consistent with a role of dopamine D1 receptors in opioid place conditioning, D1 (but not D3) receptor knockout mice failed to acquire morphine place preference (Wang et al., 2015). Likewise, opioid receptor antagonists such as naloxone, naltrexone, and CTAP have been shown to attenuate cocaine, amphetamine, and methylphenidate place preferences (Bilsky et al., 1992; Horner, Logan, Fisher, & Logue, 2017; Soderman & Unterwald, 2008; Trujillo, Belluzzi, & Stein, 1991; Zhu, Spencer, Liu-Chen, Biederman, & Bhide, 2011; but see Häggkvist, Lindholm, & Franck, 2009). Also, naloxone administered during conditioning enhanced extinction of cocaine place preference (Houdi, Bardo, & Van Loon, 1989). In contrast to the prototypical opioid receptor antagonists, BU10119, a buprenorphine analog with antagonist properties at mu and kappa opioid receptors as well as partial agonist properties at nociceptin/orphanin FQ peptide (NOP) receptors, administered during conditioning did not alter cocaine place preference (Hillhouse et al., 2021), even though it prevented reinstatement of cocaine place preference (see below).

Reinstatement of place conditioning is similar in some respects to reinstatement of drug self-administration and is also thought to reflect the extent to which drug exposure, presentation of drug-paired cues, or certain contexts induce drug-associated behaviors following a drug-free period. Compared to reinstatement of drug-maintained responding, studies on interactions between opioids and stimulants with regards to reinstatement of conditioned place preference are much more limited. One study showed that cocaine and amphetamine reinstated morphine place preference in mice (Ribeiro Do Couto, Aguilar, Rodríguez-Arias, & Miñarro, 2005), suggesting cross-reinstatement with regard to place preferences. A recent study also showed that the novel, multi-functional buprenorphine analog BU12004 (but not buprenorphine itself) reinstated cocaine place preference when administered alone (Hillhouse et al., 2021). Although studies are limited, effects of pretreatments on drug-primed reinstatement show a complicated pattern. For example, naltrexone blocked methamphetamine-primed reinstatement of methamphetamine place preference in one study (Guo et al., 2019); however, neither naloxone nor naltrexone prevented amphetamine- or cocaine-primed reinstatement of amphetamine and cocaine place preference, respectively, in other studies (Häggkvist et al., 2009; Hillhouse et al., 2021). A combination of buprenorphine and naltrexone, which alone did not elicit place conditioning, blocked cocaine primed reinstatement of cocaine place preference (Cordery et al., 2014). Buprenorphine as well as an analog having a pharmacology similar to a combination of buprenorphine and naloxone, BU10119, both attenuated cocaine-primed reinstatement, whereas naloxone and BU12004 did not (Hillhouse et al., 2021).

As with other procedures, studies using place conditioning demonstrate that stimulants can enhance the rewarding effects of opioids and vice versa. Interactions appear to depend on several factors including the temporal patterning of drug injections. Treatment regimens that result in sensitization tend to produce enhanced rewarding effects whereas those that produce tolerance tend to either have no effect or attenuate rewarding effects. Co-administration of drugs during training can also enhance apparent rewarding effects. These results indicate that the context of sequential and co-administration of stimulants and opioids can profoundly influence resulting rewarding effects and, presumably, the likelihood of co-use of opioids and stimulants.

2.5 Intracranial self-stimulation (ICSS)

ICSS is an operant conditioning procedure in which responding delivers brief pulses of electrical stimulation to specific areas of the brain. Response rates typically increase as the frequency of stimulation increases, and changes in sensitivity of responding to frequency (i.e., threshold) following administration of a drug are thought to reflect abuse-related effects. Drugs that increase responding for low stimulation frequencies (i.e., reduce the stimulation threshold) likely have potential for abuse (Negus & Miller, 2014). Interactions between opioids and stimulants have been investigated using ICSS procedures but much less frequently compared to other procedures described herein. As with other procedures, some studies reported mutual enhancement of threshold-lowering effects between opioids and stimulants. For example, in rats, both morphine and amphetamine alone dose-dependently decreased reward thresholds. Morphine and amphetamine exhibited mutual enhancement such that combinations of doses which were ineffective when given alone produced significant reductions in threshold (Hubner, Bain, & Kornetsky, 1987). Similarly, pretreatment with the dopamine releaser amfonelic acid enhanced the threshold-lowering effects of morphine (Izemwasser & Kornetsky, 1989).

Likewise, rats treated with morphine daily for 7 days prior to testing showed an enhanced response to amphetamine compared to saline-treated rats. Thus, chronic morphine appeared to produce cross-sensitization to subsequent amphetamine-induced facilitation of ICSS (Bespalov & Zvartau, 1995).

Mutual enhancement of threshold-lowering effects of opioids and stimulants suggests common or overlapping mechanisms of action; therefore, antagonist studies examined interactions further, the results of which have been mixed. For example, although naloxone attenuated the threshold-lowering effects of amphetamine, one study showed that 10-fold larger doses of naloxone were required to attenuate the effects of amphetamine as compared to effects of morphine (Schaefer & Michael, 1990), while others indicated effects of naloxone on the threshold-lowering effects of amphetamine and cocaine were not clearly dose-related (Bain & Kornetsky, 1987; Esposito, Perry, & Kornetsky, 1980). Holtzman (1976) reported that naloxone shifted the morphine dose-effect curve rightward, consistent with a competitive antagonist interaction, whereas naloxone shifted the amphetamine dose-effect curve leftward and downward, suggesting a very different interaction with amphetamine. In a later study, naltrexone administered subcutaneously via long-acting injectable formulation, blocked threshold-lowering effects of amphetamine; however, naltrexone given orally or subcutaneously was without effect (Todtenkopf et al., 2009). Moreover, other studies have also shown that blocking opioid receptors with naltrexone, given acutely or chronically and administered at doses that block mu opioid receptors, failed to alter effects of cocaine and amphetamine (e.g., Pabello et al., 1998; Sakloth & Negus, 2018).

Compared with other procedures, studies using ICSS to examine interactions between opioids and stimulants are less common. Nevertheless, results indicate evidence of mutual enhancement of rewarding effects in so far as opioids increased the potency of stimulants to lower reward thresholds and vice versa. Studies investigating interactions between opioid and dopamine systems using selective antagonists have yielded inconsistent results.

3. Conclusion

Behavioral pharmacology research highlighted in this chapter used pre-clinical self-administration, reinstatement, drug discrimination, place conditioning, and ICSS procedures to characterize complex and dynamic interactions between opioids and stimulants with regard to abuse-related effects. There is clear evidence that opioids can enhance the abuse-related effects of stimulants (and vice versa) which could have implications for co-use of opioids and stimulants. For example, many studies using drug self-administration, place conditioning, and ICSS procedures demonstrated that combinations of relatively small doses of two drugs can produce positive reinforcing or rewarding effects comparable to (and in some cases, greater than) effects of larger doses of either of the constituent drugs alone. Enhanced rewarding effects could manifest in many ways including engaging in drug seeking and taking behaviors with greater persistence, effort, and motivation. Drug discrimination studies showed a tendancy for cross-substituion between opioids and stimulants as well as mutual enhancement of discriminative stimulus effects. To the extent that discriminative stimulus effects contribute to subjective effects of drugs of abuse, these interactions might reflect a capacity for one drug to substitute for another in the case that the desired drug is unavailable and/or co-use for enhanced subjective effects. In reinstatement procedures, cross-reinstatement can occur such that a drug from one pharmacological class can occasion resumption of drug-taking behavior previously maintained by drugs from another class. In abstinent individuals, this might reflect a capacity for promoting relapse. Moreover, studies on opioid/stimulant combinations set the stage for evaluating potential pharmacological treatments for individuals who use opioids and stimulants.

While this chapter reviewed many well-conducted and comprehensive studies that can serve as examples and offer guidelines to investigators doing experiments of this nature, future work in the area of abuse-related effects of drug mixtures is still needed to advance the field, particularly with regard to the constituents of drug mixtures, dose selection, and timing of drug administration. Heroin and cocaine combinations have been researched extensively, yet a lag exists between the problems that are occurring on the streets and the published literature. For example, the specific constituents have appeared to change in popularity from heroin/cocaine to fentanyl/methamphetamine and the research has yet to catch up with this shift in large part. Similarly, there is a relatively new problem with drugs "marketed" on the street as stimulants or benzodiazepines containing adulterants such as fentanyl, often unbeknownst to the user, which can increase the risk of overdose especially if the user is opioid-naive and has not developed tolerance to the effects of opioids.

One dimension of opioid/stimulant mixtures that is potentially important is the proportions of drugs in mixtures. The strategy for selecting dose combinations varies, where in some cases a fixed dose of one drug is paired with a range of doses of another drug and in other instances the ratio of doses is fixed (e.g., 1:1). Further, the ratio for fixed doses sometimes is based on absolute dose and other times based on functional dose (e.g., ED_{50} values). The proportion of drugs in mixtures can be a determinant of drug-drug interactions and standardization of dose selection might help in integrating results across studies. Relatedly, timing of drug administration is an important variable worthy of future investigation. Drugs might be taken concurrently or in succession separated by minutes, hours, or even years, and the temporal spacing might be a relevant feature that often has not been the primary focus of studies in this area. For example, more systematic studies on the influence of drug history on abuse-related effects would be useful, especially with respect to the frequency and duration of prior drug use.

Although many studies reported enhanced abuse-related effects, results are far from unanimous as studies with each procedure have also indicated no interaction or attenuation of drug effects, with several examples of profound individual differences. Many factors come into play when studying drug-drug interactions, including pharmacodynamic and pharmacokinetic properties of the particular drugs being studied, temporal proximity of drug injections, drug history, as well as a multitude of other environmental, neurobiological, and genetic factors. This complexity underscores the need to remain diligent and rigorous when conducting such studies and to carefully consider the experimental design and analysis. Although parsing the contributions of all of these different factors is beyond the scope of this chapter, it is clear that behavioral pharmacology research has proven invaluable for elucidating these relationships using rigorous experimental designs and quantitative analyses of pharmacological and behavioral data.

Acknowledgements

Preparation of this manuscript was supported in part by NIH grant R01DA046532 (DRM).

Conflict of interest

The authors have no conflict of interest to declare.

References

Achat-Mendes, C., Valdez, G. R., Platt, D. M., Rowlett, J. K., & Spealman, R. D. (2009). Intravenous self-administration of etonitazene alone and combined with cocaine in rhesus monkeys: Comparison with heroin and antagonism by naltrexone and naloxonazine. *Psychopharmacology, 204*, 489–498.

Ahmad, F. B., Rossen, L. M., & Sutton, P. (2021). *Provisional drug overdose death counts. National Center for Health Statistics. 2021.* https://www.cdc.gov/nchs/nvss/vsrr/drug-overdose-data.htm. Accessed 30 June 2021.

Bain, G. T., & Kornetsky, C. (1987). Naloxone attenuation of the effect of cocaine on rewarding brain stimulation. *Life Sciences, 40*, 1119–1125.

Bardo, M. T., & Bevins, R. A. (2000). Conditioned place preference: What does it add to our preclinical understanding of drug reward? *Psychopharmacology, 153*, 31–43.

Bespalov, A. Y., & Zvartau, E. E. (1995). Subchronic morphine increases amphetamine-induced potentiation of brain stimulation reward: Reversal by DNQX. *European Neuropsychopharmacology, 5*, 89–93.

Bilsky, E. J., Montegut, M. J., Delong, C. L., & Reid, L. D. (1992). Opioidergic modulation of cocaine conditioned place preferences. *Life Sciences, 50*, PL85–PL90.

Blaiss, C. A., & Janak, P. H. (2006). Post-training and post-reactivation administration of amphetamine enhances morphine conditioned place preference. *Behavioural Brain Research, 171*, 329–337.

Bolin, B. L., Alcorn, J. L., Reynolds, A. R., Lile, J. A., Stoops, W. W., & Rush, C. R. (2018). Human drug discrimination: Elucidating the neuropharmacology of commonly abused illicit drugs. *Current Topics in Behavioral Neurosciences, 39*, 261–295.

Brown, E. E., Finlay, J. M., Wong, J. T., Damsma, G., & Fibiger, H. C. (1991). Behavioral and neurochemical interactions between cocaine and buprenorphine: Implications for the pharmacotherapy of cocaine abuse. *Journal of Pharmacology and Experimental Therapeutics, 256*, 119–126.

Chiang, Y. C., Hung, T. W., & Ho, I. K. (2014). Development of sensitization to methamphetamine in offspring prenatally exposed to morphine, methadone and buprenorphine. *Addiction Biology, 19*, 676–686.

Ciccarone, D. (2021). The rise of illicit fentanyls, stimulants and the fourth wave of the opioid overdose crisis. *Current Opinion in Psychiatry, 34*, 344–350.

Colpaert, F. C., Niemegeers, C. J., & Janssen, P. A. (1979). Discriminative stimulus properties of cocaine: Neuropharmacological characteristics as derived from stimulus generalization experiments. *Pharmacology Biochemistry and Behavior, 10*, 535–546.

Colpaert, F. C., Niemegeers, C. J., & Janssen, P. A. (1980). Factors regulating drug cue sensitivity: The effect of training dose in fentanyl-saline discrimination. *Neuropharmacology, 19*, 705–713.

Comer, S. D., Lac, S. T., Curtis, L. K., & Carroll, M. E. (1993). Effects of buprenorphine and naltrexone on reinstatement of cocaine-reinforced responding in rats. *Journal of Pharmacology and Experimental Therapeutics, 267*, 1470–1477.

Cook, C. D., & Picker, M. J. (1998). Dopaminergic activity and the discriminative stimulus effects of mu opioids in pigeons: Importance of training dose and attenuation by the D3 agonist (+/-)-7-OH-DPAT. *Psychopharmacology, 136*, 59–69.

Cooper, Z. D., Shi, Y. G., & Woods, J. H. (2010). Reinforcer-dependent enhancement of operant responding in opioid-withdrawn rats. *Psychopharmacology, 212*, 369–378.

Cordery, S. F., Taverner, A., Ridzwan, I. E., Guy, R. H., Delgado-Charro, M. B., Husbands, S. M., et al. (2014). A non-rewarding, non-aversive buprenorphine/naltrexone combination attenuates drug-primed reinstatement to cocaine and morphine in rats in a conditioned place preference paradigm. *Addiction Biology, 19*, 575–586.

Cornish, J. L., Lontos, J. M., Clemens, K. J., & McGregor, I. S. (2005). Cocaine and heroin ('speedball') self-administration: The involvement of nucleus accumbens dopamine and mu-opiate, but not delta-opiate receptors. *Psychopharmacology, 180*, 21–32.

Crawford, C. A., Villafranca, S. W., Cyr, M. C., Farley, C. M., Reichel, C. M., Gheorghe, S. L., et al. (2007). Effects of early methylphenidate exposure on morphine- and sucrose-reinforced behaviors in adult rats: Relationship to dopamine D2 receptors. *Brain Research, 1139*, 245–253.

Crombag, H. S., Grimm, J. W., & Shaham, Y. (2002). Effect of dopamine receptor antagonists on renewal of cocaine seeking by reexposure to drug-associated contextual cues. *Neuropsychopharmacology, 27*, 1006–1015.

Crombag, H. S., & Shaham, Y. (2002). Renewal of drug seeking by contextual cues after prolonged extinction in rats. *Behavioral Neuroscience, 116*, 169–173.

Crummy, E. A., Donckels, E. A., Baskin, B. M., Bentzley, B. S., & Ferguson, S. M. (2020). The impact of cocaine and heroin drug history on motivation and cue sensitivity in a rat model of polydrug abuse. *Psychopharmacology, 237*, 55–68.

Crummy, E. A., O'Neal, T. J., Baskin, B. M., & Ferguson, S. M. (2020). One is not enough: Understanding and modeling polysubstance use. *Frontiers in Neuroscience, 14*, 569.

de Vries, T. J., Schoffelmeer, A. N., Binnekade, R., Mulder, A. H., & Vanderschuren, L. J. (1998). Drug-induced reinstatement of heroin- and cocaine-seeking behaviour following long-term extinction is associated with expression of behavioural sensitization. *European Journal of Neuroscience, 10*, 3565–3571.

de Vries, T. J., Schoffelmeer, A. N., Binnekade, R., Raasø, H., & Vanderschuren, L. J. (2002). Relapse to cocaine- and heroin-seeking behavior mediated by dopamine D2 receptors is time-dependent and associated with behavioral sensitization. *Neuropsychopharmacology, 26*, 18–26.

de Vries, T. J., Schoffelmeer, A. N., Binnekade, R., & Vanderschuren, L. J. (1999). Dopaminergic mechanisms mediating the incentive to seek cocaine and heroin following long-term withdrawal of IV drug self-administration. *Psychopharmacology, 143*, 254–260.

de Wit, H., & Stewart, J. (1981). Reinstatement of cocaine-reinforced responding in the rat. *Psychopharmacology, 75*, 134–143.

de Wit, H., & Stewart, J. (1983). Drug reinstatement of heroin-reinforced responding in the rat. *Psychopharmacology, 79*, 29–31.

Duvauchelle, C. L., Sapoznik, T., & Kornetsky, C. (1998). The synergistic effects of combining cocaine and heroin ("speedball") using a progressive-ratio schedule of drug reinforcement. *Pharmacology Biochemistry and Behavior, 61*, 297–302.

Dykstra, L. A., Doty, P., Johnson, A. B., & Picker, M. J. (1992). Discriminative stimulus properties of cocaine, alone and in combination with buprenorphine, morphine and naltrexone. *Drug and Alcohol Dependence, 30*, 227–234.

Ellis, M. S., Kasper, Z. A., & Cicero, T. J. (2018). Twin epidemics: The surging rise of methamphetamine use in chronic opioid users. *Drug and Alcohol Dependence, 193*, 14–20.

Epstein, D. H., Preston, K. L., Stewart, J., & Shaham, Y. (2006). Toward a model of drug relapse: An assessment of the validity of the reinstatement procedure. *Psychopharmacology, 189*, 1–16.

Esposito, R. U., Perry, W., & Kornetsky, C. (1980). Effects of d-amphetamine and naloxone on brain stimulation reward. *Psychopharmacology, 69*, 187–191.

Ettenberg, A., Pettit, H. O., Bloom, F. E., & Koob, G. F. (1982). Heroin and cocaine intravenous self-administration in rats: Mediation by separate neural systems. *Psychopharmacology, 78*, 204–209.

Foltin, R. W., & Fischman, M. W. (1992). The cardiovascular and subjective effects of intravenous cocaine and morphine combinations in humans. *Journal of Pharmacology and Experimental Therapeutics, 261*, 623–632.

Foltin, R. W., Christiansen, I., Levin, F. R., & Fischman, M. W. (1995). Effects of single and multiple intravenous cocaine injections in humans maintained on methadone. *Journal of Pharmacology and Experimental Therapeutics*, *275*, 38–47.

Freeman, K. B., & Woolverton, W. L. (2011). Self-administration of cocaine and remifentanil by monkeys: Choice between single drugs and mixtures. *Psychopharmacology*, *215*, 281–290.

Gaiardi, M., Bartoletti, M., Gubellini, C., Bacchi, A., & Babbini, M. (1998). Modulation of the stimulus effects of morphine by d-amphetamine. *Pharmacology Biochemistry and Behavior*, *59*, 249–253.

Gauvin, D. V., & Young, A. M. (1989). Evidence for perceptual masking of the discriminative morphine stimulus. *Psychopharmacology*, *98*, 212–221.

Gerak, L. R., Galici, R., & France, C. P. (2008). Self administration of cocaine in monkeys receiving LAAM acutely or chronically. *Physiology and Behavior*, *93*, 20–26.

Gerak, L. R., Galici, R., & France, C. P. (2009). Self administration of heroin and cocaine in morphine-dependent and morphine-withdrawn rhesus monkeys. *Psychopharmacology*, *204*, 403–411.

Gerak, L. R., Weed, P. F., Maguire, D. R., & France, C. P. (2019). Effects of the synthetic cannabinoid receptor agonist JWH-018 on abuse-related effects of opioids in rhesus monkeys. *Drug and Alcohol Dependence*, *202*, 33–38.

Guo, L. K., Wang, Z. Y., Lu, G. Y., Wu, N., Dong, G. M., Ma, C. M., et al. (2019). Inhibition of naltrexone on relapse in methamphetamine self-administration and conditioned place preference in rats. *European Journal of Pharmacology*, *865*, 172671.

Häggkvist, J., Lindholm, S., & Franck, J. (2009). The effect of naltrexone on amphetamine-induced conditioned place preference and locomotor behaviour in the rat. *Addiction Biology*, *14*, 260–269.

Hassan, A. N., & Le Foll, B. (2019). Polydrug use disorders in individuals with opioid use disorder. *Drug and Alcohol Dependence*, *198*, 28–33.

Hedegaard, H., Miniño, A. M., & Warner, M. (2020). Drug overdose deaths in the United States, 1999-2019. *NCHS Data Brief*, *394*, 1–8. https://www.cdc.gov/nchs/products/databriefs/db394.htm.

Hemby, S. E., Co, C., Dworkin, S. I., & Smith, J. E. (1999). Synergistic elevations in nucleus accumbens extracellular dopamine concentrations during self-administration of cocaine/heroin combinations (speedball) in rats. *Journal of Pharmacology and Experimental Therapeutics*, *288*, 274–280.

Hemby, S. E., Smith, J. E., & Dworkin, S. I. (1996). The effects of eticlopride and naltrexone on responding maintained by food, cocaine, heroin and cocaine/heroin combinations in rats. *Journal of Pharmacology and Experimental Therapeutics*, *277*, 1247–1258.

Hernandez, L. L., Holohean, A. M., & Appel, J. B. (1978). Effects of opiates on the discriminative stimulus properties of dopamine agonists. *Pharmacology Biochemistry and Behavior*, *9*, 459–463.

Highfield, D., Yap, J., Grimm, J. W., Shalev, U., & Shaham, Y. (2001). Repeated lofexidine treatment attenuates stress-induced, but not drug cues-induced reinstatement of a heroin-cocaine mixture (speedball) seeking in rats. *Neuropsychopharmacology*, *25*, 320–331.

Hillhouse, T. M., Olson, K., Hallahan, J. E., Rysztak, L. G., Sears, B. F., Meurice, C., et al. (2021). The buprenorphine analogue BU10119 attenuates drug-primed and stress-induced cocaine reinstatement in mice. *Journal of Pharmacology and Experimental Therapeutics*, *378*, 287–299.

Hiranita, T., Kohut, S. J., Soto, P. L., Tanda, G., Kopajtic, T. A., & Katz, J. L. (2014). Preclinical efficacy of N-substituted benztropine analogs as antagonists of methamphetamine self-administration in rats. *Journal of Pharmacology and Experimental Therapeutics*, *348*, 174–191.

Hoffmeister, F., & Goldberg, S. R. (1973). A comparison of chlorpromazine, imipramine, morphine and d-amphetamine self-administration in cocaine-dependent rhesus monkeys. *Journal of Pharmacology and Experimental Therapeutics*, *187*, 8–14.

Hoffmeister, F., & Schlichting, U. U. (1972). Reinforcing properties of some opiates and opioids in rhesus monkeys with histories of cocaine and codeine self-administration. *Psychopharmacologia*, *23*, 55–74.

Holtzman, S. G. (1976). Comparison of the effects of morphine, pentazocine, cyclazocine and amphetamine on intracranial self-stimulation in the rat. *Psychopharmacologia*, *46*, 223–227.

Horner, K. A., Logan, M. C., Fisher, T. J., & Logue, J. B. (2017). Blockade of patch-based μ opioid receptors in the striatum attenuates methamphetamine-induced conditioned place preference and reduces activation of the patch compartment. *European Journal of Pharmacology*, *796*, 207–214.

Houdi, A. A., Bardo, M. T., & Van Loon, G. R. (1989). Opioid mediation of cocaine-induced hyperactivity and reinforcement. *Brain Research*, *497*, 195–198.

Hubner, C. B., Bain, G. T., & Kornetsky, C. (1987). The combined effects of morphine and d-amphetamine on the threshold for brain stimulation reward. *Pharmacology Biochemistry and Behavior*, *28*, 311–315.

Hursh, S. R., Galuska, C. M., Winger, G., & Woods, J. H. (2005). The economics of drug abuse: A quantitative assessment of drug demand. *Molecular Interventions*, *5*, 20–28.

Izemwasser, S., & Kornetsky, C. (1989). The effect of amfonelic acid or nisoxetine in combination with morphine on brain-stimulation reward. *Pharmacology Biochemistry and Behavior*, *32*, 983–986.

Jasinski, D. R., & Preston, K. L. (1986). Evaluation of mixtures of morphine and d-amphetamine for subjective and physiological effects. *Drug and Alcohol Dependence*, *17*, 1–13.

Joanna, L., Sylwia, T., Magdalena, G., Piotr, L., Ewa, K., Jolanta, O. G., et al. (2017). Mephedrone exposure in adolescent rats alters the rewarding effect of morphine in adults. *European Journal of Pharmacology*, *810*, 63–69.

Johanson, C. E., & Balster, R. L. (1978). A summary of the results of a drug self-administration study using substitution procedures in rhesus monkeys. *Bulletin on Narcotics*, *30*, 43–54.

Jones, C. M., Einstein, E. B., & Compton, W. M. (2018). Changes in synthetic opioid involvement in drug overdose deaths in the United States, 2010–2016. *JAMA*, *319*, 1819–1821.

Jones, C. M., & McCance-Katz, E. F. (2019). Co-occurring substance use and mental disorders among adults with opioid use disorder. *Drug and Alcohol Dependence*, *197*, 78–82.

Jones, C. M., Underwood, N., & Compton, W. M. (2020). Increases in methamphetamine use among heroin treatment admissions in the United States, 2008–17. *Addiction*, *115*, 347–353.

Kamien, J. B., & Spealman, R. D. (1991). Modulation of the discriminative-stimulus effects of cocaine by buprenorphine. *Behavioural Pharmacology*, *2*, 517–520.

Kantak, K. M., Riberdy, A., & Spealman, R. D. (1999). Cocaine-opioid interactions in groups of rats trained to discriminate different doses of cocaine. *Psychopharmacology*, *147*, 257–265.

Kariisa, M., Scholl, L., Wilson, N., Seth, P., & Hoots, B. (2019). Drug overdose deaths involving cocaine and psychostimulants with abuse potential—United States, 2003–2017. *Morbidity and Mortality Weekly Report*, *68*, 388–395.

Khroyan, T. V., Polgar, W. E., Cami-Kobeci, G., Husbands, S. M., Zaveri, N. T., & Toll, L. (2011). The first universal opioid ligand, (2S)-2-[(5R,6R,7R,14S)-N-cyclopropylmethyl-4,5-epoxy-6,14-ethano-3-hydroxy-6-methoxymorphinan-7-yl]-

3,3-dimethylpentan-2-ol (BU08028): Characterization of the in vitro profile and in vivo behavioral effects in mouse models of acute pain and cocaine-induced reward. *Journal of Pharmacology and Experimental Therapeutics*, *336*, 952–961.

Kilbey, M. M., & Ellinwood, E. H., Jr. (1979). Discriminative stimulus properties of psychomotor stimulants in the cat. *Psychopharmacology*, *63*, 151–153.

Kosten, T. A., Marby, D. W., & Nestler, E. J. (1991). Cocaine conditioned place preference is attenuated by chronic buprenorphine treatment. *Life Sciences*, *49*, PL201–PL206.

Lacy, R. T., Strickland, J. C., Brophy, M. K., Witte, M. A., & Smith, M. A. (2014). Exercise decreases speedball self-administration. *Life Sciences*, *114*, 86–92.

Lamas, X., Negus, S. S., Gatch, M. B., & Mello, N. K. (1998). Effects of heroin/cocaine combinations in rats trained to discriminate heroin or cocaine from saline. *Pharmacology Biochemistry and Behavior*, *60*, 357–364.

Lan, K. C., Chang, A. C., Liu, S. H., Ho, I. K., & Lin-Shiau, S. Y. (2009). Enhancing effects of morphine on methamphetamine-induced reinforcing behavior and its association with dopamine release and metabolism in mice. *Journal of Neurochemistry*, *109*, 382–392.

Leone, P., & Di Chiara, G. (1987). Blockade of D-1 receptors by SCH 23390 antagonizes morphine- and amphetamine-induced place preference conditioning. *European Journal of Pharmacology*, *135*, 251–254.

Leri, F., Bruneau, J., & Stewart, J. (2003). Understanding polydrug use: Review of heroin and cocaine co-use. *Addiction*, *98*, 7–22.

Leri, F., Flores, J., Rajabi, H., & Stewart, J. (2003). Effects of cocaine in rats exposed to heroin. *Neuropsychopharmacology*, *28*, 2102–2116.

Leri, F., & Stewart, J. (2001). Drug-induced reinstatement to heroin and cocaine seeking: A rodent model of relapse in polydrug use. *Experimental and Clinical Psychopharmacology*, *9*, 297–306.

Leri, F., Tremblay, A., Sorge, R. E., & Stewart, J. (2004). Methadone maintenance reduces heroin- and cocaine-induced relapse without affecting stress-induced relapse in a rodent model of poly-drug use. *Neuropsychopharmacology*, *29*, 1312–1320.

Leri, F., Zhou, Y., Goddard, B., Cummins, E., & Kreek, M. J. (2006). Effects of high-dose methadone maintenance on cocaine place conditioning, cocaine self-administration, and mu-opioid receptor mRNA expression in the rat brain. *Neuropsychopharmacology*, *31*, 1462–1474.

Lett, B. T. (1989). Repeated exposures intensify rather than diminish the rewarding effects of amphetamine, morphine, and cocaine. *Psychopharmacology*, *98*, 357–362.

Lu, L., & Dempsey, J. (2004). Cocaine seeking over extended withdrawal periods in rats: Time dependent increases of responding induced by heroin priming over the first 3 months. *Psychopharmacology*, *176*, 109–114.

Lukas, S. E., Mello, N. K., Drieze, J. M., & Mendelson, J. H. (1995). Buprenorphine-induced alterations of cocaine's reinforcing effects in rhesus monkey: A dose-response analysis. *Drug and Alcohol Dependence*, *40*, 87–98.

Lynch, W. J., Heaser, W. A., & Carroll, M. E. (1998). Effects of amphetamine, butorphanol, and morphine pretreatment on the maintenance and reinstatement of cocaine-reinforced responding. *Experimental and Clinical Psychopharmacology*, *6*, 255–263.

Maguire, D. R., Gerak, L. R., Woods, J. H., Husbands, S. M., Disney, A., & France, C. P. (2019). Long-lasting effects of methocinnamox on opioid self-administration in rhesus monkeys. *Journal of Pharmacology and Experimental Therapeutics*, *368*, 88–99.

Mahoney, J. J., 3rd, Winstanley, E. L., Lander, L. R., Berry, J. H., Marshalek, P. J., Haut, M. W., et al. (2021). High prevalence of co-occurring substance use in individuals with opioid use disorder. *Addictive Behaviors*, *114*, 106752.

Martin, T. J., Coller, M., Co, C., & Smith, J. E. (2008). Micro-opioid receptor alkylation in the ventral pallidum and ventral tegmental area, but not in the nucleus accumbens, attenuates the effects of heroin on cocaine self-administration in rats. *Neuropsychopharmacology*, *33*, 1171–1178.

Masukawa, Y., Suzuki, T., & Misawa, M. (1993). Differential modification of the rewarding effects of methamphetamine and cocaine by opioids and antihistamines. *Psychopharmacology, 111*, 139–143.
Mattox, A. J., Thompson, S. S., & Carroll, M. E. (1997). Smoked heroin and cocaine base (speedball) combinations in rhesus monkeys. *Experimental and Clinical Psychopharmacology, 5*, 113–118.
Mattson, C. L., Tanz, L. J., Quinn, K., Kariisa, M., Patel, P., & Davis, N. L. (2021). Trends and geographic patterns in drug and synthetic opioid overdose deaths—United States, 2013–2019. *Morbidity and Mortality Weekly Report, 70*, 202–207.
Mello, N. K., & Negus, S. S. (1998). The effects of buprenorphine on self-administration of cocaine and heroin "speedball" combinations and heroin alone by rhesus monkeys. *Journal of Pharmacology and Experimental Therapeutics, 285*, 444–456.
Mello, N. K., & Negus, S. S. (1999). Effects of flupenthixol and quadazocine on self-administration of speedball combinations of cocaine and heroin by rhesus monkeys. *Neuropsychopharmacology, 21*, 575–588.
Mello, N. K., Negus, S. S., Lukas, S. E., Mendelson, J. H., Sholar, J. W., & Drieze, J. (1995). A primate model of polydrug abuse: Cocaine and heroin combinations. *Journal of Pharmacology and Experimental Therapeutics, 274*, 1325–1337.
Montanari, C., Stendardo, E., De Luca, M. T., Meringolo, M., Contu, L., & Badiani, A. (2015). Differential vulnerability to relapse into heroin versus cocaine-seeking as a function of setting. *Psychopharmacology, 232*, 2415–2424.
Negus, S. S. (2005). Interactions between the reinforcing effects of cocaine and heroin in a drug-vs-food choice procedure in rhesus monkeys: A dose-addition analysis. *Psychopharmacology, 180*, 115–124.
Negus, S. S., Gatch, M. B., & Mello, N. K. (1998a). Effects of mu opioid agonists alone and in combination with cocaine and D-amphetamine in rhesus monkeys trained to discriminate cocaine. *Neuropsychopharmacology, 18*, 325–338.
Negus, S. S., Gatch, M. B., & Mello, N. K. (1998b). Discriminative stimulus effects of a cocaine/heroin "speedball" combination in rhesus monkeys. *Journal of Pharmacology and Experimental Therapeutics, 285*, 1123–1136.
Negus, S. S., & Mello, N. K. (2002). Effects of mu-opioid agonists on cocaine- and food-maintained responding and cocaine discrimination in rhesus monkeys: Role of mu-agonist efficacy. *Journal of Pharmacology and Experimental Therapeutics, 300*, 1111–1121.
Negus, S. S., & Miller, L. L. (2014). Intracranial self-stimulation to evaluate abuse potential of drugs. *Pharmacological Reviews, 66*, 869–917.
O'Connor, E. C., Chapman, K., Butler, P., & Mead, A. N. (2011). The predictive validity of the rat self-administration model for abuse liability. *Neuroscience and Biobehavioral Reviews, 35*, 912–938.
Pabello, N. G., Hubbell, C. L., Cavallaro, C. A., Barringer, T. M., Mendez, J. J., & Reid, L. D. (1998). Responding for rewarding brain stimulation: Cocaine and isradipine plus naltrexone. *Pharmacology Biochemistry and Behavior, 61*, 181–192.
Peppin, J. F., Raffa, R. B., & Schatman, M. E. (2020). The polysubstance overdose-death crisis. *Journal of Pain Research, 13*, 3405–3408.
Platt, D. M., Grech, D. M., Rowlett, J. K., & Spealman, R. D. (1999). Discriminative stimulus effects of morphine in squirrel monkeys: Stimulants, opioids, and stimulant-opioid combinations. *Journal of Pharmacology and Experimental Therapeutics, 290*, 1092–1100.
Platt, D. M., Rowlett, J. K., & Spealman, R. D. (2010). Asymmetric generalization and interaction profiles in rhesus monkeys discriminating intravenous cocaine or intravenous heroin from vehicle. *Journal of Pharmacology and Experimental Therapeutics, 332*, 985–995.
Preston, K. L., Sullivan, J. T., Strain, E. C., & Bigelow, G. E. (1996). Enhancement of cocaine's abuse liability in methadone maintenance patients. *Psychopharmacology, 123*, 15–25.

Ranaldi, R., & Munn, E. (1998). Polydrug self-administration in rats: Cocaine-heroin is more rewarding than cocaine-alone. *Neuroreport*, *9*, 2463–2466.
Ranaldi, R., & Wise, R. A. (2000). Intravenous self-administration of methamphetamine-heroin (speedball) combinations under a progressive-ratio schedule of reinforcement in rats. *Neuroreport*, *11*, 2621–2623.
Ribeiro Do Couto, B., Aguilar, M. A., Rodríguez-Arias, M., & Miñarro, J. (2005). Long-lasting rewarding effects of morphine induced by drug primings. *Brain Research*, *1050*, 53–63.
Rowlett, J. K., Platt, D. M., Yao, W. D., & Spealman, R. D. (2007). Modulation of heroin and cocaine self-administration by dopamine D1- and D2-like receptor agonists in rhesus monkeys. *Journal of Pharmacology and Experimental Therapeutics*, *321*, 1135–1143.
Rowlett, J. K., Rodefer, J. S., & Spealman, R. D. (2005). Self-Administration of cocaine-opioid combinations by rhesus monkeys: Evaluation of the role of mu receptor efficacy using labor supply analysis. *Journal of Pharmacology and Experimental Therapeutics*, *312*, 1289–1297.
Rowlett, J. K., & Spealman, R. D. (1998). Opioid enhancement of the discriminative stimulus effects of cocaine: Evidence for involvement of mu and delta opioid receptors. *Psychopharmacology*, *140*, 217–224.
Rowlett, J. K., Spealman, R. D., & Platt, D. M. (2001). Similar enhancement of the discriminative stimulus effects of cocaine and GBR 12909 by heroin in squirrel monkeys. *Psychopharmacology*, *157*, 313–319.
Rowlett, J. K., Wilcox, K. M., & Woolverton, W. L. (1998). Self-administration of cocaine-heroin combinations by rhesus monkeys: Antagonism by naltrexone. *Journal of Pharmacology and Experimental Therapeutics*, *286*, 61–69.
Rowlett, J. K., & Woolverton, W. L. (1997). Self-administration of cocaine and heroin combinations by rhesus monkeys responding under a progressive-ratio schedule. *Psychopharmacology*, *133*, 363–371.
Sakloth, F., & Negus, S. S. (2018). Naltrexone maintenance fails to alter amphetamine effects on intracranial self-stimulation in rats. *Experimental and Clinical Psychopharmacology*, *26*, 195–204.
Schaefer, G. J., & Michael, R. P. (1990). Interactions of naloxone with morphine, amphetamine and phencyclidine on fixed interval responding for intracranial self-stimulation in rats. *Psychopharmacology*, *102*, 263–268.
Schenk, S., & Partridge, B. (1999). Cocaine-seeking produced by experimenter-administered drug injections: Dose-effect relationships in rats. *Psychopharmacology*, *147*, 285–290.
Schwartz, A. S., & Marchok, P. L. (1974). Depression of morphine-seeking behaviour by dopamine inhibition. *Nature*, *248*, 257–258.
Seaman, R. W., Jr., & Collins, G. T. (2021). Impact of morphine dependence and withdrawal on the reinforcing effectiveness of fentanyl, cocaine, and methamphetamine in rats. *Frontiers in Pharmacology*, *12*, 691700.
Shalev, U., Grimm, J. W., & Shaham, Y. (2002). Neurobiology of relapse to heroin and cocaine seeking: A review. *Pharmacological Reviews*, *54*, 1–42.
Shannon, H. E., & Holtzman, S. G. (1979). Morphine training dose: A determinant of stimulus generalization to narcotic antagonists in the rat. *Psychopharmacology*, *61*, 239–244.
Shen, Y. L., Chen, S. T., Chan, T. Y., Hung, T. W., Tao, P. L., Liao, R. M., et al. (2016). Delayed extinction and stronger drug-primed reinstatement of methamphetamine seeking in rats prenatally exposed to morphine. *Neurobiology of Learning and Memory*, *128*, 56–64.
Shippenberg, T. S., Emmett-Oglesby, M. W., Ayesta, F. J., & Herz, A. (1988). Tolerance and selective cross-tolerance to the motivational effects of opioids. *Psychopharmacology*, *96*, 110–115.

Shippenberg, T. S., & Heidbreder, C. (1995). Sensitization to the conditioned rewarding effects of cocaine: Pharmacological and temporal characteristics. *Journal of Pharmacology and Experimental Therapeutics, 273*, 808–815.

Shippenberg, T. S., Heidbreder, C., & Lefevour, A. (1996). Sensitization to the conditioned rewarding effects of morphine: Pharmacology and temporal characteristics. *European Journal of Pharmacology, 299*, 33–39.

Shippenberg, T. S., & Herz, A. (1987). Place preference conditioning reveals the involvement of D1-dopamine receptors in the motivational properties of mu- and kappa-opioid agonists. *Brain Research, 436*, 169–172.

Shippenberg, T. S., & Herz, A. (1988). Motivational effects of opioids: Influence of D-1 versus D-2 receptor antagonists. *European Journal of Pharmacology, 151*, 233–242.

Shippenberg, T. S., LeFevour, A., & Thompson, A. C. (1998). Sensitization to the conditioned rewarding effects of morphine and cocaine: Differential effects of the kappa-opioid receptor agonist U69593. *European Journal of Pharmacology, 345*, 27–34.

Smith, J. E., Co, C., Coller, M. D., Hemby, S. E., & Martin, T. J. (2006). Self-administered heroin and cocaine combinations in the rat: Additive reinforcing effects-supra-additive effects on nucleus accumbens extracellular dopamine. *Neuropsychopharmacology, 31*, 139–150.

Soderman, A. R., & Unterwald, E. M. (2008). Cocaine reward and hyperactivity in the rat: Sites of mu opioid receptor modulation. *Neuroscience, 154*, 1506–1516.

Sorge, R. E., Rajabi, H., & Stewart, J. (2005). Rats maintained chronically on buprenorphine show reduced heroin and cocaine seeking in tests of extinction and drug-induced reinstatement. *Neuropsychopharmacology, 30*, 1681–1692.

Spealman, R. D., & Bergman, J. (1992). Modulation of the discriminative stimulus effects of cocaine by mu and kappa opioids. *Journal of Pharmacology and Experimental Therapeutics, 261*, 607–615.

Spyraki, C., Fibiger, H. C., & Phillips, A. G. (1983). Attenuation of heroin reward in rats by disruption of the mesolimbic dopamine system. *Psychopharmacology, 79*, 278–283.

Stewart, J. (1984). Reinstatement of heroin and cocaine self-administration behavior in the rat by intracerebral application of morphine in the ventral tegmental area. *Pharmacology Biochemistry and Behavior, 20*, 917–923.

Stewart, J. (2000). Pathways to relapse: The neurobiology of drug- and stress-induced relapse to drug-taking. *Journal of Psychiatry and Neuroscience, 25*, 125–136.

Stewart, J., & Vezina, P. (1988). A comparison of the effects of intra-accumbens injections of amphetamine and morphine on reinstatement of heroin intravenous self-administration behavior. *Brain Research, 457*, 287–294.

Strickland, J. C., Havens, J. R., & Stoops, W. W. (2019). A nationally representative analysis of "twin epidemics": Rising rates of methamphetamine use among persons who use opioids. *Drug and Alcohol Dependence, 204*, 107592.

Strickland, J. C., Stoops, W. W., Dunn, K. E., Smith, K. E., & Havens, J. R. (2021). The continued rise of methamphetamine use among people who use heroin in the United States. *Drug and Alcohol Dependence, 225*, 108750.

Substance Abuse and Mental Health Services Administration (SAMHSA). (2020). *Key substance use and mental health indicators in the United States: Results from the 2019 National Survey on Drug Use and Health (HHS Publication No. PEP20-07-01-001, NSDUH Series H-55).* Rockville, MD: Center for Behavioral Health Statistics and Quality, Substance Abuse and Mental Health Services Administration. Retrieved from https://www.samhsa.gov/data/report/2019-nsduh-annual-national-report. Accessed 19 July 2021.

Suzuki, T., Mori, T., Tsuji, M., Maeda, J., Kishimoto, Y., Misawa, M., et al. (1997). Differential effects of mu-, delta- and kappa-opioid receptor agonists on the discriminative stimulus properties of cocaine in rats. *European Journal of Pharmacology, 324*, 21–29.

Swedberg, M. D. (2016). Drug discrimination: A versatile tool for characterization of CNS safety pharmacology and potential for drug abuse. *Journal of Pharmacological and Toxicological Methods*, *81*, 295–305.

Todtenkopf, M. S., O'Neill, K. S., Kriksciukaite, K., Turncliff, R. Z., Dean, R. L., Ostrovsky-Day, I., et al. (2009). Route of administration affects the ability of naltrexone to reduce amphetamine-potentiated brain stimulation reward in rats. *Addiction Biology*, *14*, 408–418.

Trujillo, K. A., Belluzzi, J. D., & Stein, L. (1991). Naloxone blockade of amphetamine place preference conditioning. *Psychopharmacology*, *104*, 265–274.

United Nations Office on Drugs and Crime (UNODC). (2019). *World Drug Report 2019 (United Nations publication, Sales No. E.19.XI.8)*. https://wdr.unodc.org/wdr2019/. Accessed 19 July 2021.

Vanderschuren, L. J., Schoffelmeer, A. N., Mulder, A. H., & de Vries, T. J. (1999). Dopaminergic mechanisms mediating the long-term expression of locomotor sensitization following pre-exposure to morphine or amphetamine. *Psychopharmacology*, *143*, 244–253.

Wade-Galuska, T., Galuska, C. M., & Winger, G. (2011). Effects of daily morphine administration and deprivation on choice and demand for remifentanil and cocaine in rhesus monkeys. *Journal of the Experimental Analysis of Behavior*, *95*, 75–89.

Wade-Galuska, T., Winger, G., & Woods, J. H. (2007). A behavioral economic analysis of cocaine and remifentanil self-administration in rhesus monkeys. *Psychopharmacology*, *194*, 563–572.

Walsh, S. L., Sullivan, J. T., Preston, K. L., Garner, J. E., & Bigelow, G. E. (1996). Effects of naltrexone on response to intravenous cocaine, hydromorphone and their combination in humans. *Journal of Pharmacology and Experimental Therapeutics*, *279*, 524–538.

Wang, N. S., Brown, V. L., Grabowski, J., & Meisch, R. A. (2001). Reinforcement by orally delivered methadone, cocaine, and methadone-cocaine combinations in rhesus monkeys: Are the combinations better reinforcers? *Psychopharmacology*, *156*, 63–72.

Wang, Y. P., Wei, S. G., Zhu, Y. S., Zhao, B., Xun, X., & Lai, J. H. (2015). Dopamine receptor D1 but not D3 essential for morphine-induced conditioned responses. *Genetics and Molecular Research*, *14*, 180–189.

Ward, S. J., Läck, C., Morgan, D., & Roberts, D. C. (2006). Discrete-trials heroin self-administration produces sensitization to the reinforcing effects of cocaine in rats. *Psychopharmacology*, *185*, 150–159.

Ward, S. J., Morgan, D., & Roberts, D. C. S. (2005). Comparison of the reinforcing effects of cocaine and cocaine/heroin combinations under progressive ratio and choice schedules in rats. *Neuropsychopharmacology*, *30*, 286–295.

Wilson, M. C., & Schuster, C. R. (1973). The effects of stimulants and depressants on cocaine self-administration behavior in the rhesus monkey. *Psychopharmacologia*, *31*, 291–304.

Winger, G., Galuska, C. M., Hursh, S. R., & Woods, J. H. (2006). Relative reinforcing effects of cocaine, remifentanil, and their combination in rhesus monkeys. *Journal of Pharmacology and Experimental Therapeutics*, *318*, 223–229.

Winger, G., Skjoldager, P., & Woods, J. H. (1992). Effects of buprenorphine and other opioid agonists and antagonists on alfentanil- and cocaine-reinforced responding in rhesus monkeys. *Journal of Pharmacology and Experimental Therapeutics*, *261*, 311–317.

Winger, G., & Woods, J. H. (2001). The effects of chronic morphine on behavior reinforced by several opioids or by cocaine in rhesus monkeys. *Drug and Alcohol Dependence*, *62*, 181–189.

Wood, D. M., & Emmett-Oglesby, M. W. (1986). Characteristics of tolerance, recovery from tolerance and cross-tolerance for cocaine used as a discriminative stimulus. *Journal of Pharmacology and Experimental Therapeutics*, *237*, 120–125.

Woolverton, W. L., Wang, Z., Vasterling, T., & Tallarida, R. (2008). Self-administration of cocaine-remifentanil mixtures by monkeys: An isobolographic analysis. *Psychopharmacology, 198*, 387–394.

Young, A. M., Masaki, M. A., & Geula, C. (1992). Discriminative stimulus effects of morphine: Effects of training dose on agonist and antagonist effects of mu opioids. *Journal of Pharmacology and Experimental Therapeutics, 261*, 246–257.

Zhang, L., Walker, E. A., Sutherland, J., 2nd, & Young, A. M. (2000). Discriminative stimulus effects of two doses of fentanyl in rats: Pharmacological selectivity and effect of training dose on agonist and antagonist effects of mu opioids. *Psychopharmacology, 148*, 136–145.

Zhu, J., Spencer, T. J., Liu-Chen, L. Y., Biederman, J., & Bhide, P. G. (2011). Methylphenidate and μ opioid receptor interactions: A pharmacological target for prevention of stimulant abuse. *Neuropharmacology, 61*, 283–292.

Zhu, H., & Wu, L. T. (2020). Multiple drug use disorder diagnoses among drug-involved hospitalizations in the United States: Results from the 2016 National Inpatient Sample. *Drug and Alcohol Dependence, 213*, 108113.

CHAPTER TWO

In vitro and in vivo pharmacology of kratom

Takato Hiranita[a], Samuel Obeng[a,b], Abhisheak Sharma[c,d], Jenny L. Wilkerson[a], Christopher R. McCurdy[b,c,d], and Lance R. McMahon[a,*]

[a]Department of Pharmacodynamics, College of Pharmacy, University of Florida, Gainesville, FL, United States
[b]Department of Medicinal Chemistry, College of Pharmacy, University of Florida, Gainesville, FL, United States
[c]Department of Pharmaceutics, College of Pharmacy, University of Florida, Gainesville, FL, United States
[d]Translational Drug Development Core, Clinical and Translational Sciences Institute, College of Pharmacy, University of Florida, Gainesville, FL, United States
*Corresponding author: e-mail address: lance.mcmahon@cop.ufl.edu

Contents

1. Introduction 36
2. Pharmacodynamics of kratom alkaloids in vitro 38
   2.1 Opioid receptors 38
   2.2 Adrenergic and serotonergic receptors 41
3. Pharmacokinetics of kratom alkaloids 41
   3.1 Mitragynine 44
   3.2 Mitragynine metabolites and other kratom alkaloids 47
4. Behavioral effects of kratom alkaloids 50
   4.1 Antinociception 50
   4.2 I.v. drug self administration 52
   4.3 Drug discrimination 54
   4.4 Rodent locomotor activity 57
   4.5 Place conditioning 57
   4.6 Intracranial self-stimulation 60
   4.7 Respiration 60
   4.8 Tolerance 61
   4.9 Dependence and withdrawal 62
5. Conclusion 65
Acknowledgments 66
Conflicts of interests or disclaimers 66
References 66

Abstract

Kratom products have been historically and anecdotally used in south Asian countries for centuries to manage pain and opioid withdrawal. The use of kratom products has dramatically increased in the United States. More than 45 kratom alkaloids have been

Advances in Pharmacology, Volume 93
ISSN 1054-3589
https://doi.org/10.1016/bs.apha.2021.10.001

isolated, yet the overall pharmacology of the individual alkaloids is still not well characterized. The purpose of this chapter is to summarize in vitro and in vivo opioid activities of the primary kratom alkaloid mitragynine and its more potent metabolite 7-hydroxymitragynine. Following are experimental procedures described to characterize opioid receptor activity; receptor binding and functional assays, antinociceptive assays, operant conditioning assays, and respiratory plethysmography. The capacity of kratom alkaloids to confer tolerance and physical dependence as well as their pharmacokinetic properties are also summarized. The data reviewed here suggest that kratom products and mitragynine possess low efficacy agonist activity at the mu-opioid receptor in vivo. In addition, kratom products and mitragynine have been demonstrated to antagonize the effects of high efficacy mu-opioid agonists. The data further suggest that 7-hydroxymitragynine formed in vivo by metabolism of mitragynine may be minimally involved in the overall behavioral profile of mitragynine and kratom, whereas 7-hydroxymitragynine itself, at sufficiently high doses administered exogenously, shares many of the same abuse- and dependence-related behavioral effects associated with traditional opioid agonists. The apparent low efficacy of kratom products and mitragynine at mu-opioid receptors supports the development of these ligands as effective and potentially safe medications for opioid use disorder.

Abbreviations

AUC	area under curve
BCS	biopharmaceutics classification system
CYP	cytochrome P450
DEA	drug enforcement administration
DOR	δ-opioid receptor
fu	unbound fraction
i.c.v.	intracerebroventricular(li)
i.p.	intraperitoneal(ly)
i.v.	intravenous(ly)
KOR	κ-opioid receptor
log P	partition coefficient
MDCK	Madin-Darby canine kidney
MOR	μ-opioid receptor
$\mathbf{P_{app}}$	apparent permeability
P-gp	P-glycoprotein
s.c.	subcutaneous(ly)
Vd	volume of distribution

1. Introduction

Mitragyna speciosa Korth (kratom) is a medicinal plant indigenous to subtropical and tropical regions of Southeast Asia, including Thailand, Malaysia, Indonesia, Philippines, Myanmar, and New Guinea (Warner,

Kaufman, & Grundmann, 2016). Kratom belongs to the Rubiaceae family and is also referred to as krathum (Thai), or ketum and biak (Malay). Traditionally, the fresh leaves of kratom are chewed or brewed as a tea, particularly among manual laborers, to enhance energy, reduce fatigue and increase productivity. Kratom is also used to treat diseases such as cough, diarrhea, fever, anxiety, pain, depression, opioid withdrawal, and opioid use disorder (Kruegel & Grundmann, 2018).

Kratom use has increased substantially in the United States (US) where it is available in a variety of forms including raw dried leaves, capsules, tablets, energy drinks, powders, and concentrated extracts. As of 2021, it is estimated that 0.8% (2,031,803) of adults in the US used kratom within the last year (Schimmel et al., 2021). At low doses, kratom produces stimulant-like effects while at high doses it produces opioid-like effects (Adkins, Boyer, & McCurdy, 2011). Due to its opioid like effects, in 2016 the US Drug Enforcement Administration (DEA) proposed to reclassify kratom as a Schedule I drug, but later rescinded their decision due to public outcry. The DEA labeled it as a "Drug of Concern," and currently, kratom is legal and sold as a dietary supplement; however, some states have regulations or prohibitions against the possession and use of kratom (Eastlack, Cornett, & Kaye, 2020). The relative lack of regulation over the content in some kratom products may contribute to the increased harm reported with kratom use; between 2011 and 2017, there were 11 deaths associated with kratom exposure, with two of the deaths apparently linked to kratom use only (Post, Spiller, Chounthirath, & Smith, 2019). Although this is concerning, in absolute numbers this is less dramatic when compared to fatalities from commonly prescribed drugs. It is important to note that kratom can be associated with serious medical outcomes, especially when used in combination with other psychoactive substances.

To date, over 45 indole and oxindole alkaloids have been isolated from kratom. These include mitragynine (55% of total alkaloid content), paynantheine (10%), speciogynine (8%), speciociliatine (5%), 7-hydroxymitragynine (2%), corynoxine (2%), corynantheidine (<1%), 9-hydroxycorynantheidine (<1%), isocorynantheidine (<1%), corynoxine B (<1%), mitraphylline (<1%), isospeciofoline (<1%), mitragynine oxindole B (<1%), speciociliatine *N*(4)-oxide (<1%), and ajmalicine (Fig. 1) (Adkins et al., 2011). The concentrations of the individual alkaloids measured in kratom tree material vary by region, chemotypes, plant age, soil types, climates, and other environmental factors (Chear et al., 2021; Kruegel & Grundmann, 2018; Sharma et al., 2019). For instance, kratom grown in the south-central US had higher levels of mitraphylline than

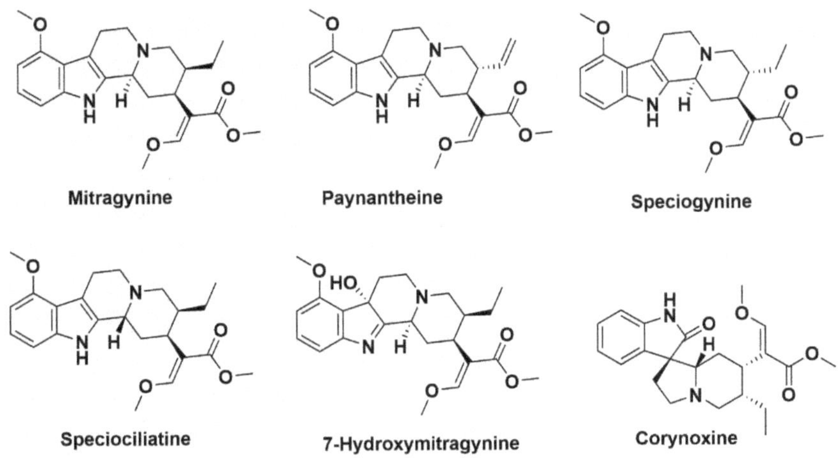

Fig. 1 Structures of kratom alkaloids with content ≥2% of total alkaloid content.

mitragynine (Leon et al., 2009). Thus, the pharmacology of kratom consumed in the US may vary based on differences in the origin of the plant material.

This chapter presents past and current research on the in vitro and in vivo pharmacodynamics and pharmacokinetics of kratom. This chapter also highlights the less explored areas of kratom's pharmacology.

2. Pharmacodynamics of kratom alkaloids in vitro

2.1 Opioid receptors

Numerous studies have been conducted to investigate the pharmacology of kratom alkaloids at the mu, kappa, and delta opioid receptors (MOR, KOR, and DOR, respectively). Mitragynine and its metabolite 7-hydroxymitragynine are the most studied kratom alkaloids at human and rodent opioid receptors. Among the kratom alkaloids and their metabolites, 7-hydroxymitragynine has the highest affinity at opioid receptors in vitro (Table 1). Mitragynine has about a 10-fold lower affinity than 7-hydroxymitragynine at the MOR (Table 1). Each of the kratom alkaloids had lower binding affinities at the DOR and KOR than at the MOR. Corynantheidine was also shown to have higher affinity at the MOR than at the DOR and KOR (Table 1) (Chakraborty et al., 2021). There are discrepancies in the binding affinities of corynoxine and corynoxine B at the human MOR in vitro. Chear et al. (2021) indicated that these two alkaloids have high affinity at the MOR ($K_i < 110\,nM$), whereas

Table 1 Reported affinities (K_i; mean ± SEM or 95% CI in nM) of kratom alkaloids at opioid receptors.

Kratom alkaloid or its metabolite	MOR	DOR	KOR
Mitragynine	161 ± 9.56[a] 709 (451—1130)[b] 233 ± 48[c] 230 ± 47[d] 740[e] 502 ± 19.4[f] 7.24 ± 3.44[g]	>10,000[a] 6800 (2980—15,900)[b] > 10,000[c] 1010 ± 50[d] 6500[e] 7910 ± 1140[f] 60.3 ± 23.1[g]	198 ± 29.5[a] 1700 (1090—2710)[b] 772 ± 207[c] 231 ± 21[d] 1300[e] 1200 ± 79.7[f] 1100 ± 436[g]
Paynantheine	410 ± 152[c] 666 ± 83[d]	>10,000[c] 4250 ± 730[d]	2560 ± 370[c] 888 ± 294[d]
Speciogynine	728 ± 61[c] 578 ± 64[d] 1,000[e]	>10,000[c] 7950 ± 950[d] > 10,000[e]	3200 ± 360[c] 2900 ± 490[d] 3600[e]
Speciociliatine	54.5 ± 4.42[a] 560 ± 168[c] 78.6 ± 10.9[d]	>10,000[a] > 10,000[c] 1160 ± 230[d]	116 ± 36.4[a] 329 ± 112[c] 649 ± 169[d]
7-Hydroxymitragynine (Metabolite of Mitragynine)	7.16 ± 0.94[a] 77.9 (45.8–152)[b] 47 ± 18[c] 36.6 ± 4.1[d] 70[e]	236 ± 5.76[a] 243 (168–355)[b] 219 ± 41[c] 90.6 ± 8.50[d] 470[e]	74.1 ± 7.78[a] 220 (162–302)[b] 188 ± 38[c] 132 ± 7.00[d] 320[e]
Corynantheidine	118 ± 11.8[a] 57.1 ± 8.3[i]	>10,000[a] 172 ± 24.5[i]	1910 ± 50[a] 385.4 ± 47[i]
9-Hydroxycorynantheidine	105 ± 0.60[a]	>10,000[a]	>10,000[a]
Corynoxine	>10,000[e] 16.4 ± 1.4[h] 140.6 ± 73.9[i]	>10,000[e] 1274 ± 226[i]	>10,000[e] 3081 ± 1728[i]
Corynoxine B	1600[e] 109.8 ± 8.1[h] 5010 ± 388[i]	7600[e] 1682 ± 261[i]	>10,000[e] > 10,000[i]

[a]Competition binding utilizing cell lines expressing human opioid receptors (Obeng et al., 2020).
[b]Competition binding utilizing cell lines expressing human opioid receptors (Obeng et al., 2021).
[c]Radioligand competition binding with cells stably expressing human MOR, DOR, and KOR conducted by the National Institute of Mental Health's Psychoactive Drug Screening Program (NIMH PDSP) (Kruegel et al., 2016).
[d]Radioligand competition binding with $[^{125}I]$BNtxA using Chinese Hamster Ovary (CHO) cells stably expressing murine clones of MOR, DOR, and KOR (Kruegel et al., 2016).
[e]Competition binding utilizing cell lines expressing human opioid receptors (Ellis et al., 2020).
[f]Competition binding using rat whole brain tissue excluding the cerebellum (Yue, Kopajtic, & Katz, 2018).
[g]Competition binding using guinea pig whole brain tissue excluding the cerebellum (Takayama et al., 2002).
[h]Competition binding utilizing cell lines expressing human opioid receptors (Chear et al., 2021).
[i]Radioligand competition binding with $[^{125}I]$BNtxA using Chinese Hamster Ovary (CHO) cells stably expressing murine clones of MOR, DOR, and KOR (Chakraborty et al., 2021).
CI, confidence interval; SEM, standard of error of mean.

Ellis et al. (2020) reported that these alkaloids have lower affinity at the MOR ($K_i > 1500$ nM). Intrinsic activity (i.e., efficacy) assessments of 7-hydroxymitragynine and mitragynine at opioid receptors indicate that they are both partial agonists at the MOR: 7-hydroxymitragynine [$EC_{50} = 34.5 \pm 4.5$ nM, $E_{max} = 47\%$ (Kruegel et al., 2016); $EC_{50} = 53 \pm 4$ nM, $E_{max} = 77 \pm 5\%$ (Varadi et al., 2016)] and mitragynine [$EC_{50} = 339 \pm 178$ nM, $E_{max} = 34\%$ (Kruegel et al., 2016), $EC_{50} = 203 \pm 13$ nM, $E_{max} = 65 \pm 2.8\%$ (Varadi et al., 2016)]. Several other alkaloids appear to have moderate or low binding affinity at MOR including paynantheine ($IC_{50} = 2200 \pm 10{,}000$ nM), speciogynine ($IC_{50} = 5700 \pm 2800$ nM), and speciociliatine ($IC_{50} = 4200 \pm 1600$ nM), and they appear to have low to negligible MOR agonist efficacy (Kruegel et al., 2016). In another study (Obeng et al., 2020), mitragynine was shown to be a partial MOR agonist in vitro ($EC_{50} = 308$ nM, $E_{max} = 45\%$), as was speciociliatine ($EC_{50} = 39.2$ nM, $E_{max} = 74\%$), whereas 7-hydroxymitragynine was shown to be a full agonist in comparison to the reference agonist peptide DAMGO ($EC_{50} = 7.60$ nM, $E_{max} = 97\%$). When the functional activities of ligands were studied in combination at MOR expressed *in vitro*, both 7-hydroxymitragynine ($EC_{50} = 43.4$ nM, $E_{max} = 41.3\%$) and mitragynine ($E_{max} = 3.46\%$) antagonized higher efficacy MOR agonists (Obeng, Wilkerson, et al., 2021). Thus, assessments of efficacy across a range of conditions generally show mitragynine and 7-hydroxymitragynine to be partial MOR agonists like buprenorphine [$E_{max} = 42.8$ (37.2–48.4)] (Obeng, Wilkerson, et al., 2021), with the precise efficacy profile determined by the receptor variant expressed in vitro (e.g., mouse, rat, and human) or different cellular assays to measure G protein activation. For instance, the efficacy studies in Varadi et al. (2016) were conducted with cell lines stably expressing murine opioid receptors while in the study by Obeng, Wilkerson, et al. (2021), the efficacy studies were conducted in cell lines expressing human opioid receptors. Mitragynine pseudoindoxyl, a metabolite of 7-hydroxymitragynine, has high affinity at opioid receptors (MOR $K_i = 0.8 \pm 0.2$ nM) and was a highly potent MOR agonist ($EC_{50} = 1.7 \pm 0.1$ nM, $E_{max} = 84 \pm 5\%$) (Varadi et al., 2016). Mitragynine, 7-hydroxymitragynine, and mitragynine pseudoindoxyl failed to recruit β-arrestin-2 at concentrations as high as 10 μM, and their bias for G-protein signaling was proposed to be due to allosteric modulation of the MOR (Varadi et al., 2016; Zhou et al., 2021). Corynantheidine

(EC_{50}= 104±4.59 nM, E_{max}=74.1%±1.24%) and corynoxine (EC_{50}= 202.8±4.4 nM, E_{max}= 136%±3.3%) were recently shown to be agonists at the MOR and both compounds did not recruit β-arrestin-2 (Chakraborty et al., 2021).

2.2 Adrenergic and serotonergic receptors

Kratom alkaloids have also been demonstrated to bind to adrenergic and serotonergic receptors in vitro. Corynantheidine was demonstrated to have the highest affinity at adrenergic receptors with an affinity of 41.7±4.7 nM at the α_{1D} receptor and 74 nM at the α_{2A} receptor (Table 2). Mitragynine also bound to adrenergic receptors albeit with lower affinity than corynantheidine at the α_{1D} adrenergic receptor (Table 2). Among the adrenergic receptors, mitragynine had the highest affinity at the α_{1A} receptor subtype (K_i=1340±100 nM). Furthermore, corynantheidine at 10 μM, produced greater than 80% displacement at the α_{1A}, α_{1B}, α_{2A}, and α_{2B} adrenergic receptors, indicating that corynantheidine may have appreciable affinity for these adrenergic receptors. Speciociliatine, at 10 μM, also produced greater than 50% displacement of bound radioligand at the above-mentioned adrenergic receptors. 9-Hydroxycorynantheidine produced greater than 50% displacement of radioligand at the α_{1A} and α_{1D} receptors. 7-Hydroxymitragynine did not displace bound radioligand at the α-adrenergic receptors, indicating that it has relatively low affinity for the adrenergic receptor subtypes (Ellis et al., 2020; Obeng et al., 2020). The kratom alkaloids speciogynine and paynantheine bound with relatively high affinity at 5-HT_{1A} and 5-HT_{2B} serotonergic receptors (Table 3). Mitragynine also bound to these serotonergic receptors, albeit with lower affinity than paynantheine and speciogynine (Table 3). 7-Hydroxymitragynine, corynoxine, and corynoxine B have low, if any, affinity for the serotonergic receptors.

3. Pharmacokinetics of kratom alkaloids

In vitro and in vivo pharmacokinetics of kratom alkaloids have been studied in various pre-clinical and clinical settings. In vivo pharmacokinetic studies were performed either after an oral dose of traditional/commercial kratom preparations (tea and organic extract) or individual kratom alkaloids.

Table 2 Reported affinities [K_i; mean ± SEM in nM] of kratom alkaloids at human adrenergic receptor subtypes.

Kratom alkaloid or its metabolite	α_{1A}	α_{1B}	α_{1D}	α_{2A}	α_{2B}	α_{2C}
Mitragynine	1340 ± 100[a]	4770 ± 120[a]	5480 ± 540[a]	4720 ± 120[a] 2300[b]	9290 ± 30[a] 4900[b]	2320 ± 140[a] 3500[b]
Speciogynine	Not determined	Not determined	Not determined	360[b]	2600[b]	680[b]
7-Hydroxymitragynine	Not determined	Not determined	Not determined	>10,000[b]	>10,000[b]	>10,000[b]
Corynantheidine	397[c]	3304[c]	41.7 ± 4.7[a]	74[c]	1539[c]	269[c]
Corynoxine	Not determined	Not determined	Not determined	>10,000[b]	8400[b]	>10,000[b]
Corynoxine B	Not determined	Not determined	Not determined	>10,000[b]	>10,000[b]	>10,000[b]

[a]Competition binding utilizing cell lines expressing human opioid receptors (Obeng et al., 2020).
[b]Competition binding utilizing cell lines expressing human opioid receptors (Ellis et al., 2020).
[c]Competition binding utilizing cell lines expressing human opioid receptors (Chakraborty et al., 2021).

Table 3 K_i values (mean ± SEM in nM) of kratom alkaloids at human serotonergic receptor subtypes.

Kratom alkaloid or its metabolite	$5\text{-}HT_{1A}$	$5\text{-}HT_{7A}$	$5\text{-}HT_{2A}$	$5\text{-}HT_{2B}$	$5\text{-}HT_{2C}$
Mitragynine	5880 ± 828[a] 5800[b]	>10,000[a]	5007 ± 1149[a] 7300[b]	1262 ± 138[a]	>10,000[a]
Speciogynine	38.5 ± 3.9[a] 95.5 ± 34.7[a] 540[b]	1600 ± 82[a]	1322 ± 365[a] 2900[b]	23.0 ± 5.7[a] 108 ± 39.5[a]	5434 ± 922[a]
Paynantheine	32.0 ± 3.5[a] 71.8 ± 13.2[a]	870 ± 72[a]	815 ± 192[a]	20.0 ± 2.8[a] 83.1 ± 32.9[a]	1766 ± 417[a]
7-Hydroxymitragynine	>10,000[b]	Not determined	>10,000[b]	Not determined	Not determined
Corynantheidine	1156[c]	Not determined	Not determined	Not determined	Not determined
Corynoxine	>10,000[b]	Not determined	>10,000[b]	Not determined	Not determined
Corynoxine B	>10,000[b]	Not determined	>10,000[b]	Not determined	Not determined

[a]Competition binding utilizing cell lines expressing human opioid receptors (León et al., 2021).
[b]Competition binding utilizing cell lines expressing human opioid receptors (Ellis et al., 2020).
[c]Competition binding utilizing cell lines expressing human opioid receptors (Chakraborty et al., 2021).

The major kratom alkaloid, mitragynine, has been the focus of most studies reported to date. The pharmacokinetics of mitragynine, along with other kratom alkaloids, will be described in this section.

3.1 Mitragynine

3.1.1 Absorption

Mitragynine is a basic compound with low aqueous solubility ($64.6 \pm 1.2\,\mu g/mL$) and high permeability across both the Caco-2 [apparent permeability (P_{app}), 24.2×10^{-6} cm/s] and Madin-Darby Canine Kidney (MDCK) (P_{app}, 15.3×10^{-6} cm/s) cell monolayers (Manda et al., 2014; Ramanathan et al., 2015). Mitragynine is not a known substrate of P-glycoprotein (P-gp, efflux ratio < 1.2), but it inhibits P-gp by down-regulating mRNA and protein expression (Manda et al., 2014; Rusli et al., 2019). During the absorption process, mitragynine can be metabolized to oxidative metabolites including 7-hydroxymitragynine through cytochrome P450 (CYP) enzymes present in the enterocytes of the intestinal epithelium (Kamble et al., 2019). Mitragynine, a biopharmaceutics classification system (BCS) Class II compound, when dosed individually, showed very fast absorption; first peak plasma concentrations (C_{max}) were observed within (T_{max}) 1.5 h post-dose in male rats, female dogs and male humans (Avery et al., 2019; Maxwell et al., 2020; Trakulsrichai et al., 2015). Mitragynine also exhibited a multiple peak phenomenon possibly due to the opioid receptor-mediated delayed gastric emptying and/or absorption through multiple sites in the gastrointestinal tract (Avery et al., 2019; Maxwell et al., 2020; Trakulsrichai et al., 2015). After an oral dose of traditional kratom drinks, the C_{max} of mitragynine was observed in ranges of 18.5–105 and 1200–2500 ng/mL in regular kratom users from Thailand and Malaysia, respectively (Trakulsrichai et al., 2015; Vicknasingam et al., 2020). Mitragynine showed faster and more extensive absorption when dosed with other kratom constituents (lyophilized tea and organic extract of kratom) compared to the equivalent oral dose of mitragynine only (Avery et al., 2019). The pharmacokinetics of any given kratom alkaloid therefore appears to depend upon the types and amounts of alkaloids contained within any given natural or commercial product.

3.1.2 Distribution

Mitragynine is lipophilic [partition coefficient (log P), 1.73] and therefore has favorable physicochemical properties to distribute throughout the body (Ramanathan et al., 2015). The volume of distribution (V_d) of mitragynine in dogs (6.3 ± 0.6 L/kg) and rats (8.0 ± 1.5 L/kg) was larger than the total blood volume in the respective species indicating widespread distribution of mitragynine into tissues (Avery et al., 2019; Maxwell et al., 2020). The mitragynine concentration-time profile exhibits biexponential decay, and a two compartmental pharmacokinetic model best describes the concentration-time data (Avery et al., 2019). Mitragynine was found at greater concentrations in highly perfused tissues than in blood. During an autopsy sample analysis, mitragynine concentrations were found to be 1.7- to 100-fold higher in the liver than in the central blood (Mata & Andera, 2020). Mitragynine crosses the blood-brain barrier and distributes throughout the brain in areas including the hippocampus, mid-brain, brainstem, and cerebellum. Concentrations of mitragynine free fraction were higher in the hippocampus than in the whole brain or in the systemic circulation (Yusof et al., 2019). Mitragynine exhibits high plasma protein binding, but species differences in plasma protein binding have been observed. A comparatively higher unbound fraction (f_u) of mitragynine is available in rat plasma (f_u, 0.21) than in human plasma (f_u, 0.02) (Obeng et al., 2020; Yusof et al., 2019).

3.1.3 Metabolism and elimination

Mitragynine is metabolized to *O*-demethylated and mono-oxidative metabolites in the liver primarily by CYP3A4 enzymes with a minor contribution of CYP2D6, CYP2C9 and CYP2C19 enzymes (Kamble et al., 2019; Le, Goggin, & Janis, 2012). Few of these metabolites were found to be further conjugated to glucuronides and/or sulfates (Fig. 2) (Philipp et al., 2009). Three glucuronide and three sulfate conjugated secondary metabolites of mitragynine have been identified in human urine (Philipp et al., 2009). A small amount of mitragynine is also excreted unchanged along with its other polar metabolites through urine (Le et al., 2012). Mitragynine metabolizes to its active metabolite 7-hydroxymitragynine through CYP3A4 enzymes (Kamble et al., 2019). Metabolite-to-parent ratio for 7-hydroxymitragynine is higher when mitragynine is dosed orally, as opposed to intravenously (i.v.), due to the CYP3A4 mediated intestinal metabolism of mitragynine (Hiranita et al., 2020). Among the 22 identified metabolites, 7-hydroxymitragynine, mitragynine acid, and 9-hydroxycorynantheidine (Fig. 2) are the three major metabolites of mitragynine (Kamble et al., 2019). The exposure of 7-hydroxymitragynine formed after the metabolism of mitragynine in beagle dogs was equivalent to a 0.24 mg/kg dose of

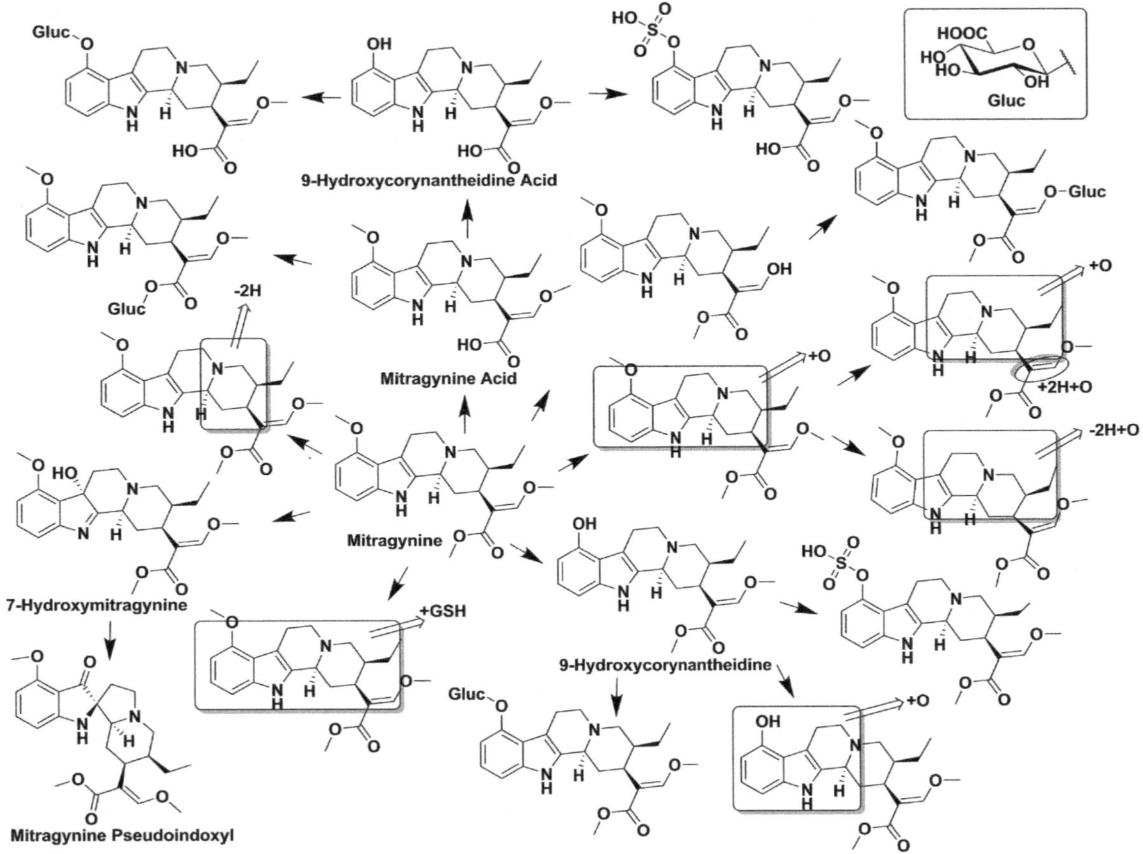

Fig. 2 Metabolism pathway of mitragynine (Kamble et al., 2019; Le et al., 2012; Philipp et al., 2009).

7-hydroxymitragynine, and it corresponds to a 23.1% conversion of mitragynine to 7-hydroxymitragynine in vivo (Maxwell et al., 2020, 2021).

Following an oral dose of a traditional kratom drink, mitragynine showed a long elimination half-life (23.2 ± 16.1 h) in regular kratom users. There is no clearance or bioavailability data available for mitragynine in humans, but it showed 1.7 ± 0.1 and 1.8 ± 0.4 L/h/kg (Tables 4 and 5) clearance in male rats and female dogs, respectively. The oral bioavailability of mitragynine ranged from 3.0% to 52.7% in rats and was 69.6% in female beagle dogs. A significant effect of sex, species, salt form used for formulation, and type of formulation (individual versus kratom extract) on the oral bioavailability of mitragynine was observed (Avery et al., 2019; de Moraes et al., 2009; Kamble et al., 2021; Parthasarathy et al., 2010). Mitragynine showed higher oral bioavailability in rats when administered as an active ingredient in lyophilized tea (1.5-fold) or as an organic extract (1.8-fold) of kratom compared to when mitragynine was administered alone at an equivalent dose of 20 mg/kg (Avery et al., 2019).

3.2 Mitragynine metabolites and other kratom alkaloids

Apart from mitragynine, there is some, albeit more limited information in the literature regarding the preclinical pharmacokinetics of 7-hydroxymitragynine, corynantheidine, paynantheine, speciociliatine and speciogynine. Studies were performed either after administration of kratom products or as individual alkaloids. When administered exogenously, 7-hydroxymitragynine, an oxidative metabolite of mitragynine, showed very rapid absorption in female beagle dogs, and the C_{max} occurred within 15 min post-dose. Compared with mitragynine and the other kratom alkaloids that have been studied, 7-hydroxymitragynine has lower plasma protein binding (90%) and a limited capability to cross the blood-brain barrier (Obeng et al., 2020; Yusof et al., 2019). The systemic exposure for 7-hydroxymitragynine is also 2.5-fold lower than mitragynine when dosed orally (Maxwell et al., 2021). Similar to female beagle dogs, a short elimination half-life ($T_{1/2}$, 0.4 ± 0.1 h) of 7-hydroxymitragynine was observed in male rats after intravenous administration of 7-hydroxymitragynine (Vuppala et al., 2013). Clearance of 7-hydroxymitragynine (2.6 ± 0.3 L/h/kg) is lower than the total hepatic blood flow (4.8 L/h/kg) in male rats (Vuppala et al., 2013). 7-Hydroxymitragynine is unstable in human plasma and converts further to the more potent MOR agonist, mitragynine pseudoindoxyl (Fig. 2) (Kamble et al., 2020). Most of the studied kratom alkaloids, including

Table 4 Pharmacokinetic parameters of kratom alkaloids in rats (Avery et al., 2019; Berthold et al., 2021; de Moraes, Moretti, Furr 3rd, McCurdy, & Lanchote, 2009; Kamble et al., 2021; King et al., 2020; Leon et al., 2021; Parthasarathy et al., 2010; Vuppala, Jamalapuram, Furr, McCurdy, & Avery, 2013).

	Mitragynine		Speciociliatine		Corynantheidine		7-Hydroxymitragynine	Paynantheine	Speciogynine
Parameter	**Oral**	**I.V.**	**Oral**	**I.V.**	**Oral**	**I.V.**	**I.V.**	**I.V.**	**I.V.**
C_{max}/Dose (ng/mL/mg/kg)	22.9–44.2	–	63.3 ± 15.0	–	10.7 ± 2.0	–	–	–	–
T_{max} (h)	1.4–3.8	–	1.0 ± 0.4	–	4.1 ± 1.3	–	–	–	–
Clearance (L/h/kg)	–	1.7 ± 0.1	–	0.7 ± 0.2	–	3.5 ± 0.1	2.6 ± 0.3	5.3 ± 0.2	3.2 ± 0.0
V_d (L/kg)	–	6.3 ± 1.4	–	6.2 ± 2.3	–	32.0 ± 4.8	1.7 ± 0.2	71.9 ± 6.5	30.1 ± 8.4
$T_{1/2}$ (h)	2.9–3.3	6.0 ± 1.5	3.8 ± 1.2	6.3 ± 2.0	–	6.9 ± 0.0	0.4 ± 0.1	9.4 ± 0.8	6.6 ± 1.8
Bioavailability (%)	3.0–52.7	–	20.7	–	49.9	–	–	–	–

Abbreviations: I.V., intravenous; C_{max}, peak plasma concentration; T_{max}, time to reach C_{max}; $T_{1/2}$, elimination half-life; V_d, volume of distribution.

Table 5 Pharmacokinetic parameters of kratom alkaloids in beagle dogs (Maxwell et al., 2020; Maxwell et al., 2021).

	Mitragynine		7-Hydroxymitragynine
Parameters	**Oral**	**I.V.**	**Oral**
C_{max}/Dose (ng/mL/mg/kg)	55.6 ± 9.5	–	56.4 ± 1.6
T_{max} (h)	0.3 ± 0.1	–	0.14 ± 0.1
Clearance (L/h/kg)	–	1.8 ± 0.4	–
V_d (L/kg)	–	6.3 ± 0.6	–
$T_{1/2}$ (h)	8.7 ± 0.2	2.7 ± 0.6	3.6 ± 0.5
Bioavailability (%)	69.6	–	–

Abbreviations: I.V., intravenous; C_{max}, peak plasma concentration; T_{max}, time to reach C_{max}; $T_{1/2}$, elimination half-life; V_d, volume of distribution.

mitragynine, 7-hydroxymitragynine, and speciociliatine showed rapid absorption, but corynantheidine demonstrated prolonged absorption in male rats. Corynantheidine exhibited flip-flop kinetics and the C_{max} was observed after 4.1 ± 1.3 h (T_{max}) post-dose (King et al., 2020). Similar to mitragynine, corynantheidine exhibited high plasma protein binding (f_u, 0.02) (Obeng et al., 2020). Corynantheidine showed high clearance (3.5 ± 0.1 L/h/kg), a large V_d (32.0 ± 4.8 L/kg) and adequate oral bioavailability (49.9% ± 16.4%) in rats. Corynantheidine can cross the blood-brain barrier and is localized in the corpus callosum and hippocampal regions of the brain (King et al., 2020).

Speciociliatine, a diastereomer (i.e., four isomers possible based on the presence of two chiral centers in the molecule) of mitragynine, showed rapid absorption; the C_{max} occurred within 1.0 ± 0.4 h (T_{max}) post-dose in rats. Speciociliatine exhibited a large V_d (6.2 ± 2.3 L/kg) and low clearance (0.7 ± 0.2 L/h/kg) in male rats. It exhibited a moderate elimination half-life (3.8 ± 1.2 h) with an oral bioavailability of 20.7%. Paynantheine and speciogynine, two kratom alkaloids with high affinity for 5-HT_{1A} and 5-HT_{2B} receptors, exhibited a large V_d (71.9 ± 6.5 and 30.1 ± 8.4 L/kg) like other kratom alkaloids in rats. Clearance of speciogynine (3.2 ± 0.0 L/h/kg) was comparatively lower than paynantheine (5.3 ± 0.2 L/h/kg) in rats (Leon et al., 2021). Of the various kratom alkaloids that have been studied to date, including corynantheidine, mitragynine, 7-hydroxymitragynine, paynantheine and speciogynine, speciociliatine exhibited the highest systemic exposure [area under curve (AUC)/Dose] with the lowest clearance in male rats (Berthold et al., 2021) (Table 4). Speciociliatine is also one of four kratom alkaloids (the others being mitragynine, 7-hydroxymitragynine and corynantheidine) available systemically after an oral dose of either traditional or commercial kratom products in male rats (Kamble et al., 2021).

4. Behavioral effects of kratom alkaloids

4.1 Antinociception

Publications dating back to 1930 report that kratom possesses analgesic properties and opioid-like effects (Boyer, Babu, Adkins, McCurdy, & Halpern, 2008; Burkill & Haniff, 1930; Jansen & Prast, 1988; Swogger et al., 2015). Despite these claims, relatively few preclinical studies have been conducted to explore the analgesic potential of the various kratom alkaloids. The most widely utilized preclinical acute nociceptive pain models to examine kratom alkaloids have been noxious stimuli applied to the tail (i.e., heat, pinch) and the hot plate test. The tail nociception assays measure the latency for a rodent to move its tail away from a noxious stimulus, whereas the hot plate test measures the latency for a rodent to respond via lifting paws or jumping, after being placed on a heated surface. Although both assays capture response times to noxious stimulus, acute nociceptive signaling in the hot plate assay is regulated largely via the spinothalamic tract (Smith et al., 2017), whereas acute nociceptive responses produced by tail nociception assays are mediated by spinally driven reflexes (Irwin, Houde, Bennett, Hendershot, & Seevers, 1951). To date mitragynine, 7-hydroxymitragynine, corynanthidine, corynoxine, mitraciliatine, isopaynantheine, speciociliatine, various preparations of mixed kratom alkaloids, as well as derivatives of mitragynine and corynanthidine have shown analgesic activity in preclinical pain models. The analgesic potential of other kratom alkaloids has not been explored.

4.1.1 Mitragynine

Mitragynine has been to produce antinociceptive effects in preclinical acute nociceptive pain models. In both rats and mice, systemic administration of mitragynine produced antinociception in the hot plate assay but was only a partially antinociceptive when compared to prototypical opioid agonists (Carpenter et al., 2016; Hiranita et al., 2019; Obeng, Hiranita, Leon, McMahon, & McCurdy, 2021; Shamima et al., 2012). Mitragynine-induced hot plate antinociception was antagonized by both naltrexone and naltrindole, indicative of mediation by opioid receptors (Carpenter et al., 2016; Hiranita et al., 2019; Shamima et al., 2012). When delivered via an intracerebroventricular (i.c.v.) injection in mice, mitragynine produced significant antinociception in both tail nociception and hot plate tests (Matsumoto et al., 1996). As with systemic mitragynine, this antinociception was also not as robust as that observed from i.c.v. administered prototypical opioids (Matsumoto et al., 1996).

Limited reports have detailed the effects of mitragynine in chronic, pathological pain models. Recently, Foss and colleagues found that systemic mitragynine reversed mechanical allodynia, or light touch sensitivity, in a rat chemotherapeutic neuropathy model (Foss et al., 2020). This reversal was significantly reduced by naltrexone as well as by the adrenergic α_2 receptor antagonist yohimbine and the adrenergic α_1 receptor antagonist prazosin, suggesting antiallodynic activity of mitragynine through a combination of opioid and adrenergic receptors (Foss et al., 2020). In contrast to acute pain models, mitragynine was more effective in attenuating mechanical allodynia. As with the hot plate assay, mechanical allodynia is mediated via the spinothalamic tract, but the two behaviors have different underlying cellular mechanisms (Otsubo et al., 2012).

4.1.2 7-Hydroxymitragynine

7-Hydroxymitragynine produces antinociceptive effects in preclinical acute nociceptive pain models. When delivered systemically in mice and rats, 7-hydroxymitragynine produced significant opioid receptor-mediated antinociception and was more potent than morphine in both tail nociception and hot plate tests (Matsumoto et al., 2004; Obeng et al., 2020).

4.1.3 Other kratom alkaloids

When administered i.v. in female and male Sprague-Dawley rats, both speciociliatine and corynoxine produced robust antinociceptive effects in the hotplate test (Chear et al., 2021; Obeng et al., 2020). In addition, i.c.v. corynoxine produced robust antinociceptive effects under a warm-water tail-withdrawal assay at 55 °C in male C57BL/6J mice, and the antinociceptive effects of i.c.v. corynoxine was significant but lower in MOR knockout mice than in their wildtype littermates (Chakraborty et al., 2021).

Robust antinociception under the warm-water tail-withdrawal assay at 55 °C was also produced by i.c.v. injection of corynanthidine, mitraciliatine, and isopaynantheine in male C57BL/6J mice and the antinociceptive effects of i.c.v. administered corynanthidine, mitraciliatine, and isopaynantheine were attenuated in MOR knockout mice (Chakraborty et al., 2021).

4.1.4 Mixed kratom alkaloid preparations

Several different kratom preparations of various alkaloid mixtures and percentages have been studied in preclinical antinociception models. When administered systemically or orally, these preparations have shown, in mice and rats, to produce anticonception in both tail nociception and hot plate assays (Carpenter et al., 2016; Reanmongkol, Keawpradub, & Sawangjaroen, 2007; Sabetghadam, Ramanathan, & Mansor, 2010). In mice, orally administered lyophilized kratom tea has been found to produce μ- and κ-opioid receptor mediated antinociception in tail nociception assays (Wilson et al., 2020).

4.1.5 Mitragynine and corynanthidine derivatives

Pseudoindoxyl derivatives of both mitragynine and corynanthidine have been made and subsequently shown to exert considerable opioid activity (Takayama et al., 2002; Varadi et al., 2016). When administered orally, systemically and i.c.v. these compounds have been found to produce significant antinociception in both tail nociception and hot plate tests, comparable to morphine (Takayama et al., 2002; Varadi et al., 2016; Wilson et al., 2021). Matsumoto and colleagues have produced a series of mitragynine derivatives which possess antinociceptive properties. One compound in this series, MGM-9, dosed both orally and systemically, produced potent μ- and κ-opioid receptor mediated antinociception in mice in both the tail nociception and hot plate assays, as well as in the acetic acid-induced writhing chemical nociception model (Matsumoto et al., 2008). In this model, acetic acid is administered intraperitoneally (i.p.), which produces discomfort to the animal, and the number of writhing-related behaviors is counted (Gawade, 2012). Another mitragynine derivative, MGM-16, dosed orally, attenuated partial sciatic nerve-induced mechanical allodynia in mice, and this attenuation appeared to be mediated by both μ- and δ-opioid receptor mechanisms (Matsumoto et al., 2014).

4.2 I.v. drug self administration

This procedure is generally thought to be the gold standard for assessment of the abuse liability of drugs of abuse, and is often used to assess abuse potential of novel compounds and preclinical efficacy to treat substance use disorders (see reviews by Grabowski, Shearer, Merrill, & Negus, 2004; Horton,

Potter, & Mead, 2013; Katz, Hiranita, Hong, Job, & McCurdy, 2017; O'Connor, Chapman, Butler, & Mead, 2011). An experimental animal is placed in an operant conditioning chamber and an i.v. injection of test compound through a chronic indwelling catheter is scheduled to be given upon completion of an operant response (e.g., lever-pressing behavior). The rate of responding is compared to that when vehicle is substituted for the training compound.

Using this procedure under fixed-ratio schedules of reinforcement, two studies have assessed the abuse-related effects of mitragynine and 7-hydroxymitragynine. Consistent with the in vitro receptor binding data at MOR (Kruegel et al., 2019; Obeng, Wilkerson, et al., 2021), 7-hydroxymitragynine maintained self-administration responding above vehicle levels in male rats when substituted for morphine (Fischer 344 strain) or methamphetamine (Sprague-Dawley strain) as well as in male naïve rats (Fischer 344 strain) (Hemby, McIntosh, Leon, Cutler, & McCurdy, 2019; Yue et al., 2018). When substituted for morphine, the responding maintained by a fixed dose of 7-hydroxymitragynine was decreased dose-dependently by naloxonazine, a MOR antagonist, as well as naltrindole, a DOR antagonist (Hemby et al., 2019). Due to the doses that were studied, it could not be determined whether the decreases in 7-hydroxymitragynine self-administration were due to a leftward (i.e., potentiation), rightward (i.e., antagonism), or downward shift of the inverted u-shaped 7-hydroxymitragynine self-administration dose-effect function. In contrast, mitragynine failed to maintain self-administration responding above vehicle levels in male rats when substituted for morphine or methamphetamine (Hemby et al., 2019; Yue et al., 2018). Thus, by comparing the robust self-administration of 7-hydroxymitragynine, a known in vivo metabolite of mitragynine, to the absence of any self-administration of mitragynine, it may be speculated that conversion of mitragynine to 7-hydroxymitragynine does not confer abuse-related effects.

When pretreated i.p., mitragynine dose-dependently produced downward shifts in the dose-effect function of heroin substitution for methamphetamine (Yue et al., 2018). In addition, the attenuation of heroin self-administration by mitragynine was relatively selective because mitragynine was more potent in decreasing responding maintained by heroin than in decreasing responding maintained by methamphetamine (Yue et al., 2018). The insurmountable and specific antagonism of heroin self-administration with mitragynine suggests the potential development of mitragynine to treat opioid use disorder. However, a mechanism underlying the insurmountable antagonism remains to be elucidated. Given that pretreatment with MOR agonists and antagonists can result in insurmountable and surmountable antagonism of self-administration of MOR agonists, respectively (Hiranita et al., 2014; Hiranita, Soto, Tanda, Kopajtic, & Katz, 2013; Tanda et al., 2016), it appears that the insurmountable antagonism of heroin self-administration with mitragynine is due to partial MOR agonist activity of mitragynine and/or 7-hydroxymitragynine converted from mitragynine. However, this pattern of substitution and pretreatment effects of mitragynine is inconsistent from the profile produced by pretreatment with the partial MOR agonist buprenorphine. Buprenorphine produced insurmountable antagonism of self-administration of the MOR agonist alfentanil as well as the dopamine uptake inhibitor cocaine in rhesus monkeys self-administering alfentanil and cocaine, respectively (Winger, Skjoldager, & Woods, 1992). In addition, buprenorphine maintained self-administration responding above vehicle levels when substituted for alfentanil in rhesus monkeys self-administering alfentanil (Winger et al., 1992). Currently the mechanism underlying the inconsistency in the effects of mitragynine and buprenorphine remains to be elucidated. Given that mitragynine pseudoindoxyl is an active and potent metabolite of 7-hydromitragynine, abuse potential of mitragynine pseudoindoxyl and its effects on self-administration of opioids remain to be elucidated. In addition, given that only male subjects have been used for the i.v. self-administration, the impact of biological sex on the abuse potential and preclinical efficacy of mitragynine, 7-hydroxymitragynine, and mitragynine pseudoindoxyl to decrease self-administration of opioids remains to be elucidated. Moreover, while fixed-ratio schedules of reinforcement are useful to assess the presence or absence of reinforcing effects of test compounds, the relative reinforcing strength of kratom alkaloids cannot be easily measured with these procedures. Thus, assessment of the reinforcing strength of mitragynine and 7-hydroxymitragynine remains to be elucidated. The reinforcing strength can be compared using an i.v. drug self-administration procedure using progressive-ratio schedules of drug reinforcement (Roberts & Bennett, 1993) and choice procedures (Townsend, Schwienteck, Robinson, Lawson, & Banks, 2021).

4.3 Drug discrimination

Whereas drug discrimination assays are not directly employed to assess the abuse potential of test compounds, these assays have considerable pharmacological selectivity and can be used to identify the receptor mechanism of action of test compounds by comparing their effects to reference compounds (i.e., training drugs) that have a well-established receptor mechanism of action (e.g., Holtzman, 1985; Katz et al., 2017; Schuster & Johanson, 1988). An experimental animal is placed in an operant conditioning chamber typically with two levers on which the animal is conditioned to press for delivery of food or water. Allocation of responses to one of the two levers is established with an injection of the training compound as a discriminative stimulus (Catania, 2013). In one type of training session, the completion of operant responding on one lever is assigned as correct (i.e., is reinforced by food delivery) when preceded by an injection of a training drug (i.e., drug training). In the second type of training session, responding on the second lever is assigned as correct (i.e., is reinforced by food delivery) when preceded by an injection of vehicle (i.e., vehicle training). Once trained to meet predetermined learning criteria, the animals are considered to be able to discriminate the presence of the training drug from its absence. Trained animals can be tested with various doses and pretreatment times of the training drug, or doses or varying pretreatment times of other compounds. In these test session the percentage of responding on the drug-appropriate lever is used as an indication of the extent to which the test and training drugs share interoceptive effects and a pharmacological mechanism of action. Additionally, antagonists can be tested to for their capacity to attenuate the effects of a training and/or test drug; attenuation is evidenced by a shift in responding from the drug-appropriate lever to the vehicle-appropriate lever. A shift down or rightward of the dose-effect function of the training or testing compound by an antagonist is evidence of functional or competitive antagonism, respectively (Hiranita et al., 2014; Hiranita, Soto, Tanda, & Katz, 2011; Kohut et al., 2014), although care must be taken to rule out other interpretations (i.e., perceptual masking).

Using this procedure, only two studies assessed discriminative-stimulus effects of mitragynine and 7-hydroxymitragynine. In male Sprague-Dawley rats, mitragynine (15 mg/kg, i.p.) served as a discriminative stimulus (Harun, Hassan, Navaratnam, Mansor, & Shoaib, 2015). In male and female Sprague-Dawley rats, 32 mg/kg mitragynine (i.p.) also served as a discriminative stimulus (Obeng, Wilkerson, et al., 2021). 7-Hydroxymitragynine substituted for 32 mg/kg mitragynine (Obeng, Wilkerson, et al., 2021). The extent to which 7-hydroxymitragynine may substitute for 15 mg/kg mitragynine was not assessed (Harun et al., 2015). In both studies (Harun et al., 2015; Obeng, Wilkerson, et al., 2021), another group of rats was trained with morphine (5.0 and 3.2 mg/kg, i.p., respectively). 7-hydroxymitragynine substituted for morphine regardless of the training doses of morphine (Harun et al., 2015; Obeng, Wilkerson, et al., 2021). 7-Hydroxymitragynine substitution for morphine was antagonized by the opioid receptor antagonists naloxone (0.3 mg/kg) and naltrexone (0.032 mg/kg) (Harun et al., 2015; Obeng, Wilkerson, et al., 2021). However, it appears that the studies of mitragynine substitution for morphine resulted in a marked asymmetric pattern. For example, regardless of sex, no dose of mitragynine (up to 56 mg/kg which was the largest dose that did not disrupt operant responding or produce marked adverse effects) produced greater than 80% morphine-lever responding when tested in animals discriminating 3.2 mg/kg morphine (Obeng, Wilkerson, et al., 2021). The cross-substitution patterns of mitragynine and morphine differs from that of the partial MOR agonist buprenorphine. For example, buprenorphine substituted for mitragynine as well as morphine. Naltrexone shifted the dose-effect function of mitragynine discrimination rightward and downward (Obeng, Wilkerson, et al., 2021). In rats trained with the higher dose of morphine (Harun et al., 2015), greater than 80% morphine lever responding was obtained with 15, but not a higher dose 30 mg/kg of mitragynine. No dose of naloxone (0.1, 0.3, and 1.0 mg/kg) significantly antagonized the discriminative-stimulus effects of 15 mg/kg mitragynine (Harun et al., 2015). However, only 0.3 mg/kg of naloxone, but not a higher dose of 1.0 mg/kg, antagonized the discriminative-stimulus effects of 5.0 mg/kg morphine (Harun et al., 2015). The extent to which substitution of 15 mg/kg mitragynine for 5.0 mg/kg morphine could be antagonized by 0.3 mg/kg naloxone was not assessed. A plausible explanation for lack of morphine antagonism at a low and not high dose of naloxone is not clear (Harun et al., 2015). In general, these findings suggest that full substitution of mitragynine for morphine is not consistently obtained across the few studies that have been conducted. In addition, mitragynine can produce its discriminative-stimulus effects in a manner sensitive to naltrexone. Given that the antinociceptive and antiallodynic effects of mitragynine were antagonized by the adrenergic α_2 receptor antagonists (Foss et al., 2020; Matsumoto et al., 1996), sensitivity of mitragynine discrimination to an adrenergic α_2 receptor antagonist remains to be assessed.

In mitragynine-trained rats substitution tests were conducted with several ligands that have little, if any, affinity at MOR; these include KOR agonist U69,593, DOR agonist SNC 80, and the monoamine transporter inhibitor cocaine. However, no dose of these compounds produced greater than 80% mitragynine lever responding (Harun et al., 2015; Obeng, Wilkerson, et al., 2021). Thus, none of these non-MOR receptor mechanisms can fully explain mitragynine pharmacology.

4.4 Rodent locomotor activity

Whereas morphine has well-established locomotor stimulant effects in rodents, no dose of mitragynine (5–30 mg/kg, i.p.) increased locomotor activity counts in male Sprague-Dawley rats and male ddY and ICR mice, and these negative outcomes were not dependent on whether animals had been habituated to the activity chambers or not (Apryani, Hidayat, Moklas, Fakurazi, & Idayu, 2010; Japarin, Yusoff, Hassan, Muller, & Harun, 2021; Matsumoto et al., 1997; Yusoff, Mansor, Muller, & Hassan, 2017, 2018). No increase in locomotor activity counts was obtained with a methanolic extract and alkaloid-enriched fractions of *M. speciosa* in male ICR and C57BL/6 mice (Cheaha et al., 2017; Gutridge et al., 2020; Reanmongkol et al., 2007). However, 7-hydroxymitragynine did increase locomotor activity counts in male ddY and C57BL/6 mice (Gutridge et al., 2020; Matsumoto et al., 2008). The marked differences in locomotor stimulant effects of 7-hydroxymitragynine *versus* mitragynine as well as the methanolic extract and alkaloid-enriched fractions of *M. speciosa* provide further evidence that there is little, if any, contribution of 7-hydroxymitragynine converted from mitragynine to the in vivo activity of mitragynine.

As with mitragynine, robust increases in locomotor activity counts were not produced by i.c.v. injection of corynoxine or mitraciliatine in male C57BL/6J mice (Chakraborty et al., 2021).

4.5 Place conditioning

Typically, rodents are placed in a chamber with at least two compartments, each with distinct features such as different tactile flooring patterns (grids or mesh), wall decorations (solid or stripes), or types of bedding. During "preconditioning" sessions, experimental subjects are initially allowed to habituate throughout the different compartments, and their allocation of time in each compartment is recorded as baseline. Some studies exclude experimental subjects that spend significantly more time in one compartment *versus* the other (e.g., greater than 80% of preconditioning period) so that only experimental subjects exhibiting no initial "place preference" are selected (unbiased conditioning). During subsequent conditioning sessions, a compound of interest is injected and the experimental subject is restricted to one compartment. Vehicle injections typically precede daily conditioning sessions in which the subject is confined to the alternate compartment. These conditioning sessions are conducted to affect a Pavlovian (classical) conditioning of the distinctive stimuli of the compartment with the experimental subjective effect of compound of interest. During a subsequent drug-free post-conditioning assessment, the experimental subject is given concurrent access to both compartments as in baseline (pre-conditioning) sessions, and time allocation in each compartment is again recorded. An increase compared to baseline in time allocated to the compound-paired compartment is considered an indication of an effective place conditioning (i.e., place preference), with the distinctive features of the compound-paired compartment as the conditional stimuli and the compound effect as the unconditional stimulus. Allocation of greater time in post- compared to pre-conditioning may be considered a result of reinforcing effects of the conditional stimulus which result in the increase in time allocation. The increase in time allocation is thought to provide an indication of the abuse liability and abuse potential of the compound (Hutchinson et al., 2012; Northcutt et al., 2015). Alternatively, a decrease in time allocated to the compound-paired compartment is also considered an indication of an effective place conditioning (i.e., place aversion) reflecting a noxious effect of the conditional stimuli associated with an unconditional noxious effect of the compound. Some studies intentionally use experimental subjects exhibiting initial "place preference" and the preferred compartment is paired with vehicle. Thus, the subject assignment allows to assess if the positive reinforcing effects of compound can overcome the initial "preference" (biased conditioning). Assessments of the literature utilizing this procedure have indicated that it has reasonable predictive validity for drugs of abuse, though it has its share of false positives and negatives (e.g., Bardo & Bevins, 2000; Carr, Fibiger, & Phillips, 1989).

In general, kratom products lack a place-conditioning effect. For example, a methanol extract of *M. speciosa* produced no place-conditioning effect in male Sprague-Dawley rats up to 300 mg/kg (i.p.) under a biased conditioning design with four compound-vehicle pairings (Sufka et al., 2014). Lyophilized kratom tea also produced no place-conditioning effect in male C57BL/6J mice up to 1 g/kg (p.o.) under only one compound-vehicle pairing (Wilson et al., 2020). As with the methanol extract of *M. speciosa*, no place-conditioning effect was observed up to 75 mg/kg dose (i.p.) of an alkaloid-enriched fraction of *M. speciosa* in male Sprague-Dawley rats under a biased conditioning design with four compound-vehicle pairings

(Sufka et al., 2014). However, a lower 30 mg/kg dose (i.p.) of an alkaloid-enriched fraction of *M. speciosa* produced a place preference in male C57BL/6NHsd mice under an unbiased conditioning design with four compound-vehicle pairings (Gutridge et al., 2020). It is not yet clear whether the inconsistency in the place conditioning effects of alkaloid-enriched fractions of *M. speciosa* might have resulted from doses tested, rodent species, and/or species strain. In male Sprague-Dawley rats under an unbiased or biased conditioning design with four compound-vehicle pairings, a place preference was observed with 5, 10 and 30 mg/kg doses of mitragynine (i.p.) in some studies, but not observed with 10 and 30 mg/kg doses (i.p.) in other studies (Japarin et al., 2021; Sufka et al., 2014; Yusoff et al., 2016; Yusoff et al., 2017, 2018). These inconsistent results suggest that kratom products and mitragynine are not consistently effective to produce a reliable positive place conditioning effect. In addition, 7-hydroxymitragynine produced place preference at 2 (subcutaneously, s.c.) and 3 (i.p.) mg/kg in male ddY and C57BL/6NHsd mice under an unbiased conditioning design with three or four compound-vehicle pairings (Gutridge et al., 2020; Matsumoto et al., 2008). In male CD1 mice under an unbiased conditioning design with two compound-vehicle pairings, mitragynine pseudoindoxyl produced no significant place conditioning effect up to a 3.2 mg/kg dose (i.p.), though two compound-vehicle pairings and the particular dose tested might not be comprehensive enough to firmly conclude that there is a lack of place-conditioning effects with mitragynine pseudoindoxyl (Varadi et al., 2016).

One study assessed pretreatment effects of a methanolic extract of *M. speciosa* on place conditioning effects of ethanol. In male Swiss mice, the expression of ethanol-induced place preference was reduced by 50 and 75 but not 100 mg/kg doses (p.o.) of the methanolic extract of *M. speciosa* (Vijeepallam, Pandy, Murugan, & Naidu, 2019). The lack of a monotonic dose-dependency of the methanolic extract of *M. speciosa* requires further assessment. As with other experimental procedures, these studies employing place conditioning procedures used only male subjects. Thus, the impact of biological sex on the place conditioning effects of kratom products, mitragynine, 7-hydroxymitragynine, and mitragynine pseudoindoxyl remain to be assessed in studies using both sexes. As with outcomes from the i.v. drug self-administration and drug discrimination procedures, the lack of place conditioning effects of kratom products and mitragynine suggests that the contribution of 7-hydroxymitragynine converted from mitragynine to the *in vivo* activity of mitragynine is negligible.

4.6 Intracranial self-stimulation

Typically, rats are implanted with an electrode in a brain region of interest, and the frequency and threshold to respond to an electrical stimulus is measured. Acute administration of drugs of abuse can increase the frequency and decrease the threshold for an electrical stimulus (Esposito, Motola, & Kornetsky, 1978; Esposito, Perry, & Kornetsky, 1980; Igari et al., 2014). In contrast, drugs of abuse can increase the frequency and the threshold for an electrical stimulus during an acute withdrawal period (Bruijnzeel et al., 2006; Cryan, Hoyer, & Markou, 2003; Epping-Jordan, Watkins, Koob, & Markou, 1998).

Using a self-stimulation procedure, a single study assessed the impact of mitragynine and 7-hydroxymitragynine on the threshold for an electrical stimulus into the medial forebrain bundle in female and male Sprague-Dawley rats (Behnood-Rod et al., 2020). No dose of either mitragynine or 7-hydroxymitragynine affected the threshold regardless of sex, whereas morphine decreased the threshold for the electrical stimulus, as would be expected of a drug of abuse (Behnood-Rod et al., 2020). Intracranial self-stimulation procedures may prove useful to assess withdrawal like properties of kratom products and their alkaloids.

4.7 Respiration

Incidents of respiratory arrest following intake of kratom products have been reported (Abdullah, Haq, & Lamfers, 2019; Eggleston, Stoppacher, Suen, Marraffa, & Nelson, 2019; Overbeek, Abraham, & Munzer, 2019; Post et al., 2019). However, there is little literature characterizing the impact of kratom products and related alkaloids using experimental animals under carefully controlled conditions.

Non-invasive whole body plethysmography (WBP) in unrestrained, non-anesthetized, rodents is a common preclinical method for assessing respiratory depression (Crowley et al., 2021; Goineau, Rompion, Guillaume, & Picard, 2010; van den Hoogen & Colpaert, 1986). Advantages of this method are that it omits the need for anesthesia, which profoundly alters respiration (Svorc, Petrasova, & Svorc Jr., 2018), and the need for handling of the experimental animal prior to assessment (e.g., to administer an intraperitoneal injection), which can yield inconsistent hyperventilation and variable breathing and control data across animals (Goineau et al., 2010).

Using WBP, a single study assessed the impact of mitragynine pseudoindoxyl, a metabolite of 7-hydroxymitragynine, on respiration.

For example, 3 mg/kg mitragynine pseudoindoxyl (s.c.) failed to decrease respiratory frequency in male CD1 mice (Varadi et al., 2016). Using another automated, closed-air comprehensive lab animal monitoring system (CLAMS), 1 g/kg of lyophilized kratom tea (p.o.) decreased respiratory frequency in male C57BL/6J mice, but not in mice lacking μ-opioid receptor (Wilson et al., 2020). Using the CLAMS, corynoxine and mitraciliatine increased rather than decreased respiratory frequency in male C57BL/6J mice (Chakraborty et al., 2021). Using an Anderson glass inspirometer, the impact of mitragynine on respiration was assessed in dogs (unspecified strain and sex); mitragynine (unspecified dose, i.v.) increased rather than *decreased* tidal volume (Macko, Weisbach, & Douglas, 1972). In addition, a methanol extract of *M. africanus* stembark (100–6400 mg/kg, i.p.) has been reported to disrupt respiration in Wistar rats regardless of sex (Aji, Onyeyili, & Osunkwo, 2001). Collectively, these results might suggest that kratom products can produce respiratory depression through receptor mechanisms independent from MORs though the non-MOR mechanism remains to be elucidated. Also, corynoxine and mitraciliatine can produce respiratory stimulation rather than depression. However, given high vulnerability of respiratory parameters with a subtle change in experimental conditions, it appears too early to conclude the impact of kratom products and their alkaloids on respiration due to the scarcity of available literature.

4.8 Tolerance

Given the in vitro and in vivo activity of kratom alkaloids at the MORs as described throughout this review, the development of tolerance to MOR-mediated effects is an area of concern. The extent to which repeated administration of kratom products and related metabolites confers tolerance has been assessed preclinically using antinociceptive assays. For example, hotplate response latency (50 °C) in male ICR mice was compared prior to and after daily injections of mitragynine (15 and 25 mg/kg, i.p.) for 9 days; in this study, antinociceptive tolerance to mitragynine did not develop (Fakurazi et al., 2013). In a follow-up ex vivo study, there was no increase in cAMP production in the cortex and thalamus following repeated injections of mitragynine whereas antinociceptive tolerance and increases in cAMP production were observed following repeated injections of a low dose of morphine (5 mg/kg, i.p.) (Fakurazi et al., 2013). The in vivo and in vitro effects of morphine were blocked when morphine was treated with both doses (15 and 25 mg/kg, i.p.) of mitragynine (Fakurazi et al., 2013).

The doses of mitragynine in vivo and ex vivo might not have been sufficient to cause tolerance. In contrast, there is in vitro evidence that tolerance may develop to mitragynine; one study demonstrated that 24-h incubation of mitragynine (10 and 50 μM) increased forskolin-induced production of cAMP using human neuroblastoma SK–N–SH cells (Jamil, Subki, Lan, Majid, & Adenan, 2013). Chronic exposure of experimental cells to opioid agonists results in cAMP overshoot or super-activation, a cellular adaptation thought to be associated with the development of tolerance (Koob & Bloom, 1988; Nestler & Aghajanian, 1997; Sharma, Klee, & Nirenberg, 1977). Because high concentrations of mitragynine produced a cAMP overshoot, the lack of in vivo tolerance observed for mitragynine could indicate that only ineffective doses of mitragynine have been tested.

In marked contrast to mitragynine, tolerance to the in vivo effects of 7-hydroxymitragynine has been demonstrated. Antinociceptive tolerance in male ddY mice using a tail flick assay was demonstrated following two s.c. injection regimens of 7-hydroxymitragynine (10 mg/kg for 10 days and 2 mg/kg, b.i.d. for 5 days) (Matsumoto et al., 2005, 2008). Furthermore, 7-hydroxymitragynine (10 mg/kg, s.c.) produced cross-tolerance to the antinociceptive effects of morphine (Matsumoto et al., 2005). Daily injections of a methanolic extract of *M. speciosa* (400 mg/kg, p.o. for 15 days) in male Wistar rats resulted in tolerance to an inhibitory effect in the intestinal transit (Chittrakarn, Sawangjaroen, Prasettho, Janchawee, & Keawpradub, 2008). As with respiration, it appears too early to conclude with certainty whether tolerance can develop to kratom products and mitragynine, although tolerance to 7-hydroxymitragynine appears to be robust. In addition, the impact of sex on the capacity of kratom products and their alkaloids to produce tolerance to their opioid activity remains to be assessed.

4.9 Dependence and withdrawal

Kratom products have been reported to attenuate withdrawal symptoms in opioid-dependent subjects, though the available information has not been obtained from controlled clinical studies (Boyer et al., 2008). In addition, withdrawal symptoms following use of kratom products in humans adults has been described (Ahmad & Aziz, 2012; Bin Abdullah, 2020; Bowe & Kerr, 2020; Buresh, 2018; Diep et al., 2018; Eggleston et al., 2019; Galbis-Reig, 2016; Giancola, Caplan, & McKnight, 2021; Grundmann, 2017; Kalin, Dakhlalla, & Bhardwaj, 2020; Khazaeli, Jerry, & Vazirian, 2018; Kucharik, Gupta, Averkiou, Luck, & Ross, 2019; Lei, Butz, &

Valentino, 2021; McWhirter & Morris, 2010; Muller, Hillemacher, & Muller, 2020; Post et al., 2019; Sablaban & Gautam, 2021; Saingam, Assanangkornchai, Geater, & Lerkiatbundit, 2014, 2016; Singh, Narayanan, Muller et al., 2018; Singh, Narayanan, Vicknasingam et al., 2018; Singh, Muller, & Vicknasingam, 2014; Smid, Charles, Gordon, & Wright, 2018; Swogger et al., 2015; Trakulsrichai et al., 2013; Vento et al., 2021; Vicknasingam, Narayanan, Beng, & Mansor, 2010; Weiss & Douglas, 2021). There is limited evidence to suggest that kratom use in pregnant mothers may result in a neonatal withdrawal syndrome (Davidson, Rawat, Stojanovski, & Chandrasekharan, 2019; Post et al., 2019; Wright, Ginsberg, Parkison, Dubose, & Shores, 2021). However, it has been suggested that the withdrawal symptoms are generally not severe in human adults (Garcia-Romeu, Cox, Smith, Dunn, & Griffiths, 2020; Vicknasingam et al., 2020). Some degree of a withdrawal syndrome from kratom products in clinical studies is generally consistent with outcomes from preclinical studies using rodents. For example, increases in global withdrawal scores were demonstrated in Sprague-Dawley rats within 24h following daily injections of mitragynine regardless of sex (Hassan, Othman, Mansor, Muller, & Hassan, 2021; Sabetghadam, Ramanathan, Sasidharan, & Mansor, 2013; Yusoff et al., 2016). However, abrupt discontinuation of mitragynine treatment is not consistently reported to result in a withdrawal syndrome; food-maintained behavior under a fixed-ratio schedule of food delivery was not decreased approximately 24h after the last mitragynine dose in male Sprague-Dawley rats (Harun, Johari, Mansor, & Shoaib, 2020). In male C57BL/6J mice, withdrawal-like behaviors (e.g., jumping and wet-dog shakes) were not precipitated with an injection of a relatively high dose of naloxone (10mg/kg, i.p.) following escalating doses of mitragynine (10–75mg/kg, i.p.) (Wilson et al., 2021). The inconsistency in the capacity of repeated treatment with mitragynine and its abrupt discontinuation to result in a withdrawal syndrome might reflect differences in the experimental methods employed (i.e., direct observation of unconditioned withdrawal signs *versus* disruptions in operant behavior) and/or animal species.

The preclinical effectiveness of mitragynine to attenuate spontaneous and naloxone-precipitated withdrawal-like behaviors from morphine has been consistently reported in male Sprague-Daley rats (Harun et al., 2020; Hassan et al., 2020), male C57BL/6J and Swiss mice (Cheaha et al., 2017; Wilson et al., 2020, 2021), and female and male zebrafish (Khor, Jamil, Adenan, & Shu-Chien, 2011). An ex vivo study demonstrated that mitragynine can inhibit naloxone-induced contraction of Guinea pig ilea previously treated with morphine (Watanabe, Yano, Horie, & Yamamoto, 1997). As with mitragynine, repeated treatment with 7-hydroxymitragynine conferred a withdrawal syndrome (e.g., jumping), as evidenced in male ddY mice treated with escalating doses of 7-hydroxymitragynine followed by a naloxone (3 mg/kg, s.c.) challenge (Matsumoto et al., 2005).

The capacity of repeated treatment with mitragynine pseudoindoxyl, an active metabolite of 7-hydroxymitragynine, to produce a withdrawal syndrome (e.g., jumping) was also assessed following administration of naloxone. For example, a low dose of naloxone (1 mg/kg) failed to produce jumping in male CD1 mice treated with a dose two-fold higher than the ED50 of mitragynine pseudoindoxyl to produce antinociception (no greater than 1.0 mg/kg, b.i.d., s.c.) for 29 consecutive days and the authors concluded that the lack of withdrawal-like behaviors was due to mitragynine pseudoindoxyl not recruiting β-arrestin-2 (Varadi et al., 2016). However, a higher dose of naloxone (10 mg/kg, s.c.) produced significant jumping in male C57BL/6J mice treated with escalating doses (1–35 mg/kg, p.o.) of mitragynine pseudoindoxyl (Wilson et al., 2021). The different outcomes obtained with repeated mitragynine pseudoindoxyl treatment and naloxone challenge might be due to various differences in the experimental parameters (e.g., mouse strain). However, given the 10-fold difference in naloxone doses used and 35-fold difference in doses of mitragynine pseudoindoxyl (Varadi et al., 2016; Wilson et al., 2021), it appears that the doses of naloxone and mitragynine pseudoindoxyl are primary factors in determining the extent to which antagonist-induced withdrawal is obtained with mitragynine pseudoindoxyl treatment in male mice. Mitragynine pseudoindoxyl was reported to attenuate naloxone-precipitated withdrawal in male C57BL/6J mice that had received repeated morphine treatment (Wilson et al., 2020, 2021).

In contrast to mitragynine, 7-hydroxymitragynine, and mitragynine pseudoindoxyl, dosing with either kratom tea or a mixture of kratom alkaloids does not appear to produce physical dependence. For example, naloxone (10 mg/kg, s.c.) did not produce jumping in male C57BL/6J mice treated with lyophilized kratom tea and methanolic extract of kratom alkaloids (escalating doses 30–125 mg/kg, p.o., each) (Wilson et al., 2020; Wilson et al., 2021). Lyophilized kratom tea (40 mg/kg, p.o.) was reported to attenuate naloxone-precipitated withdrawal in male C57BL/6J mice receiving repeated morphine treatment (Wilson et al., 2020; Wilson et al., 2021). In addition, an alkaloid enriched fraction of *M. speciosa* (60, 80, and 100 mg/kg, p.o.) attenuated naloxone-induced (5 mg/kg, s.c.) jumping in male ICR mice treated with escalating doses of morphine (Cheaha et al., 2017). The alkaloid enriched fraction of *M. speciosa* (80 mg/kg, p.o.) attenuated spontaneous withdrawal-like events [gamma oscillation (30.5–45 Hz) and increased activity counts] in male Wistar rats withdrawn from escalating doses of ethanol (Cheaha, Keawpradub, Sawangjaroen, Phukpattaranont, & Kumarnsit, 2015). These demonstrations of the capacity of kratom products to attenuate withdrawal-like behaviors from morphine indicates their potential development as a medication for opioid use disorder. However, the impact of sex on the opioid withdrawal attenuating effects of kratom products remains to be assessed.

5. Conclusion

Kratom products are used in Southeastern Asian countries to reportedly manage pain and opioid withdrawal. There has been a marked increase in the use of kratom products in the US. The high MOR affinity and efficacy of 7-hydroxymitragynine, an in vivo metabolite of mitragynine, and the lower affinity and efficacy of mitragynine at MOR, suggest that kratom alkaloids need to be assessed carefully for opioid-like therapeutic versus adverse effects. The pharmacology of the dozens of kratom alkaloids identified to date has not been adequately characterized, and there is much progress that needs to be made. From preclinical data collected thus far and summarized in this chapter, it appears that mitragynine and some of its related kratom alkaloids exert a profile of in vivo activity consistent with low efficacy agonism at MOR. There is little evidence to suggest that in vivo conversion of mitragynine to 7-hydroxymitragynine is important for the behavioral profile of mitragynine, and the amounts of 7-hydroxymitragynine measured in plant material or as a consequence of post-harvesting handling are not so large as to suggest that 7-hydroxymitragynine plays a fundamental role in the effects of natural products. The low efficacy MOR agonist profile of mitragynine and kratom products may suggest that, as is the case with other FDA approved low efficacy MOR agonists (e.g., buprenorphine), there is great potential to develop mitragynine and related alkaloids as medications for the treatment of pain and opioid use disorder.

Acknowledgments

The authors would like to thank Ms. Samantha N. Hart at the College of Pharmacy, University of Florida, for administrative assistance. This study was supported by National Institute of Health (NIH) grants [DA25267, DA48353 and UG3 DA048353 01], University of Florida Foundation and University of Florida Department of Pharmacodynamics Funding.

Conflicts of interests or disclaimers

None.

References

Abdullah, H. M. A., Haq, I., & Lamfers, R. (2019). Cardiac arrest in a young healthy male patient secondary to kratom ingestion: Is this 'legal high' substance more dangerous than initially thought ? *BML Case Reports*, *12*(7). https://doi.org/10.1136/bcr-2019-229778.

Adkins, J. E., Boyer, E. W., & McCurdy, C. R. (2011). Mitragyna speciosa, a psychoactive tree from Southeast Asia with opioid activity. *Current Topics in Medicinal Chemistry*, *11*(9), 1165–1175. https://doi.org/10.2174/156802611795371305.

Ahmad, K., & Aziz, Z. (2012). Mitragyna speciosa use in the northern states of Malaysia: A cross-sectional study. *Journal of Ethnopharmacology*, *141*(1), 446–450. https://doi.org/10.1016/j.jep.2012.03.009.

Aji, B. M., Onyeyili, P. A., & Osunkwo, U. A. (2001). The central nervous effects of Mitragyna africanus (Willd) stembark extract in rats. *Journal of Ethnopharmacology*, *77*(2–3), 143–149. https://doi.org/10.1016/s0378-8741(01)00267-7.

Apryani, E., Hidayat, M. T., Moklas, M. A., Fakurazi, S., & Idayu, N. F. (2010). Effects of mitragynine from Mitragyna speciosa Korth leaves on working memory. *Journal of Ethnopharmacology*, *129*(3), 357–360. https://doi.org/10.1016/j.jep.2010.03.036.

Avery, B. A., Boddu, S. P., Sharma, A., Furr, E. B., Leon, F., Cutler, S. J., et al. (2019). Comparative pharmacokinetics of mitragynine after oral administration of Mitragyna speciosa (kratom) leaf extracts in rats. *Planta Medica*, *85*(4), 340–346. https://doi.org/10.1055/a-0770-3683.

Bardo, M. T., & Bevins, R. A. (2000). Conditioned place preference: What does it add to our preclinical understanding of drug reward? *Psychopharmacology*, *153*(1), 31–43.

Behnood-Rod, A., Chellian, R., Wilson, R., Hiranita, T., Sharma, A., Leon, F., et al. (2020). Evaluation of the rewarding effects of mitragynine and 7-hydroxymitragynine in an intracranial self-stimulation procedure in male and female rats. *Drug and Alcohol Dependence*, *215*, 108235. https://doi.org/10.1016/j.drugalcdep.2020.108235.

Berthold, E. C., Kamble, S. H., Raju, K. S., King, T. I., Popa, R., Sharma, A., et al. (2021). Preclinical pharmacokinetic study of speciociliatine, a kratom alkaloid, in rats using an UPLC-MS/MS method. *Journal of Pharmaceutical and Biomedical Analysis*, *194*, 113778. https://doi.org/10.1016/j.jpba.2020.113778.

Bin Abdullah, M. (2020). Kratom dependence and treatment options: A comprehensive review of the literature. *Current Drug Targets*, *21*(15), 1566–1579. https://doi.org/10.2174/1389450121666200719011653.

Bowe, A., & Kerr, P. L. (2020). A complex case of kratom dependence, depression, and chronic pain in opioid use disorder: Effects of buprenorphine in clinical management. *Journal of Psychoactive Drugs*, *52*(5), 447–452. https://doi.org/10.1080/02791072.2020.1773586.

Boyer, E. W., Babu, K. M., Adkins, J. E., McCurdy, C. R., & Halpern, J. H. (2008). Self-treatment of opioid withdrawal using kratom (Mitragynia speciosa korth). *Addiction, 103*(6), 1048–1050. https://doi.org/10.1111/j.1360-0443.2008.02209.x.

Bruijnzeel, A. W., Lewis, B., Bajpai, L. K., Morey, T. E., Dennis, D. M., & Gold, M. (2006). Severe deficit in brain reward function associated with fentanyl withdrawal in rats. *Biological Psychiatry, 59*(5), 477–480. https://doi.org/10.1016/j.biopsych.2005.07.020.

Buresh, M. (2018). Treatment of kratom dependence with buprenorphine-naloxone maintenance. *Journal of Addiction Medicine, 12*(6), 481–483. https://doi.org/10.1097/ADM.0000000000000428.

Burkill, I., & Haniff, M. (1930). Malay village medicine. In *Vol. 6 (6-10). The Garden's bulletin stairs settlements* (p. 207).

Carpenter, J. M., Criddle, C. A., Craig, H. K., Ali, Z., Zhang, Z., Khan, I. A., et al. (2016). Comparative effects of Mitragyna speciosa extract, mitragynine, and opioid agonists on thermal nociception in rats. *Fitoterapia, 109*, 87–90. https://doi.org/10.1016/j.fitote.2015.12.001.

Carr, G. D., Fibiger, H. C., & Phillips, A. G. (1989). *Conditioned place preference as a measure of drug reward.*

Catania, A. (2013). *Learning* (5th ed.). USA: Sloan Publishing, Cornwall on Hudson, NY, ISBN:978-1-59738-023-2.

Chakraborty, S., Uprety, R., Daibani, A. E., Rouzic, V. L., Hunkele, A., Appourchaux, K., et al. (2021). Kratom alkaloids as probes for opioid receptor function: Pharmacological characterization of minor indole and Oxindole alkaloids from kratom. *ACS Chemical Neuroscience*. https://doi.org/10.1021/acschemneuro.1c00149.

Cheaha, D., Keawpradub, N., Sawangjaroen, K., Phukpattaranont, P., & Kumarnsit, E. (2015). Effects of an alkaloid-rich extract from Mitragyna speciosa leaves and fluoxetine on sleep profiles, EEG spectral frequency and ethanol withdrawal symptoms in rats. *Phytomedicine, 22*(11), 1000–1008. https://doi.org/10.1016/j.phymed.2015.07.008.

Cheaha, D., Reakkamnuan, C., Nukitram, J., Chittrakarn, S., Phukpattaranont, P., Keawpradub, N., et al. (2017). Effects of alkaloid-rich extract from Mitragyna speciosa (Korth.) Havil. on naloxone-precipitated morphine withdrawal symptoms and local field potential in the nucleus accumbens of mice. *Journal of Ethnopharmacology, 208*, 129–137. https://doi.org/10.1016/j.jep.2017.07.008.

Chear, N. J., Leon, F., Sharma, A., Kanumuri, S. R. R., Zwolinski, G., Abboud, K. A., et al. (2021). Exploring the chemistry of alkaloids from Malaysian Mitragyna speciosa (kratom) and the role of oxindoles on human opioid receptors. *Journal of Natural Products, 84*(4), 1034–1043. https://doi.org/10.1021/acs.jnatprod.0c01055.

Chittrakarn, S., Sawangjaroen, K., Prasettho, S., Janchawee, B., & Keawpradub, N. (2008). Inhibitory effects of kratom leaf extract (Mitragyna speciosa Korth.) on the rat gastrointestinal tract. *Journal of Ethnopharmacology, 116*(1), 173–178. https://doi.org/10.1016/j.jep.2007.11.032.

Crowley, M. L., Restrepo, L. F., Gamez-Jimenez, L. R., Patel, A., Braun, T., Pallares, V. L. C., et al. (2021). The use of hypercapnic conditions to assess opioid-induced respiratory depression in rats. *Journal of Pharmacological and Toxicological Methods*, 107101. https://doi.org/10.1016/j.vascn.2021.107101.

Cryan, J. F., Hoyer, D., & Markou, A. (2003). Withdrawal from chronic amphetamine induces depressive-like behavioral effects in rodents. *Biological Psychiatry, 54*(1), 49–58. https://doi.org/10.1016/s0006-3223(02)01730-4.

Davidson, L., Rawat, M., Stojanovski, S., & Chandrasekharan, P. (2019). Natural drugs, not so natural effects: Neonatal abstinence syndrome secondary to 'kratom'. *Journal of Neonatal-Perinatal Medicine, 12*(1), 109–112. https://doi.org/10.3233/NPM-1863.

de Moraes, N. V., Moretti, R. A., Furr, E. B., 3rd, McCurdy, C. R., & Lanchote, V. L. (2009). Determination of mitragynine in rat plasma by LC-MS/MS: Application to pharmacokinetics. *Journal of Chromatography. B, Analytical Technologies in the Biomedical and Life Sciences, 877*(24), 2593–2597. https://doi.org/10.1016/j.jchromb.2009.06.023.

Diep, J., Chin, D. T., Gupta, S., Syed, F., Xiong, M., & Cheng, J. (2018). Kratom, an emerging drug of abuse: A case report of overdose and management of withdrawal. *A&A practice, 10*(8), 192–194. https://doi.org/10.1213/XAA.0000000000000658.

Eastlack, S. C., Cornett, E. M., & Kaye, A. D. (2020). Kratom-pharmacology, clinical implications, and outlook: A comprehensive review. *Pain and therapy, 9*(1), 55–69. https://doi.org/10.1007/s40122-020-00151-x.

Eggleston, W., Stoppacher, R., Suen, K., Marraffa, J. M., & Nelson, L. S. (2019). Kratom use and toxicities in the United States. *Pharmacotherapy, 39*(7), 775–777. https://doi.org/10.1002/phar.2280.

Ellis, C. R., Racz, R., Kruhlak, N. L., Kim, M. T., Zakharov, A. V., Southall, N., et al. (2020). Evaluating kratom alkaloids using PHASE. *PLoS One, 15*(3), e0229646. https://doi.org/10.1371/journal.pone.0229646.

Epping-Jordan, M. P., Watkins, S. S., Koob, G. F., & Markou, A. (1998). Dramatic decreases in brain reward function during nicotine withdrawal. *Nature, 393*(6680), 76–79. https://doi.org/10.1038/30001.

Esposito, R. U., Motola, A. H., & Kornetsky, C. (1978). Cocaine: Acute effects on reinforcement thresholds for self-stimulation behavior to the medial forebrain bundle. *Pharmacology, Biochemistry, and Behavior, 8*(4), 437–439. https://doi.org/10.1016/0091-3057(78)90082-5.

Esposito, R. U., Perry, W., & Kornetsky, C. (1980). Effects of d-amphetamine and naloxone on brain stimulation reward. *Psychopharmacology, 69*(2), 187–191. https://doi.org/10.1007/BF00427648.

Fakurazi, S., Rahman, S. A., Hidayat, M. T., Ithnin, H., Moklas, M. A., & Arulselvan, P. (2013). The combination of mitragynine and morphine prevents the development of morphine tolerance in mice. *Molecules, 18*(1), 666–681. https://doi.org/10.3390/molecules18010666.

Foss, J. D., Nayak, S. U., Tallarida, C. S., Farkas, D. J., Ward, S. J., & Rawls, S. M. (2020). Mitragynine, bioactive alkaloid of kratom, reduces chemotherapy-induced neuropathic pain in rats through alpha-adrenoceptor mechanism. *Drug and Alcohol Dependence, 209*, 107946. https://doi.org/10.1016/j.drugalcdep.2020.107946.

Galbis-Reig, D. (2016). A case report of kratom addiction and withdrawal. *WMJ, 115*(1), 49–52. quiz 53.

Garcia-Romeu, A., Cox, D. J., Smith, K. E., Dunn, K. E., & Griffiths, R. R. (2020). Kratom (Mitragyna speciosa): User demographics, use patterns, and implications for the opioid epidemic. *Drug and Alcohol Dependence, 208*, 107849. https://doi.org/10.1016/j.drugalcdep.2020.107849.

Gawade, S. P. (2012). Acetic acid induced painful endogenous infliction in writhing test on mice. *Journal of Pharmacology and Pharmacotherapeutics, 3*(4), 348. https://doi.org/10.4103/0976-500X.103699.

Giancola, N. B., Caplan, J. P., & McKnight, C. A. (2021). "A kratom Konundrum": Management of kratom withdrawal with gabapentin in a patient with a left ventricular assist device. *Journal of the Academy of Consultation-Liaison Psychiatry, 62*(3), 368–369. https://doi.org/10.1016/j.psym.2020.10.004.

Goineau, S., Rompion, S., Guillaume, P., & Picard, S. (2010). Ventilatory function assessment in safety pharmacology: Optimization of rodent studies using normocapnic or hypercapnic conditions. *Toxicology and Applied Pharmacology, 247*(3), 191–197. https://doi.org/10.1016/j.taap.2010.06.012.

Grabowski, J., Shearer, J., Merrill, J., & Negus, S. S. (2004). Agonist-like, replacement pharmacotherapy for stimulant abuse and dependence. *Addictive Behaviors, 29*(7), 1439–1464. https://doi.org/10.1016/j.addbeh.2004.06.018.

Grundmann, O. (2017). Patterns of kratom use and health impact in the US-results from an online survey. *Drug and Alcohol Dependence*, *176*, 63–70. https://doi.org/10.1016/j.drugalcdep.2017.03.007.

Gutridge, A. M., Robins, M. T., Cassell, R. J., Uprety, R., Mores, K. L., Ko, M. J., et al. (2020). G protein-biased kratom-alkaloids and synthetic carfentanil-amide opioids as potential treatments for alcohol use disorder. *British Journal of Pharmacology*, *177*(7), 1497–1513. https://doi.org/10.1111/bph.14913.

Harun, N., Hassan, Z., Navaratnam, V., Mansor, S. M., & Shoaib, M. (2015). Discriminative stimulus properties of mitragynine (kratom) in rats. *Psychopharmacology*, *232*(13), 2227–2238. https://doi.org/10.1007/s00213-015-3866-5.

Harun, N., Johari, I. S., Mansor, S. M., & Shoaib, M. (2020). Assessing physiological dependence and withdrawal potential of mitragynine using schedule-controlled behaviour in rats. *Psychopharmacology*, *237*(3), 855–867. https://doi.org/10.1007/s00213-019-05418-6.

Hassan, R., Othman, N., Mansor, S. M., Muller, C. P., & Hassan, Z. (2021). Proteomic analysis reveals brain Rab35 as a potential biomarker of mitragynine withdrawal in rats. *Brain Research Bulletin*, *172*, 139–150. https://doi.org/10.1016/j.brainresbull.2021.04.018.

Hassan, R., Pike See, C., Sreenivasan, S., Mansor, S. M., Muller, C. P., & Hassan, Z. (2020). Mitragynine attenuates morphine withdrawal effects in rats-a comparison with methadone and buprenorphine. *Frontiers in Psychiatry*, *11*, 411. https://doi.org/10.3389/fpsyt.2020.00411.

Hemby, S. E., McIntosh, S., Leon, F., Cutler, S. J., & McCurdy, C. R. (2019). Abuse liability and therapeutic potential of the Mitragyna speciosa (kratom) alkaloids mitragynine and 7-hydroxymitragynine. *Addiction Biology*, *24*(5), 874–885. https://doi.org/10.1111/adb.12639.

Hiranita, T., Kohut, S. J., Soto, P. L., Tanda, G., Kopajtic, T. A., & Katz, J. L. (2014). Preclinical efficacy of N-substituted benztropine analogs as antagonists of methamphetamine self-administration in rats. *The Journal of Pharmacology and Experimental Therapeutics*, *348*(1), 174–191. https://doi.org/10.1124/jpet.113.208264.

Hiranita, T., Leon, F., Felix, J. S., Restrepo, L. F., Reeves, M. E., Pennington, A. E., et al. (2019). The effects of mitragynine and morphine on schedule-controlled responding and antinociception in rats. *Psychopharmacology*, *236*(9), 2725–2734. https://doi.org/10.1007/s00213-019-05247-7.

Hiranita, T., Sharma, A., Oyola, F., Obeng, S., Reeves, M., Restrepo, L., et al. (2020). Potential contribution of 7-hydroxymitragynine, a metabolite of the primary kratom (Mitragyna Speciosa) alkaloid mitragynine, to the μ-opioid activity of mitragynine in rats. *The FASEB Journal*, *34*(S1), 1.

Hiranita, T., Soto, P. L., Tanda, G., & Katz, J. L. (2011). Lack of cocaine-like discriminative-stimulus effects of sigma-receptor agonists in rats. *Behavioural Pharmacology*, *22*(5–6), 525–530. https://doi.org/10.1097/FBP.0b013e328349ab22.

Hiranita, T., Soto, P. L., Tanda, G., Kopajtic, T. A., & Katz, J. L. (2013). Stimulants as specific inducers of dopamine-independent sigma agonist self-administration in rats. *The Journal of Pharmacology and Experimental Therapeutics*, *347*(1), 20–29. https://doi.org/10.1124/jpet.113.207522.

Hiranita, T., Wilkinson, D. S., Hong, W. C., Zou, M. F., Kopajtic, T. A., Soto, P. L., et al. (2014). 2-Isoxazol-3-phenyltropane derivatives of cocaine: Molecular and atypical system effects at the dopamine transporter. *The Journal of Pharmacology and Experimental Therapeutics*, *349*(2), 297–309. https://doi.org/10.1124/jpet.113.212738.

Holtzman, S. G. (1985). Drug discrimination studies. *Drug and Alcohol Dependence*, *14*(3–4), 263–282.

Horton, D. B., Potter, D. M., & Mead, A. N. (2013). A translational pharmacology approach to understanding the predictive value of abuse potential assessments. *Behavioural Pharmacology*, *24*(5–6), 410–436. https://doi.org/10.1097/FBP.0b013e3283644d2e.

Hutchinson, M. R., Northcutt, A. L., Hiranita, T., Wang, X., Lewis, S. S., Thomas, J., et al. (2012). Opioid activation of toll-like receptor 4 contributes to drug reinforcement. *The Journal of Neuroscience*, *32*(33), 11187–11200. https://doi.org/10.1523/JNEUROSCI.0684-12.2012.

Igari, M., Alexander, J. C., Ji, Y., Qi, X., Papke, R. L., & Bruijnzeel, A. W. (2014). Varenicline and cytisine diminish the dysphoric-like state associated with spontaneous nicotine withdrawal in rats. *Neuropsychopharmacology*, *39*(2), 455–465. https://doi.org/10.1038/npp.2013.216.

Irwin, S., Houde, R. W., Bennett, D. R., Hendershot, L. C., & Seevers, M. H. (1951). The effects of morphine methadone and meperidine on some reflex responses of spinal animals to nociceptive stimulation. *The Journal of Pharmacology and Experimental Therapeutics*, *101*(2), 132–143.

Jamil, M. F., Subki, M. F., Lan, T. M., Majid, M. I., & Adenan, M. I. (2013). The effect of mitragynine on cAMP formation and mRNA expression of mu-opioid receptors mediated by chronic morphine treatment in SK-N-SH neuroblastoma cell. *Journal of Ethnopharmacology*, *148*(1), 135–143. https://doi.org/10.1016/j.jep.2013.03.078.

Jansen, K. L., & Prast, C. J. (1988). Ethnopharmacology of kratom and the Mitragyna alkaloids. *Journal of Ethnopharmacology*, *23*(1), 115–119. https://doi.org/10.1016/0378-8741(88)90121-3.

Japarin, R. A., Yusoff, N. H., Hassan, Z., Muller, C. P., & Harun, N. (2021). Cross-reinstatement of mitragynine and morphine place preference in rats. *Behavioural Brain Research*, *399*, 113021. https://doi.org/10.1016/j.bbr.2020.113021.

Kalin, S., Dakhlalla, S., & Bhardwaj, S. (2020). Treatment for kratom abuse in a contingency-management-based MAT setting: A case series. *Journal of Opioid Management*, *16*(5), 391–394. https://doi.org/10.5055/jom.2020.0594.

Kamble, S. H., Berthold, E. C., King, T. I., Raju Kanumuri, S. R., Popa, R., Herting, J. R., et al. (2021). Pharmacokinetics of eleven kratom alkaloids following an oral dose of either traditional or commercial kratom products in rats. *Journal of Natural Products*, *84*(4), 1104–1112. https://doi.org/10.1021/acs.jnatprod.0c01163.

Kamble, S. H., Leon, F., King, T. I., Berthold, E. C., Lopera-Londono, C., Siva Rama Raju, K., et al. (2020). Metabolism of a kratom alkaloid metabolite in human plasma increases its opioid potency and efficacy. *ACS Pharmacology & Translational Science*, *3*(6), 1063–1068. https://doi.org/10.1021/acsptsci.0c00075.

Kamble, S. H., Sharma, A., King, T. I., Leon, F., McCurdy, C. R., & Avery, B. A. (2019). Metabolite profiling and identification of enzymes responsible for the metabolism of mitragynine, the major alkaloid of Mitragyna speciosa (kratom). *Xenobiotica*, *49*(11), 1279–1288. https://doi.org/10.1080/00498254.2018.1552819.

Katz, J. L., Hiranita, T., Hong, W. C., Job, M. O., & McCurdy, C. R. (2017). A role for sigma receptors in stimulant self-administration and addiction. *Handbook of Experimental Pharmacology*, *244*, 177–218. https://doi.org/10.1007/164_2016_94.

Khazaeli, A., Jerry, J. M., & Vazirian, M. (2018). Treatment of kratom withdrawal and addiction with buprenorphine. *Journal of Addiction Medicine*, *12*(6), 493–495. https://doi.org/10.1097/ADM.0000000000000435.

Khor, B. S., Jamil, M. F., Adenan, M. I., & Shu-Chien, A. C. (2011). Mitragynine attenuates withdrawal syndrome in morphine-withdrawn zebrafish. *PLoS One*, *6*(12), e28340. https://doi.org/10.1371/journal.pone.0028340.

King, T. I., Sharma, A., Kamble, S. H., Leon, F., Berthold, E. C., Popa, R., et al. (2020). Bioanalytical method development and validation of corynantheidine, a kratom alkaloid, using UPLC-MS/MS, and its application to preclinical pharmacokinetic studies. *Journal of Pharmaceutical and Biomedical Analysis*, *180*, 113019. https://doi.org/10.1016/j.jpba.2019.113019.

Kohut, S. J., Hiranita, T., Hong, S. K., Ebbs, A. L., Tronci, V., Green, J., et al. (2014). Preference for distinct functional conformations of the dopamine transporter alters the relationship between subjective effects of cocaine and stimulation of mesolimbic dopamine. *Biological Psychiatry*, *76*(10), 802–809. https://doi.org/10.1016/j.biopsych.2014.03.031.

Koob, G. F., & Bloom, F. E. (1988). Cellular and molecular mechanisms of drug dependence. *Science*, *242*(4879), 715–723. https://doi.org/10.1126/science.2903550.

Kruegel, A. C., Gassaway, M. M., Kapoor, A., Varadi, A., Majumdar, S., Filizola, M., et al. (2016). Synthetic and receptor signaling explorations of the Mitragyna alkaloids: Mitragynine as an atypical molecular framework for opioid receptor modulators. *Journal of the American Chemical Society*, *138*(21), 6754–6764. https://doi.org/10.1021/jacs.6b00360.

Kruegel, A. C., & Grundmann, O. (2018). The medicinal chemistry and neuropharmacology of kratom: A preliminary discussion of a promising medicinal plant and analysis of its potential for abuse. *Neuropharmacology*, *134*(Pt. A), 108–120. https://doi.org/10.1016/j.neuropharm.2017.08.026.

Kruegel, A. C., Uprety, R., Grinnell, S. G., Langreck, C., Pekarskaya, E. A., Le Rouzic, V., et al. (2019). 7-Hydroxymitragynine is an active metabolite of mitragynine and a key mediator of its analgesic effects. *ACS Central Science*, *5*(6), 992–1001. https://doi.org/10.1021/acscentsci.9b00141.

Kucharik, M., Gupta, A., Averkiou, P., Luck, G. R., & Ross, A. S. (2019). Complicated postoperative course secondary to kratom withdrawal: A case report. *Journal of Surgery Case Reports*, *2019*(11), rjz309. https://doi.org/10.1093/jscr/rjz309.

Le, D., Goggin, M. M., & Janis, G. C. (2012). Analysis of mitragynine and metabolites in human urine for detecting the use of the psychoactive plant kratom. *Journal of Analytical Toxicology*, *36*(9), 616–625. https://doi.org/10.1093/jat/bks073.

Lei, J., Butz, A., & Valentino, N. (2021). Management of kratom dependence with buprenorphine/naloxone in a veteran population. *Substance Abuse*, 1–11. https://doi.org/10.1080/08897077.2021.1878086.

Leon, F., Habib, E., Adkins, J. E., Furr, E. B., McCurdy, C. R., & Cutler, S. J. (2009). Phytochemical characterization of the leaves of Mitragyna speciosa grown in U.S.A. *Natural Product Communications*, *4*(7), 907–910.

Leon, F., Obeng, S., Mottinelli, M., Chen, Y., King, T. I., Berthold, E. C., et al. (2021). Activity of Mitragyna speciosa ("kratom") alkaloids at serotonin receptors. *Journal of Medicinal Chemistry*. https://doi.org/10.1021/acs.jmedchem.1c00726.

León, F., Obeng, S., Mottinelli, M., Chen, Y., King, T. I., Berthold, E. C., et al. (2021). Activity of Mitragyna Speciosa ('kratom') alkaloids at serotonin receptors. *Journal of Medicinal Chemistry*. Submitted.

Macko, E., Weisbach, J. A., & Douglas, B. (1972). Some observations on the pharmacology of mitragynine. *Archives Internationales de Pharmacodynamie et de Thérapie*, *198*(1), 145–161.

Manda, V. K., Avula, B., Ali, Z., Khan, I. A., Walker, L. A., & Khan, S. I. (2014). Evaluation of in vitro absorption, distribution, metabolism, and excretion (ADME) properties of mitragynine, 7-hydroxymitragynine, and mitraphylline. *Planta Medica*, *80*(7), 568–576. https://doi.org/10.1055/s-0034-1368444.

Mata, D., & Andera, K. (2020). Case series: Mitragynine blood and tissue concentrations in fatalities from 2017 to 2018 in Orange County, CA, USA. *Forensic Chemistry*, *17*, 100205.

Matsumoto, K., Horie, S., Ishikawa, H., Takayama, H., Aimi, N., Ponglux, D., et al. (2004). Antinociceptive effect of 7-hydroxymitragynine in mice: Discovery of an orally active opioid analgesic from the Thai medicinal herb Mitragyna speciosa. *Life Sciences*, *74*(17), 2143–2155. https://doi.org/10.1016/j.lfs.2003.09.054.

Matsumoto, K., Horie, S., Takayama, H., Ishikawa, H., Aimi, N., Ponglux, D., et al. (2005). Antinociception, tolerance and withdrawal symptoms induced by 7-hydroxymitragynine, an alkaloid from the Thai medicinal herb Mitragyna speciosa. *Life Sciences, 78*(1), 2–7. https://doi.org/10.1016/j.lfs.2004.10.086.

Matsumoto, K., Mizowaki, M., Suchitra, T., Murakami, Y., Takayama, H., Sakai, S., et al. (1996). Central antinociceptive effects of mitragynine in mice: Contribution of descending noradrenergic and serotonergic systems. *European Journal of Pharmacology, 317*(1), 75–81. https://doi.org/10.1016/s0014-2999(96)00714-5.

Matsumoto, K., Mizowaki, M., Takayama, H., Sakai, S., Aimi, N., & Watanabe, H. (1997). Suppressive effect of mitragynine on the 5-methoxy-N,N-dimethyltryptamine-induced head-twitch response in mice. *Pharmacology, Biochemistry, and Behavior, 57*(1–2), 319–323. https://doi.org/10.1016/s0091-3057(96)00314-0.

Matsumoto, K., Narita, M., Muramatsu, N., Nakayama, T., Misawa, K., Kitajima, M., et al. (2014). Orally active opioid mu/delta dual agonist MGM-16, a derivative of the indole alkaloid mitragynine, exhibits potent antiallodynic effect on neuropathic pain in mice. *The Journal of Pharmacology and Experimental Therapeutics, 348*(3), 383–392. https://doi.org/10.1124/jpet.113.208108.

Matsumoto, K., Takayama, H., Narita, M., Nakamura, A., Suzuki, M., Suzuki, T., et al. (2008). MGM-9 [(E)-methyl 2-(3-ethyl-7a,12a-(epoxyethanoxy)-9-fluoro-1,2,3,4,6,7,12,12b-octahydro-8-methoxy indolo[2,3-a]quinolizin-2-yl)-3-methoxyacrylate], a derivative of the indole alkaloid mitragynine: A novel dual-acting mu- and kappa-opioid agonist with potent antinociceptive and weak rewarding effects in mice. *Neuropharmacology, 55*(2), 154–165. https://doi.org/10.1016/j.neuropharm.2008.05.003.

Maxwell, E. A., King, T. I., Kamble, S. H., Raju, K. S. R., Berthold, E. C., Leon, F., et al. (2020). Pharmacokinetics and safety of mitragynine in beagle dogs. *Planta Medica, 86*(17), 1278–1285. https://doi.org/10.1055/a-1212-5475.

Maxwell, E. A., King, T. I., Kamble, S. H., Raju, K. S. R., Berthold, E. C., Leon, F., et al. (2021). Oral pharmacokinetics in beagle dogs of the mitragynine metabolite, 7-hydroxymitragynine. *European Journal of Drug Metabolism and Pharmacokinetics, 46*(3), 459–463. https://doi.org/10.1007/s13318-021-00684-2.

McWhirter, L., & Morris, S. (2010). A case report of inpatient detoxification after kratom (Mitragyna speciosa) dependence. *European Addiction Research, 16*(4), 229–231. https://doi.org/10.1159/000320288.

Muller, E., Hillemacher, T., & Muller, C. P. (2020). Kratom instrumentalization for severe pain self-treatment resulting in addiction—a case report of acute and chronic subjective effects. *Heliyon, 6*(7), e04507. https://doi.org/10.1016/j.heliyon.2020.e04507.

Nestler, E. J., & Aghajanian, G. K. (1997). Molecular and cellular basis of addiction. *Science, 278*(5335), 58–63. https://doi.org/10.1126/science.278.5335.58.

Northcutt, A. L., Hutchinson, M. R., Wang, X., Baratta, M. V., Hiranita, T., Cochran, T. A., et al. (2015). DAT isn't all that: Cocaine reward and reinforcement require Toll-like receptor 4 signaling. *Molecular Psychiatry, 20*(12), 1525–1537. https://doi.org/10.1038/mp.2014.177.

Obeng, S., Hiranita, T., Leon, F., McMahon, L. R., & McCurdy, C. R. (2021). Novel approaches, drug candidates, and targets in pain drug discovery. *Journal of Medicinal Chemistry, 64*(10), 6523–6548. https://doi.org/10.1021/acs.jmedchem.1c00028.

Obeng, S., Kamble, S. H., Reeves, M. E., Restrepo, L. F., Patel, A., Behnke, M., et al. (2020). Investigation of the adrenergic and opioid binding affinities, metabolic stability, plasma protein binding properties, and functional effects of selected indole-based kratom alkaloids. *Journal of Medicinal Chemistry, 63*(1), 433–439. https://doi.org/10.1021/acs.jmedchem.9b01465.

Obeng, S., Wilkerson, J. L., Leon, F., Reeves, M. E., Restrepo, L. F., Gamez-Jimenez, L. R., et al. (2021). Pharmacological comparison of mitragynine and 7-hydroxymitragynine: in vitro affinity and efficacy for mu-opioid receptor and opioid-like behavioral effects in rats. *The Journal of Pharmacology and Experimental Therapeutics*, *376*(3), 410–427. https://doi.org/10.1124/jpet.120.000189.

O'Connor, E. C., Chapman, K., Butler, P., & Mead, A. N. (2011). The predictive validity of the rat self-administration model for abuse liability. *Neuroscience and Biobehavioral Reviews*, *35*(3), 912–938.

Otsubo, Y., Satoh, Y., Kodama, M., Araki, Y., Satomoto, M., Sakamoto, E., et al. (2012). Mechanical allodynia but not thermal hyperalgesia is impaired in mice deficient for ERK2 in the central nervous system. *Pain*, *153*(11), 2241–2252. https://doi.org/10.1016/j.pain.2012.07.020.

Overbeek, D. L., Abraham, J., & Munzer, B. W. (2019). Kratom (mitragynine) ingestion requiring naloxone reversal. *Clinical Practice and Cases in Emergency Medicine*, *3*(1), 24–26. https://doi.org/10.5811/cpcem.2018.11.40588.

Parthasarathy, S., Ramanathan, S., Ismail, S., Adenan, M. I., Mansor, S. M., & Murugaiyah, V. (2010). Determination of mitragynine in plasma with solid-phase extraction and rapid HPLC-UV analysis, and its application to a pharmacokinetic study in rat. *Analytical and Bioanalytical Chemistry*, *397*(5), 2023–2030. https://doi.org/10.1007/s00216-010-3707-7.

Philipp, A. A., Wissenbach, D. K., Zoerntlein, S. W., Klein, O. N., Kanogsunthornrat, J., & Maurer, H. H. (2009). Studies on the metabolism of mitragynine, the main alkaloid of the herbal drug kratom, in rat and human urine using liquid chromatography-linear ion trap mass spectrometry. *Journal of Mass Spectrometry*, *44*(8), 1249–1261. https://doi.org/10.1002/jms.1607.

Post, S., Spiller, H. A., Chounthirath, T., & Smith, G. A. (2019). Kratom exposures reported to United States poison control centers: 2011-2017. *Clinical Toxicology (Philadelphia, Pa.)*, *57*(10), 847–854. https://doi.org/10.1080/15563650.2019.1569236.

Ramanathan, S., Parthasarathy, S., Murugaiyah, V., Magosso, E., Tan, S. C., & Mansor, S. M. (2015). Understanding the physicochemical properties of mitragynine, a principal alkaloid of Mitragyna speciosa, for preclinical evaluation. *Molecules*, *20*(3), 4915–4927. https://doi.org/10.3390/molecules20034915.

Reanmongkol, W., Keawpradub, N., & Sawangjaroen, K. (2007). Effects of the extracts from Mitragyna speciosa Korth. leaves on analgesic and behavioral activities in experimental animals. *Songklanakarin. Journal of Science and Technology*, *29*(Suppl. 1), 39–48.

Roberts, D. C., & Bennett, S. A. (1993). Heroin self-administration in rats under a progressive ratio schedule of reinforcement. *Psychopharmacology*, *111*(2), 215–218. https://doi.org/10.1007/BF02245526.

Rusli, N., Amanah, A., Kaur, G., Adenan, M. I., Sulaiman, S. F., Wahab, H. A., et al. (2019). The inhibitory effects of mitragynine on P-glycoprotein in vitro. *Naunyn-Schmiedeberg's Archives of Pharmacology*, *392*(4), 481–496. https://doi.org/10.1007/s00210-018-01605-y.

Sabetghadam, A., Ramanathan, S., & Mansor, S. M. (2010). The evaluation of antinociceptive activity of alkaloid, methanolic, and aqueous extracts of Malaysian Mitragyna speciosa Korth leaves in rats. *Pharmacognosy Research*, *2*(3), 181–185. https://doi.org/10.4103/0974-8490.65514.

Sabetghadam, A., Ramanathan, S., Sasidharan, S., & Mansor, S. M. (2013). Subchronic exposure to mitragynine, the principal alkaloid of Mitragyna speciosa, in rats. *Journal of Ethnopharmacology*, *146*(3), 815–823. https://doi.org/10.1016/j.jep.2013.02.008.

Sablaban, I. M., & Gautam, M. (2021). The diagnosis of severe obsessions in the setting of kratom withdrawal and treatment with lorazepam: Case report. *Journal of Addictive Diseases*, *39*(1), 138–139. https://doi.org/10.1080/10550887.2020.1813357.

Saingam, D., Assanangkornchai, S., Geater, A. F., & Lerkiatbundit, S. (2014). Validation of Krathom (Mitragyna speciosa Korth.) dependence scale (KDS): A dependence screen for internationally emerging psychoactive substance. *Substance Abuse*, *35*(3), 276–283. https://doi.org/10.1080/08897077.2014.924464.

Saingam, D., Assanangkornchai, S., Geater, A. F., & Lerkiatbundit, S. (2016). Factor analytical investigation of Krathom (Mitragyna speciosa Korth.) withdrawal syndrome in Thailand. *Journal of Psychoactive Drugs*, *48*(2), 76–85. https://doi.org/10.1080/02791072.2016.1156791.

Schimmel, J., Amioka, E., Rockhill, K., Haynes, C. M., Black, J. C., Dart, R. C., et al. (2021). Prevalence and description of kratom (Mitragyna speciosa) use in the United States: A cross-sectional study. *Addiction*, *116*(1), 176–181. https://doi.org/10.1111/add.15082.

Schuster, C. R., & Johanson, C. E. (1988). Relationship between the discriminative stimulus properties and subjective effects of drugs. *Psychopharmacology Series*, *4*, 161–175.

Shamima, A. R., Fakurazi, S., Hidayat, M. T., Hairuszah, I., Moklas, M. A., & Arulselvan, P. (2012). Antinociceptive action of isolated mitragynine from Mitragyna Speciosa through activation of opioid receptor system. *International Journal of Molecular Sciences*, *13*(9), 11427–11442. https://doi.org/10.3390/ijms130911427.

Sharma, A., Kamble, S. H., Leon, F., Chear, N. J., King, T. I., Berthold, E. C., et al. (2019). Simultaneous quantification of ten key kratom alkaloids in Mitragyna speciosa leaf extracts and commercial products by ultra-performance liquid chromatography-tandem mass spectrometry. *Drug Testing and Analysis*, *11*(8), 1162–1171. https://doi.org/10.1002/dta.2604.

Sharma, S. K., Klee, W. A., & Nirenberg, M. (1977). Opiate-dependent modulation of adenylate cyclase. *Proceedings of the National Academy of Sciences of the United States of America*, *74*(8), 3365–3369. https://doi.org/10.1073/pnas.74.8.3365.

Singh, D., Muller, C. P., & Vicknasingam, B. K. (2014). Kratom (Mitragyna speciosa) dependence, withdrawal symptoms and craving in regular users. *Drug and Alcohol Dependence*, *139*, 132–137. https://doi.org/10.1016/j.drugalcdep.2014.03.017.

Singh, D., Narayanan, S., Muller, C. P., Swogger, M. T., Rahim, A. A., Leong Bin Abdullah, M. F. I., et al. (2018). Severity of kratom (Mitragyna speciosa Korth.) psychological withdrawal symptoms. *Journal of Psychoactive Drugs*, *50*(5), 445–450. https://doi.org/10.1080/02791072.2018.1511879.

Singh, D., Narayanan, S., Vicknasingam, B. K., Prozialeck, W. C., Ramanathan, S., Zainal, H., et al. (2018). Severity of pain and sleep problems during kratom (Mitragyna speciosa Korth.) cessation among regular kratom users. *Journal of Psychoactive Drugs*, *50*(3), 266–274. https://doi.org/10.1080/02791072.2018.1443234.

Smid, M. C., Charles, J. E., Gordon, A. J., & Wright, T. E. (2018). Use of kratom, an opioid-like traditional herb, in pregnancy. *Obstetrics & Gynecology*, *132*(4), 926–928. https://doi.org/10.1097/AOG.0000000000002871.

Smith, M. D., Woodhead, J. H., Handy, L. J., Pruess, T. H., Vanegas, F., Grussendorf, E., et al. (2017). Preclinical comparison of mechanistically different antiseizure, antinociceptive, and/or antidepressant drugs in a battery of rodent models of nociceptive and neuropathic pain. *Neurochemical Research*, *42*(7), 1995–2010. https://doi.org/10.1007/s11064-017-2286-9.

Sufka, K. J., Loria, M. J., Lewellyn, K., Zjawiony, J. K., Ali, Z., Abe, N., et al. (2014). The effect of *Salvia divinorum* and Mitragyna speciosa extracts, fraction and major constituents on place aversion and place preference in rats. *Journal of Ethnopharmacology*, *151*(1), 361–364. https://doi.org/10.1016/j.jep.2013.10.059.

Svorc, P., Petrasova, D., & Svorc, P., Jr. (2018). Arterial pH and blood gas values in rats under three types of general anesthesia: A chronobiological study. *Physiological Research*, *67*(5), 721–728. https://doi.org/10.33549/physiolres.933692.

Swogger, M. T., Hart, E., Erowid, F., Erowid, E., Trabold, N., Yee, K., et al. (2015). Experiences of kratom users: A qualitative analysis. *Journal of Psychoactive Drugs, 47*(5), 360–367. https://doi.org/10.1080/02791072.2015.1096434.

Takayama, H., Ishikawa, H., Kurihara, M., Kitajima, M., Aimi, N., Ponglux, D., et al. (2002). Studies on the synthesis and opioid agonistic activities of mitragynine-related indole alkaloids: Discovery of opioid agonists structurally different from other opioid ligands. *Journal of Medicinal Chemistry, 45*(9), 1949–1956. https://doi.org/10.1021/jm010576e.

Tanda, G., Mereu, M., Hiranita, T., Quarterman, J. C., Coggiano, M., & Katz, J. L. (2016). Lack of specific involvement of (+)-naloxone and (+)-naltrexone on the reinforcing and neurochemical effects of cocaine and opioids. *Neuropsychopharmacology, 41*(11), 2772–2781. https://doi.org/10.1038/npp.2016.91.

Townsend, E. A., Schwienteck, K. L., Robinson, H. L., Lawson, S. T., & Banks, M. L. (2021). A drug-vs-food "choice" self-administration procedure in rats to investigate pharmacological and environmental mechanisms of substance use disorders. *Journal of Neuroscience Methods, 354*, 109110. https://doi.org/10.1016/j.jneumeth.2021.109110.

Trakulsrichai, S., Sathirakul, K., Auparakkitanon, S., Krongvorakul, J., Sueajai, J., Noumjad, N., et al. (2015). Pharmacokinetics of mitragynine in man. *Drug Design, Development and Therapy, 9*, 2421–2429. https://doi.org/10.2147/DDDT.S79658.

Trakulsrichai, S., Tongpo, A., Sriapha, C., Wongvisawakorn, S., Rittilert, P., Kaojarern, S., et al. (2013). Kratom abuse in Ramathibodi poison center, Thailand: A five-year experience. *Journal of Psychoactive Drugs, 45*(5), 404–408. https://doi.org/10.1080/02791072.2013.844532.

van den Hoogen, R. H., & Colpaert, F. C. (1986). Respiratory effects of morphine in awake unrestrained rats. *The Journal of Pharmacology and Experimental Therapeutics, 237*(1), 252–259.

Varadi, A., Marrone, G. F., Palmer, T. C., Narayan, A., Szabo, M. R., Le Rouzic, V., et al. (2016). Mitragynine/corynantheidine pseudoindoxyls as opioid analgesics with Mu agonism and delta antagonism, which do not recruit beta-arrestin-2. *Journal of Medicinal Chemistry, 59*(18), 8381–8397. https://doi.org/10.1021/acs.jmedchem.6b00748.

Vento, A. E., de Persis, S., De Filippis, S., Schifano, F., Napoletano, F., Corkery, J. M., et al. (2021). Case report: Treatment of kratom use disorder with a classical tricyclic antidepressant. *Frontiers in Psychiatry, 12*, 640218. https://doi.org/10.3389/fpsyt.2021.640218.

Vicknasingam, B., Chooi, W. T., Rahim, A. A., Ramachandram, D., Singh, D., Ramanathan, S., et al. (2020). Kratom and pain tolerance: A randomized, placebo-controlled, Double-Blind Study. *Yale Journal of Biology and Medicine, 93*(2), 229–238.

Vicknasingam, B., Narayanan, S., Beng, G. T., & Mansor, S. M. (2010). The informal use of ketum (Mitragyna speciosa) for opioid withdrawal in the northern states of peninsular Malaysia and implications for drug substitution therapy. *The International Journal on Drug Policy, 21*(4), 283–288. https://doi.org/10.1016/j.drugpo.2009.12.003.

Vijeepallam, K., Pandy, V., Murugan, D. D., & Naidu, M. (2019). Methanolic extract of Mitragyna speciosa Korth leaf inhibits ethanol seeking behaviour in mice: Involvement of antidopaminergic mechanism. *Metabolic Brain Disease, 34*(6), 1713–1722. https://doi.org/10.1007/s11011-019-00477-2.

Vuppala, P. K., Jamalapuram, S., Furr, E. B., McCurdy, C. R., & Avery, B. A. (2013). Development and validation of a UPLC-MS/MS method for the determination of 7-hydroxymitragynine, a mu-opioid agonist, in rat plasma and its application to a pharmacokinetic study. *Biomedical Chromatography, 27*(12), 1726–1732. https://doi.org/10.1002/bmc.2986.

Warner, M. L., Kaufman, N. C., & Grundmann, O. (2016). The pharmacology and toxicology of kratom: From traditional herb to drug of abuse. *International Journal of Legal Medicine, 130*(1), 127–138. https://doi.org/10.1007/s00414-015-1279-y.

Watanabe, K., Yano, S., Horie, S., & Yamamoto, L. T. (1997). Inhibitory effect of mitragynine, an alkaloid with analgesic effect from Thai medicinal plant Mitragyna speciosa, on electrically stimulated contraction of isolated Guinea-pig ileum through the opioid receptor. *Life Sciences, 60*(12), 933–942. https://doi.org/10.1016/s0024-3205(97)00023-4.

Weiss, S. T., & Douglas, H. E. (2021). Treatment of kratom withdrawal and dependence with buprenorphine/naloxone: A case series and systematic literature review. *Journal of Addiction Medicine, 15*(2), 167–172. https://doi.org/10.1097/ADM.0000000000000721.

Wilson, L. L., Chakraborty, S., Eans, S. O., Cirino, T. J., Stacy, H. M., Simons, C. A., et al. (2021). Kratom alkaloids, natural and semi-synthetic, show less physical dependence and ameliorate opioid withdrawal. *Cellular and Molecular Neurobiology, 41*(5), 1131–1143. https://doi.org/10.1007/s10571-020-01034-7.

Wilson, L. L., Harris, H. M., Eans, S. O., Brice-Tutt, A. C., Cirino, T. J., Stacy, H. M., et al. (2020). Lyophilized kratom tea as a therapeutic option for opioid dependence. *Drug and Alcohol Dependence, 216*, 108310. https://doi.org/10.1016/j.drugalcdep.2020.108310.

Winger, G., Skjoldager, P., & Woods, J. H. (1992). Effects of buprenorphine and other opioid agonists and antagonists on alfentanil- and cocaine-reinforced responding in rhesus monkeys. *The Journal of Pharmacology and Experimental Therapeutics, 261*(1), 311–317.

Wright, M. E., Ginsberg, C., Parkison, A. M., Dubose, M., & Shores, E. (2021). Outcomes of mothers and newborns to prenatal exposure to kratom: A systematic review. *Journal of Perinatology*. https://doi.org/10.1038/s41372-021-00952-8.

Yue, K., Kopajtic, T. A., & Katz, J. L. (2018). Abuse liability of mitragynine assessed with a self-administration procedure in rats. *Psychopharmacology, 235*(10), 2823–2829. https://doi.org/10.1007/s00213-018-4974-9.

Yusof, S. R., Mohd Uzid, M., Teh, E. H., Hanapi, N. A., Mohideen, M., Mohamad Arshad, A. S., et al. (2019). Rate and extent of mitragynine and 7-hydroxymitragynine blood-brain barrier transport and their intra-brain distribution: The missing link in pharmacodynamic studies. *Addiction Biology, 24*(5), 935–945. https://doi.org/10.1111/adb.12661.

Yusoff, N. H. M., Mansor, S. M., Muller, C. P., & Hassan, Z. (2017). Opioid receptors mediate the acquisition, but not the expression of mitragynine-induced conditioned place preference in rats. *Behavioural Brain Research, 332*, 1–6. https://doi.org/10.1016/j.bbr.2017.05.059.

Yusoff, N. H. M., Mansor, S. M., Muller, C. P., & Hassan, Z. (2018). Baclofen blocks the acquisition and expression of mitragynine-induced conditioned place preference in rats. *Behavioural Brain Research, 345*, 65–71. https://doi.org/10.1016/j.bbr.2018.02.039.

Yusoff, N. H., Suhaimi, F. W., Vadivelu, R. K., Hassan, Z., Rumler, A., Rotter, A., et al. (2016). Abuse potential and adverse cognitive effects of mitragynine (kratom). *Addiction Biology, 21*(1), 98–110. https://doi.org/10.1111/adb.12185.

Zhou, Y., Ramsey, S., Provasi, D., El Daibani, A., Appourchaux, K., Chakraborty, S., et al. (2021). Predicted mode of binding to and allosteric modulation of the mu-opioid receptor by Kratom's alkaloids with reported antinociception in vivo. *Biochemistry, 60*(18), 1420–1429. https://doi.org/10.1021/acs.biochem.0c00658.

CHAPTER THREE

Human behavioral pharmacology of stimulant drugs: An update and narrative review

Ashley Strzelecki[a], Jessica Weafer[a], and William W. Stoops[a,b,c,d,*]
[a]University of Kentucky, Department of Psychology, Lexington, KY, United States
[b]University of Kentucky, Department of Behavioral Science, Lexington, KY, United States
[c]University of Kentucky, Department of Psychiatry, Lexington, KY, United States
[d]University of Kentucky, Center on Drug and Alcohol Research, Lexington, KY, United States
*Corresponding author: e-mail address: william.stoops@uky.edu

Contents

1. Introduction 78
   1.1 Stimulant use epidemiology 78
   1.2 Basic neuropharmacology of stimulants 79
   1.3 Purpose of this chapter 79
2. Human behavioral pharmacology of cocaine 80
   2.1 Subjective effects 80
   2.2 Reinforcing effects 83
   2.3 Cognitive/behavioral effects 86
   2.4 Discriminative stimulus effects 87
3. Human behavioral pharmacology of amphetamine 87
   3.1 Subjective effects 87
   3.2 Reinforcing effects 91
   3.3 Cognitive/behavioral effects 92
4. Conclusion 94
Conflict of interest 96
References 96

Abstract

Stimulant use disorders present an enduring public health concern. Chronic stimulant use is associated with a range of health problems, with notable increases in stimulant overdose that disproportionately affect marginalized populations. With these persistent problems, it is important to understand the behavioral and pharmacological factors that contribute to stimulant use in humans. The purpose of this chapter is to provide an update and narrative review on recent human laboratory research that has evaluated the behavioral pharmacology of stimulant drugs. We focus on two prototypic stimulants: cocaine as a prototype monoamine reuptake inhibitor and d-amphetamine as a prototype monoamine releaser. As such, placebo controlled human laboratory studies

Advances in Pharmacology, Volume 93
ISSN 1054-3589
https://doi.org/10.1016/bs.apha.2021.07.001

that involved administration of doses of cocaine or d-amphetamine and were published in peer reviewed journals within the last 10 years (i.e., since 2011) are reviewed. Primary outcomes from these studies are subjective effects, reinforcing effects, cognitive/behavioral effects, and discriminative stimulus effects. Both cocaine and d-amphetamine produce classical stimulant-like behavioral effects (e.g., increase positive subjective effects, function as reinforcers), but there are notable gaps in the literature including understanding sex differences in response to stimulant drugs, cognitive-behavioral effects of stimulants, and influence of use history (e.g., relatively drug naïve vs drug experienced) on stimulant effects.

Abbreviations

kg kilogram
mg milligram

1. Introduction

1.1 Stimulant use epidemiology

Stimulant use disorders present an enduring public health concern. Data from the National Survey on Drug Use and Health indicate that approximately 2 million Americans over 12 years of age report current (i.e., past month) cocaine use, making cocaine the most widely used stimulant in the United States (Substance Abuse and Mental Health Services Administration, 2020). That same survey indicated that approximately 1.2 million Americans report current methamphetamine use and that 1.6 million Americans report current nonmedical use of prescription stimulants, including d-amphetamine and mixed amphetamine salts. Of the individuals reporting illicit use, 1 million people met stimulant use disorder criteria for cocaine and another 1 million people met stimulant use disorder criteria for methamphetamine. Approximately 558,000 Americans met stimulant use disorder criteria for prescription stimulants.

Chronic stimulant use produces a number of direct health problems like cardiovascular toxicity, malnutrition, or miscarriage in pregnant women (Chen, Scheier, & Kandel, 1996; Hando, Howard, & Zibert, 1997; Hando, Topp, & Hall, 1997; Richards et al., 1999; Schwartz, Rezkalla, & Kloner, 2010; Vearrier, Greenberg, Miller, Okaneku, & Haggerty, 2012). Stimulant use also increases risks for other health issues including smoking cigarettes, comorbid psychological disorders, and acquiring and transmitting sexually transmitted infections (Hando, Howard, et al., 1997; Hando, Topp, et al., 1997; Liu et al., 2017; Rounsaville et al., 1991;

Substance Abuse and Mental Health Services Administration, 2010; Van Tieu & Koblin, 2009). Lastly, stimulant overdoses are increasing, which appears to be a wave that is following the opioid crisis in the United States (Cano & Huang, 2021; Kariisa, Scholl, Wilson, Seth, & Hoots, 2019). There are clear health disparities in stimulant overdose (i.e., increased overdose rates in Black and Hispanic Americans; Cano & Huang, 2021; Cano, Oh, Salas-Wright, & Vaughn, 2020; Shiels, Freedman, Thomas, & Berrington de Gonzalez, 2018), making the dangers posed by stimulant use even more evident. With these persistent problems, it is important to understand the behavioral and pharmacological factors that contribute to stimulant use in humans. Carefully controlled human laboratory studies that administer doses of stimulants, the focus of this chapter, can provide this information.

1.2 Basic neuropharmacology of stimulants

Stimulant drugs produce their behavioral and physiological effects via interaction with monoamine transporters (dopamine, norepinephrine, and serotonin) (reviewed in Fleckenstein, Gibb, & Hanson, 2000; Johanson & Fischman, 1989; Rothman & Glowa, 1995). Based on *in vitro* studies, stimulants can be broadly categorized into two categories by their mechanism of action at these transporters: monoamine reuptake inhibitors or monoamine releasers. Stimulants like cocaine and methylphenidate bind to monoamine transporters and prevent their reuptake back into the presynaptic terminal (Iversen, 2006; Shellenberg, Stoops, Lile, & Rush, 2020). Amphetamines, by contrast, act as a substrate for monoamine transporters and are transported into the nerve terminal where they promote the release of monoamines into the synapse by preventing the accumulation of neurotransmitter in storage vesicles and also by carrier-mediated exchange (Reith & Gnegy, 2020; Simmler & Liechti, 2018). Amphetamines also usually function as transporter blockers, although they are less potent at inhibiting reuptake compared to their ability to act as transporter substrates (Rothman et al., 2001). Thus, although they may have different pharmacological mechanisms of action, the administration of stimulant drugs ultimately results in increased synaptic levels of dopamine, serotonin, and norepinephrine.

1.3 Purpose of this chapter

The purpose of this chapter is to provide an update and narrative review on recent human laboratory research that has evaluated the behavioral pharmacology of stimulant drugs. We focus on two prototypic stimulants: cocaine as a prototype monoamine reuptake inhibitor and d-amphetamine as a prototype monoamine releaser. We chose d-amphetamine over methamphetamine because the behavioral pharmacological effects of both drugs overlap to a large extent and more human laboratory research has been published with d-amphetamine than with methamphetamine. Placebo controlled human laboratory studies that involved administration of doses of cocaine or d-amphetamine and were published in peer reviewed journals within the last 10 years (i.e., since 2011) are reviewed below. Primary outcomes from these studies are subjective effects, reinforcing effects, cognitive/behavioral effects, and discriminative stimulus effects. For work published more than 10 years ago, we refer readers to several reviews of older studies evaluating the behavioral pharmacology of stimulants in humans (Johanson & Fischman, 1989 ; Romach, Schoedel, & Sellers, 2014; Rush, Stoops, & Ling, 2009).

2. Human behavioral pharmacology of cocaine

2.1 Subjective effects

Much of the work that evaluated the subjective effects of cocaine was conducted before 2011, so the general results of these studies will be described before we then describe the findings of studies that qualified for inclusion in this chapter. Cocaine has been administered across numerous routes in controlled human laboratory studies, including orally, intranasally (i.e., "snorted"), intravenously, and smoked. Intravenous and smoked cocaine typically produce rapid and robust increases in subjective responses (e.g., Foltin & Fischman, 1991), with intranasal dosing resulting in a slower onset, longer lasting, and blunted response relative to intravenous and smoked doses (Cone, 1995). Orally administered cocaine results in the slowest onset and longest lasting effects, but it can produce subjective effects comparable to or greater than those of intranasal cocaine (Johnson, Herrmann, Sweeney, LeComte, & Johnson, 2017; Smith, Jones, & Griffiths, 2001; Van Dyke, Jatlow, Ungerer, Barash, & Byck, 1978). Regardless of route, cocaine produces time and dose dependent increases in prototypic "positive" (e.g., ratings of liking, good effects) and general (e.g., ratings of high or any effect) subjective drug effects (Foltin & Fischman, 1991; Foltin & Haney, 2004; Smith et al., 2001). Recent studies have evaluated how individual differences might impact the subjective effects of cocaine.

Studies have found no relationship between reported years of cocaine use, age, or endogenous butyrylcholinesterase levels and subjective response to smoked cocaine (Askalsky, Kalapatapu, Foltin, & Comer, 2015; Kalapatapu et al., 2012), whereas one study indicated that greater family and social dysfunction reported on the Addiction Severity Index were correlated with subjective response to intravenous cocaine (Grasing, Mathur, Newton, & Desouza, 2013). The focus of more recent research with cocaine has largely been to understand how pharmacological manipulations impact the subjective effects of cocaine, described below.

2.1.1 Pharmacological manipulations of the subjective effects of cocaine

Given that cocaine primarily exerts its effects through brain monoamine systems, controlled human laboratory studies have determined how manipulations of these systems or administration of compounds that interact with these systems influence the subjective response to cocaine. In one study, human subjects with a history of cocaine use were assigned to undergo tryptophan depletion or to a control condition and then received 1.0 mg/kg intranasal cocaine (Cox et al., 2011). Tryptophan depletion, which reduces serotonin transmission, resulted in increased ratings of cocaine-induced drug wanting, but did not alter other subjective effects (e.g., ratings of drug liking or high). Another study determined how acute administration of 10 mg oral lorcaserin, a serotonin 2c receptor agonist, impacted subjective response to 0.23 or 0.46 mg/kg intravenous cocaine (Pirtle et al., 2019). Although lorcaserin reduced ratings of cocaine wanting after intravenous placebo, it enhanced ratings of high and stimulated following administration of 0.23 mg/kg intravenous cocaine. Verrico and colleagues found that treatment with the SSRI escitalopram (20 mg/day) did not change subjective response to 20 mg intravenous cocaine (Verrico et al., 2014).

Maintenance on 20 mg/day buspirone, which has agonist/partial agonist activity at numerous serotonin receptors and antagonist activity at dopamine D2-like receptors, did not change subjective effects of 15 or 45 mg intranasal cocaine (Bolin et al., 2016). Three studies have evaluated how pretreatment with aripiprazole, a partial agonist at D2-like dopamine and serotonin 1A receptors and antagonist at serotonin 2 receptors, influenced subjective response to cocaine (Haney, Rubin, & Foltin, 2011; Lile, Stoops, Glaser, Hays, & Rush, 2011; Lofwall, Nuzzo, Campbell, & Walsh, 2014). In one study, acute pretreatment with 15 mg oral aripiprazole attenuated stimulant-like and positive subjective effects of 100 mg oral cocaine (Lile et al., 2011). However, in studies that evaluated aripiprazole maintenance dosing, 15 mg oral aripiprazole/day decreased the amount of money subjects indicated they would be willing to pay for a 25 mg dose of smoked cocaine, but otherwise did not change subjective responding (Haney et al., 2011). In the most recent study, neither acute nor chronic dosing with 2 or 10 mg oral aripiprazole/day significantly influenced the subjective effects of 20 or 40 mg/70 kg intravenous cocaine (Lofwall et al., 2014).

Other work has determined how administration of relatively selective dopamine agonists impact subjective responding to cocaine. For example, in one study, acute pretreatment with the dopamine reuptake inhibitor bupropion (100 or 200 mg, oral) enhanced a range of subjective responses to 15 and 45 mg of intranasal cocaine, including ratings of willing to take again and liking (Stoops, Lile, Glaser, Hays, & Rush, 2012b). In another study, maintenance on 30 or 60 mg oral d-amphetamine reduced subjective response (e.g., ratings of willing to pay for or willing to take again) to a range of doses of intravenous cocaine (Lile et al., 2020). Lastly, maintenance on oral phendimetrazine 70–210 mg/day, a prodrug for phenmetrazine (a dopamine and norepinephrine releaser), did not alter any subjective responses to intranasal cocaine across two studies (Stoops et al., 2019, 2016).

Aside from manipulating monoaminergic systems, human laboratory studies have also determined how agents that alter glutamate (i.e., modafinil, ketamine, *n*-acetylcysteine) or acetylcholine (i.e., huperzine A; rivastigmine) function influence the subjective effects of cocaine. Two studies have evaluated modafinil/cocaine interactions (Foltin, Haney, Bedi, & Evans, 2016; Verrico et al., 2014). In the more recent study, maintenance on 300 mg oral modafinil/day did not change subjective drug effect ratings following administration of 25 mg smoked cocaine (Foltin et al., 2016). In the earlier study, maintenance on 200 mg oral modafinil/day attenuated ratings of any effect, high, good effects, and stimulated following administration of 20 mg intravenous cocaine (Verrico et al., 2014). Interestingly, in that study, combining modafinil and 20 mg/day oral escitalopram, did not result in any changes of the effects of modafinil on cocaine. Another study showed that intravenous ketamine, a glutamate *N*-methyl-D-aspartate (NMDA) receptor antagonist, (0.11 mg/kg in a 2 min bolus, followed by 0.60 mg/kg in saline over 50 min) did not alter any subjective responses to 25 mg smoked cocaine (Dakwar, Hart, Levin, Nunes, & Foltin, 2017). Maintenance on 2.4 g oral *n*-acetylcysteine/day, which restores glutamate homeostasis by enhancing activity of the cystine/glutamate exchanger and glutamate transporter, generally did not change the subjective effects of 30 or 60 mg intranasal cocaine, although significant reductions were observed for two items: ratings of euphoria and stimulated (Bolin et al., 2017). Maintenance on oral huperzine A, an acetylcholinesterase inhibitor and NMDA receptor antagonist, (0.4 mg/day) blunted ratings of any effect, high, bad effects, anxious, willing to pay, and stimulated following administration of 40 mg intravenous cocaine (De La Garza, Verrico, Newton, Mahoney, & Thompson-Lake, 2015). A higher dose of huperzine A (0.8 mg/day) only attenuated ratings of stimulated produced by intravenous cocaine. Finally, maintenance on 3 or 6 mg oral rivastigmine did not alter the subjective effects of 40 mg intravenous cocaine (Patel, Verrico, & De La Garza, 2019).

A final approach has been to determine how manipulating hormone levels, namely, progesterone, impacts the subjective effects of cocaine (Reed, Evans, Bedi, Rubin, & Foltin, 2011). In that study, maintenance on oral micronized progesterone (150 mg twice daily) during the follicular phase of the menstrual cycle did not alter the subjective effects of a range of doses of 12–50 mg smoked cocaine.

Taken together, the findings of these studies demonstrate that pharmacologically manipulating systems impacted by cocaine can alter cocaine's subjective effects. It may be the case that serotonin systems influence cocaine craving/wanting, as indicated by the findings with serotonin depletion or lorcaserin administration described above (Cox et al., 2011; Pirtle et al., 2019), whereas subchronic treatment with more potent indirect-acting monoamine agonists like d-amphetamine reduce the subjective effects of cocaine, perhaps by increasing tolerance (Lile et al., 2020). Less potent indirect-acting monoamine agonists or partial agonists have not reliably influenced subjective response to cocaine, particularly following subchronic maintenance (Haney et al., 2011; Lile et al., 2011; Lofwall et al., 2014; Stoops et al., 2019, 2016). However, mixed findings (e.g., the findings with modafinil; Foltin et al., 2016; Verrico et al., 2014) and the diversity of subjective effects measured/altered (e.g., liking type ratings, drug strength type ratings, craving type ratings) in the studies described above, require caution in interpretation of results.

2.2 Reinforcing effects

As with studies assessing the subjective effects of cocaine, much of the work that evaluated the reinforcing effects of cocaine was conducted before 2011, so general findings will be described before we then describe the findings of studies that qualified for inclusion in this chapter. Cocaine, administered across various routes in controlled human laboratory studies (intranasal, intravenous, and smoked), is a robust reinforcer. Earlier research has demonstrated that human subjects reliably self-administer active cocaine doses to a greater degree than placebo across a number of arrangements (e.g., drug vs alternative reinforcer choice, progressive ratio schedules; Foltin & Fischman, 1992; Stoops, Lile, & Rush, 2010; Walsh, Donny, Nuzzo, Umbricht, & Bigelow, 2010). Although cocaine self-administration outcomes can be dose-dependent (e.g., Matuskey et al., 2012; Walsh et al., 2010), this is not always the case (e.g., Stoops, Lile, Glaser, Hays, & Rush, 2010), which is potentially due to the limited dose range that can be tested in humans. The results of one recent study show that sleep changes in early abstinence from cocaine use were negatively corelated with self-administration of 32mg/70kg intravenous cocaine (Angarita, Canavan, Forselius, Bessette, & Morgan, 2014), but the focus of most recent research with cocaine has largely been to understand how pharmacological and behavioral manipulations impact the reinforcing effects of cocaine, described below.

2.2.1 Pharmacological manipulations of the reinforcing effects of cocaine

As with subjective effects, many studies that have evaluated pharmacological manipulation of cocaine self-administration have focused on manipulation of monoaminergic systems. In fact, many of the studies that are described above in the Subjective Effects section also evaluated cocaine self-administration. This section is thus organized in a similar fashion, reviewing studies that administered drugs that target monoamine systems, glutamate systems, acetylcholine systems, and hormones.

Pirtle and colleagues found that while acute treatment with lorcaserin (10mg, oral) prolonged the time it took for subjects to choose an intravenous cocaine dose over money, it did not alter overall cocaine self-administration (Pirtle et al., 2019). Maintenance on buspirone (30mg, oral) also did not change the reinforcing effects of intranasal cocaine on concurrent progressive ratio schedules of money vs drug availability (Bolin et al., 2016). Studies that assessed the effects of maintenance on oral aripiprazole found that it did not change self-administration of intravenous cocaine (Lofwall et al., 2014) but that it enhanced self-administration of smoked cocaine (Haney et al., 2011) under drug vs money choice arrangements.

Two studies have found that treatment with relatively more potent indirect-acting monoamine agonists reduced the reinforcing effects of cocaine.

Specifically, acute pretreatment with oral bupropion (100 or 200 mg) reduced choice of intranasal cocaine over money (Stoops et al., 2012b) and maintenance on oral d-amphetamine also reduced choice of intravenous cocaine over money (Lile et al., 2020). Maintenance on a less potent and selective indirect-acting monoamine agonist, phendimetrazine (210 mg, oral), did not change the reinforcing effects of intranasal cocaine (Stoops et al., 2019).

Maintenance on modafinil (300 mg, oral) reduced smoked cocaine self-administration when the response requirement for drug was high and the alternative reinforcer available was large (Foltin et al., 2016), but maintenance on a lower modafinil dose (i.e., 200 mg, oral) failed to change intravenous cocaine self-administration when administered alone or combined with escitalopram (Verrico et al., 2014). Treatment with ketamine also reduced smoked cocaine self-administration (Dakwar et al., 2017) whereas maintenance on *n*-acetylcysteine reduced intranasal cocaine self-administration, dependent upon maintenance order (i.e., choice of cocaine over money was attenuated across maintenance conditions in subjects assigned to receive *n*-acetylcysteine first in a crossover study whereas no change was observed in subjects assigned to receive placebo first; Bolin et al., 2017). Neither maintenance on huperzine A nor rivastigmine affected intravenous cocaine self-administration (De La Garza et al., 2015; Patel et al., 2019). Lastly, maintenance on oral micronized progesterone did not affect the reinforcing effects of smoked cocaine (Reed et al., 2011).

Taken together, the results of these studies further demonstrate the robust reinforcing effects of cocaine in that they are difficult to change with pharmacological pretreatment (e.g., in one study, administration of modafinil only reduced cocaine self-administration when other parameters like response cost for cocaine were high; Foltin et al., 2016). Importantly, though, treatment with bupropion, d-amphetamine, and ketamine all reduced cocaine taking, which is consistent with the effects of these drugs in clinical trials for cocaine use disorder (e.g., Dakwar et al., 2019; Grabowski et al., 2004; Poling et al., 2006).

2.2.2 Behavioral manipulations of the reinforcing effects of cocaine

As indicated above, behavioral manipulations can also alter the reinforcing effects of cocaine (e.g., Foltin et al., 2016). This effect is most clearly shown in studies demonstrating that increasing the value/magnitude of a mutually exclusive alternative reinforcer, typically money, reduced choice for cocaine (Foltin et al., 2015; Greenwald, Ledgerwood, Lundahl, & Steinmiller, 2014; Lile et al., 2016). In one of those studies, probabilistic alternative reinforcers produced similar decreases in cocaine self-administration to that of a higher value certain alternative reinforcer (Greenwald et al., 2014). Increasing the response requirements to earn cocaine doses also reduced cocaine self-administration (Foltin et al., 2015) whereas increasing the response requirements to earn alternative reinforcers, relative to the response requirements to earn cocaine, increased cocaine self-administration (Stoops, Lile, Glaser, Hays, & Rush, 2012a). In contrast to many of the studies of pharmacological manipulation, these studies demonstrate that behavioral manipulations reliably change cocaine self-administration, which mirrors the reliable effectiveness of contingency management/abstinence reinforcement procedures to reduce cocaine taking in clinical trials for cocaine use disorder (Schierenberg, van Amsterdam, van den Brink, & Goudriaan, 2012). These consistent findings are even more remarkable considering that these effects have been observed across a range of routes of administration (i.e., intranasal, smoked, and intravenous).

2.3 Cognitive/behavioral effects

Earlier research with cocaine indicated that it can enhance performance on cognitive tasks, but it appears that this effect is not particularly pronounced or consistent (e.g., it increased correct responses on a Rapid Visual Information Processing task, but not on a Digit Symbol Substitution Task in rested subjects; Johnson et al., 1998). Compared to the number of studies that have evaluated the subjective and reinforcing effects of cocaine, relatively few recent studies have evaluated the influence of controlled cocaine administration on cognitive or behavioral performance outcomes. Johnson and colleagues evaluated how administration of 0, 125 and 250 mg/70 kg oral cocaine impacted hypothetical sexual risk delay discounting, as well as monetary delay and probability discounting in individuals with cocaine use disorder. Cocaine dose-dependently decreased the likelihood participants would endorse condom usage when condom availability was delayed or when it was uncertain whether the hypothetical partner had a sexually transmitted infection (Johnson et al., 2017). Cocaine did not change monetary delay or probability discounting.

A series of other publications evaluated how 300 mg oral cocaine influenced a range of cognitive/behavioral performance outcomes in individuals who reported regular cocaine use, but who did not necessarily meet criteria for cocaine use disorder (Hutten et al., 2018; Ramaekers, van Wel, Spronk, Franke, et al., 2016; Ramaekers, van Wel, Spronk,

Toennes, et al., 2016; van Wel et al., 2013). Those studies indicated that although acute cocaine administration can enhance performance on psychomotor function, attention, and prospective memory tasks, it also increased errors and impaired impulse control. One of those studies showed that the impulsivity enhancing effects of cocaine may be tied to low activity dopamine-beta-hydroxylase genotypes (Ramaekers, van Wel, Spronk, Franke, et al., 2016). The performance enhancing effects of cocaine may also be tied to severity of use because other research did not show that intranasal or oral cocaine changed psychomotor performance in individuals with cocaine use disorder (Lile et al., 2011; Stoops et al., 2012b).

2.4 Discriminative stimulus effects

Very little work has been conducted since 2011 that has evaluated the discriminative stimulus effects of cocaine. A number of earlier studies established cocaine's ability to function as a discriminative stimulus across routes of administration (Johanson, Lundahl, Lockhart, & Schubiner, 2006; Oliveto, Rosen, Woods, & Kosten, 1995), although the discriminative stimulus effects of intranasal cocaine appear to be peripherally mediated (Schuh, Schubiner, & Johanson, 2000). Lile and colleagues evaluated the influence of oral aripiprazole pretreatment (15 mg) on the discriminative stimulus effects of oral cocaine (0, 25, 50, 100 and 200 mg; Lile et al., 2011). Cocaine alone dose-dependently increased drug appropriate responding, which was attenuated by aripiprazole administration and matched the subjective effects outcomes described above. The decline in the use of drug discrimination measures in recent years may be tied to questions about its clinical relevance (McMahon, 2015), although it is clear that this method provides a robust measure of the neuropharmacological effects of centrally acting drugs (Kelly, Stoops, Perry, Prendergast, & Rush, 2003).

3. Human behavioral pharmacology of amphetamine

3.1 Subjective effects

Like cocaine, the majority of controlled human laboratory studies investigating subjective responses to amphetamine were conducted prior to 2011 and will be summarized briefly. Of note, we use the term "amphetamine" throughout this section to refer specifically to d-amphetamine. In many of these studies, amphetamine was administered orally, which mirrors how amphetamine and other prescription stimulants are used medically and illicitly

(Teter, McCabe, LaGrange, Cranford, & Boyd, 2006). Amphetamine produces similar subjective effects to cocaine, including euphoria, arousal, increased alertness and energy, and reduced drowsiness (Chou, Talledo, Lamb, Thompson, & Swerdlow, 2013; Fischman & Foltin, 1991; Heal, Smith, Gosden, & Nutt, 2013). It also has generally positive impacts on mood (de Wit, Ulhenhuth, & Johanson, 1986; Rasmussen, 2015). These prototypic positive drug effects are thought to play an important role in the abuse potential of amphetamine (de Wit & Phillips, 2012). As such, there has been significant effort dedicated to determining who may be at risk for experiencing heightened subjective responses to amphetamine (more so than for cocaine), as well as identifying potential pharmacological and behavioral manipulations for reducing sensitivity to the drug's subjective effects.

3.1.1 Predictors of individual differences in the subjective effects of amphetamine

Individuals differ markedly in their subjective responses to amphetamine, both in terms of the quality of the response (i.e., positive or negative) and the magnitude of the response. Given that individuals who are more sensitive to positive subjective drug effects are more likely to develop a substance use disorder (de Wit & Phillips, 2012), researchers have begun to examine individual difference factors that may predict increased sensitivity to amphetamine's subjective effects. Amphetamine studies are particularly well-suited to provide this information because they typically involve stimulant-naïve individuals, allowing for investigation of initial subjective responses (prior to the development of any tolerance or sensitization). These studies typically test the degree to which known risk factors for amphetamine use (e.g., high impulsivity, reward sensitivity) are associated with heightened subjective responses to the drug, with the hypothesis that this increased risk for amphetamine use may be due in part to enhanced sensitivity to subjective effects. Below we review the findings of this literature over the past 10 years.

A number of studies have reported associations between behavioral and self-report measures of impulsivity and subjective responses to amphetamine. For example, individuals high in self-reported trait impulsivity report greater subjective euphoria and arousal following amphetamine (Kirkpatrick, Johanson, & de Wit, 2013). Similarly, individuals high in sensation seeking report greater sensitivity to the subjective effects of amphetamine, including ratings of good effect and any effect (Harvanko, Martin, Lile, Kryscio, & Kelly, 2016). Miller and colleagues reported a positive association between sensation seeking and drug liking, but the association was observed in men only (Miller, Badger, Heil, Higgins, & Sigmon, 2015). Individual differences in behavioral measures of impulsivity and attention are also predictive of subjective responses to amphetamine. Specifically, individuals with poor inhibitory control (assessed as an impaired ability to inhibit motor responses), report greater euphoria and stimulation from amphetamine (Weafer & de Wit, 2013; Weafer, Gorka, et al., 2017). By contrast, inattention (assessed as deviation in reaction time on a simple reaction time task), is *negatively* associated with ratings of drug liking and feel drug following amphetamine (Lake & Meck, 2013; Weafer & de Wit, 2013).

Behavioral and self-report measures of reward sensitivity have also been linked to subjective effects of amphetamine. For instance, individuals who choose to consume caffeine over placebo (an index of sensitivity to caffeine reward) report more positive subjective effects of amphetamine (e.g., ratings of drug liking and well-being) (Sigmon & Griffiths, 2011). Similarly, preference for a sweet taste reward (i.e., liking highly sweet concentrations), is associated with greater euphoria from amphetamine, specifically in women (Weafer, Lyon, Hedeker, & de Wit, 2017). Greater sensitivity to the rewarding effects of physical activity is also associated with positive mood and arousal following amphetamine (Pester, Kirkpatrick, Geary, & Leventhal, 2018). Additionally, questionnaire measures of trait reward sensitivity are related to subjective effects of amphetamine. For example, higher scores on the achievement and social potency subscales of the Multidimensional Personality Questionnaire-BF positively predict euphoria following amphetamine, whereas higher scores on the physical fearlessness scale predict arousal (Kirkpatrick et al., 2013). Finally, greater trait anticipatory pleasure (i.e., a heightened tendency for excitement and motivation to engage in pleasurable experiences) is associated with greater positive mood from amphetamine (Kirkpatrick et al., 2016).

Trait measures of emotional functioning have also been examined in relation to subjective responses to amphetamine. Specifically, greater anxious distress, as measured by the Mood and Anxiety Symptom Questionnaire is associated with greater increase in positive mood following amphetamine (Kirkpatrick et al., 2016). By contrast, hypomania, as assessed by the Mood Disorder Questionnaire, is associated with *dampened* stimulation and euphoria following amphetamine (Schepers, Arndt, Rogers, Hedeker, & de Wit, 2019).

Taken together, subjective responses to amphetamine are generally positive and can be predicted by multiple factors, including impulsivity, inattention, reward sensitivity, and emotional functioning. Increased impulsivity, sensation seeking, and reward sensitivity are all associated with increased ratings of positive subjective effects of amphetamine (Harvanko et al., 2016; Kirkpatrick et al., 2016, 2013; Miller et al., 2015; Pester et al., 2018; Sigmon & Griffiths, 2011; Weafer & de Wit, 2013; Weafer, Gorka, et al., 2017). As such, the increased risk for amphetamine use associated with these risk factors could be due in part to an enhanced sensitivity to the positive effects of amphetamine. By contrast, inattention and hypomania are associated with dampened subjective responses to amphetamine and may serve as protective factors against amphetamine use.

3.1.2 Pharmacological manipulations of the subjective effects of amphetamine

Two recent human laboratory studies investigated the degree to which pharmacological manipulations served to reduce subjective responses to amphetamine. In one study (published just prior to our 2011 cutoff date), Reed, Levin, and Evans (2010) tested the effects of 200mg progesterone pretreatment compared to placebo on amphetamine responses in healthy, naturally-cycling women in the follicular phase of the menstrual cycle. Contrary to hypothesis, progesterone *increased* positive subjective effects (i.e., positive mood, arousal, vigor, elation, and friendliness) produced by 10 and 20mg amphetamine. In a second study, Marks and colleagues examined the effects of 50mg naltrexone, a mu opioid receptor antagonist, and 0.5mg alprazolam, a positive modulator of GABA type A receptors, alone and in combination on amphetamine responses in nontreatment-seeking stimulant-using adults (Marks, Lile, Stoops, & Rush, 2014). Both naltrexone and alprazolam alone decreased some subjective responses to 15 and 30mg amphetamine (i.e., any effect and rush for naltrexone; energy, good effect, and rush for alprazolam). Additionally, the combination of naltrexone and alprazolam reduced a larger number of subjective responses to amphetamine than either drug on its own, particularly subjective high, which neither drug alone impacted. Taken together, these findings suggest that the subjective effects of amphetamine can be pharmacologically manipulated, with progesterone enhancing positive effects and naltrexone and alprazolam dampening positive effects.

3.2 Reinforcing effects

Like cocaine, amphetamine is a powerful reinforcer. A number of human laboratory studies conducted prior to 2011 have shown that individuals reliably self-administer amphetamine over placebo. This is true both for drug choice procedures, in which participants are given a choice between amphetamine or placebo (de Wit et al., 1986; Johanson & Uhlenhuth, 1980; Stoops, 2008) and for progressive-ratio procedures, where subjects work for amphetamine and/or placebo (Rush, Essman, Simpson, & Baker, 2001; Stoops, Glaser, Fillmore, & Rush, 2004). Given the well-established reinforcing effects of amphetamine, recent studies have focused on identifying individual difference factors that predict sensitivity to these effects, as well as potential manipulations that could serve to reduce the drug's reinforcing effects.

3.2.1 Predictors of individual differences in the reinforcing effects of amphetamine

Initial studies have investigated sensation seeking as a predictor of sensitivity to amphetamine reinforcement. Harvanko et al. (2016) found an association between sensation seeking and amphetamine self-administration in healthy young adults. Specifically, high sensation seekers earned significantly more 1 and 2 mg amphetamine capsules in a modified progressive-ratio task than did low sensation seekers. Similarly, Miller et al. (2015) observed an association between greater sensation seeking and increased choice for 5, 10, and 20 mg amphetamine over placebo. However, in this study the relationship was observed in men only.

3.2.2 Associations between the subjective and reinforcing effects of amphetamine

There is initial evidence to suggest a positive association between the subjective and reinforcing effects of amphetamine. For instance, amphetamine self-administration on a progressive-ratio task is positively associated with multiple subjective effects (Bolin, Reynolds, Stoops, & Rush, 2013). That is, individuals who reported higher ratings of positive subjective effects (i.e., drug liking, high, willingness to pay for drug, and willingness to take the drug again) during a sampling session self-administered larger total doses of amphetamine in a separate session. Similar associations have also been reported between amphetamine choice and positive subjective ratings (Murray, Li, Weafer, & de Wit, 2021). In this study, subjects were classified as amphetamine choosers or nonchoosers based on their choice of amphetamine or placebo after four sampling sessions of 20 mg amphetamine. Amphetamine choosers reported higher ratings of positive subjective effects (i.e., positive mood, elation, drug liking, and willingness to pay for drug) during the sampling sessions compared to amphetamine nonchoosers. Taken together, individuals who report greater positive subjective effects from amphetamine are more likely to self-administer larger amounts of amphetamine over placebo in a laboratory setting.

3.2.3 Behavioral manipulations of the reinforcing effects of amphetamine

Since 2011, only one study has investigated the degree to which a behavioral manipulation can alter the reinforcing effects of amphetamine. In this study, male subjects sampled doses of amphetamine (12 and 50 mg) and received a single, alternate monetary reinforcer (either $5 or $20; Kirkpatrick et al., 2012). Following each sample day, the subjects underwent a choice session in which they could work for some or all of either the drug or money that they received in the previous session. When compared to alternate monetary reinforcers, increasing amphetamine doses were chosen more than the small monetary reward ($5). However, amphetamine self-administration diminished with larger monetary rewards ($20), suggesting that the reinforcing effects of amphetamine are malleable in the presence of other reinforcers.

3.3 Cognitive/behavioral effects

Amphetamine has historically been used as a cognitive enhancer in order to increase performance and productivity. Earlier studies on the cognitive effects of amphetamine found that it enhances psychomotor functioning, perceptual speed, attention (Silber, Croft, Papafotiou, & Stough, 2006), and vigilance (Koelega, 1993). However, some reviews suggest that amphetamine improves performance on simple tasks only (Advokat, 2010) or that it enhances motor output rather than cognition (Solanto, 1998). Amphetamine has generally inconsistent results on memory, although there is evidence that it may improve some aspects (i.e., consolidation and retention; Advokat, 2010).

Recent studies provide some support for the cognitive and behavioral performance-enhancing properties of amphetamine in healthy adults. Relative to placebo, amphetamine improves response inhibition and attention (Weafer & de Wit, 2013; Weyandt et al., 2018), and increases psychomotor task speed and willingness to exert effort for reward (Wardle,

Treadway, Mayo, Zald, & de Wit, 2011). Amphetamine also reduces behavioral reactivity to errors, as inferred by less posterror slowing compared to placebo (Wardle, Yang, & de Wit, 2012). Chou et al. (2013) found that amphetamine increases neurocognitive functioning as measured by composite scores on the MATRICS Consensus Cognitive Battery. However, this enhanced performance was only observed in those with poor baseline performance, raising the possibility of regression to the mean. In contrast to studies showing positive effects of amphetamine on performance, Ilieva, Boland, and Farah (2013) found that amphetamine has no impact on 13 dimensions of cognitive functioning (e.g., memory, inhibitory control, creativity, and intelligence), despite subjects' perceived increased performance following the drug.

One specific aspect of cognitive functioning for which amphetamine effects have been studied in more detail is memory. Amphetamine increased memory of studied word lists compared to placebo in the Deese/Roediger-McDermott paradigm (Ballard, Gallo, & de Wit, 2012). Additionally, amphetamine administered prior to encoding enhanced memory for emotional pictures (Ballard, Gallo, & de Wit, 2013). However, when encoding occurred in a drug-free state and amphetamine was given just before retrieval, amphetamine impaired memory for emotional images (Ballard, Gallo, & de Wit, 2014). Amphetamine may also impair working memory, as Weyandt et al. (2018) found that amphetamine significantly reduced digit recall on the Digit Span Forward test (Weschler, 2008). Another study found no effect of amphetamine on memory encoding or retrieval of positive, negative, or neutral emotional images (Weafer, Gallo, & de Wit, 2014). Overall, findings have been inconsistent regarding amphetamine effects on memory in healthy adults.

Finally, several studies have assessed the effects of amphetamine on emotional reactivity. In one study, amphetamine increased reactions to negative but not positive emotional stimuli and lowered the threshold needed to identify emotions compared to placebo on the Dynamic Emotional Identification Task (Wardle et al., 2012). In a second study by this group, amphetamine increased positive self-reported responses and facial muscle reactivity to emotional stimuli (Wardle & de Wit, 2012). Similarly, Dolder and colleagues found that amphetamine increased empathy for positive stimuli, as measured by the Multifaceted Empathy Test, compared to placebo (Dolder, Strajhar, Vizeli, Odermatt, & Liechti, 2018).

Taken together, amphetamine exerts clear effects on cognitive, behavioral, and emotional performance; however, the direction of these effects is inconsistent across studies. Multiple studies have shown that amphetamine improves aspects of cognitive functioning, including psychomotor task speed, willingness to exert effort, attention, inhibitory control, and reactivity to errors (Wardle et al., 2011, 2012; Weafer & de Wit, 2013; Weyandt et al., 2018). However, others have found that these improvements occur only in those with lower baseline cognitive performance (Chou et al., 2013) or that amphetamine has no impact on cognitive functioning (Ilieva et al., 2013). There are similar inconsistencies for amphetamine's impact on memory, with some evidence that amphetamine improves memory (Ballard et al., 2012, 2013) and some evidence that amphetamine impairs or has no impact on memory (Ballard et al., 2014; Ilieva et al., 2013; Weafer et al., 2014; Weyandt et al., 2018). Finally, recent research suggests that amphetamine impacts emotional reactivity by making emotions easier to identify and increasing reactivity to positive and negative stimuli (Dolder et al., 2018; Wardle et al., 2012).

4. Conclusion

Recent findings from human laboratory studies have provided considerable advances in our knowledge and understanding of the behavioral pharmacology of prototypic stimulant drugs (i.e., cocaine and d-amphetamine). Early studies established the robust reinforcing and positive subjective effects of these drugs, along with their ability to improve some aspects of cognitive and behavioral function. In the last 10 years, these findings have been extended to identify: (1) individual difference factors that predict responses to stimulant drugs; (2) successful pharmacological and behavioral manipulations of stimulant drug effects; and (3) additional effects of stimulants on cognitive, behavioral, and emotional performance. Specifically, the studies reviewed here suggest that individual difference factors related to impulsivity, reward seeking, and emotional functioning predict subjective and reinforcing effects of stimulants. Additionally, initial evidence suggests that pretreatment with potent indirect-acting monoamine agonist and serotonergic drugs can successfully reduce stimulant self-administration. Finally, recent findings suggest that these drugs have complicated effects on various aspects of cognitive and behavioral functioning, including memory, impulsivity, and emotional processing.

One of the most consistent findings across studies of both cocaine and amphetamine is that their reinforcing effects can be manipulated behaviorally and pharmacologically. Specifically, behavioral manipulations (typically involving the availability of mutually exclusive monetary reinforcement) reliably reduce the reinforcing properties of both cocaine and amphetamine. Although evidence for pharmacological manipulation is mixed, there is some data to suggest that serotonergic drugs, indirect-acting monoamine agonists, and opioid antagonists can reduce the positive subjective and reinforcing effects of stimulant drugs. Given that these manipulations successfully reduce reports of positive subjective effects and actual drug self-administration in the lab, it is possible that they may also reduce excessive or problematic stimulant use outside of the lab. As such, these findings have important implications regarding treatment of stimulant use disorders in humans, and they encourage future studies that translate these human behavioral pharmacology lab findings to large-scale clinical trials. Medications that are likely to be affective are those that reduce drug taking, typically under choice procedures, in nonhuman animals and humans (Czoty, Stoops, & Rush, 2016); such medications also need to be shown to be safe and tolerable when combined with the target drug of abuse before advancement to clinical trials.

An important distinction between the cocaine and amphetamine studies reviewed here involves the samples typically recruited to assess the effects of each drug. Studies involving cocaine administration tend to recruit people actively engaged in cocaine use, including both recreational users and individuals with cocaine use disorder. By contrast, studies involving amphetamine administration tend to recruit healthy volunteers, with or without any stimulant drug experience. As such, findings from cocaine and amphetamine studies may provide information regarding different phases of stimulant drug addiction. That is, d-amphetamine studies are highly useful in providing information on risk factors for stimulant use (i.e., identifying those individuals who, based on initial drug responses, might be most at risk for using and abusing stimulant drugs). Thus, these studies may be most useful for informing prevention efforts. On the other hand, cocaine studies are useful in providing information on potential manipulations to reduce drug use among individuals with a history of moderate to heavy use. As a result, these studies may be most useful for informing treatment efforts.

Despite important advances in this literature over the past 10 years, clear gaps remain. First, there has been little recent work investigating sex differences in the behavioral pharmacology of stimulant drugs. Past research has shown that women tend to be more sensitive to the subjective and reinforcing effects of stimulant drugs than men, and that ovarian hormones influence responses to stimulants in women (Fattore, Altea, & Fratta, 2008).

However, of the studies reviewed here, only two reported on sex differences (Miller et al., 2015; Weafer, Lyon, et al., 2017), and only two assessed the influence of sex hormones (both from the same research group; Reed et al., 2011, 2010). As such, it will be important for future, sufficiently-powered studies to examine sex differences in individual difference factors that predict drug responses, as well as in the efficacy of pharmacological and behavioral manipulations in reducing drug effects. Second, as mentioned above, little is known regarding cocaine effects in naive users or amphetamine effects in experienced users. As such, it will be important for future studies to assess risk factors for cocaine in healthy volunteers and potential manipulations of amphetamine response in regular users. Finally, data regarding the cognitive/behavioral effects of stimulant drugs are still quite mixed, likely due to variable sample characteristics, drug doses, and tasks administered across studies. Future studies are needed to systematically assess these cognitive effects across standardized measures and doses, and within both novice and experienced users.

Conflict of interest

The authors declare no relevant conflicts of interest.

References

Advokat, C. (2010). What are the cognitive effects of stimulant medications? Emphasis on adults with attention-deficit/hyperactivity disorder (ADHD). *Neuroscience & Biobehavioral Reviews*, *34*(8), 1256–1266.

Angarita, G. A., Canavan, S. V., Forselius, E., Bessette, A., & Morgan, P. T. (2014). Correlates of polysomnographic sleep changes in cocaine dependence: Self-administration and clinical outcomes. *Drug and Alcohol Dependence*, *143*, 173–180.

Askalsky, P., Kalapatapu, R. K., Foltin, R. W., & Comer, S. D. (2015). Butyrylcholinesterase levels and subjective effects of smoked cocaine in healthy cocaine users. *The American Journal of Drug and Alcohol Abuse*, *41*(2), 161–165.

Ballard, M. E., Gallo, D. A., & de Wit, H. (2012). Psychoactive drugs and false memory: Comparison of dextroamphetamine and δ-9-tetrahydrocannabinol on false recognition. *Psychopharmacology*, *219*(1), 15–24.

Ballard, M. E., Gallo, D. A., & de Wit, H. (2013). Pre-encoding administration of amphetamine or THC preferentially modulates emotional memory in humans. *Psychopharmacology*, *226*(3), 515–529.

Ballard, M. E., Gallo, D. A., & de Wit, H. (2014). Amphetamine increases errors during episodic memory retrieval. *Journal of Clinical Psychopharmacology*, *34*(1), 85–93.

Bolin, B. L., Alcorn, J. L., 3rd, Lile, J. A., Rush, C. R., Rayapati, A. O., Hays, L. R., et al. (2017). N-acetylcysteine reduces cocaine-cue attentional bias and differentially alters cocaine self-administration based on dosing order. *Drug and Alcohol Dependence*, *178*, 452–460.

Bolin, B. L., Lile, J. A., Marks, K. R., Beckmann, J. S., Rush, C. R., & Stoops, W. W. (2016). Buspirone reduces sexual risk-taking intent but not cocaine self-administration. *Experimental and Clinical Psychopharmacology*, *24*(3), 162–173.

Bolin, B. L., Reynolds, A. R., Stoops, W. W., & Rush, C. R. (2013). Relationship between oral d-amphetamine self-administration and ratings of subjective effects: Do subjective-effects ratings correspond with a progressive-ratio measure of drug-taking behavior? *Behavioural Pharmacology*, *24*(5–6), 533–542.

Cano, M., & Huang, Y. (2021). Overdose deaths involving psychostimulants with abuse potential, excluding cocaine: State-level differences and the role of opioids. *Drug and Alcohol Dependence*, *218*, 108384.

Cano, M., Oh, S., Salas-Wright, C. P., & Vaughn, M. G. (2020). Cocaine use and overdose mortality in the United States: Evidence from two national data sources, 2002-2018. *Drug and Alcohol Dependence*, *214*, 108148.

Chen, K., Scheier, L. M., & Kandel, D. B. (1996). Effects of chronic cocaine use on physical health: A prospective study in a general population sample. *Drug and Alcohol Dependence*, *43*(1–2), 23–37.

Chou, H., Talledo, J. A., Lamb, S. N., Thompson, W. K., & Swerdlow, N. R. (2013). Amphetamine effects on MATRICS consensus cognitive battery performance in healthy adults. *Psychopharmacology*, *227*(1), 165–176.

Cone, E. J. (1995). Pharmacokinetics and pharmacodynamics of cocaine. *Journal of Analytical Toxicology*, *19*(6), 459–478.

Cox, S. M., Benkelfat, C., Dagher, A., Delaney, J. S., Durand, F., Kolivakis, T., et al. (2011). Effects of lowered serotonin transmission on cocaine-induced striatal dopamine response: PET [^{11}C]raclopride study in humans. *The British Journal of Psychiatry: the Journal of Mental Science*, *199*(5), 391–397.

Czoty, P. W., Stoops, W. W., & Rush, C. R. (2016). Evaluation of the "pipeline" for development of medications for cocaine use disorder: A review of translational preclinical, human laboratory and clinical trial research. *Pharmacological Reviews*, *68*, 533–562.

Dakwar, E., Hart, C. L., Levin, F. R., Nunes, E. V., & Foltin, R. W. (2017). Cocaine self-administration disrupted by the N-methyl-D-aspartate receptor antagonist ketamine: A randomized, crossover trial. *Molecular Psychiatry*, *22*(1), 76–81.

Dakwar, E., Nunes, E. V., Hart, C. L., Foltin, R. W., Mathew, S. J., Carpenter, K. M., et al. (2019). A single ketamine infusion combined with mindfulness-based behavioral modification to treat cocaine dependence: A randomized clinical trial. *The American Journal of Psychiatry*, *176*(11), 923–930.

De La Garza, R., 2nd, Verrico, C. D., Newton, T. F., Mahoney, J. J., 3rd, & Thompson-Lake, D. G. (2015). Safety and preliminary efficacy of the acetylcholinesterase inhibitor Huperzine a as a treatment for cocaine use disorder. *The International Journal of Neuropsychopharmacology*, *19*(3), pyv098.

de Wit, H., & Phillips, T. J. (2012). Do initial responses to drugs predict future use or abuse? *Neuroscience and Biobehavioral Reviews*, *36*(6), 1565–1576.

de Wit, H., Ulhenhuth, E. H., & Johanson, C. E. (1986). Individual differences in the reinforcing and subjective effects of amphetamine and diazepam. *Drug and Alcohol Dependence*, *16*(4), 341–360.

Dolder, P. C., Strajhar, P., Vizeli, P., Odermatt, A., & Liechti, M. E. (2018). Acute effects of lisdexamfetamine and d-amphetamine on social cognition and cognitive performance in a placebo-controlled study in healthy subjects. *Psychopharmacology*, *235*(5), 1389–1402.

Fattore, L., Altea, S., & Fratta, W. (2008). Sex differences in drug addiction: A review of animal and human studies. *Women's Health (London, England)*, *4*, 51–65.

Fischman, M. W., & Foltin, R. W. (1991). Utility of subjective effects measurements in assessing abuse liability of drugs in humans. *British Journal of Addiction*, *86*(12), 1563–1570.

Fleckenstein, A. E., Gibb, J. W., & Hanson, G. R. (2000). Differential effects of stimulants on monoaminergic transporters: Pharmacological consequences and implications for neurotoxicity. *European Journal of Pharmacology*, *406*(1), 1–13.

Foltin, R. W., & Fischman, M. W. (1991). Smoked and intravenous cocaine in humans: Acute tolerance cardiovascular and subjective effects. *The Journal of Pharmacology and Experimental Therapeutics*, *257*(1), 247–261.

Foltin, R. W., & Fischman, M. W. (1992). Self-administration of cocaine by humans: Choice between smoked and intravenous cocaine. *The Journal of Pharmacology and Experimental Therapeutics*, *261*(3), 841–849.

Foltin, R. W., & Haney, M. (2004). Intranasal cocaine in humans: Acute tolerance, cardiovascular and subjective effects. *Pharmacology, Biochemistry, and Behavior*, *78*(1), 93–101.

Foltin, R. W., Haney, M., Bedi, G., & Evans, S. M. (2016). Modafinil decreases cocaine choice in human cocaine smokers only when the response requirement and the alternative reinforcer magnitude are large. *Pharmacology, Biochemistry, and Behavior*, *150-151*, 8–13.

Foltin, R. W., Haney, M., Rubin, E., Reed, S. C., Vadhan, N., Balter, R., et al. (2015). Development of translational preclinical models in substance abuse: Effects of cocaine administration on cocaine choice in humans and non-human primates. *Pharmacology, Biochemistry, and Behavior*, *134*, 12–21.

Grabowski, J., Rhoades, H., Stotts, A., Cowan, K., Kopecky, C., Dougherty, A., et al. (2004). Agonist-like or antagonist-like treatment for cocaine dependence with methadone for heroin dependence: Two double-blind randomized clinical trials. *Neuropsychopharmacology*, *29*(5), 969–981.

Grasing, K., Mathur, D., Newton, T. F., & Desouza, C. (2013). Individual predictors of the subjective effects of intravenous cocaine. *Psychiatry Research*, *208*(3), 245–251.

Greenwald, M. K., Ledgerwood, D. M., Lundahl, L. H., & Steinmiller, C. L. (2014). Effect of experimental analogs of contingency management treatment on cocaine seeking behavior. *Drug and Alcohol Dependence*, *139*, 164–168.

Hando, J., Howard, J., & Zibert, E. (1997). Risky drug practices and treatment needs of youth detained in New South Wales juvenile justice Centres. *Drug and Alcohol Review*, *16*(2), 137–145.

Hando, J., Topp, L., & Hall, W. (1997). Amphetamine-related harms and treatment preferences of regular amphetamine users in Sydney, Australia. *Drug and Alcohol Dependence*, *46*(1–2), 105–113.

Haney, M., Rubin, E., & Foltin, R. W. (2011). Aripiprazole maintenance increases smoked cocaine self-administration in humans. *Psychopharmacology*, *216*(3), 379–387.

Harvanko, A., Martin, C., Lile, J., Kryscio, R., & Kelly, T. H. (2016). Individual differences in the reinforcing and subjective effects of d-amphetamine: Dimensions of impulsivity. *Experimental and Clinical Psychopharmacology*, *24*(6), 436–446.

Heal, D. J., Smith, S. L., Gosden, J., & Nutt, D. J. (2013). Amphetamine, past and present – A pharmacological and clinical perspective. *Journal of Psychopharmacology*, *27*(6), 479–496.

Hutten, N. R., Kuypers, K. P., van Wel, J. H., Theunissen, E. L., Toennes, S. W., Verkes, R. J., et al. (2018). A single dose of cocaine enhances prospective memory performance. *Journal of Psychopharmacology*, *32*(8), 883–892.

Ilieva, I., Boland, J., & Farah, M. J. (2013). Objective and subjective cognitive enhancing effects of mixed amphetamine salts in healthy people. *Neuropharmacology*, *64*, 496–505.

Iversen, L. (2006). Neurotransmitter transporters and their impact on the development of psychopharmacology. *British Journal of Pharmacology*, *147*(Suppl 1), S82–S88.

Johanson, C.-E., & Fischman, M. W. (1989). The pharmacology of cocaine related to its abuse. *Pharmacological Reviews*, *41*(1), 3–52.

Johanson, C. E., Lundahl, L. H., Lockhart, N., & Schubiner, H. (2006). Intravenous cocaine discrimination in humans. *Experimental and Clinical Psychopharmacology*, *14*(2), 99–108.

Johanson, C. E., & Uhlenhuth, E. H. (1980). Drug preference and mood in humans: Repeated assessment of d-amphetamine. *Pharmacology, Biochemistry & Behavior*, *14*, 159–163.

Johnson, M. W., Herrmann, E. S., Sweeney, M. M., LeComte, R. S., & Johnson, P. S. (2017). Cocaine administration dose-dependently increases sexual desire and decreases condom use likelihood: The role of delay and probability discounting in connecting cocaine with HIV. *Psychopharmacology, 234*(4), 599–612.
Johnson, B., Overton, D., Wells, L., Kenny, P., Abramson, D., Dhother, S., et al. (1998). Effects of acute intravenous cocaine on cardiovascular function, human learning, and performance in cocaine addicts. *Psychiatry Research*, 77(1), 35–42.
Kalapatapu, R. K., Bedi, G., Haney, M., Evans, S. M., Rubin, E., & Foltin, R. W. (2012). The subjective effects of cocaine: Relationship to years of cocaine use and current age. *The American Journal of Drug and Alcohol Abuse, 38*(6), 530–534.
Kariisa, M., Scholl, L., Wilson, N., Seth, P., & Hoots, B. (2019). Drug overdose deaths involving cocaine and psychostimulants with Abuse potential - United States, 2003-2017. *Morbidity and Mortality Weekly Report, 68*(17), 388–395.
Kelly, T. H., Stoops, W. W., Perry, A. S., Prendergast, M. A., & Rush, C. R. (2003). Clinical neuropharmacology of drugs of abuse: A comparison of drug-discrimination and subject-report measures. *Behavioral and Cognitive Neuroscience Reviews, 2*(4), 227–260.
Kirkpatrick, M. G., Goldenson, N. I., Kapadia, N., Kahler, C. W., de Wit, H., Swift, R. M., et al. (2016). Emotional traits predict individual differences in amphetamine-induced positive mood in healthy volunteers. *Psychopharmacology, 233*(1), 89–97.
Kirkpatrick, M. G., Gunderson, E. W., Johanson, C., Levin, F. R., Foltin, R. W., & Hart, L. (2012). Comparison of intranasal methamphetamine and d-amphetamine self-administration by humans. *Addiction, 107*(4), 783–791.
Kirkpatrick, M. G., Johanson, C., & de Wit, H. (2013). Personality and the acute subjective effects of d-amphetamine in humans. *Journal of Psychopharmacology, 27*(3), 256–264.
Koelega, H. S. (1993). Stimulant drugs and vigilance performance: A review. *Psychopharmacology, 111*, 1–16.
Lake, J. I., & Meck, W. H. (2013). Differential effects of amphetamine and haloperidol on temporal reduction: Dopaminergic regulation of attention and clock speed. *Neuropsychologia, 51*(2), 284–292.
Lile, J. A., Johnson, A. R., Banks, M. L., Hatton, K. W., Hays, L. R., Nicholson, K. L., et al. (2020). Pharmacological validation of a translational model of cocaine use disorder: Effects of d-amphetamine maintenance on choice between intravenous cocaine and a nondrug alternative in humans and rhesus monkeys. *Experimental and Clinical Psychopharmacology, 28*(2), 169–180.
Lile, J. A., Stoops, W. W., Glaser, P. E., Hays, L. R., & Rush, C. R. (2011). Discriminative stimulus, subject-rated and cardiovascular effects of cocaine alone and in combination with aripiprazole in humans. *Journal of Psychopharmacology, 25*(11), 1469–1479.
Lile, J. A., Stoops, W. W., Rush, C. R., Negus, S. S., Glaser, P. E., Hatton, K. W., et al. (2016). Development of a translational model to screen medications for cocaine use disorder II: Choice between intravenous cocaine and money in humans. *Drug and Alcohol Dependence, 165*, 111–119.
Liu, D., Jiang, Z., Xiu, C., Li, Z., Song, Q., & Wang, Z. (2017). Sexually transmitted infection prevalence and related risk factors among heterosexual male methamphetamine users in China. *International Journal of STD & AIDS, 28*(12), 1208–1214.
Lofwall, M. R., Nuzzo, P. A., Campbell, C., & Walsh, S. L. (2014). Aripiprazole effects on self-administration and pharmacodynamics of intravenous cocaine and cigarette smoking in humans. *Experimental and Clinical Psychopharmacology, 22*(3), 238–247.
Marks, K. R., Lile, J. A., Stoops, W. W., & Rush, C. R. (2014). Separate and combined impact of acute naltrexone and alprazolam on subjective and physiological effects of oral d-amphetamine in stimulant users. *Psychopharmacology, 231*(14), 2741–2750.
Matuskey, D., Pittman, B., Chen, J. I., Wanyiri, J., Nadim, H., Jatlow, P., et al. (2012). A single-day paradigm of self-regulated human cocaine administration. *Pharmacology, Biochemistry, and Behavior, 103*(1), 95–101.

McMahon, L. R. (2015). The rise (and fall?) of drug discrimination research. *Drug and Alcohol Dependence*, *151*, 284–288.

Miller, M. E., Badger, G. J., Heil, S. H., Higgins, S. T., & Sigmon, S. C. (2015). Associations between sensation seeking and d-amphetamine reinforcement. *The American Journal of Addictions*, *24*(5), 435–442.

Murray, C. H., Li, J., Weafer, J., & de Wit, H. (2021). Subjective responses predict d-amphetamine choice in healthy volunteers. *Pharmacology, Biochemistry and Behavior*, *204*, 173158.

Oliveto, A. H., Rosen, M. I., Woods, S. W., & Kosten, T. R. (1995). Discriminative stimulus, self-reported and cardiovascular effects of orally administered cocaine in humans. *The Journal of Pharmacology and Experimental Therapeutics*, *272*(1), 231–241.

Patel, M., Verrico, C. D., & De La Garza, R., 2nd. (2019). Rivastigmine does not alter cocaine-induced subjective effects or self-administration. *Pharmacology, Biochemistry, and Behavior*, *185*, 172758.

Pester, M. S., Kirkpatrick, M. G., Geary, B. A., & Leventhal, A. M. (2018). Rewarding effects of physical activity predict sensitivity to the acute subjective effects of d-amphetamine in healthy volunteers. *Journal of Psychopharmacology*, *32*(3), 302–308.

Pirtle, J. L., Hickman, M. D., Boinpelly, V. C., Surineni, K., Thakur, H. K., & Grasing, K. W. (2019). The serotonin-2C agonist lorcaserin delays intravenous choice and modifies the subjective and cardiovascular effects of cocaine: A randomized, controlled human laboratory study. *Pharmacology, Biochemistry, and Behavior*, *180*, 52–59.

Poling, J., Oliveto, A., Petry, N., Sofuoglu, M., Gonsai, K., Gonzalez, G., et al. (2006). Six-month trial of bupropion with contingency management for cocaine dependence in a methadone-maintained population. *Archives of General Psychiatry*, *63*(2), 219–228.

Ramaekers, J. G., van Wel, J. H., Spronk, D., Franke, B., Kenis, G., Toennes, S. W., et al. (2016). Cannabis and cocaine decrease cognitive impulse control and functional corticostriatal connectivity in drug users with low activity DBH genotypes. *Brain Imaging and Behavior*, *10*(4), 1254–1263.

Ramaekers, J. G., van Wel, J. H., Spronk, D. B., Toennes, S. W., Kuypers, K. P., Theunissen, E. L., et al. (2016). Cannabis and tolerance: Acute drug impairment as a function of cannabis use history. *Scientific Reports*, *6*, 26843.

Rasmussen, N. (2015). Amphetamine-type stimulants: The early history of their medical and non-medical uses. *International Review of Neurobiology*, *120*, 9–25.

Reed, S. C., Evans, S. M., Bedi, G., Rubin, E., & Foltin, R. W. (2011). The effects of oral micronized progesterone on smoked cocaine self-administration in women. *Hormones and Behavior*, *59*(2), 227–235.

Reed, S. C., Levin, F. R., & Evans, S. M. (2010). The effects of progesterone pretreatment on the response to oral d-amphetamine in women. *Hormones and Behavior*, *58*(3), 533–543.

Reith, M., & Gnegy, M. E. (2020). Molecular mechanisms of amphetamines. *Handbook of Experimental Pharmacology*, *258*, 265–297.

Richards, J. R., Bretz, S. W., Johnson, E. B., Turnipseed, S. D., Brofeldt, B. T., & Derlet, R. W. (1999). Methamphetamine abuse and emergency department utilization. *The Western Journal of Medicine*, *170*(4), 198–202.

Romach, M. K., Schoedel, K. A., & Sellers, E. M. (2014). Human abuse liability evaluation of CNS stimulant drugs. *Neuropharmacology*, *87*, 81–90.

Rothman, R. B., Baumann, M. H., Dersch, C. M., Romero, D. V., Rice, K. C., Carroll, F. I., et al. (2001). Amphetamine-type central nervous system stimulants release norepinephrine more potently than they release dopamine and serotonin. *Synapse*, *39*(1), 32–41.

Rothman, R. B., & Glowa, J. R. (1995). A review of the effects of dopaminergic agents on humans, animals, and drug-seeking behavior, and its implications for medication development. Focus on GBR 12909. *Molecular Neurobiology*, *11*(1–3), 1–19.

Rounsaville, B. J., Anton, S. F., Carroll, K., Budde, D., Prusoff, B. A., & Gawin, F. (1991). Psychiatric diagnoses of treatment-seeking cocaine abusers. *Archives of General Psychiatry*, *48*(1), 43–51.

Rush, C. R., Essman, W., Simpson, C. A., & Baker, R. W. (2001). Reinforcing and subject-rated effects of methylphenidate and d-amphetamine in non-drug-abusing humans. *Journal of Clinical Psychopharmacology*, *21*(3), 273–286.

Rush, C. R., Stoops, W. W., & Ling, W. (2009). Behavioral pharmacology and psychiatric consequences of methamphetamine. In J. M. Roll, R. A. Rawson, W. Ling, & S. Shoptaw (Eds.), *Methamphetamine addiction: From basic science to treatment* (pp. 92–116). The Guilford Press.

Schepers, S. T., Arndt, D. L., Rogers, R. D., Hedeker, D., & de Wit, H. (2019). Subjective responses to amphetamine in young adults with previous mood elevation experiences. *Psychopharmacology*, *236*(11), 3363–3370.

Schierenberg, A., van Amsterdam, J., van den Brink, W., & Goudriaan, A. E. (2012). Efficacy of contingency management for cocaine dependence treatment: A review of the evidence. *Current Drug Abuse Reviews*, *5*(4), 320–331.

Schuh, K. J., Schubiner, H., & Johanson, C. E. (2000). Discrimination of intranasal cocaine. *Behavioural Pharmacology*, *11*(6), 511–515.

Schwartz, B. G., Rezkalla, S., & Kloner, R. A. (2010). Cardiovascular effects of cocaine. *Circulation*, *122*(24), 2558–2569.

Shellenberg, T. P., Stoops, W. W., Lile, J. A., & Rush, C. R. (2020). An update on the clinical pharmacology of methylphenidate: Therapeutic efficacy, abuse potential and future considerations. *Expert Review of Clinical Pharmacology*, *13*(8), 825–833.

Shiels, M. S., Freedman, N. D., Thomas, D., & Berrington de Gonzalez, A. (2018). Trends in U.S. drug overdose deaths in non-Hispanic black, Hispanic, and non-Hispanic White persons, 2000-2015. *Annals of Internal Medicine*, *168*(6), 453–455.

Sigmon, S. C., & Griffiths, R. R. (2011). Caffeine choice prospectively predicts positive subjective effects of caffeine and d-amphetamine. *Drug and Alcohol Dependence*, *111*(2–3), 341–348.

Silber, B. Y., Croft, R. J., Papafotiou, K., & Stough, C. (2006). The acute effects of *d*-amphetamine and methamphetamine on attention and psychomotor performance. *Psychopharmacology*, *187*, 154–169.

Simmler, L. D., & Liechti, M. E. (2018). Pharmacology of MDMA- and amphetamine-like new psychoactive substances. *Handbook of Experimental Pharmacology*, *252*, 143–164.

Smith, B. J., Jones, H. E., & Griffiths, R. R. (2001). Physiological, subjective and reinforcing effects of oral and intravenous cocaine in humans. *Psychopharmacology*, *156*(4), 435–444.

Solanto, M. V. (1998). Neuropsychopharmacological mechanisms of stimulant drug action in attention-deficit hyperactivity disorder: A review and integration. *Behavioural Brain Research*, *94*(1), 127–152.

Stoops, W. W. (2008). Reinforcing effects of stimulants in humans: Sensitivity of progressive-ratio schedules. *Experimental and Clinical Psychopharmacology*, *16*(6), 503–512.

Stoops, W. W., Glaser, P. E. A., Fillmore, M. T., & Rush, C. R. (2004). Reinforcing, subject-rated, performance and physiological effects of methylphenidate and d-amphetamine in stimulant abusing humans. *Journal of Psychopharmacology*, *18*(4), 534–543.

Stoops, W. W., Lile, J. A., Glaser, P. E., Hays, L. R., & Rush, C. R. (2010). Intranasal cocaine functions as reinforcer on a progressive ratio schedule in humans. *European Journal of Pharmacology*, *644*(1–3), 101–105.

Stoops, W. W., Lile, J. A., Glaser, P. E., Hays, L. R., & Rush, C. R. (2012a). Alternative reinforcer response cost impacts cocaine choice in humans. *Progress in Neuropsychopharmacology & Biological Psychiatry*, *36*(1), 189–193.

Stoops, W. W., Lile, J. A., Glaser, P. E., Hays, L. R., & Rush, C. R. (2012b). Influence of acute bupropion pre-treatment on the effects of intranasal cocaine. *Addiction*, *107*, 1140–1147.

Stoops, W. W., Lile, J. A., & Rush, C. R. (2010). Monetary alternative reinforcers more effectively decrease intranasal cocaine choice than food alternative reinforcers. *Pharmacology, Biochemistry, and Behavior, 95*(2), 187–191.

Stoops, W. W., Strickland, J. C., Alcorn, J. L., III, Hays, L. R., Rayapati, A. O., Lile, J. A., et al. (2019). Influence of phendimetrazine maintenance on the reinforcing, subjective, performance, and physiological effects of intranasal cocaine. *Psychopharmacology, 236*(9), 2569–2577.

Stoops, W. W., Strickland, J. C., Hays, L. R., Rayapati, A. O., Lile, J. A., & Rush, C. R. (2016). Safety and tolerability of intranasal cocaine during phendimetrazine maintenance. *Psychopharmacology, 233*(11), 2055–2063.

Substance Abuse and Mental Health Services Administration. (2010). *Results from the 2009 National Survey on drug use and health.* Rockville, MD: National FindingsOffice of Applied Studies.

Substance Abuse and Mental Health Services Administration. (2020). *The National Survey on drug use and health: 2019.* Rockville, MD: Office of Applied Studies.

Teter, C. J., McCabe, S. E., LaGrange, K., Cranford, J. A., & Boyd, C. J. (2006). Illicit use of specific prescription stimulants among college students: Prevalence, motives, and routes of administration. *Pharmacotherapy, 26*(10), 1505–1510.

Van Dyke, C., Jatlow, P., Ungerer, J., Barash, P. G., & Byck, R. (1978). Oral cocaine: Plasma concentrations and central effects. *Science, 200*(4338), 211–213.

Van Tieu, H., & Koblin, B. A. (2009). HIV, alcohol, and noninjection drug use. *Current Opinion in HIV and AIDS, 4*(4), 314–318.

van Wel, J. H., Kuypers, K. P., Theunissen, E. L., Toennes, S. W., Spronk, D. B., Verkes, R. J., et al. (2013). Single doses of THC and cocaine decrease proficiency of impulse control in heavy cannabis users. *British Journal of Pharmacology, 170*(7), 1410–1420.

Vearrier, D., Greenberg, M. I., Miller, S. N., Okaneku, J. T., & Haggerty, D. A. (2012). Methamphetamine: History, pathophysiology, adverse health effects, current trends, and hazards associated with the clandestine manufacture of methamphetamine. *Disease-a-month: DM, 58*(2), 38–89.

Verrico, C. D., Haile, C. N., Mahoney, J. J., III, Thompson-Lake, D. G. Y., Newton, T. F., & De La Garza, R., II. (2014). Treatment with modafinil and escitalopram, alone and in combination, on cocaine-induced effects: A randomized, double blind, placebo-controlled human laboratory study. *Drug and Alcohol Dependence, 141*, 72–78.

Walsh, S. L., Donny, E. C., Nuzzo, P. A., Umbricht, A., & Bigelow, G. E. (2010). Cocaine abuse versus cocaine dependence: Cocaine self-administration and pharmacodynamic response in the human laboratory. *Drug and Alcohol Dependence, 106*(1), 28–37.

Wardle, M. C., & de Wit, H. (2012). Effects of amphetamine on reactivity to emotional stimuli. *Psychopharmacology, 220*(1), 143–153.

Wardle, M. C., Treadway, M. T., Mayo, L. M., Zald, D. H., & de Wit, H. (2011). Amping up efforts: Effects of d-amphetamine on human effort-based decision-making. *The Journal of Neuroscience, 31*(46), 16597–16602.

Wardle, M. C., Yang, A., & de Wit, H. (2012). Effect of d-amphetamine on post-error slowing in healthy volunteers. *Psychopharmacology, 220*(1), 109–115.

Weafer, J., & de Wit, H. (2013). Inattention, impulsive action, and subjective response to D-amphetamine. *Drug and Alcohol Dependence, 133*(1), 127–133.

Weafer, J., Gallo, D. A., & de Wit, H. (2014). Amphetamine fails to alter cued recollection of emotional images: Study of encoding, retrieval, and state-dependency. *PLoS One, 9*(2), 90423.

Weafer, J., Gorka, S. M., Hedeker, D., Dzemidzic, M., Kareken, D. V., Phan, K. L., et al. (2017). Associations between behavioral and neural correlates of inhibitory control and amphetamine sensitivity. *Neuropsychopharmacology, 42*(9), 1905–1913.

Weafer, J., Lyon, N., Hedeker, D., & de Wit, H. (2017). Sweet taste liking is associated with subjective response to amphetamine in women but not men. *Psychopharmacology, 234*(21), 3185–3194.

Weschler, D. (2008). *Weschler Adult Intelligence Scale* (4th ed.). Pearson: San Antonio, TX, USA.

Weyandt, L. L., White, T. L., Gugmundsdottir, B. G., Nitenson, A. Z., Rathkey, E. S., De Leon, K. A., et al. (2018). Neurocognitive, autonomic, and mood effects of Adderall: A pilot study of healthy college students. *Pharmacy: Journal of Pharmacy Education and Practice, 6*(5), 58.

CHAPTER FOUR

Human behavioral pharmacology of psychedelics

Justin C. Strickland and Matthew W. Johnson*
Department of Psychiatry and Behavioral Sciences, Johns Hopkins University School of Medicine, Baltimore, MD, United States
*Corresponding author: e-mail address: mwj@jhu.edu

Contents

1. Introduction 106
2. Classic psychedelics 107
3. Special considerations 108
   3.1 Set and setting 108
   3.2 The mystical experience 110
   3.3 Blinding and placebos 110
   3.4 Abuse-related effects of classic psychedelics 111
4. Psilocybin 113
   4.1 Subjective and physiological effects 113
   4.2 Clinical research 117
5. LSD 119
   5.1 Subjective and physiological effects 120
   5.2 Clinical effects 122
6. DMT 123
   6.1 Subjective and physiological effects 123
   6.2 Clinical effects 125
7. Conclusion 125
Funding 126
Conflicts of interest 126
References 126

Abstract

The past decade has witnessed a rapid growth of research on the basic science and clinical understanding of psychedelics. This chapter provides an overview of the human behavioral pharmacology of psychedelics focusing on three prototypic classic psychedelics—psilocybin, lysergic acid diethylamide (LSD), and dimethyltryptamine (DMT). A brief historical overview of the classic psychedelics and naming and drug classification is first specified. Next, special considerations in the conduct of human behavioral pharmacology work with psychedelics is described including the role of set and setting, mystical experience measurement, the use of effective blinding and placebos, and the abuse liability of psychedelics. Following, a description of the subjective,

Advances in Pharmacology, Volume 93
ISSN 1054-3589
https://doi.org/10.1016/bs.apha.2021.10.003

physiological, and clinical effects of psilocybin, LSD, and DMT is provided. This body of work clearly documents a unique and complex collection of subjective effects following psychedelic use, both during acute drug administration and as related to long-term behavior change following use. Clinical research demonstrates potential therapeutic utility with early phase clinical trials showing positive and enduring effects in many difficult-to-treat conditions including treatment-resistant depression, alcohol use disorder, and cigarette smoking. Future work in this newly reemerged field is needed to reveal mechanisms of behavior change in psychedelic drug action. Behavioral pharmacology is ultimately well served to provide this direction answering questions at the intersection of environment and pharmacology.

Abbreviations

5-HT2AR serotonin 2A receptor
DMT dimethyltryptamine
LSD lysergic acid diethylamide
MDMA 3,4-methylenedioxymethamphetamine

1. Introduction

Psychedelics (sometimes referred to as hallucinogens; see Section 2 for a history of naming conventions) are a collection of psychoactive compounds that act as agonists or partial agonists at the serotonin 2A receptor (5-HT2AR). Interest in psychedelics has grown in recent years given their marked potential as clinical therapeutics, a utility that was first speculated during the 1950s and 1960s and was freshly renewed in focus over the past decade following a period of relative research dormancy.

During mid-20th century, the scientific evaluation of psychedelics and the treatment of tens of thousands of patients with psychedelics was described in some of the leading medical and scientific journals. The basic science of psychedelics drugs, including the remarkable potency of lysergic acid diethylamide (LSD), added to the emerging biobehavioral model of brain function supplanting the existing dominance of psychodynamic models. At the same time, clinical applications were evaluated to include the treatment of addictive behaviors by psychedelics (Johnson & Griffiths, 2017).

However, human laboratory and clinical research on psychedelics largely came to a halt in the early 1970s. This was due to a combination of factors to include increasing marginalization owing to use of psychedelics outside clinical research settings, regulatory changes surrounding FDA scheduling, halted production of LSD and termination of access to the LSD drug master file by the pharmaceutical company Sandoz, and psychedelic's association with ongoing counter-culture movements. Although ethical and responsible human research occurred during this time by scientific pioneers like Abram Hoffer, Humphry Osmond, and Sidney Cohen, others (e.g., Timothy Leary) who eventually abandoned the scientific approach were highlighted as rationales for wider restrictions and scientific prohibitions.

It was not until the 1990s that human subjects research began anew, first by a small number of investigators in the United States and Europe and now within an increasingly widescale network of laboratory science and clinical trials. In these decades since, researchers have established and closely followed safety guidelines for administering psychedelics (Johnson, Richards, & Griffiths, 2008) that involve careful screening and preparation before drug administration sessions, close monitoring during these sessions, and follow-up care involving both clinically supportive discussion of session experiences and assessment for any adverse effects resulting from drug administration. Compared to the earlier era, modern psychedelic science has increasingly used novel methods and technological approaches including double-blind designs and neuroscience techniques (e.g., brain imaging). With these advances have come newly identified challenges in isolating the behavioral and therapeutic contributions of psychedelics and identifying the mechanisms of action in clinical practice.

This chapter will provide summary of the human behavioral pharmacology of psychedelics. We focus on three prototypic or "classic" (5-HT2AR agonist) psychedelics including psilocybin (a compound present in many species of mushrooms), LSD, and dimethyltryptamine (DMT). First, we provide a brief overview of classic psychedelics, including naming conventions and drug classification. Second, we describe some of the special considerations and current challenges when conducting human behavioral pharmacology research with psychedelics. Third, we overview existing human behavioral pharmacology research that has evaluated the subjective, physiological, and clinical effects of each compound. Finally, we provide a summative state of the field and key future directions.

2. Classic psychedelics

Nomenclature has historically been inconsistently applied within the field of psychedelic science with alternative labels like hallucinogen or entactogen often used to identify various compounds. For example, the previously popular, and sometimes still used, label hallucinogen is considered less accurate and potentially misleading when referring to these drugs given that not all effects of 5-HT2AR agonists are strict hallucinations or confined to perceptual effects alone. Presently, the term psychedelic, first coined by Humphrey Osmond in 1957 referring to the class of drugs that he considered "mind-manifesting," is considered preferred by many given its suggestion of a class of compounds that produce more general, non-ordinary forms of consciousness and/or altered states of self upon use (Dyck, 2006).

Classic psychedelics typically refer to two structural categories of 5-HT2AR agonists, indoleamines and phenylalkylamines. The indoleamines include psilocybin, DMT, and LSD while the phenylalkylamines include mescaline (the psychoactive component of peyote and San Pedro cactus), and a variety of synthetic compounds such as 2,5-dimethoxy-4-iodoamphetamine (DOI) and 2,5-dimethoxy-4-methylamphetamine (DOM). Although differing somewhat in chemical structures, these classic psychedelics are categorically grouped based on a shared primary action as agonists (or partial agonists) at the 5-HT2AR and their substitution for the prototypic compounds DOM or DOI in drug discrimination assays. More recently, classification structures have sometimes included atypical compounds such as ketamine, salvinorin A, and 3,4-methylenedioxymethamphetamine (MDMA) within the larger grouping of psychedelic drugs. Although these substances are known to produce phenomenologically experiences somewhat similar to classic psychedelics and some have shown clinical efficacy in similar arrangements (e.g., Grunebaum et al., 2018; Mitchell et al., 2021), their primary mechanisms of action as well as distinct constellation of subjective effects set them apart from the classic psychedelics.

3. Special considerations

Several special considerations are present in the conduct of human behavioral pharmacology and clinical psychopharmacology research involving psychedelics. In this section, we briefly review four key considerations, the role of set and setting, "mystical experience," drug blinding, and abuse liability.

3.1 Set and setting

Psychedelic science has long recognized the centrality of set (i.e., psychological state of a person) and setting (i.e., a person's environmental context) when determining the behavioral and clinical effects of 5-HT2AR compounds (Eisner, 1997; Hartogsohn, 2016; Johnson et al., 2008). Specifically, the subjective experience of psychedelic drug effects is thought greatly influenced by the intention or expectancy surrounding the event as well as the context in which the person may use the substance. This overall relevance of set and setting has partly contributed to the design of standardized and widely used psychedelic therapy for 5-HT2AR agonist administration in humans.

The notion of set and setting is not dissimilar from other work in behavioral pharmacology describing the role of expectancy (a specific form of set) on drug effects. For example, research using the balanced-placebo design has shown that the manipulation of pharmacological dose (e.g., active vs placebo) and expectation (e.g., told receiving active vs placebo) can isolate the role of expectancies in drug effects (Rohsenow & Marlatt, 1981; Ross, Krugman, Lyerly, & Clyde, 1962). An important and consistent finding of these studies is that the belief that alcohol is administered irrespective of actual content results in subjective changes like increased craving and aggressive behavior as well as interactions with dose that impact reaction time and cognitive-behavioral task performance (Marlatt & Rohsenow, 1980; Testa et al., 2006). Consistent independent or interactive effects involving expectancy have been observed across a variety of drugs and drug classes, including cannabinoids, stimulants, and opioids (Atlas et al., 2012; Lotshaw, Bradley, & Brooks, 1996; Metrik et al., 2012, 2009; Ross et al., 1962). Similarly, work in behavioral pharmacology at large has shown how the environment in which a substance is used can influence drug effects. For example, preclinical and clinical research has shown how the effects of cocaine are considered more positive and preferred in non-home environments while those of heroin are greater for in-home environments (e.g., Caprioli et al., 2009).

It is thought that set and setting may be specifically relevant for psychedelics with some hypotheses that a partial mechanism of drug action is amplification of set and setting characteristics. For example, typical laboratory contexts containing white walls, medical equipment, or other "sterile" stimuli are posited to increase the likelihood of negative drug effects (Studerus, Gamma, Kometer, & Vollenweider, 2012). Early observations similarly suggested that psychological or environmental factors such as the number of people present during drug administration sessions and feeling socially supported or not throughout the drug administration process could have an important influence on psilocybin effects (Leary, Litwin, & Metzner, 1963). We recently described how randomized manipulations of music played during psilocybin sessions for smoking cessation did not directly impact subjective experience or long-term clinical outcomes, although a slight advantage was observed for a non-traditional "overtone-based" playlist compared to a classical-music based one (Strickland, Garcia-Romeu, & Johnson, 2020). Consideration of set and setting in the design of psychedelic studies as well as future research experimentally testing implicit assumptions of these recommendations are needed.

3.2 The mystical experience

An additional unique consideration in the human behavioral pharmacology of psychedelics is the measurement and (often) focus on the mystical experience. The majority of human laboratory and clinical work involving psychedelics has operationalized and measured mystical experiences (or similar constructs such as oceanic boundlessness; Dittrich, 1998) as a key subjective drug effect with posited clinical significance The Mystical Experience Questionnaire (MEQ-30), for instance, is a widely used, validated, and modern scale of these experiences which considers features involving: (1) unity, noetic quality, and sacredness, (2) positive mood, (3) transcendence of time and space, and (4) ineffability (difficulty communicating or describing the experience) (Barrett, Johnson, & Griffiths, 2015; MacLean, Leoutsakos, Johnson, & Griffiths, 2012).

As described in greater detail in the following sections, several studies have demonstrated a positive relationship between greater mystical experiences and improved therapeutic outcomes following psychedelic-assisted treatment. Debate exists, however, about the extent to which these kinds of subjective experiences are necessary for therapeutic drug effects or may be epiphenomenal to other changes (e.g., neurotropic or neuroplastic changes) mediating positive clinical outcomes (Olson, 2020; Yaden & Griffiths, 2020). Several study designs have been proposed to test these hypotheses such as the use of general anesthesia to prevent waking recollection of drug effect during acute drug action. However, such studies have not yet been published making the role of mystical experiences (or subjective experience in general) an open question. In the meantime, it is likely there will be a continued focus on this subjective experience possibly underlying psychedelics' unique behavioral and clinical profile.

3.3 Blinding and placebos

Laboratory work and clinical designs using psychedelics have employed several different placebo conditions to include true placebos, low dose placebos (e.g., 1 mg psilocybin), or active placebos (e.g., niacin or methylphenidate) in the attempt to effectively blind psychedelic administration. Debate about the integrity of these blinding procedures, particularly in randomized clinical trials, is evident (see discussion in Gukasyan and Nayak (2021), Hartogsohn (2016), Nayak and Johnson (2021), Olson, Suissa-Rocheleau, Lifshitz, Raz, and Veissière (2020)). Limited data on the integrity of such blinding attempts emphasizes possible concerns. For instance, therapists in older studies were able to distinguish a patient receiving LSD from placebo in 86% of cases and from ephedrine in 95% (Smart, Storm, Baker, & Solursh, 1966; Soskin, 1973). Broken blinds are potentially problematic in clinical settings where they may lead to an exaggerated poor clinical response in the placebo group due to broken expectancy of receiving active drug.

A solution to blinding and placebos for psychedelic studies awaits further investigation. On one side, evaluation of drugs better matched on subjective experience (e.g., dextromethorphan or high doses of THC) may help to improve blinding albeit at the possible expense of producing therapeutic effects themselves in clinical contexts. On the other side, embracing the difficulty or impossibility of designing an effective placebo could encourage exploration of innovative clinical trial designs that can demonstrate causal inference in the absence of a traditional placebo-controlled randomized designs (see discussion of this in the context of psychotherapy in Nayak and Johnson (2021)).

3.4 Abuse-related effects of classic psychedelics

Prior to reviewing the subjective and clinical data surrounding psychedelics, it is important to understand their unique status as drugs of abuse. As described in the following, a variety of psychedelic compounds, such as mushrooms containing psilocybin, have been used in religious or spiritual rituals with documentation of these activities as early as the sixteenth century and probable use dating back centuries further (Johnson, Hendricks, Barrett, & Griffiths, 2019; Tylš, Páleníček, & Horáček, 2014). Contemporary use of psychedelics in Western cultures is sometimes attributed to similar "spiritual" intent in settings and rituals inspired by these historical uses (an additional specific set and setting of psychedelic use). Psychedelics at the same time also are drugs used for casual, unsupervised experimentation in non-clinical or non-traditional settings (Carbonaro et al., 2016; Center for Behavioral Health Statistics and Quality, 2020). These forms of use include cases in which the safety or well-being of the person or others may be jeopardized, for instance, if driving while acutely impaired. While these forms of abuse are evident, a comprehensive review of abuse liability of the prototypic psychedelic psilocybin found generally low abuse and no physical dependence potential (Johnson, Griffiths, Hendricks, & Henningfield, 2018). Psychedelics including psilocybin and LSD have failed to show overt signs of dependence and are not typically considered drugs of dependence in that they do not engender compulsive drug seeking or produce a known withdrawal symptom (Johnson et al., 2018). Similar observations are observed preclinically where these drugs are not reliably self-administered in non-human animals (Fantegrossi, Woods, & Winger, 2004; Johnson et al., 2018; Poling & Bryceland, 1979). A pooled analysis conducted by Studerus and colleagues (2011) further found that following use of psilocybin in laboratory settings, the large majority of participants (~90%) reported no change in their psilocybin use. In contrast, those that did report changes in use reported a decreased consumption with more participants reporting using it *less* often after their laboratory sessions (5.6% of all participants) than more often (3.3% of all participants). These findings collectively highlight that while psychedelics may be abused, many of the well characterized features relevant to other drugs of abuse and DSM-5 substance use disorder such as dependence and withdrawal are absent. Other factors, therefore, may motivate continued use (Carbonaro, Johnson, & Griffiths, 2020).

In the following sections, we review human laboratory and clinical work involving three classic psychedelics, psilocybin, LSD, and DMT. The focus on these three drugs is provided due to their: (1) uniform classification as classic psychedelics with mechanisms of actions primarily as 5-HT2AR agonists, (2) emerging relevance for similar clinical conditions as therapeutics, and (3) well characterized status within the human laboratory relative to other classic psychedelics. This overview focuses largely on contemporary human research given the advances in behavioral and neuroscience techniques present in this work, which can better isolate and study the effects of psychedelic compounds. However, summaries of older work are also provided for their historical or practical significance. Important to note is that the effects of many of the drugs are largely overlapping, varying most distinctly in the duration and intensity of effect rather than the subjective nature of their effects. Nonetheless, action at other receptors than the 5-HT receptors that is distinct or of differing relative potencies across these compounds may contribute to some of the unique effects or pharmacodynamics described hereafter. For these reasons, we focus our detailed discussion of prototypic effects of classic psychedelics when describing psilocybin given the larger breadth of research as the most widely used of these compounds in the modern era of psychedelic human behavioral pharmacology and clinical psychopharmacology.

4. Psilocybin

Psilocybin (sometimes referred to informally as "shrooms" or "magic mushrooms") is the primary active constituent present in a variety of mushroom species, most notably those from the genus *Psilocybe*. Albert Hoffman first isolated psilocybin from mushrooms in 1957, and first synthesized psilocybin in 1958 (Passie, Seifert, Schneider, & Emrich, 2002). Psilocybin when ingested is metabolized into an active metabolite psilocin, which is an agonist at the 5-HT2AR among other serotonergic sites (Nichols, 2016). Anthropological evidence suggests that psilocybin has been used by various indigenous people for religious and healing ceremonies for centuries (Stamets, 1996; Wasson, 1980). Modern research with psilocybin began soon after cultural anthropologist Wasson (1957) provided one of the first descriptions of these kinds of psilocybin-induced spiritual experiences, describing it as one of "holy communion…poised in space, a disembodied eye, invisible, incorporeal, seeing but not seen." Since these initial Western descriptions and isolation from the *Psilocybe* mushroom in the late 1950s, psilocybin has been evaluated in human laboratory settings for its unique profile of subjective effects characteristic of classic psychedelics.

4.1 Subjective and physiological effects

Psilocybin and its active metabolite psilocin generally exhibit low toxicity and are physiologically well-tolerated (Gable, 2004; Johnson et al., 2018; Nichols, 2016; Passie et al., 2002; Tylš et al., 2014). For example, preclinical studies suggest that that the median lethal dose (LD50) of psilocybin in rodents is approximately 2000 to 3000 times the usual human dose used on a mg/kg basis, comparing favorably with drugs such as caffeine. In fact, in a review and analysis of safety ratios calculated for 20 psychoactive compounds that compared lethal doses to commonly used doses found that psilocybin was associated with the lowest toxicity (Gable, 2004). These findings are generally consistent with other analyses describing the relative harms of commonly abused drugs and finding psilocybin low or the lowest in these rank orders (Nutt, King, Phillips, & Independent Scientific Committee on Drugs, 2010).

Human data have similarly shown psilocybin to have a broadly safe physiological profile. Several research studies have demonstrated this physiological safety in a variety of populations including cancer patients, people with and without prior psychedelic use, and treatment-seeking cigarette smokers (Carbonaro, Johnson, Hurwitz, & Griffiths, 2018;

Griffiths et al., 2016, 2018, 2011; Johnson, Garcia-Romeu, Cosimano, & Griffiths, 2014; Studerus et al., 2012; Studerus, Kometer, Hasler, & Vollenweider, 2011). Minor adverse physiological effects are generally dose dependent and include dizziness, nausea, vomiting, muscle twitching, and transient headaches of mild to moderate severity (Johnson, Sewell, & Griffiths, 2012; Tylš et al., 2014). Physiological effects of psilocybin also include moderate cardiovascular increases in heart rate and blood pressure that are similarly dose dependent. Peak effects typically occur within 2–3 h of oral use (the dominant route of use, for concerns with unsupervised intravenous use see Giancola, Korson, Caplan, and McKnight (2021)) with overt effects dissipating by approximately 6–7 h.

Some of the first modern studies of the subjective and physiological effects of psilocybin were conducted in the late 1990s. For example, one study evaluated the effects of oral psilocybin (0.25 mg/kg) in healthy adults (Vollenweider, Vollenweider-Scherpenhuyzen, Bäbler, Vogel, & Hell, 1998). Psilocybin produced changes in measures of altered state of consciousness (e.g., increased "oceanic boundlessness") that were dose-dependently prevented by pretreatment with the 5-HT2AR antagonist ketanserin, suggesting mediation of these effects by activity at this receptor. Additional studies conducted at this time and since have replicated this role of the 5-HT2AR in the prototypic effects of psychedelics by showing attenuation or prevention of these effects following ketanserin pretreatment (Kometer et al., 2012; Kometer, Schmidt, Jäncke, & Vollenweider, 2013; Quednow, Kometer, Geyer, & Vollenweider, 2012). Further evidence for the role of the 5-HT2AR is provided by PET imaging research in humans (Stenbæk et al., 2021).

Another study randomized healthy participants to receive oral doses of psilocybin (0.2 mg/kg up to 15 mg), 3,4-methylenedioxyethylamphetamine (MDE; 2 mg/kg up to 140 mg), d-methamphetamine (0.2 mg/kg up to 17.5 mg), or matched placebo (Gouzoulis-Mayfrank et al., 1999). Compared to placebo, psilocybin produced robust alterations in perception and affect to again include increases in various subjective effects and increases in both positive and negative mood. A pooled analysis of eight double-blind studies conducted in healthy participants ($N = 110$) from 1999 to 2008 corroborated these findings with observed dose-dependent changes in mood and subjective effects that were rated as positive during acute drug experience as well as in retrospective reflection in long-term follow-up (Studerus et al., 2011).

One double-blind, active comparator study evaluated the acute and long-term effects of higher doses of psilocybin (30 mg/70 kg) compared to methylphenidate (40 mg/70 kg) in psychedelic-naïve adults (Griffiths, Richards, McCann, & Jesse, 2006). This experiment was designed as a replication and extension of the first experimental study of psychedelics, the Good Friday experiment (Doblin, 1991; Pahnke, 1963), to address experimental limitations of that early work. Psilocybin produced higher subjective drug effects than methylphenidate as assessed by blinded monitors during the study session (e.g., higher ratings of overall drug effect and "distance from ordinary reality") and retrospective accounts by the participant of the study session 7 h after administration (e.g., higher ratings of mystical experience). Two months after the session, participants receiving psilocybin reported positive mood and attitudinal changes attributed to the experience that were supported by community observers with many participants rating the experience as one of the top five most personally meaningful experiences of their life. Notably, a secondary analysis of these data found that greater subjective mystical experience during the study session was associated with a greater likelihood of ascribing personal meaning to the session at long-term follow-up (i.e., up to 14 months later; Griffiths, Richards, Johnson, McCann, & Jesse, 2008).

These general effects of psilocybin on subjective well-being have been replicated in other studies conducted with healthy participants (Griffiths et al., 2018, 2011; Nicholas et al., 2018). For example, a later dose-effect, within-subject study evaluated psilocybin (5, 10, 20, and 30 mg/70 kg) and placebo under double-blind conditions in healthy adults (Griffiths et al., 2011). Similar acute perceptual and subjective effects were observed in that study and were generally dose-orderly with the highest observations of mystical experiences observed at the two highest doses and, subsequently, greatest attributions of personal significance reported at these doses. Physiological effects were also dose-dependent with greater increases in systolic blood pressure, diastolic blood pressure, and heart rate observed with higher doses (although these increases were considered within levels that were clinically safe and tolerable).

A secondary analysis recently conducted by our group evaluated the relationship between weight-adjusted doses of psilocybin and subjective drug effects including mystical experience and overall drug intensity (Garcia-Romeu, Barrett, Carbonaro, Johnson, & Griffiths, 2021). Data were pooled from 10 studies conducted at Johns Hopkins University

School of Medicine between 2001 and 2018 in which participants were administered psilocybin doses from 20 mg/70 kg to 30 mg/70 kg (total $N = 288$). Separate multivariable regression analyses examined the relationships between demographic variables including body weight and subjective effects in participants receiving 20 mg/70 kg ($n = 120$), those receiving 30 mg/70 kg ($n = 182$), and those whose weight-adjusted dose was approximately 25 mg (to approximate the fixed dose that is currently being evaluated in several clinical trials) ($n = 103$). In each weight-adjusted group, and in the fixed dose group, no significant associations were found between subjective effects and demographic variables including body weight (across a range of 49–113 kg) or sex. These findings suggest that body weight is not a major factor influencing the subjective effects of psilocybin across a range of populations and dosing structures.

Other work has evaluated psilocybin relative to non-classic psychedelics, including the non-competitive NMDA receptor antagonist dextromethorphan (DXM) (Barrett, Carbonaro, Hurwitz, Johnson, & Griffiths, 2018; Carbonaro et al., 2020, 2018). Although DXM is clinically used at low doses as an over-the-counter cough suppressant, at high doses DXM can function as a dissociative anesthetic (robotripping) and produce perpetual and cognitive effects like classic psychedelics. One study compared a single acute dose of DXM (400 mg/70 kg) to psilocybin (10, 20, and 30 mg/70 kg) and placebo using a double-blind, within-subject design in healthy, psychedelic-naïve participants (Barrett et al., 2018; Carbonaro et al., 2020, 2018). Psilocybin produced dose-orderly effects on cognitive tasks including alterations in psychomotor performance, working memory, episodic memory, associative learning, and visual perception with similar effects observed for DXM on psychomotor performance, visual perception, and associative learning as compared to the moderate to high doses of psilocybin (20–30 mg/70 kg). High doses of both drugs produced similar increases in participant ratings of peak overall drug effect strength, with similar times to maximal effect and time-course. Psilocybin also produced orderly dose-related increases on expected subjective measures and cardiovascular increases that were observed with the DXM dose. With respect to differences, psilocybin produced somewhat greater ratings of mystical experience and psychological insight compared to DXM while DXM produced greater effects on measures of light-headedness, disembodiment, and nausea/emesis. A secondary analysis of these data compared these reported experiences that may contribute to motives for psychedelic use including liking, visual effects, positive mood, insight, positive social effects, increased awareness of beauty (both visual and music), awe/amazement, meaningfulness, and mystical experience (Carbonaro et al., 2020). That analysis found that across these domains, both psilocybin and DXM produced effects greater than placebo, but that DXM ratings were significantly lower than those for the two highest doses of psilocybin on most items. Greater ratings in each of these domains is broadly consistent with the higher use rates of psilocybin for its psychedelic drug effects in the general population as well as data from the study showing greater self-reported desire to take the blinded psilocybin drug condition again compared to blinded DXM. These data provide possible insight into component features that may contribute to the motivational aspects of psychedelic use (despite the relatively low rates of reinforcement and lack of overt dependence or withdrawal as noted in Section 3.4).

4.2 Clinical research

The therapeutic effects of psilocybin have more recently been evaluated in contemporary clinical trials (see review in Johnson et al., 2019). These studies have tested the potential positive clinical benefit of psilocybin for a variety of indications to include depression and anxiety related to cancer and other life-threatening illness (Griffiths et al., 2016; Grob et al., 2011; Ross et al., 2016), major depressive disorder (Carhart-Harris et al., 2016, 2021; Davis et al., 2021), smoking cessation (Johnson et al., 2014; Johnson, Garcia-Romeu, & Griffiths, 2017), and alcohol use disorder (Bogenschutz et al., 2015).

Research on depression and anxiety in patients with cancer and other life-threatening illness was some of the first clinical work conducted in this modern era of psychedelic clinical psychopharmacology. An initial pilot study conducted in 2011 found that a moderate dose of psilocybin (0.2 mg/kg) relative to a niacin comparator showed a trend towards reducing depression and anxiety severity at a 2-week follow-up (Grob et al., 2011). Later larger trials using higher doses of psilocybin (21–30 mg/70 kg) found immediate and sustained improvements in depression and anxiety at 5-week and 6-month follow-ups (Griffiths et al., 2016; Ross et al., 2016). In both of these studies, ratings of mystical experience during the study session mediated the positive clinical effects of psilocybin, suggesting a mechanism of clinical benefit.

Other research has evaluated the role of psilocybin in major depressive disorder. An initial open-label pilot study of treatment-resistant depression found that two doses of psilocybin (10 and 25 mg fixed dose) separated by 1 week reduced depressive symptoms at follow-up, including at 6 months post-treatment (Carhart-Harris, Bolstridge, et al., 2016). A follow-up study to this pilot used a comparative efficacy, double dummy design to evaluate participants randomized to receive active psilocybin (25 mg fixed dose in two sessions) or escitalopram (a selective serotonin-reuptake inhibitor) with 1 mg psilocybin doses in study sessions (Carhart-Harris et al., 2021). Participants randomized to the active psilocybin group showed no significant difference from the escitalopram on the primary outcome (although numerically greater deceases in depression with psilocybin), but significantly improved clinical outcomes were observed for the psilocybin group in most secondary measures of depression, well-being, and quality of life. Another study used a randomized wait-list control design and evaluated the effect of two psilocybin sessions (20 mg/70 kg, 30 mg/70 kg across sequential sessions) in immediate and delayed treatment groups (Davis et al., 2021). Robust decreases in depression scores were observed in that study in the immediate treatment group relative to waitlist control group (who had not yet received treatment) with reductions observed in both groups after receiving the psilocybin intervention. For example, 17 of 24 participants that completed the full intervention showed a clinically significant response ($\geq$50% reduction in GRID-HAMD score) 4 weeks following their first psilocybin session.

Other work has evaluated the impact of psilocybin in the treatment of addictive behaviors. Following up on older studies that showed promise in using LSD to treat alcoholism (Krebs & Johansen, 2012), Bogenschutz et al. (2015) conducted the first research using psilocybin to treat alcohol use disorder. This study was an open-label design in which treatment-seeking participants with alcohol use disorder received one or two doses of psilocybin (0.3 and 0.4 mg/kg) along with supportive motivational interviewing. Significant reductions in drinking days and heavy drinking days (i.e., $\geq$5 drinks for men, $\geq$4 drinks for women; an FDA clinical trial endpoint for alcohol use disorder pharmacotherapy trials) were observed following the first psilocybin session with lower drinking sustained 36 weeks after treatment. For example, the mean percentage of heavy drinking days decreased from approximately 26% in the 4 weeks of treatment preceding the psilocybin sessions, to approximately 8% in the 4 weeks following the psilocybin session and remained at approximately 13% at the final follow-up period 21–32 weeks later.

Our research group has similarly evaluated the role of psilocybin-assisted treatment in smoking cessation. We first demonstrated the safety, feasibility, and potential efficacy of the approach in an open-label design wherein treatment-seeking smokers received psilocybin (20 mg/70 kg) on a target quit date while receiving cognitive behavioral therapy for cigarette cessation (Johnson et al., 2014). Two additional sessions at 30 mg/70 kg were then completed 2 and 8 weeks after the target quit date. Robust decreases in smoking were observed with biologically verified abstinence in 80% of participants 6 months post-target quit date and in 60% at approximately 2.5 years post quit date (Johnson et al., 2014, 2017). At this long-term follow-up (mean of approximately 2.5 years), participants were also qualitatively interviewed regarding their experience in the study (Noorani, Garcia-Romeu, Swift, Griffiths, & Johnson, 2018). Participants described the psilocybin sessions as leading to insights into self-identity and reasons for smoking, and a lasting sense of interconnectedness, awe, and curiosity. These psilocybin effects were reported to have overshadowed tobacco withdrawal symptoms. Moreover, aside from smoking, participants reported increases in other pro-social behavior and esthetic appreciation.

Collectively, these findings underscore the potential clinical utility of psilocybin-assisted treatment for a variety of conditions. Important to emphasize is that these studies have been conducted with an underlying psychotherapy or other behavioral intervention supporting the therapeutic administration of psychedelics (e.g., the preparation and interpersonal support described in Johnson et al. (2008)). Recent work has hypothesized that psychedelics may uniquely facilitate common factors of psychotherapy through their effects on meaning, relationship, and emotional skills making this interaction of psychedelic administration and psychotherapeutic support key to intervention success (Nayak & Johnson, 2021). Interactions of this kind may be considered a specific example of the role of set and setting in the effects of psychedelics (see discussion in *Special Considerations* above). Future work is needed to better interrogate these component processes to evaluate those necessary and those sufficient for the clinical effects of psychedelics with a goal of optimizing treatment.

5. LSD

The synthetic psychedelic LSD was first synthesized in 1938 with its psychoactive properties (accidentally) identified by Albert Hofmann in 1943. LSD is more potent than psilocybin or DMT at the 5-HT2AR where it acts as a partial agonist (Rickli, Moning, Hoener, & Liechti, 2016). In addition to this 5-HT2AR activity, LSD also has dopaminergic and adrenergic effects at higher doses (Kyzar, Nichols, Gainetdinov, Nichols, & Kalueff, 2017; Nichols, 2016). Compared to psilocybin, LSD has a longer duration of action with peak effects occurring approximately 2–3 h after oral dosing but lasting for up to 12 h, for example, after oral use of 200 mg (Dolder et al., 2017). LSD in real-world contexts is typically consumed orally.

5.1 Subjective and physiological effects

A series of placebo-controlled, crossover design studies during the modern research era have evaluated the subjective and physiological effects of LSD in healthy adults. One study evaluated 200 mg of oral LSD compared to placebo in healthy adults using a double-blind, crossover design (Schmid et al., 2015). LSD produced similar overt subjective effects as psilocybin including increases in subjective well-being and experience of altered states of consciousness. Physiological effects were also similar with increases in blood pressure and heart rate following dosing. A role for the 5-HT2AR in these acute effects has similarly been demonstrated with pretreatment with ketanserin blocking LSD-induced changes in subjective effects including positive affect (Kraehenmann et al., 2017; Preller et al., 2017). Another study administered a dose of 100 mg of oral LSD to an additional cohort of participants and compared the pharmacokinetic and pharmacodynamic effects of this dose to those of 200 mg in previous participants in the Schmid et al. (2015) study (Dolder et al., 2017). Increases in positive subjective effects and heart rate were dose-orderly with greater increases with the 200 mg dose. Similar to long-term changes observed with psilocybin, 12-month follow-up with participants receiving 200 mg of LSD indicated benefits for well-being and positive mood with attribution to the LSD experience as one of the most meaningful life experiences (Schmid & Liechti, 2018).

A recent dose-response study was conducted with oral LSD evaluating LSD (25, 50, 100, and 200 mg) and placebo in healthy adults (Holze et al., 2021). Participants completed experimental sessions with at least 10 days separating each and pharmacokinetic and pharmacodynamic parameters measured. Duration of effect was dose-dependent ranging from 6.7 to 11 h for the 25–200 mg doses. Dose-dependent increases in the aforementioned subjective effects were observed, although a possible ceiling effect for good drug effects were found with no difference between 100 and 200 mg doses. In contrast, a subjective measure of "ego dissolution" and anxiety were higher with the 200 mg dose. Heart rate and blood pressure increases were also dose-dependently observed with higher LSD doses.

Pretreatment with ketanserin (40 mg) prior to the 200 mg dose attenuated the subjective effects and prevented the heart rate increases, further emphasizing the 5-HT2AR mediation of these outcomes.

A comparative pharmacology study was also recently conducted evaluating the physiological and subjective effects of oral LSD (100 mg), MDMA (125 mg), d-amphetamine (40 mg), and placebo in heathy adults (Holze et al., 2020). At these doses, LSD produced greater peak ratings on subjective measures of drug effect and mystical experience than MDMA or d-amphetamine as well as had a longer time course with overt effects lasting until 10–11 h post administration (as compared to 6–7 h for the other two drugs). These findings indicate a unique profile of subjective experience (or at least unique intensity of those experiences) for LSD compared to the entactogen MDMA or the psychomotor stimulant d-amphetamine when observed under blinded conditions.

Although not commonly used recreationally, studies with intravenous LSD administration have also been conducted with human participants. For example, one study evaluated 75 mg of intravenous LSD compared to placebo (saline infusion) in healthy adults (Carhart-Harris et al., 2016). LSD produced marked changes in visual perception and increases in positive mood in addition to higher scores on a "psychosis-like" scale (owing to effects on cognitive disorganization and paranoia). Notably, changes in personality were observed 2 weeks following dosing with increases in optimism and trait openness following LSD administration. These findings are consistent with studies involving psilocybin showing long-term increases in trait openness following psilocybin administration, which are similarly positively related to greater within-session mystical experience scores (MacLean, Johnson, & Griffiths, 2011).

Other studies have evaluated the phenomenon of microdosing using laboratory designs. Microdosing refers to the process of repeated use of very low doses of a psychedelic, like LSD, that is anecdotally reported to improve mood, cognition, and well-being. One of these studies evaluated low doses of oral LSD (6.5, 13, and 26 mg) or placebo in healthy young adults using a double-blind, within-subject design and acute administration (Bershad, Schepers, Bremmer, Lee, & de Wit, 2019). Cognition, physiological, and most measures of mood were not impacted by LSD administration. Drug effects, however, were observed with ratings of "feel drug," "feel high," and "like drug" all dose-dependently increased (although of a relatively small magnitude even at the highest dose). Another study similarly found that with doses of LSD (5, 10, and 20 mg) administered to healthy adults in a double-blind, crossover design, subjective effects were reported starting at the 10 mg dose with effects lasting approximately 4 h (Holze et al., 2021). A recent observational study found that increased self-reported well-being and reductions in anxiety/depression were observed following induction of a weekly microdosing regiment (Kaertner et al., 2021). However, positive expectancies collected at baseline in that study predicted the positive clinical response reported, suggesting that these effects may be related to a placebo/expectancy response rather than pharmacologically mediated one.

5.2 Clinical effects

An early focus of psychedelic research from the 1950s to early 1970s was using LSD in the treatment of clinical disorders. Research led by Humphry Osmond and Abram Hoffer was among the first to study addiction treatment using psychedelics, specifically using LSD and mescaline to treat alcoholism (the clinical diagnosis at the time) (Chwelos, Blewett, Smith, & Hoffer, 1959). This work was informed by data indicating that sobriety was often achieved following the experience of delirium tremens during alcohol withdrawal with the premise that psychedelics may offer a safe model for psychosis (i.e., a safer delirium without the fatal risks of delirium tremens). Subsequent randomized trials conducted during this period provided non-significant trends that tended to favor improved outcome for LSD. A contemporary meta-analysis of six of these studies comprising 536 participants randomized to LSD (in doses from 210 to 800 mg) or control conditions found improvements in alcohol misuse in LSD groups with odd ratio effect sizes of approximately 2 at 1 month post-treatment (Krebs & Johansen, 2012).

Other research during this older era evaluated LSD in the context of opioid use (Savage & McCabe, 1973). This study used a residential design of persons with heroin dependence and found that those in an LSD group (receiving 300–450 mg of LSD) showed lower biologically confirmed heroin use compared to control groups up to 12-months post-treatment. A similar series of studies evaluated LSD as a therapeutic for pain relief (Kast, 1967; Kast & Collins, 1964). These studies identified reductions following acute LSD administration that were comparable to opioid analgesics with a longer duration of action (Kast, 1967; Kast & Collins, 1964). Moreover, moderate reductions in pain were observed after acute LSD sessions that persisted for approximately 3 weeks (Kast, 1967).

Modern therapeutic research with LSD, however, is more limited. One of the only trials evaluated LSD for patients with anxiety related to cancer and other life-threatening illness (Gasser et al., 2014; Gasser, Kirchner, & Passie, 2015). Participants were first assigned to receive either 200 mg of LSD ($N=8$) or a low dose (20 mg; $N=3$) in two double-blind sessions followed by the option for open-label cross-over to the 200 mg dose. Reductions in anxiety were observed in the randomized treatment group that were not observed in the control group (although the small N precluded powered statistical testing). Long-term positive outcomes were also observed with lasting reductions in anxiety at a 12-month follow-up.

6. DMT

Richard Manske first synthesized DMT in 1931 (Manske, 1931). DMT is the psychedelic constituent of ayahuasca, a tea historically used by indigenous people of the Amazon basin as well as organized religious groups in sacramental ceremonies. DMT is not active orally unless co-administered with a monoamine oxidase inhibitor (MAOI) because it is rapidly metabolized after oral administration. DMT naturally occurs in several species of plants (e.g., *Psychotria viridis*) and is combined with plants containing naturally occurring MAOIs (e.g., *Banisteriopsis caapi*) in ayahuasca brews to produce psychedelic effects on consumption. DMT is also commonly used via inhalation of snuffs where an MAOI is not necessary to produce the subjective or physiological effects. Compared to other classic psychedelics, DMT is short acting and can produce effects in less than a minute after inhaled use with effects dissipating within 15–30 min (thus referred to as a "businessman's trip"). DMT is also an agonist at 5-HT2AR and like other classic psychedelics this is believed to be the primary site at which psychedelic drug effects are mediated. DMT, although structurally and phenomenological similar, is distinct from the related psychedelic 5-methoxy-*N*,*N*-dimethyltryptamine (5-MeO-DMT), which is found in the skin and venom of the *Bufo alavarius* toad as well as in a large number of plants (Ott, 2001).

6.1 Subjective and physiological effects

Beginning in the early 1990s, a series of systematic studies evaluating the effects of DMT in human participants were conducted (Strassman, 1996). The first of these studies evaluated intravenous DMT (0.05, 0.1, 0.2, and 0.4 mg/kg) and placebo under double-blind conditions in healthy adults with a history of psychedelic use (Strassman & Qualls, 1994). Peak effects occurred within 2 min of drug administration and subsided by 30 min. Dose-dependent increases in blood pressure and heart rate were observed like those effects of other classic psychedelics albeit in a more constrained timecourse. A companion study evaluated subjective effects with two doses of DMT (0.04 and 0.4 mg/kg) under non-blinded conditions to develop a systematic view of DMT drug effects (Strassman, Qualls, Uhlenhuth, & Kellner, 1994). Subjective effects similarly occurred rapidly, peaking within 1.5–2 min of administration, and subsiding within 30 min. Pronounced visual effects were reported as were overwhelming feelings of euphoria intermixed with anxiety. A follow-up study evaluated tolerance to these subjective and physiological effects of DMT following repeated administration of 0.3 mg/kg intravenous doses at 30-min intervals (Strassman, Qualls, & Berg, 1996). Acute tolerance to heart rate increases were observed after repeated administration whereas minimal tolerance was observed to the subjective effects of DMT, which remained high and stable across the repeated dosing.

Other work has evaluated the subjective effects of DMT via oral dosing, most typical in the form of ayahuasca preparations. One study evaluated encapsulated doses of freeze-dried ayahuasca (0.5, 0.75, and 1.0 mg DMT/kg) and placebo in male healthy adults using a single-blind, crossover design (Riba et al., 2001). Dose-dependent increases in overt drug effects (e.g., "good effect") as well as those specific to psychedelics (e.g., a Hallucinogen Rating Scale) were observed. These effects began at approximately 30–60 min with peak occurring at 1–2 h and resolution of drug effects by 4 h. Relative to intravenous dosing, these effects were longer in duration, but were lower in overall magnitude. A related study evaluated oral doses of 0.6 and 0.85 mg/kg DMT in a larger sample of healthy male and female adults (Riba et al., 2003). A similar dose-effect relationship and time course were observed. A more recent comparative study evaluated oral and smoked DMT (25 mg) administration in healthy adults (Riba, McIlhenny, Bouso, & Barker, 2015). Notably, DMT was delivered *without* concurrent MAOI administration because the primary focus of that study was to evaluate drug metabolites via these different routes in the absence of MAOI administration. Expectedly, then, DMT via the oral route produced minimal subjective effects (1 participants reported a low intensity effect) whereas smoked administration produced robust increases on a Hallucinogen Rating Scale.

The role of the 5-HT2AR in DMT effects has also been evaluated in a double-blind, placebo-controlled study of ayahuasca (0.75 mg/kg DMT) using ketanserin (40 mg) pretreatment in a fully crossed, within-subject design (Valle et al., 2016). Antagonism of 5-HT2AR attenuated some of the subjective effects of ayahuasca, although complete reduction was not observed. Interestingly, pretreatment with the serotonin 5-HT1A receptor antagonist pindolol in another study enhanced the subjective effects of DMT, which is possibly related to an inhibitory role of 5-HT1A in the psychedelic effects of DMT (DMT is an equally or more potent agonist at 5-HT1A receptors) and/or unopposed 5-HT2A agonism (Strassman, 1996).

6.2 Clinical effects

Experimental studies evaluating the clinical effects of DMT are more limited. One open-label study of ayahuasca (0.8 mg/mL DMT content) in six patients with recurrent major depressive disorder found significant and substantial reductions in depressive symptoms at 1, 7 and 21-days post administration (Osório Fde et al., 2015). These findings were replicated in another open-label trial in a larger sample of 17 patients with similar reductions in depressive symptoms observed (Sanches et al., 2016). A subsequent double-blind, placebo-controlled randomized clinical trial for treatment-resistant depression was conducted with participants randomized to receive ayahuasca (0.36 mg/kg DMT) or placebo (Palhano-Fontes et al., 2019). Patients receiving the ayahuasca intervention showed significant and sustained reductions in depression that differed from placebo at 1, 2, and 7-days post intervention (with the largest difference observed at the 7-day timepoint). Future work is needed to evaluate these findings further as well as the potential clinical utility of alternative routes of administration (e.g., inhaled and intravenous DMT).

7. Conclusion

This chapter provided an overview of current and future directions in the human behavioral pharmacology of psychedelics. As emphasized throughout, classic psychedelics such as psilocybin, LSD, and DMT produce a distinct and complex profile of subjective mood states and a pattern of use that markedly differs from other substances of abuse. Strong signals of positive clinical benefits across a variety of conditions underscore the need for more information about the mechanisms of health change mediated by psychedelics. Behavioral pharmacology, given its tools to address those questions at the interaction of environment and pharmacology, is uniquely positioned to advance these directions for the future of psychedelic science.

Funding

Support for effort by M.W.J. was provided by the Johns Hopkins Center for Psychedelics and Consciousness Research which is funded by the Steven and Alexandra Cohen Foundation and the Tim Ferriss, Matt Mullenweg, Craig Nerenberg, and Blake Mycoskie Collaborative. Support for effort by J.C.S. was provided by the National Institute on Drug Abuse Grant T32DA07209.

Conflicts of interest

M.W.J. has served as a paid consultant for AJNA Labs LLC, AWAKN Life Sciences Inc., Beckley Psychedelic Ltd., Entheogen Biomedical Corp., Field Trip Psychedelics Inc., Mind Medicine Inc., Otsuka Pharmaceutical Development & Commercialization Inc., and Silo Pharma, Inc. J.C.S. has no conflicts of interest to declare.

References

Atlas, L. Y., Whittington, R. A., Lindquist, M. A., Wielgosz, J., Sonty, N., & Wager, T. D. (2012). Dissociable influences of opiates and expectations on pain. *Journal of Neuroscience*, *32*(23), 8053–8064.

Barrett, F. S., Carbonaro, T. M., Hurwitz, E., Johnson, M. W., & Griffiths, R. R. (2018). Double-blind comparison of the two hallucinogens psilocybin and dextromethorphan: Effects on cognition. *Psychopharmacology*, *235*(10), 2915–2927.

Barrett, F. S., Johnson, M. W., & Griffiths, R. R. (2015). Validation of the revised mystical experience questionnaire in experimental sessions with psilocybin. *Journal of Psychopharmacology*, *29*(11), 1182–1190.

Bershad, A. K., Schepers, S. T., Bremmer, M. P., Lee, R., & de Wit, H. (2019). Acute subjective and behavioral effects of microdoses of lysergic acid diethylamide in healthy human volunteers. *Biological Psychiatry*, *86*(10), 792–800.

Bogenschutz, M. P., Forcehimes, A. A., Pommy, J. A., Wilcox, C. E., Barbosa, P. C., & Strassman, R. J. (2015). Psilocybin-assisted treatment for alcohol dependence: A proof-of-concept study. *Journal of Psychopharmacology*, *29*(3), 289–299.

Caprioli, D., Celentano, M., Dubla, A., Lucantonio, F., Nencini, P., & Badiani, A. (2009). Ambience and drug choice: Cocaine- and heroin-taking as a function of environmental context in humans and rats. *Biological Psychiatry*, *65*(10), 893–899.

Carbonaro, T. M., Bradstreet, M. P., Barrett, F. S., MacLean, K. A., Jesse, R., Johnson, M. W., et al. (2016). Survey study of challenging experiences after ingesting psilocybin mushrooms: Acute and enduring positive and negative consequences. *Journal of Psychopharmacology*, *30*(12), 1268–1278.

Carbonaro, T. M., Johnson, M. W., & Griffiths, R. R. (2020). Subjective features of the psilocybin experience that may account for its self-administration by humans: A double-blind comparison of psilocybin and dextromethorphan. *Psychopharmacology*, *237*(8), 2293–2304.

Carbonaro, T. M., Johnson, M. W., Hurwitz, E., & Griffiths, R. R. (2018). Double-blind comparison of the two hallucinogens psilocybin and dextromethorphan: Similarities and differences in subjective experiences. *Psychopharmacology*, *235*(2), 521–534.

Carhart-Harris, R. L., Bolstridge, M., Rucker, J., Day, C. M., Erritzoe, D., Kaelen, M., et al. (2016). Psilocybin with psychological support for treatment-resistant depression: An open-label feasibility study. *Lancet Psychiatry*, *3*(7), 619–627.

Carhart-Harris, R., Giribaldi, B., Watts, R., Baker-Jones, M., Murphy-Beiner, A., Murphy, R., et al. (2021). Trial of psilocybin versus escitalopram for depression. *New England Journal of Medicine*, *384*(15), 1402–1411.

Carhart-Harris, R. L., Kaelen, M., Bolstridge, M., Williams, T. M., Williams, L. T., Underwood, R., et al. (2016). The paradoxical psychological effects of lysergic acid diethylamide (LSD). *Psychological Medicine*, *46*(7), 1379–1390.

Center for Behavioral Health Statistics and Quality. (2020). *Results from the 2019 National Survey on drug use and health: Detailed tables*. Rockville, MD: Substance Abuse and Mental Health Services Administration.

Chwelos, N., Blewett, D. B., Smith, C. M., & Hoffer, A. (1959). Use of d-lysergic acid diethylamide in the treatment of alcoholism. *Quarterly Journal of Studies on Alcohol*, *20*, 577–590.

Davis, A. K., Barrett, F. S., May, D. G., Cosimano, M. P., Sepeda, N. D., Johnson, M. W., et al. (2021). Effects of psilocybin-assisted therapy on major depressive disorder: A randomized clinical trial. *JAMA Psychiatry*, *78*(5), 481–489.

Dittrich, A. (1998). The standardized psychometric assessment of altered states of consciousness (ASCs) in humans. *Pharmacopsychiatry*, *31*(Suppl 2), 80–84.

Doblin, R. (1991). Pahnke's "good Friday experiment": A long-term follow-up and methodological critique. *Journal of Transpersonal Psychology*, *23*(1), 1–28.

Dolder, P. C., Schmid, Y., Steuer, A. E., Kraemer, T., Rentsch, K. M., Hammann, F., et al. (2017). Pharmacokinetics and pharmacodynamics of lysergic acid diethylamide in healthy subjects. *Clinical Pharmacokinetics*, *56*(10), 1219–1230.

Dyck, E. (2006). 'Hitting highs at rock bottom': LSD treatment for alcoholism, 1950–1970. *Social History of Medicine*, *19*(2), 313–329.

Eisner, B. (1997). Set, setting, and matrix. *Journal of Psychoactive Drugs*, *29*(2), 213–216.

Fantegrossi, W. E., Woods, J. H., & Winger, G. (2004). Transient reinforcing effects of phenylisopropylamine and indolealkylamine hallucinogens in rhesus monkeys. *Behavioural Pharmacology*, *15*(2), 149–157.

Gable, R. S. (2004). Comparison of acute lethal toxicity of commonly abused psychoactive substances. *Addiction*, *99*(6), 686–696.

Garcia-Romeu, A., Barrett, F. S., Carbonaro, T. M., Johnson, M. W., & Griffiths, R. R. (2021). Optimal dosing for psilocybin pharmacotherapy: Considering weight-adjusted and fixed dosing approaches. *Journal of Psychopharmacology*, *35*(4), 353–361.

Gasser, P., Holstein, D., Michel, Y., Doblin, R., Yazar-Klosinski, B., Passie, T., et al. (2014). Safety and efficacy of lysergic acid diethylamide-assisted psychotherapy for anxiety associated with life-threatening diseases. *The Journal of Nervous and Mental Disease*, *202*(7), 513–520.

Gasser, P., Kirchner, K., & Passie, T. (2015). LSD-assisted psychotherapy for anxiety associated with a life-threatening disease: A qualitative study of acute and sustained subjective effects. *Journal of Psychopharmacology*, *29*(1), 57–68.

Giancola, N. B., Korson, C. J., Caplan, J. P., & McKnight, C. A. (2021). A "trip" to the intensive care unit: An intravenous injection of psilocybin. *Journal of the Academy of Consultation-Liaison Psychiatry*, *62*(3), 370–371.

Gouzoulis-Mayfrank, E., Thelen, B., Habermeyer, E., Kunert, H. J., Kovar, K. A., Lindenblatt, H., et al. (1999). Psychopathological, neuroendocrine and autonomic effects of 3,4-methylenedioxyethylamphetamine (MDE), psilocybin and d-methamphetamine in healthy volunteers. Results of an experimental double-blind placebo-controlled study. *Psychopharmacology*, *142*(1), 41–50.

Griffiths, R. R., Johnson, M. W., Carducci, M. A., Umbricht, A., Richards, W. A., Richards, B. D., et al. (2016). Psilocybin produces substantial and sustained decreases in depression and anxiety in patients with life-threatening cancer: A randomized double-blind trial. *Journal of Psychopharmacology*, *30*(12), 1181–1197.

Griffiths, R. R., Johnson, M. W., Richards, W. A., Richards, B. D., Jesse, R., MacLean, K. A., et al. (2018). Psilocybin-occasioned mystical-type experience in combination with meditation and other spiritual practices produces enduring positive changes in psychological functioning and in trait measures of prosocial attitudes and behaviors. *Journal of Psychopharmacology*, *32*(1), 49–69.

Griffiths, R. R., Johnson, M. W., Richards, W. A., Richards, B. D., McCann, U., & Jesse, R. (2011). Psilocybin occasioned mystical-type experiences: Immediate and persisting dose-related effects. *Psychopharmacology*, *218*(4), 649–665.
Griffiths, R., Richards, W., Johnson, M., McCann, U., & Jesse, R. (2008). Mystical-type experiences occasioned by psilocybin mediate the attribution of personal meaning and spiritual significance 14 months later. *Journal of Psychopharmacology*, *22*(6), 621–632.
Griffiths, R. R., Richards, W. A., McCann, U., & Jesse, R. (2006). Psilocybin can occasion mystical-type experiences having substantial and sustained personal meaning and spiritual significance. *Psychopharmacology*, *187*(3), 268–283.
Grob, C. S., Danforth, A. L., Chopra, G. S., Hagerty, M., McKay, C. R., Halberstadt, A. L., et al. (2011). Pilot study of psilocybin treatment for anxiety in patients with advanced-stage cancer. *Archives of General Psychiatry*, *68*(1), 71–78.
Grunebaum, M. F., Galfalvy, H. C., Choo, T.-H., Keilp, J. G., Moitra, V. K., Parris, M. S., et al. (2018). Ketamine for rapid reduction of suicidal thoughts in major depression: A midazolam-controlled randomized clinical trial. *American Journal of Psychiatry*, *175*(4), 327–335.
Gukasyan, N., & Nayak, S. M. (2021). Psychedelics, placebo effects, and set and setting: Insights from common factors theory of psychotherapy. *Transcultural Psychiatry*. https://doi.org/10.1177/1363461520983684.
Hartogsohn, I. (2016). Set and setting, psychedelics and the placebo response: An extra-pharmacological perspective on psychopharmacology. *Journal of Psychopharmacology*, *30*(12), 1259–1267.
Holze, F., Liechti, M. E., Hutten, N., Mason, N. L., Dolder, P. C., Theunissen, E. L., et al. (2021). Pharmacokinetics and pharmacodynamics of lysergic acid diethylamide microdoses in healthy participants. *Clinical Pharmacology & Therapeutics*, *109*(3), 658–666.
Holze, F., Vizeli, P., Ley, L., Müller, F., Dolder, P., Stocker, M., et al. (2021). Acute dose-dependent effects of lysergic acid diethylamide in a double-blind placebo-controlled study in healthy subjects. *Neuropsychopharmacology*, *46*(3), 537–544.
Holze, F., Vizeli, P., Müller, F., Ley, L., Duerig, R., Varghese, N., et al. (2020). Distinct acute effects of LSD, MDMA, and D-amphetamine in healthy subjects. *Neuropsychopharmacology*, *45*(3), 462–471.
Johnson, M. W., Garcia-Romeu, A., Cosimano, M. P., & Griffiths, R. R. (2014). Pilot study of the 5-HT2AR agonist psilocybin in the treatment of tobacco addiction. *Journal of Psychopharmacology*, *28*(11), 983–992.
Johnson, M. W., Garcia-Romeu, A., & Griffiths, R. R. (2017). Long-term follow-up of psilocybin-facilitated smoking cessation. *American Journal of Drug and Alcohol Abuse*, *43*(1), 55–60.
Johnson, M. W., & Griffiths, R. R. (2017). Potential therapeutic effects of psilocybin. *Neurotherapeutics*, *14*(3), 734–740.
Johnson, M. W., Griffiths, R. R., Hendricks, P. S., & Henningfield, J. E. (2018). The abuse potential of medical psilocybin according to the 8 factors of the controlled substances act. *Neuropharmacology*, *142*, 143–166.
Johnson, M. W., Hendricks, P. S., Barrett, F. S., & Griffiths, R. R. (2019). Classic psychedelics: An integrative review of epidemiology, therapeutics, mystical experience, and brain network function. *Pharmacology & Therapeutics*, *197*, 83–102.
Johnson, M., Richards, W., & Griffiths, R. (2008). Human hallucinogen research: Guidelines for safety. *Journal of Psychopharmacology*, *22*(6), 603–620.
Johnson, M. W., Sewell, R. A., & Griffiths, R. R. (2012). Psilocybin dose-dependently causes delayed, transient headaches in healthy volunteers. *Drug and Alcohol Dependence*, *123*(1–3), 132–140.
Kaertner, L. S., Steinborn, M. B., Kettner, H., Spriggs, M. J., Roseman, L., Buchborn, T., et al. (2021). Positive expectations predict improved mental-health outcomes linked to psychedelic microdosing. *Scientific Reports*, *11*(1), 1941.

Kast, E. (1967). Attenuation of anticipation: A therapeutic use of lysergic acid diethylamide. *Psychiatric Quarterly, 41*(4), 646–657.
Kast, E. C., & Collins, V. J. (1964). Study of lysergic acid diethylamide as an analgesic agent. *Anesthesia & Analgesia, 43*, 285–291.
Kometer, M., Schmidt, A., Bachmann, R., Studerus, E., Seifritz, E., & Vollenweider, F. X. (2012). Psilocybin biases facial recognition, goal-directed behavior, and mood state toward positive relative to negative emotions through different serotonergic subreceptors. *Biological Psychiatry, 72*(11), 898–906.
Kometer, M., Schmidt, A., Jäncke, L., & Vollenweider, F. X. (2013). Activation of serotonin 2A receptors underlies the psilocybin-induced effects on α oscillations, N170 visual-evoked potentials, and visual hallucinations. *Journal of Neuroscience, 33*(25), 10544–10551.
Kraehenmann, R., Pokorny, D., Aicher, H., Preller, K. H., Pokorny, T., Bosch, O. G., et al. (2017). LSD increases primary process thinking via serotonin 2a receptor activation. *Frontiers in Pharmacology, 8*, 814.
Krebs, T. S., & Johansen, P. (2012). Lysergic acid diethylamide (LSD) for alcoholism: Meta-analysis of randomized controlled trials. *Journal of Psychopharmacology, 26*(7), 994–1002.
Kyzar, E. J., Nichols, C. D., Gainetdinov, R. R., Nichols, D. E., & Kalueff, A. V. (2017). Psychedelic drugs in biomedicine. *Trends in Pharmacological Sciences, 38*(11), 992–1005.
Leary, T., Litwin, G. H., & Metzner, R. (1963). Reactions to psilocybin administered in a supportive environment. *Journal of Nervous and Mental Disorders, 137*, 561–573.
Lotshaw, S. C., Bradley, J. R., & Brooks, L. R. (1996). Illustrating caffeine's pharmacological and expectancy effects utilizing a balanced placebo design. *Journal of Drug Education, 26*(1), 13–24.
MacLean, K. A., Johnson, M. W., & Griffiths, R. R. (2011). Mystical experiences occasioned by the hallucinogen psilocybin lead to increases in the personality domain of openness. *Journal of Psychopharmacology, 25*(11), 1453–1461.
MacLean, K. A., Leoutsakos, J. M., Johnson, M. W., & Griffiths, R. R. (2012). Factor analysis of the mystical experience questionnaire: A study of experiences occasioned by the hallucinogen psilocybin. *Journal of the Scientific Study of Religion, 51*(4), 721–737.
Manske, R. H. F. (1931). A synthesis of the methyltryptamines and some derivatives. *Canadian Journal of Research, 5*(5), 592–600.
Marlatt, G. A., & Rohsenow, D. J. (1980). Cognitive processes in alcohol use: Expectancy and the balanced placebo design. *Advances in Substance Abuse: Behavioral biological research, 1*, 159–199.
Metrik, J., Kahler, C. W., Reynolds, B., McGeary, J. E., Monti, P. M., Haney, M., et al. (2012). Balanced placebo design with marijuana: Pharmacological and expectancy effects on impulsivity and risk taking. *Psychopharmacology, 223*(4), 489–499.
Metrik, J., Rohsenow, D. J., Monti, P. M., McGeary, J., Cook, T. A., de Wit, H., et al. (2009). Effectiveness of a marijuana expectancy manipulation: Piloting the balanced-placebo design for marijuana. *Experimental & Clinical Psychopharmacology, 17*(4), 217–225.
Mitchell, J. M., Bogenschutz, M., Lilienstein, A., Harrison, C., Kleiman, S., Parker-Guilbert, K., et al. (2021). MDMA-assisted therapy for severe PTSD: A randomized, double-blind, placebo-controlled phase 3 study. *Nature Medicine, 27*(6), 1025–1033.
Nayak, S., & Johnson, M. W. (2021). Psychedelics and psychotherapy. *Pharmacopsychiatry, 54*(4), 167–175.
Nicholas, C. R., Henriquez, K. M., Gassman, M. C., Cooper, K. M., Muller, D., Hetzel, S., et al. (2018). High dose psilocybin is associated with positive subjective effects in healthy volunteers. *Journal of Psychopharmacology, 32*(7), 770–778.
Nichols, D. E. (2016). Psychedelics. *Pharmacological Reviews, 68*(2), 264–355.

Noorani, T., Garcia-Romeu, A., Swift, T. C., Griffiths, R. R., & Johnson, M. W. (2018). Psychedelic therapy for smoking cessation: Qualitative analysis of participant accounts. *Journal of Psychopharmacology, 32*(7), 756–769.

Nutt, D. J., King, L. A., Phillips, L. D., & Independent Scientific Committee on Drugs. (2010). Drug harms in the UK: A multicriteria decision analysis. *Lancet, 376*(9752), 1558–1565.

Olson, D. E. (2020). The subjective effects of psychedelics may not be necessary for their enduring therapeutic effects. *ACS Pharmacology & Translational Science, 4*(2), 563–567.

Olson, J. A., Suissa-Rocheleau, L., Lifshitz, M., Raz, A., & Veissière, S. P. L. (2020). Tripping on nothing: Placebo psychedelics and contextual factors. *Psychopharmacology, 237*(5), 1371–1382.

Osório Fde, L., Sanches, R. F., Macedo, L. R., Santos, R. G., Maia-de-Oliveira, J. P., Wichert-Ana, L., et al. (2015). Antidepressant effects of a single dose of ayahuasca in patients with recurrent depression: A preliminary report. *Brazilian Journal of Psychiatry, 37*(1), 13–20.

Ott, J. (2001). Pharmepena-psychonautics: Human intranasal, sublingual and oral pharmacology of 5-methoxy-N, N-dimethyl-tryptamine. *Journal of Psychoactive Drugs, 33*(4), 403–407.

Pahnke, W. N. (1963). *Drugs and mysticism: An analysis of the relationship between psychedelic drugs and the mystical consciousness: A thesis.*

Palhano-Fontes, F., Barreto, D., Onias, H., Andrade, K. C., Novaes, M. M., Pessoa, J. A., et al. (2019). Rapid antidepressant effects of the psychedelic ayahuasca in treatment-resistant depression: A randomized placebo-controlled trial. *Psychological Medicine, 49*(4), 655–663.

Passie, T., Seifert, J., Schneider, U., & Emrich, H. M. (2002). The pharmacology of psilocybin. *Addiction Biology, 7*(4), 357–364.

Poling, A., & Bryceland, J. (1979). Voluntary drug self-administration by nonhumans: A review. *Journal of Psychedelic Drugs, 11*(3), 185–190.

Preller, K. H., Herdener, M., Pokorny, T., Planzer, A., Kraehenmann, R., Stämpfli, P., et al. (2017). The fabric of meaning and subjective effects in LSD-induced states depend on serotonin 2a receptor activation. *Current Biology, 27*(3), 451–457.

Quednow, B. B., Kometer, M., Geyer, M. A., & Vollenweider, F. X. (2012). Psilocybin-induced deficits in automatic and controlled inhibition are attenuated by ketanserin in healthy human volunteers. *Neuropsychopharmacology, 37*(3), 630–640.

Riba, J., McIlhenny, E. H., Bouso, J. C., & Barker, S. A. (2015). Metabolism and urinary disposition of N,N-dimethyltryptamine after oral and smoked administration: A comparative study. *Drug Testing and Analysis, 7*(5), 401–406.

Riba, J., Rodríguez-Fornells, A., Urbano, G., Morte, A., Antonijoan, R., Montero, M., et al. (2001). Subjective effects and tolerability of the south American psychoactive beverage Ayahuasca in healthy volunteers. *Psychopharmacology, 154*(1), 85–95.

Riba, J., Valle, M., Urbano, G., Yritia, M., Morte, A., & Barbanoj, M. J. (2003). Human pharmacology of ayahuasca: Subjective and cardiovascular effects, monoamine metabolite excretion, and pharmacokinetics. *Journal of Pharmacology and Experimental Theapeutics, 306*(1), 73–83.

Rickli, A., Moning, O. D., Hoener, M. C., & Liechti, M. E. (2016). Receptor interaction profiles of novel psychoactive tryptamines compared with classic hallucinogens. *European Neuropsychopharmacology, 26*(8), 1327–1337.

Rohsenow, D. J., & Marlatt, G. A. (1981). The balanced placebo design: Methodological considerations. *Addictive Behaviors, 6*(2), 107–122.

Ross, S., Bossis, A., Guss, J., Agin-Liebes, G., Malone, T., Cohen, B., et al. (2016). Rapid and sustained symptom reduction following psilocybin treatment for anxiety and depression in patients with life-threatening cancer: A randomized controlled trial. *Journal of Psychopharmacology, 30*(12), 1165–1180.

Ross, S., Krugman, A. D., Lyerly, S. B., & Clyde, D. J. (1962). Drugs and placebos: A model design. *Psychological Reports, 10*(2), 383–392.
Sanches, R. F., de Lima Osório, F., Dos Santos, R. G., Macedo, L. R., Maia-de-Oliveira, J. P., Wichert-Ana, L., et al. (2016). Antidepressant effects of a single dose of ayahuasca in patients with recurrent depression: A SPECT study. *Journal of Clinical Psychopharmacology, 36*(1), 77–81.
Savage, C., & McCabe, O. L. (1973). Residential psychedelic (LSD) therapy for the narcotic addict. A controlled study. *Archives of General Psychiatry, 28*(6), 808–814.
Schmid, Y., Enzler, F., Gasser, P., Grouzmann, E., Preller, K. H., Vollenweider, F. X., et al. (2015). Acute effects of lysergic acid diethylamide in healthy subjects. *Biological Psychiatry, 78*(8), 544–553.
Schmid, Y., & Liechti, M. E. (2018). Long-lasting subjective effects of LSD in normal subjects. *Psychopharmacology, 235*(2), 535–545.
Smart, R. G., Storm, T., Baker, E. F., & Solursh, L. (1966). A controlled study of lysergide in the treatment of alcoholism. 1. The effects on drinking behavior. *Quarterly Journal of Studies on Alcohol, 27*(3), 469–482.
Soskin, R. A. (1973). The use of LSD in time-limited psychotherapy. *Journal of Nervous and Mental Disorders, 157*(6), 410–419.
Stamets, P. (1996). *Psilocybin mushrooms of the world*. Berkeley, CA: Ten Speed Press.
Stenbæk, D. S., Madsen, M. K., Ozenne, B., Kristiansen, S., Burmester, D., Erritzoe, D., et al. (2021). Brain serotonin 2A receptor binding predicts subjective temporal and mystical effects of psilocybin in healthy humans. *Journal of Psychopharmacology, 35*(4), 459–468.
Strassman, R. J. (1996). Human psychopharmacology of N,N-dimethyltryptamine. *Behavioural Brain Research, 73*(1–2), 121–124.
Strassman, R. J., & Qualls, C. R. (1994). Dose-response study of N,N-dimethyltryptamine in humans. I. Neuroendocrine, autonomic, and cardiovascular effects. *Archives of General Psychiatry, 51*(2), 85–97.
Strassman, R. J., Qualls, C. R., & Berg, L. M. (1996). Differential tolerance to biological and subjective effects of four closely spaced doses of N,N-dimethyltryptamine in humans. *Biological Psychiatry, 39*(9), 784–795.
Strassman, R. J., Qualls, C. R., Uhlenhuth, E. H., & Kellner, R. (1994). Dose-response study of N,N-dimethyltryptamine in humans. II. Subjective effects and preliminary results of a new rating scale. *Archives of General Psychiatry, 51*(2), 98–108.
Strickland, J. C., Garcia-Romeu, A., & Johnson, M. W. (2020). Set and setting: A randomized study of different musical genres in supporting psychedelic therapy. *ACS Pharmacology & Translational Science, 4*(2), 472–478.
Studerus, E., Gamma, A., Kometer, M., & Vollenweider, F. X. (2012). Prediction of psilocybin response in healthy volunteers. *PLoS One, 7*(2), e30800.
Studerus, E., Kometer, M., Hasler, F., & Vollenweider, F. X. (2011). Acute, subacute and long-term subjective effects of psilocybin in healthy humans: A pooled analysis of experimental studies. *Journal of Psychopharmacology, 25*(11), 1434–1452.
Testa, M., Fillmore, M. T., Norris, J., Abbey, A., Curtin, J. J., Leonard, K. E., et al. (2006). Understanding alcohol expectancy effects: Revisiting the placebo condition. *Alcoholism: Clinical and Experimental Research, 30*(2), 339–348.
Tylš, F., Páleníček, T., & Horáček, J. (2014). Psilocybin- -summary of knowledge and new perspectives. *European Neuropsychopharmacology, 24*(3), 342–356.
Valle, M., Maqueda, A. E., Rabella, M., Rodríguez-Pujadas, A., Antonijoan, R. M., Romero, S., et al. (2016). Inhibition of alpha oscillations through serotonin-2A receptor activation underlies the visual effects of ayahuasca in humans. *European Neuropsychopharmacology, 26*(7), 1161–1175.
Vollenweider, F. X., Vollenweider-Scherpenhuyzen, M. F., Bäbler, A., Vogel, H., & Hell, D. (1998). Psilocybin induces schizophrenia-like psychosis in humans via a serotonin-2 agonist action. *Neuroreport, 9*(17), 3897–3902.

Wasson, R. G. (1957). Seeking the magic mushroom. *Life*, *42*(19), 100–120.

Wasson, R. G. (1980). *The wondrous mushroom. Mycolatry in mesoamerica.* New York, NY: McGraw-Hill Book Company.

Yaden, D. B., & Griffiths, R. R. (2020). The subjective effects of psychedelics are necessary for their enduring therapeutic effects. *ACS Pharmacology & Translational Science*, *4*(2), 568–572.

CHAPTER FIVE

Stimulus functions of nicotine

Mark G. LeSage[a,b,*]
[a]Hennepin Healthcare Research Institute, Minneapolis, MN, United States
[b]Departments of Medicine, Pharmacology, and Psychology, University of Minnesota, Minneapolis, MN, United States
*Corresponding author: e-mail address: lesag002@umn.edu

Contents

1. Introduction 134
2. Stimulus functions of nicotine 137
  2.1 Respondent stimulus functions 138
  2.2 Operant stimulus functions: Nicotine as a consequent stimulus 143
  2.3 Operant stimulus functions: Nicotine as an antecedent stimulus 150
3. Role of stimulus functions in tobacco use theory 157
4. Conclusion 159
Acknowledgments 161
Conflict of interest statement 161
References 161

Abstract

Behavioral pharmacology has made vital contributions to the concepts and methods used in tobacco and other drug use research, and is largely responsible for the now generally accepted notion that nicotine is the primary component in tobacco that engenders and maintains tobacco use. One of the most important contributions of behavioral pharmacology to the science of drug use is the notion that drugs can act as environmental stimuli that control behavior in many of the same ways as other stimuli (e.g., visual, gustatory, olfactory). The purpose of this chapter is to provide an overview of research that illustrates the respondent and operant stimulus functions of nicotine, using a contemporary taxonomy of stimulus functions as a general framework. Each function is formally defined and examples from research on the behavioral pharmacology of nicotine are presented. Some of the factors that modulate each function are also discussed. The role of nicotine's stimulus functions in operant and respondent theories of tobacco use is examined and some suggestions for future research are presented. The chapter illustrates how a taxonomy of stimulus functions can guide conceptions of tobacco use and direct research and theory accordingly.

Advances in Pharmacology, Volume 93
ISSN 1054-3589
https://doi.org/10.1016/bs.apha.2021.11.001

Abbreviations

ACTH adrenocorticotropic hormone
AO abolishing operation
CORT corticosterone
CPA conditioned place aversion
CPP conditioned place preference
CR conditioned response
CS conditioned stimulus
CTA conditioned taste aversion
EO establishing operation
FI fixed interval
FR fixed ratio
i.p. intraperitoneal
i.v. intravenous
ICSS intracranial self-stimulation
MO motivating operation
NSA nicotine self-administration
PR progressive ratio
s.c. subcutaneous
S^{Δ} S-delta, an antecedent stimulus correlated the absence of a consequence
S^{D} discriminative stimulus
S^{D-} discriminative stimulus correlated with punishment
S^{D+} discriminative stimulus correlated with reinforcement
UC unconditioned conditioner
UR unconditioned response
US unconditioned stimulus
VI variable interval

1. Introduction

Worldwide, 1.1 billion adults smoke cigarettes (WHO, 2019), and 14% (34.1 million) of adults in the United States currently smoked cigarettes in 2019 (Cornelius, Wang, Jamal, Loretan, & Neff, 2020). Although smoking initiation in youth has been declining since 2011, 4.6% of high school and 1.6% of middle school students still smoke cigarettes (Gentzke et al., 2019, 2020). Each day, 1,600 youth in the United States try their first cigarette (SAMHSA, 2020). In addition, there has been a marked rise in use of electronic nicotine delivery systems (ENDS, i.e., electronic cigarettes) over the past decade, especially among youth. For example, past 30-day ENDS use increased by over 11-fold (from 1.5% to 16%) among adolescents in the U.S. between 2011–2015, and nearly doubled between 2017–2018

(Miech, Johnston, O'Malley, Bachman, & Patrick, 2019; NIDA, 2018). This 1-year rise in ENDS use was greater than that for any other drug of abuse in the history of NIDA's Monitoring the Future survey (45 years), and ENDS use now surpasses combustible cigarette, alcohol, marijuana, and other substance use in youth (Miech et al., 2019; NIDA, 2018; Singh et al., 2016; Stratton, Kwan, & Eaton, 2018). More recent reports show some decline in ENDS use among high school students from 2019 to 2020 (27.5–19.6%, respectively), but use remains high (Wang et al., 2021). Although the harm of ENDS is not yet fully understood, harm from combusted tobacco products is clear. Cigarette smoking causes numerous diseases, including cardiovascular disease, stroke, type 2 diabetes, chronic obstructive pulmonary disease, and numerous forms of cancer (USDHHS, 2010, 2014). Consequently, combusted tobacco use in the United States is associated with over 450,000 deaths and over $300 billion in healthcare spending annually (Xu, Bishop, Kennedy, Simpson, & Pechacek, 2015). In light of these issues, research on use of both combusted tobacco products and ENDS remains a major public health priority.

Behavioral pharmacology has made critical contributions to our current understanding of tobacco and other drug use (Henningfield, Buchhalter, & Fant, 2016; Henningfield, Smith, Kleykamp, Fant, & Donny, 2016). The field of behavioral pharmacology emerged in the mid-1950s from a merger of the concepts and methods of the experimental analysis of behavior and traditional pharmacology to explain the behavioral effects of drugs. Discussions of the details of its emergence and specific features are provided elsewhere and are beyond the scope of this chapter (Branch, 1991; Pickens, 1977; Poling & Byrne, 2000; Thompson & Schuster, 1968). Briefly, behavioral pharmacology borrows several methodological principles from the experimental analysis of behavior, such as use of within-subjects designs, direct and repeated measures of behavior, experimental rather than statistical control of extraneous variables, and preference for visual rather than statistical analysis of data (Poling & Byrne, 2000). Concepts and methods borrowed from pharmacology include recognizing that drugs have multiple effects, the pharmacokinetics of a drug are powerful determinants of those effects, drug effects are dose dependent, and that comprehensive understanding of drug effects therefore requires analysis of dose-response relationship of those effects. A vital feature of behavioral pharmacology is its fundamental tenet that the behavioral effects of drugs are interesting and important in their own right, not as a sign of underlying cognitive or neuropharmacological processes. The primary interests of behavioral pharmacologists are elucidating a drugs behavioral mechanisms of action and the environmental variables that modulate the behavioral effects of drugs (Poling & Byrne, 2000; Thompson & Schuster, 1968).

Behavioral mechanisms of action refer to how a drug interacts with normal or ongoing behavioral processes (not physiological or neuropharmacological ones), including the respondent (i.e., Pavlovian or classical) and operant conditioning processes that engender and maintain the behavior of organisms (Catania, 1992; Mazur, 1990). One of the most influential contributions of behavioral pharmacology is the concept that drugs can serve as environmental stimuli that control behavior in the same ways as other types of stimuli (e.g., visual, auditory, Thompson & Pickens, 1971). The procedures developed to demonstrate this concept (e.g., drug self-administration, drug discrimination) have been widely adopted in other fields (e.g., neuroscience (Koob & Volkow, 2010)). They are also routinely used by pharmaceutical companies for medication development, and government agencies like the FDA and Drug Enforcement Agency (DEA) rely on them to regulate medications, controlled substances, and tobacco products (Food and Drug Administration, 2017). Research on the stimulus functions of nicotine is also largely responsible for the now generally-accepted notion that nicotine is the primary constituent in tobacco products responsible for their use (Donny et al., 2012; Goldberg, Spealman, Risner, & Henningfield, 1983; Henningfield, Buchhalter, et al., 2016; Henningfield & Goldberg, 1983a; LeSage, Smethells, & Harris, 2018; Stolerman & Jarvis, 1995). Review of this research is not the focus of this chapter, as excellent reviews of it have already been provided (Stolerman & Jarvis, 1995). The purpose of this chapter is to provide an overview of research demonstrating the various stimulus functions of nicotine and illustrate how delineating those functions has shaped conceptions of tobacco use and guided research and theory accordingly.

Although the scope of stimulus functions covered in this chapter is broad, the scope of discussing each function is necessarily limited. Because the concepts and principles of behavioral pharmacology are the springboard for this review, the neuropharmacological mechanisms mediating nicotine's stimulus functions are especially beyond the scope of this review. Where appropriate, readers are directed to more exhaustive reviews of the literature on a particular stimulus function. The primary focus will be on preclinical research in nonhumans, where more stimulus functions have been studied under controlled experimental conditions. Given that scientists in other fields (e.g., neuroscience) often use some of the procedures described in this chapter, one purpose of this chapter is to familiarize those scientists with the broader scope of the concepts and methods used to study the stimulus functions of drugs. Another purpose is to provide an overview of research in this area to behavioral pharmacologists with an interest in the stimulus functions of drugs, but who may not keep abreast of the nicotine and tobacco use literature. The chapter is also intended to acquaint readers who are interested in the behavioral effects of drugs generally, but may not be familiar with the concept of stimulus functions and the terminology used to describe them. The author assumes readers have some familiarity with the basic methods used in behavioral pharmacology (e.g., schedules of reinforcement).

2. Stimulus functions of nicotine

A current taxonomy used by behavior analysts to categorize the stimulus functions of non-drug stimuli provides a basis for the following framework for categorizing the stimulus functions of nicotine (Laraway, Snycerski, Michael, & Poling, 2003; Michael, 1995, 2004; Schlinger & Blakely, 1994). It includes the same functions that have been formally reviewed previously (Thompson & Pickens, 1971), but extends the analysis to other ones that have been clarified more recently (e.g., motivating operations, Laraway et al., 2003). Within this framework, stimuli are defined as energy changes that affect an organism through its receptors. In other words, they are the afferent neural input to and within the central nervous system (Eikelboom & Stewart, 1982; Michael, 2004). Responses are defined as the action of an organisms effectors, which include striated muscles, smooth muscles, and glands. In other words, they are the activity of non-neural tissue (Eikelboom & Stewart, 1982; Michael, 2004).

Stimulus functions of nicotine will be categorized based on (a) the type of behavior involved (respondent or operant), (b) their provenance of control (whether a conditioning/learning history is required), and (c) their effect on behavior (increase or decrease). Respondent and operant behaviors are distinguished according to the relative importance of the stimuli that precede (antecedent) or follow the behavior (consequence). That is, respondent behavior is primarily controlled by antecedent stimuli and relatively insensitive to its consequences, whereas operant behavior is primarily controlled by its consequences. Although antecedent stimuli play an important role in operant behavior, they acquire their control by being correlated with the consequences of behavior. Each stimulus function will be formally defined, then illustrated by examples from research on the behavioral pharmacology of nicotine and tobacco. Some of the factors that modulate each stimulus function will also be discussed.

2.1 Respondent stimulus functions

2.1.1 Unconditioned stimulus (US)

A US is a stimulus that elicits a response without a learning (i.e., conditioning) history. The response that a US elicits is an unconditioned response (UR). The functional relation between a US and UR is referred to as an unconditioned reflex. For example, a puff of air to the eye is a US that elicits an eyeblink UR in humans with no learning history required. Similarly, acute nicotine or smoking is a US that can elicit numerous URs in humans and nonhumans, including an increase in blood pressure and heart rate (Nishikawa & Tsujimoto, 1975; Tsai, Byun, Shin, & Alexander, 2020), nausea and vomiting (McMahon, 2019; Seyler, Pomerleau, Fertig, Hunt, & Parker, 1986; Spealman, 1983; Spealman & Goldberg, 1982), tremors (Kunisawa et al., 2017, 2018; Shiffman et al., 1983), and seizures (Faulcon, Rudy, Limpert, Wang, & Murphy, 2020; Miner & Collins, 1989; Spealman & Goldberg, 1982; Tunock et al., 2001). In rodents, nicotine also decreases locomotor activity in nicotine-naïve rodents exposed to a novel environment (Bevins & Besheer, 2001; Clarke & Kumar, 1983; Stolerman, Garcha, & Mirza, 1995; Walter & Kuschinsky, 1989). Nicotine administration or smoking also elicits adrenal gland secretion of corticosterone (CORT), beta-endorphin and growth hormone (Caggiula et al., 1998; Tweed, Hsia, Lutfy, & Friedman, 2012; Xue et al., 2010), as well as pituitary gland secretion of prolactin and adrenocorticotropic hormone (ACTH, (Tweed et al., 2012).

Several factors modulate the qualitative and quantitative effect of a nicotine US. The likelihood of URs to non-drug USs is dependent on the intensity of the US. For example, higher acid concentrations of a solution on the tongue have a higher likelihood eliciting salivation (Catania, 1992). Similarly, the likelihood of nicotine-elicited URs is dependent upon the nicotine dose, nicotine content of cigarettes smoked, or number of cigarettes smoked (Arbol et al., 2000; Tweed et al., 2012; Xue et al., 2010). In addition, the dose required to elicit a UR differs between URs. For example, higher doses elicit seizures (2 mg/kg i.p.) than those that elicit tremors (1 mg/kg i.p.) or changes in locomotor activity in rats (0.1–0.4 mg/kg s.c., (Bevins, Besheer, & Pickett, 2001; Kunisawa et al., 2016; Tunock et al., 2001). Different nicotine doses can also elicit opposite URs. For example, relatively low nicotine doses associated with smoking elicit increases in heart rate and blood pressure, but high doses associated with toxicity (i.e., "green tobacco sickness") have the opposite effect on those responses (Benowitz, 2008; McMahon, 2019). The direction of the UR can be dependent on the history of exposure to nicotine or history of exposure to the test environment. As noted above, acute nicotine injection decreases locomotor activity in a novel environment in nicotine naïve rats, but increases locomotor activity in rats with a history of nicotine exposure or habituation to the test environment (Benwell & Balfour, 1992; Clarke & Kumar, 1983; Lobina et al., 2011). Finally, the magnitude of nicotine's CORT releasing effect is dependent on the history of nicotine exposure in the environment in which nicotine is administered. CORT release is relatively robust when nicotine is administered in a novel environment, but relatively weak in an environment in which repeated nicotine exposure has occurred (i.e., conditioned tolerance to CORT release occurs, (Caggiula et al., 1991).

2.1.2 Unconditioned conditioner (UC)

A US can alter the function of other stimuli through the process of respondent (i.e., Pavlovian or classical) conditioning. In respondent conditioning, pairing a neutral stimulus with a US results in the neutral stimulus becoming a conditioned stimulus (CS) that elicits a conditioned response (CR) that is often similar to the UR elicited by the US. The CR can also be opposite to the UR under certain conditions. The resulting relationship between a CS and CR is a conditioned reflex. The stimulus function of the US that establishes a CS in respondent conditioning is referred to as a UC (Michael, 1995, 2004). This terminology allows a taxonomic distinction between the function-altering effect of a stimulus, as a UC, from its response-eliciting effect, as a US. Nicotine has been shown to be a UC for engendering several types of neutral stimuli as CSs. For example, pairing a buzzer with intravenous nicotine injections (16 μg/kg) established the buzzer as a CS that could elicit conditioned increases in heart rate and blood pressure in dogs (Rush & Lang, 1970). In addition, pairing a unique environment with subcutaneous nicotine injections (e.g. 0.6 mg/kg) that elicit hyperactivity in rats established the environment as CS that alone could elicit hyperactivity (Bevins et al., 2001; Reid, Ho, & Berger, 1996; Walter & Kuschinsky, 1989). Pairing a complex stimulus with smoking under experimentally-controlled conditions can establish that stimulus as a CS that elicits increased heart rate (Lazev, Herzog, & Brandon, 1999). This supports the notion that the natural history of pairing certain stimuli with smoking (e.g., sight/smell/

taste of a cigarette, environments in which smoking usually occurs) establishes those stimuli as CSs capable of eliciting URs similar to those elicited by smoking itself. In addition, such CSs can serve operant stimulus functions, such as conditioned reinforcing or discriminative stimulus functions (discussed below). However, it is important to note that responses to a nicotine CS such as craving, urges, liking, or wanting are not CRs. These types of responses are verbal behaviors (vocal or textual self-report measures) that are controlled by (i.e., describe) the private stimuli (i.e., feelings) that co-occur with the CRs, not the CRs themselves (e.g., endocrine system activation). An extensive operant learning history shapes the verbal behaviors people emit in response to private events, and they are largely dependent on the presence of a listener (Skinner, 1957).

Conditioned place preference (CPP) and conditioned place aversion (CPA) are two popular preclinical models that illustrate another way that nicotine can serve as a UC (see (Bardo & Bevins, 2000). They are unique from the examples above, because, although they involve stimulus-stimulus pairings, they do not involve conditioning of a reflex per se. Although specific procedures vary between studies, a CPP model generally involves differentially pairing two distinct environments with the presence or absence of nicotine. The environments are typically two compartments of a rectangular box, in which different stimuli are present in each compartment (e.g., different flooring material, wall colors or patterns, or olfactory cues). Conditioning involves sessions during which a rodent is exposed to nicotine while contained in one compartment alternating with sessions during which the subject is contained in the other compartment without nicotine (i.e., saline is administered). Following several pairings, the subject is given access to both compartments in a drug-free state and the time spent in each compartment is measured. Several studies using this procedure have shown that rodents increase the amount of time spent in the nicotine-paired compartment relative to the other compartment, indicating a preference for the stimuli in the nicotine-paired compartment (Fudala, Teoh, & Iwamoto, 1985; Shoaib, Stolerman, & Kumar, 1994; Vastola, Douglas, Varlinskaya, & Spear, 2002). This is typically considered by scientists who use this model as evidence that nicotine has "rewarding/pleasurable" effects because it is typical for organisms to approach and maintain contact with stimuli that have been associated with "rewarding/pleasurable" events.

As mentioned above, it is important to note that CPP differs from other respondently conditioned behaviors because it is not a conditioned reflex per se. That is, time spent in the nicotine-paired compartment is not a UR that is conditioned to be elicited by a CS (the nicotine-paired compartment), because nicotine as US does not elicit that form of response. The time spent in a compartment is only a proxy or sign of the quality of the sensory effects (i.e., afferent input) of nicotine. Therefore, what is presumably conditioned in a CPP assay is the ability of the nicotine-paired stimuli to elicit "rewarding" sensory/perceptual effects similar to nicotine (cf. conditioned visual or auditory sensations, (Ellson, 1941; Powers, Mathys, & Corlett, 2017), not a response per se (i.e., action of an effector, Eikelboom & Stewart, 1982).

The same procedures for CPP can be used for CPA to study the aversive effects of nicotine. In this case, a decrease in time spent in the nicotine-paired compartment indicates a conditioned aversion to the nicotine-paired stimuli (Jorenby, Steinpreis, Sherman, & Baker, 1990; Risinger & Oakes, 1995). This presumably indicates nicotine has aversive sensory effects, because organisms typically avoid stimuli associated with aversive events. Nicotine-induced conditioned taste aversion (CTA) is another example of nicotine serving as a UC to study aversive effects of nicotine (for review see Verendeev & Riley, 2012). In this model, a subject is provided access to a novel solution to taste/consume, followed by administration of nicotine. After several such pairings, the subject avoids consuming the solution in a drug-free state, presumably because the prior pairing with nicotine conditions the taste (and other correlated stimuli) to elicit aversive sensory effects (not a CR per se) similar to that elicited by nicotine (Iwamoto & Williamson, 1984; Rinker, Busse, & Riley, 2008).

Several factors can modulate the UC effects of nicotine. The nicotine dose determines whether a CPP (relatively low doses) or CPA (relatively high doses) is conditioned (Risinger & Oakes, 1995), and whether conditioned hyperactivity can be established (Bevins et al., 2001; Bevins & Palmatier, 2003). Preexposure to nicotine has been shown to facilitate development of CPP and conditioned hyperactivity (Bevins & Palmatier, 2003; Shoaib et al., 1994) but weaken CTA (Iwamoto & Williamson, 1984). The temporal relation between a CS and nicotine influences development of conditioned hyperactivity. For example, nicotine administered 15 min after placement in the chamber CS is ineffective at conditioning hyperactivity, whereas conditioning was weak or strongest when nicotine was administered 15 min or immediately before the placement in the chamber, respectively (Bevins, Eurek, & Besheer, 2005). Finally, exposure to a previously nicotine-paired CS that elicits hyperactivity enhances conditioning and slows extinction of a second nicotine-paired CS (Bevins & Palmatier, 2003).

2.1.3 Conditioned stimulus (CS)

A CS is a stimulus that elicits a response only after a learning history. That learning history is the same respondent or Pavlovian conditioning process described above. To establish nicotine as a CS, nicotine would initially need to be a neutral stimulus that *does not* elicit the UR of interest. After nicotine is paired with a US that *does* elicit the UR of interest, if nicotine alone elicits the UR, then nicotine would be considered a CS and the response to it a CR. Much less research has been done on the CS function of nicotine compared to other stimulus functions. The way it is typically studied is by use of a goal-tracking assay (for review see, Bevins & Palmatier, 2004). In this assay, rats are exposed to nicotine or saline in alternating sessions. During nicotine sessions, rats are placed in chamber after nicotine administration and receive intermittent deliveries of a sucrose solution from a liquid dipper. During saline sessions, rats are placed in the chamber after saline administration and no sucrose is delivered. After several sessions, the rate of dipper entries (goal tracking) prior to the first sucrose delivery is significantly higher during nicotine sessions compared to saline sessions. Dipper entries during nicotine sessions decline when sucrose is no longer presented (extinctions occurs), is sensitive to nicotine dose and pre-session injection interval, and partially generalizes to other stimulant drugs (Besheer, Palmatier, Metschke, & Bevins, 2004). The interpretation of these findings is that, via respondent conditioning, pairing nicotine with a sucrose US establishes nicotine as a CS for the dipper entry CR (Bevins & Palmatier, 2004).

However, an interpretation of these findings should not be solely in terms of respondent conditioning. In the presence of nicotine, the putative UR/CR (dipper entry) necessarily occurs immediately before the the putative US (taste of sucrose) when the US is delivered. This relationship, the basis of the conditioning, is not a reflex because the dipper entry response precedes the US (taste of sucrose). One cannot establish a conditioned reflex without an unconditioned reflex. Other sensory modalities of sucrose delivery (e.g., sound of the dipper motor) might be a US for head entry initially (as approaching a novel sound), but habituation occurs without sucrose (as occurs during saline sessions). It is possible that dipper entries are, at least in part, an operant behavior adventitiously reinforced by sucrose delivery, and that nicotine becomes a discriminative stimulus for dipper entries (see below). Indeed, scientists have long acknowledged a joint role of respondent and operant conditioning in goal tracking behavior (Holland, 1979). Although research using the goal tracking assay to study the CS function of nicotine has made vital contributions to understanding the stimulus functions of nicotine, further research in this area requires clearer examples involving unambiguous US–UR reflexes. For example, perhaps a dose of nicotine that normally doesn't elicit changes in respiration might come to suppress respiration after being paired with a stimulus (e.g., opioid administration) that does elicit that response (cf. Revusky, Davey, & Zagorski, 1989).

2.1.4 Conditioned conditioner (CC)

Like a US, a CS can alter the function of other stimuli that are paired with it. In this case, higher-order respondent conditioning takes place, in which pairing a neutral stimulus with an established CS in turn establishes the neutral stimulus as another CS that elicits the same CR. The resulting relationship between the new CS and CR is a second-order conditioned reflex. Because the conditioning function of the CS in higher-order conditioning requires a learning history, this stimulus function is referred to as a CC. As noted above for the UC function, the CC term allows a taxonomic distinction between the function-altering effect of a stimulus, as a CC, from its response-eliciting effect, as a CS. To the present author's knowledge, such higher-order conditioning with a nicotine CS has not been demonstrated. Using the example above, if pairing an auditory stimulus with a nicotine CS that has been conditioned to elicit respiratory depression (by virtue of being paired with an opioid infusion) comes to elicit respiratory depression itself, nicotine would be considered a CC.

2.2 Operant stimulus functions: Nicotine as a consequent stimulus

2.2.1 Unconditioned reinforcer

An unconditioned reinforcer is a stimulus that, when presented (or removed/reduced in intensity) after a response, produces an increase in the frequency of that response without a learning (i.e., conditioning) history. Reinforcers that are presented after a response are referred to as positive reinforcers, while those that are removed/reduced after a response are called negative reinforcers. The most common way of demonstrating nicotine's positive reinforcing effects is with an intravenous nicotine self-administration (NSA) assay, in which subjects emit a response (e.g., lever press) that results in an intravenous infusion of nicotine. Initial evidence of nicotine reinforcement was mixed (Dougherty, Miller, Todd, & Kostenbauder, 1981; Henningfield & Goldberg, 1983b), but with refinements in procedures and experimental design, it became clearer that nicotine can serve as a positive

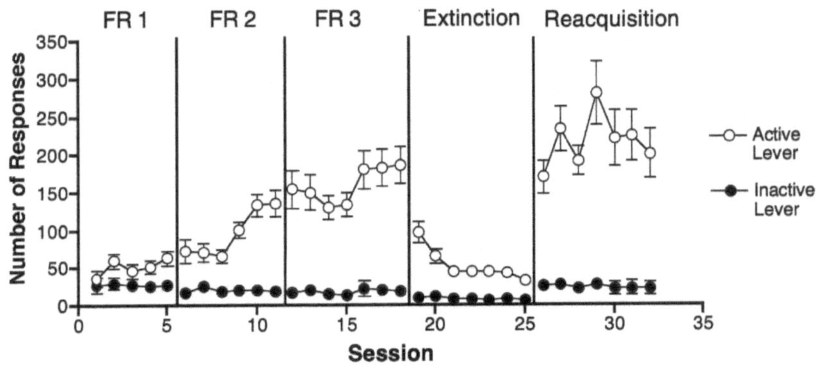

Fig. 1 Mean (±SEM) response rates for intravenous infusions of nicotine (0.01 mg/kg per infusion) in rats with access to nicotine 23 h/day. Open circles represent response rates on an active lever that produced nicotine infusions. Closed circles represent rates on an inactive lever that had no programmed consequence. The number of responses required per infusion is indicated by the fixed ratio (FR) value, which remained at FR 3 during extinction and reacquisition. *Data are redrawn from LeSage, M. G., Keyler, D. E., Shoeman, D., Raphael, D., Collins, G., & Pentel, P. R. (2002). Continuous nicotine infusion reduces nicotine self-administration in rats with 23-h/day access to nicotine. Pharmacology, Biochemistry, and Behavior, 72(1–2), 279–289 with permission of the publisher.*

reinforcer in a wide range of species, including rats, mice, dogs, monkeys, baboons, and humans (Henningfield & Goldberg, 1983b; Matta et al., 2007). For example, Fig. 1 shows data from a study in rats self-administering nicotine (0.01 mg/kg/infusion, i.v.) with relatively unlimited (23 h/day) access to the drug (LeSage et al., 2002). Pressing an active lever produced nicotine infusions, while pressing an inactive lever had no programmed consequence. Initially, a single lever press was required to produce an infusion (i.e., a fixed ratio (FR) 1 schedule was in effect). As robust active lever pressing developed the response requirement was gradually increased to two (FR 2) and three (FR 3) responses per infusion. Then, after active lever responding stabilized, extinction was arranged by substituting saline for nicotine. Nicotine was then reintroduced after responding stabilized during extinction.

Three features of these data demonstrate that nicotine was serving as a positive reinforcer. First, higher rates of responding were emitted on the active lever than the inactive lever. Second, response rates differentially increased on the active lever as the response requirement increased. Third, active lever pressing was significantly lower in the absence of nicotine than when nicotine was available (i.e., extinction was evident). Decreases in NSA also occur when nicotine's effects are blocked pharmacologically by administering the nicotinic acetylcholine receptor antagonist mecamylamine (Corrigall & Coen, 1989; Spealman & Goldberg, 1982). The differential changes in response rate on the active lever is perhaps the most critical evidence that nicotine is serving as a reinforcer, as it shows that responding was not changing due to other plausible mechanisms, like nicotine-elicited increases in locomotor activity, which can't be ruled out by an extinction effect alone.

Several factors can modulate the positive reinforcing function of nicotine. For example, NSA varies with the unit nicotine dose, exhibiting an inverted-U shaped dose-response curve. Fig. 2 shows the nicotine dose-response curve for rats using the same i.v. NSA procedures as for Fig. 1, except that rats were trained with a higher unit dose (0.06 mg/kg) and the unit dose was then gradually decreased (weekly) until extinction was evident (Grebenstein, Burroughs, Roiko, Pentel, & LeSage, 2015). A clear inverted-U shape curve is evident with marked (>10-fold) variability between subjects in the threshold (lowest) reinforcing dose that maintains responding above saline levels. Across low to moderate doses, the reinforcing effect of nicotine increases to a peak near 0.01 mg/kg. Further

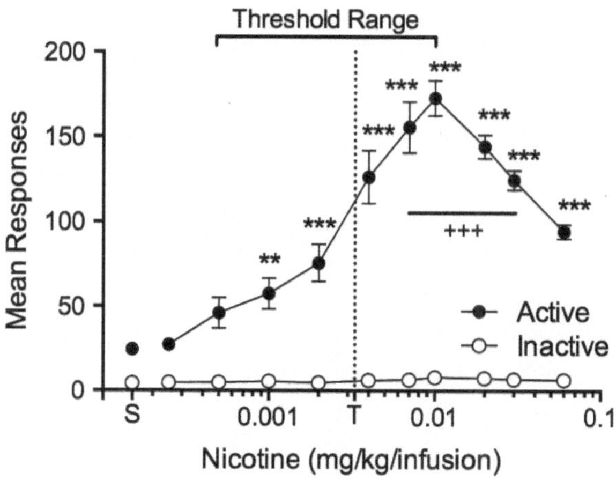

Fig. 2 Mean (±SEM) number of responses on the active and inactive levers in rats trained to self-administer 0.06 mg/kg/infusion i.v. The unit dose for NSA was reduced weekly until responding was within range of responding during saline extinction (S). The vertical dotted line indicates the mean threshold reinforcing unit dose (T). Significant differences from saline, ** $P < 0.01$, *** $P < 0.001$. Significant differences from 0.06 mg/kg baseline, +++ $P < 0.001$. *Data are from Grebenstein, P. E., Burroughs, D., Roiko, S. A., Pentel, P. R., & LeSage, M. G. (2015). Predictors of the nicotine reinforcement threshold, compensation, and elasticity of demand in a rodent model of nicotine reduction policy. Drug and Alcohol Dependence, 151, 181–193 with permission of the publisher.*

increases result in a decrease in responding because fewer infusions are needed to maintain brain nicotine concentrations at a reinforcing level and/or aversive effects of very high nicotine doses/brain concentrations punish responding. However, the dose-response curve can be relatively flat under other conditions (e.g., prior food training, (Corrigall & Coen, 1989; Donny, Caggiula, Knopf, & Brown, 1995). The dose range within which nicotine serves as a positive reinforcer is very similar across species, including humans (e.g., 0.01–0.03 mg/kg/infusion, i.v., (Matta et al., 2007; Rose & Corrigall, 1997). Longer infusion durations (i.e., delayed reinforcement) of the same dose can decrease NSA (Wing & Shoaib, 2013); but see (Sorge & Clarke, 2009). Other factors, such as food deprivation or prior training of the response (i.e., "food training"), have been shown to facilitate acquisition of NSA in nonhumans, but they are not necessary for nicotine to serve as a positive reinforcer (e.g., Donny et al., 1998; Garcia, Lê, & Tyndale, 2014; Shoaib, Schindler, & Goldberg, 1997). Finally, the presence of exteroceptive stimuli paired with nicotine infusions can significantly enhance acquisition and maintenance of NSA in rats and monkeys (Caggiula et al., 2002; Goldberg, Spealman, & Goldberg, 1981; Sorge, Pierre, & Clarke, 2009). This finding is thought to reflect multiple stimulus functions of nicotine acting simultaneously (Caggiula et al., 2009), as will be discussed in Section 3.

A nicotine reinforcer can establish patterns of behavior similar to other drug and non-drug reinforcers under various schedules of reinforcement. For example, typical post-reinforcement pauses followed by high steady running rates can develop under FR schedules (Goldberg et al., 1983; Risner & Goldberg, 1983; Shoaib, et al., 1997), post-reinforcement pauses followed by an accelerating ("scallop-like") pattern of responding can develop under fixed interval (FI) schedules (Ator & Griffiths, 1983; Spealman & Goldberg, 1982), and persistent high rates of responding can be maintained under second-order schedules (Goldberg et al., 1981; Spealman & Goldberg, 1982; Wing & Shoaib, 2010b). Finally, despite plentiful evidence that nicotine can serve as positive reinforcer, it is also clear that nicotine exhibits lower reinforcing efficacy compared to other drugs of abuse, as indicated by lower breaking points under progressive ratio (PR) schedules, lower preference under concurrent choice procedures, and lower economic demand for nicotine compared to cocaine (Koffarnus & Winger, 2015; Manzardo, Rio, Stein, & Belluzzi, 2001; Risner & Goldberg, 1983). Given this relatively weak reinforcing function, acquisition and maintenance of robust nicotine self-administration can hinge on certain procedural variables (e.g., pairing infusions with a visual stimulus).

The aforementioned work by Goldberg and colleagues examining NSA under second-order schedules is particularly noteworthy. Under the second-order schedule they empoyed, a non-drug stimulus (e.g., illumination of a light) was presented under a unit schedule (FR 10) and nicotine delivery occurred with the non-drug stimulus when the unit schedule was completed after a fixed interval of time (FI 1 minute). By virtue of being paired with nicotine delivery, the non-drug stimulus acquired a conditioned reinforcing function that, alone, was capable of maintaining responding. Consequently, long sequences of responding could be maintained at high rates with minimal nicotine delivery, and responding was especially resistant to extinction when the nicotine-paired stimuli continued to be presented in the absence of nicotine. Given that smoking occurs under complex schedules of nicotine and non-drug stimulus delivery (e.g., visual, gustatory, and olfactory stimuli) and is quite resistant to extinction when the nicotine content in cigarettes is reduced (Donny et al., 2015; Donny, Houtsmuller, & Stitzer, 2007), NSA under second-order schedules of nicotine self-administration are thought to be more clinically relevant to smoking than simpler schedules (Schindler, Panlilio, & Goldberg, 2002). This work was pioneering and played a pivotal role in the scientific case that nicotine met criteria to be considered addictive (Stolerman & Jarvis, 1995) and provided a basis for current theories of tobacco use (see below). The importance of Goldberg's work has been discussed further by others (Henningfield, Smith, et al., 2016).

Nicotine can also serve as a negative reinforcer, in which case the removal or reduction in nicotine exposure following a response increases the frequency of that response. For example, Spealman (1983) showed that monkeys could learn to press a lever to suspend a schedule of response-independent i.v. nicotine delivery (30–56 μg/kg/infusion every 20 s, 30 injection limit) for 60 s. Rates and patterns of lever pressing were similar to those maintained by suspension of a similar schedule of electric shock delivery. Intravenous nicotine also served as a negative reinforcer in humans under a similar schedule of i.v. nicotine delivery (Henningfield & Goldberg, 1983a). To the author's knowledge, no other studies have directly examined the negative reinforcing function of nicotine. Numerous studies show that nicotine self-administration or smoking can reduce nicotine withdrawal signs or symptoms, and this can be mistakenly considered evidence of a negative reinforcing function of nicotine. However, it is the withdrawal state (an interoceptive stimulus), not nicotine, that is the negative reinforcer in such studies, because that is the stimulus being removed/reduced. Nicotine still serves as a positive reinforcer in these cases.

2.2.2 Conditioned reinforcer

A conditioned reinforcer is a stimulus that, when presented (or removed/reduced) after a response, produces an increase in the frequency of that response only after a learning history that involves pairing the stimulus with delivery of an established reinforcer. For example, if presentation of a neutral auditory stimulus has been repeatedly paired with (i.e., followed by) food delivery to a rat, and subsequent presentation of that stimulus alone after a lever press increases the frequency of lever pressing, the auditory stimulus would be considered a conditioned reinforcer. For nicotine to be considered a conditioned reinforcer, a nicotine dose that is normally is not self-administered (i.e., not reinforcing) would need to be repeatedly paired with an established reinforcer and subsequently shown to increase a behavior that leads to its delivery alone (i.e., to be self-administered).

To the author's knowledge, no preclinical studies have shown that a *non-reinforcing* nicotine dose can be established as a conditioned reinforcer. However, one preclinical study has shown that pairing a *reinforcing* dose of nicotine with another unconditioned reinforcer (sucrose) can enhance the reinforcing efficacy of nicotine (Charntikov, Pittenger, Swalve, Barrett, & Bevins, 2020). In that study, rats were trained to press a lever to self-administer nicotine alone or nicotine paired with sucrose delivery (another primary reinforcer). Then, they were trained to emit a different response (nose poke) for nicotine alone under a PR schedule. Breaking points under the PR schedule were higher in rats trained with nicotine-sucrose than those trained with nicotine alone, suggesting that nicotine had acquired some degree of a conditioned reinforcing function in addition to its unconditioned reinforcing function by virtue of being paired with another reinforcer. Demonstration of this stimulus function may be difficult, because non-reinforcing doses of nicotine might also not be detectable (i.e., salient or discriminable).

2.2.3 Unconditioned punisher

An unconditioned punisher is a stimulus that, when presented (or removed/reduced) after a response, produces a decrease in the frequency of that response without a learning history. Punishers that are presented after a response are referred to as positive punishers, while those that are removed/reduced after a response are called negative punishers. The first preclinical demonstration of nicotine's punishing function was by Goldberg and Spealman (Goldberg & Spealman, 1983; Goldberg & Spealman, 1982). In that study, lever pressing by squirrel monkeys was maintained under a two-component multiple schedule. In one component (unpunished component), a green light was illuminated and responding was reinforced with food under an FR 30 schedule. In the other component (punished component), a red light was illuminated and the same FR 30 schedule was in effect, except that the first response in each FR also produced an i.v. infusion of saline or nicotine. When saline was delivered, response rates were similar between components. When nicotine was delivered (10–30 μg/kg/infusion), response rates were significantly reduced in the punished component but not in the unpunished component, indicating that nicotine served as a punisher. Patterns of responding were comparable to those produced under a similar schedule employing electric shock in the punished component. Others replicated this finding and also showed that the punishing effects of nicotine were similar to those of other drugs like histamine and β-carbolines (Takada, Barrett, Allen, Cook, & Katz, 1992). Nicotine has also been shown to punish remifentanil self-administration under a choice procedure (Koffarnus & Winger, 2015). Note that the punishing doses in these studies are similar to the same doses that served as a positive reinforcer in monkeys. The implication of these divergent effects will be discussed later in the chapter.

To the author's knowledge, no studies have been published that demonstrate nicotine serving a negative punisher function, in which a response removes or reduces access to nicotine and the frequency of that response decreases. This might be demonstrated by switching the contingencies used by LeSage (2009), in which reduced access to sucrose was a negative punisher for NSA in rats. In that study, rats were trained on a two component multiple FR 3 nicotine (0.03 mg/kg/infusion) FR 1 sucrose schedule. Responses on one lever produced nicotine while responses on another lever produced sucrose pellets. After responding stabilized, a concurrent FR 3 nicotine FR 1 sucrose schedule was arranged with the additional contingency that each lever press for nicotine postponed access to sucrose (another contingency was operative but not relevant here). This reduced lever pressing for nicotine, indicating that sucrose was a negative punisher of NSA. This contingency could simply be reversed to demonstrate a negative punishment effect of nicotine if postponing access to nicotine punished lever pressing for sucrose.

2.2.4 Conditioned punisher

A conditioned punisher is a stimulus that, when presented (or removed/reduced) after a response, produces a decrease in the frequency of that response only after a learning history that involves pairing the stimulus with delivery of an established punisher. For example, if a neutral auditory stimulus has been repeatedly paired with electric shock delivery to a rat and subsequent presentation of that stimulus alone after a lever press decreases the frequency of lever pressing, the auditory stimulus would be considered a conditioned punisher. To the author's knowledge, this stimulus function has not been studied with nicotine. In order to demonstrate it, a neutral dose of nicotine would need to be paired with an established punisher (e.g., electric shock delivery) and subsequently shown to reduce the frequency of a behavior that produces that nicotine dose. This could be demonstrated using procedures similar to Goldberg & Spealman (1982). After showing that an i. v. nicotine dose (e.g., 3 μg/kg/infusion) has no effect on food-maintained lever pressing in the punished component of the multiple schedule, punishing electric shocks could be paired with nicotine delivery in that component for several sessions. Subsequently, if nicotine delivery alone suppresses responding in that component, it would be evidence of a conditioned punishing effect of nicotine. However, this sort of study may be problematic, because known non-punishing nicotine doses in monkeys (e.g., ≥3 μg/kg/infusion i.v. (Goldberg & Spealman, 1983) are also below the known discrimination threshold for that species (Moerke, Zhu, Tyndale, Javors, & McMahon, 2017; Takada, Hagen, Cook, Goldberg, & Katz, 1988; Takada, Swedberg, Goldberg, & Katz, 1989). Thus, novel methods may be required to demonstrate this stimulus function, at least in monkeys.

2.3 Operant stimulus functions: Nicotine as an antecedent stimulus

2.3.1 Discriminative stimulus

A discriminative stimulus (S^D) is an antecedent stimulus that increases (or decreases) the frequency of a response because, in the past, that response has been reinforced (or punished) in the presence of that stimulus, and not reinforced (or punished) in the absence of that stimulus. Those S^Ds correlated with reinforcement can be symbolized S^{D+}, while those correlated with punishment can be symbolized S^{D-}. Antecedent stimuli correlated with the absence of a consequence (i.e., extinction) is typically symbolized S^{Δ}. For example, if a food-deprived rat has a history of receiving food when it presses a lever while a light is on (S^{D+}) but not when the light is off (S^{Δ}), and the frequency of lever pressing subsequently increases whenever the light is turned on and decreases when the light is turned off, the onset of the light would be considered an S^{D+}. Conversely, if a history of being shocked when the lever is pressed while the light is on (S^{D-}) but not when the light is off (S^{Δ}) leads to a decrease in lever pressing whenever the light is on and an increase when the light is off, the onset of the light would be considered an S^{D-}. The light off in both cases would be an S^{Δ}. As Poling and Byrne explain (Poling & Byrne, 2000), two conditions must be met for a drug to serve as an S^{D}: (1) the drug's effects must be detectable by the organism receiving it, and (2) that organism must have a history of being differentially reinforced (or punished) in the presence and absence of those drug effects.

Nicotine can be established as an S^{D+} using the drug discrimination assay. This assay was initially developed by Overton (Overton, 1991) using maze-running procedures. Morrison and Stephenson (Morrison & Stephenson, 1969) were the first to use an operant choice model to demonstrate nicotine as an S^{D+}. In this procedure, one response (e.g., right lever press) is differentially reinforced (e.g., with food or water) in the presence of nicotine (e.g., the interoceptive effects following nicotine administration) and a different response (e.g., left lever press) is reinforced in the absence of nicotine (i.e., vehicle administration). If, under extinction conditions, this history of differential reinforcement results in the subject emitting the nicotine-associated response more often following nicotine administration and emitting the vehicle-associated response more often following vehicle administration, then the interoceptive stimulus arising from nicotine administration can be said to be serving as an S^{D+}. Nicotine has been established as an S^{D+} in mice, rats, monkeys and humans using similar experimental procedures (for review, see Shoaib & Perkins, 2020; Smith & Stolerman, 2009).

After the discrimination is trained, other doses of the training drug can be substituted to obtain a generalization gradient. For example, Fig. 3 shows the percentage of responding on the nicotine lever in rats at the nicotine training dose (0.4 mg/kg, s.c.) and a range of lower doses that were substituted for the training dose (LeSage, Shelley, Ross, Carroll, & Corrigall, 2009). As the dose is decreased, the magnitude or salience of nicotine's interoceptive sensory effects become weaker and the percentage of responding shifts accordingly from the nicotine lever to the saline lever, and very low nicotine doses have little or no interoceptive effects (i.e., they "felt" like saline). Similarly, to the extent that substituting a different drug for nicotine evokes the same level of responding on the nicotine-paired lever, it indicates that drug produces similar interoceptive effects (i.e., that their effects "feel" similar to nicotine). Such drugs include other tobacco constituents (e.g., nornicotine, anabasine, anatabine (Caine et al., 2014), the smoking cessation drugs bupropion and varenicline (LeSage et al., 2009; Young & Glennon, 2002), and other

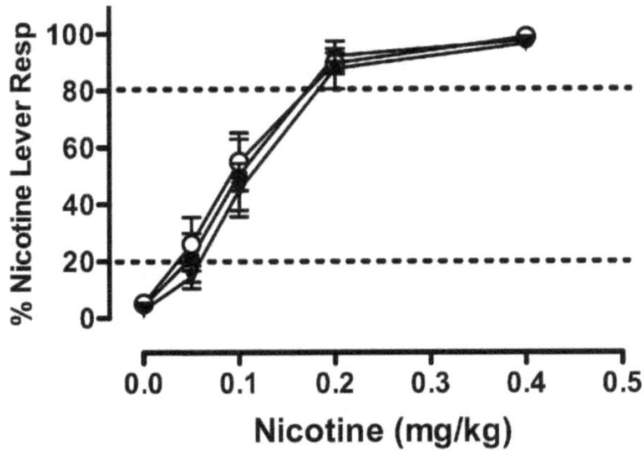

Fig. 3 Mean (±SEM) percentage of lever presses on the nicotine associated lever in rats trained to discriminate 0.4 mg/kg s.c. nicotine from saline at each of the indicated nicotine doses that were substituted for the training dose. Each dose-response curve was obtained in the same subjects prior to or after pretreatment with other drugs, indicating the stability of the discrimination across baseline phases. *Data are from LeSage, M. G., Shelley, D., Ross, J. T., Carroll, F. I., & Corrigall, W. A. (2009). Effects of the nicotinic receptor partial agonists varenicline and cytisine on the discriminative stimulus effects of nicotine in rats. Pharmacology, Biochemistry, and Behavior, 91(3), 461–467 with permission of the publisher.*

stimulants like cocaine and amphetamine (Gasior, Shoaib, Yasar, Jaszyna, & Goldberg, 1999; Stolerman & Garcha, 1989). Conversely, drugs that fail to substitute for nicotine are considered to have interoceptive stimulus effects that differ from nicotine, such as morphine (Stolerman, 1989), or possibly no interoceptive effects at all. The neuropharmacological mechanisms through which nicotine produces its discriminative stimulus effects are quite specific, and the nicotine discrimination assay has played a vital role in discovering the neural mechanisms mediating nicotine's subjective effects (Smith & Stolerman, 2009).

Numerous factors modulate the discriminative stimulus effects of nicotine (for an in-depth review, see (Smith & Stolerman, 2009). For example, lower training doses shift the nicotine dose-response curve to the left (lower ED_{50}), indicating an increase in sensitivity to the interoceptive stimulus effects of nicotine (Smith & Stolerman, 2009; Stolerman, Garcha, Pratt, & Kumar, 1984; Stolerman, Naylor, Elmer, & Goldberg, 1999). Longer pretreatment intervals (time between nicotine injection and discrimination testing) result in weaker discrimination, but rats can still exhibit some discriminative control of nicotine-lever responding (subjective effects) up to 60–120 min after a dose of 0.4 mg/kg (Hirschhorn & Rosecrans, 1974). Research on the effects of dose and pretreatement interval have suggested that the plasma nicotine concentration associated with the threshold discriminable (ED_{50}) nicotine dose in rats is 48 ng/mL, which is within range of concentrations reported in human smokers (10–50 ng/mL, (Hukkanen, Jacob, & Benowitz, 2005; Pratt, Stolerman, Garcha, Giardini, & Feyerabend, 1983) and those associated with reinforcing doses of nicotine in nonhumans (Donny et al., 2012; LeSage et al., 2002; Matta et al., 2007; Sofuoglu & LeSage, 2012). Nicotine is about an order of magnitude less potent for producing discriminative stimulus effects via the transdermal route compared to other routes (Craft & Howard, 1988). Finally, the schedule of reinforcement can modulate the nature of the nicotine discrimination dose-response curve. For example, nicotine discrimination in rats can be less sensitive to dose (i.e. dose-response curves are flatter) under FR schedules compared to variable interval (VI) schedules, and lower doses appear to maintain nicotine discrimination in monkeys trained under a schedule of electric shock avoidance compared to those trained under a schedule of food delivery (Moerke et al., 2017; Takada et al., 1988, 1989).

2.3.2 Motivating operation (MO)

The ability of a consequent stimulus to be reinforcing (or punishing) is not static. It can vary significantly over time in the same context or across contexts. The environmental events that alter the effectiveness of reinforcers (or punishers) are referred to as motivating operations (Laraway et al., 2003; Michael, 1993; Poling, Lotfizadeh, & Edwards, 2017). In contrast to an S^D, an MO alters the effectiveness of a reinforcer (or punisher), but is not correlated with its availability. As Schlinger (1993) explains, S^Ds and MOs are similar in that behavior is reinforceable (or punishable) in their presence and consequently can evoke (or suppress) behavior. But behavior must be extinguished in the absence of S^Ds for them to acquire and maintain control over behavior. Behavior can't be extinguished in the absence of an MO, because it's not reinforceable (or punishable). Hence, an S^D (and reinforcer/punisher) can only be effective when a relevant MO is operative. As Poling et al. (2017) explain in everyday terms, "MOs influence what an organism currently wants [or loathes] and discriminative stimuli indicate what is currently available to it." As such, nicotine can be an MO if it influences what an organism currently wants or loathes. MOs are categorized as establishing or abolishing operations, based on the direction in which they influence the effectiveness of the relevant consequence.

2.3.2.1 Establishing operation (EO)

An EO is a change in the environment that increases the momentary effectiveness of a reinforcer (or punisher) and increases (or decreases) any behavior that in the past has produced that reinforcer (or punisher). For example, water deprivation increases the reinforcing effectiveness of water and increases behaviors that in the past have produced water. The evidence of an increase in reinforcing effectiveness of water could include an increase in rate of water-maintained responding, choice of water over other reinforcers, breaking point under a PR schedule of water delivery, behavioral economic demand for water (i.e., resistance of consumption to increases in unit price of water), or rate of acquiring a new behavior that produces water, among others (Poling et al., 2017).

Many studies show that nicotine administration can be an EO for the reinforcing effectiveness of visual stimuli in rats. For example, noncontingent nicotine exposure increased response rate for a visual stimulus (cue light onset/house light offset) produced by lever pressing in rats under a FR schedule without affecting lever pressing that didn't produce the visual stimulus, indicating the increased response rate was not due to locomotor stimulant effects of nicotine (Constantin & Clarke, 2018; Donny et al., 2003; Wright, Ren, Constantin, & Clarke, 2018). Nicotine pretreatment also increased response rate for a visual stimulus in rats across a wide range of FR schedules (FR 1-32) and, consequently, increased several parameters of economic demand for the visual stimulus (Barrett & Bevins, 2012). Increased response rate for a visual stimulus has also been produced by nicotine pretreatment in rats under second-order and observing-response schedules (Raiff & Dallery, 2006, 2009; Wing & Shoaib, 2010a). Nicotine also facilitates acquisition of a new response with a complex visual-auditory conditioned reinforcer previously paired with a water reinforcer, as well as a visual conditioned reinforcer previously paired with nicotine (Olausson, Jentsch, & Taylor, 2004; Palmatier, Liu, et al., 2007). This EO function of nicotine can be observed with stimuli that are either unconditioned or conditioned reinforcers, and the magnitude of the effect of a nicotine EO is directly related to the baseline reinforcing effectiveness of a visual-auditory stimulus (Olausson et al., 2004; Palmatier, Matteson, et al., 2007; Raiff & Dallery, 2006; Wing & Shoaib, 2010a).

Nicotine can also be an EO for other types of stimuli. Numerous studies have shown that moderate doses of nicotine (0.1–0.3 mg/kg, s.c.) reduce the magnitude (milliampere of current) of electrical brain stimulation required to reinforce a wheel-turning response under a discrete-trial intracranial self-stimulation (ICSS) schedule in rats, indicating that nicotine can increase the reinforcing potency of electrical brain stimulation (Harris et al., 2015; Harrison, Gasparini, & Markou, 2002). Some studies suggest nicotine is an EO for sucrose reinforcement in rats, as indicated by an increase in breaking point under a PR schedule, which is directly related to the magnitude of the sucrose reinforcer (Kirshenbaum et al., 2015; Palmatier, O'Brien, & Hall, 2012). Nicotine has also been shown to increase the reinforcing efficacy of social stimuli in rats, as indicated by a higher breaking point under a PR schedule of social stimulus presentation compared to sucrose, and greater preference for social stimuli over sucrose in a choice assay (Martin et al., 2018). Smoking served as an EO for the punishing effect of point loss under an operant schedule of point delivery in humans, as indicated by a nicotine-dose related decrease in punished responding (Cherek & Bennett, 1991). Such punishment enhancing effects of nicotine have also been reported in rodents under schedules of electric shock punishment (Glowa, 1986; Morrison, 1969). Finally, administration of punishing i.v. nicotine doses can serve as an EO for its own removal/reduction as a negative reinforcer (Spealman, 1983), similar to how other forms of aversive stimulation (e.g., pain) increase the effectiveness of their removal as a negative reinforcer.

Nicotine deprivation (i.e., withdrawal) is an EO that increases the reinforcing effectiveness of nicotine. For example, intermittent periods of suspending NSA sessions results in higher rates of NSA compared to when NSA sessions are uninterrupted (O'Dell & Koob, 2007). Similarly, smoking deprivation (i.e., abstinence) in humans increases the number of cigarettes smoked (Griffiths & Henningfield, 1982; Zacny & Stitzer, 1985), number of puffs per cigarette (Rose, Jarvik, & Ananda, 1984), preference for higher nicotine concentrations in cigarettes (Rose et al., 1984), and preference for a nicotine inhaler over a placebo inhaler (Perkins, Grobe, Weiss, Fonte, & Caggiula, 1996). Nicotine withdrawal can also be an EO for non-nicotine reinforcers. For example, it can increase operant responding for and intake of food in rats and humans (Bunney, Burroughs, Hernandez, & LeSage, 2016; Epstein, Bulik, Perkins, Caggiula, & Rodefer, 1991; Grebenstein, Burroughs, Hernandez, & LeSage, 2015; Perkins, Epstein, Sexton, & Pastor, 1990; Spring, 2003; Spring, Wurtman, Gleason, Wurtman, & Kessler, 1991).

Nicotine deprivation can produce interoceptive effects (withdrawal symptoms) that can have stimulus functions of their own. For example, they can serve as a respondent US/UC in the CPA model discussed above. In this case, after the two environments in that model are differentially paired with nicotine withdrawal (precipitated by mecamylamine during chronic nicotine exposure), rodents will spend less time in the withdrawal-paired compartment than the unpaired compartment when they are not in withdrawal (Jackson, Martin, Changeux, & Damaj, 2008; Suzuki, Ise, Tsuda, Maeda, & Misawa, 1996), indicating the withdrawal-paired stimuli serve as a CS that elicits conditioned aversive sensory effects. Similarly, neutral stimuli (light/tone onset) paired with antagonist-precipitated withdrawal (US) in the ICSS model (increase in threshold for brain stimulation reinforcement) can come to serve as a CS that alone can elicit this form of withdrawal (Kenny & Markou, 2005). In this case, nicotine withdrawal could also be considered an abolishing operation for brain stimulation reinforcement, as discussed below.

2.3.2.2 Abolishing operation (AO)

An AO is a change in the environment that decreases the effectiveness of a reinforcer (or punisher) and decreases (or increases) any behavior that in the past has produced that reinforcer (or punisher). For example, nicotine administration is an AO that decreases the reinforcing effectiveness of nicotine. Acute or continuous nicotine administration decreases NSA in rats (Corrigall & Coen, 1989; LeSage, Keyler, Collins, & Pentel, 2003; LeSage et al., 2002), and nicotine administration by several routes (e.g., i. v., transdermal, oral, inhaled) decreases smoking in humans (Benowitz & Jacob, 1990; Hatsukami et al., 2007; Nemeth-Coslett, Henningfield, O'Keeffe, & Griffiths, 1987; Perkins, Grobe, Stiller, Fonte, & Goettler, 1992). Nicotine administration can serve as an AO for food reinforcement, as some studies show it can reduce operant responding for or intake of food in humans and nonhumans under certain conditions (Bunney et al., 2016; Bunney, Hansen, & LeSage, 2018; Grunberg, 1982; O'Dell et al., 2007; Perkins, 1992; Perkins, Epstein, et al., 1992). As mentioned above, nicotine deprivation can act as an AO for reinforcing electrical brain stimulation in rats, as indicated by an increase in the electrical current required to reinforce responding in the ICSS model (Harris et al., 2015; Harrison et al., 2002). As mentioned above, a stimulus paired with nicotine withdrawal in the ICSS model can come to elicit withdrawal itself (Kenny & Markou, 2005). In this case, the tone/light could be considered a conditioned AO (Laraway et al., 2003; Michael, 1993), because it's presentation reduces the reinforcing effectiveness of electrical brain stimulation only after a learning history of being paired with an unconditioned AO, nicotine deprivation.

3. Role of stimulus functions in tobacco use theory

Current theories of tobacco use recognize the multiple stimulus functions of nicotine. For example, the dual-reinforcement model proposed by Caggiula and colleagues (Caggiula et al., 2009, 2001) is based on their findings from the NSA studies mentioned above and others showing that NSA was synergistically increased when an environmental stimulus with weak reinforcing effects of its' own accompanied nicotine delivery. That is, the rate of NSA was more than the sum of the response rates maintained by nicotine or the environmental stimulus alone. In addition, studies showed that noncontingent nicotine administration could increase the reinforcing effects of an environmental stimulus, and that neutral stimuli can acquire a conditioned reinforcer function by being paired with nicotine delivery. These findings were in agreement with the aforementioned pioneering work of Goldberg and colleagues showing that nicotine-paired stimuli can promote persistent high rates of NSA under second-order schedules (Goldberg et al., 1981; Spealman & Goldberg, 1982). Based on these findings, Caggiula et al. proposed a model positing that nicotine engenders and maintains self-administration (and smoking) by serving as (1) a primary reinforcer, (2) a primary reinforcer that, through Pavlovian conditioning, can establish neutral environmental stimuli as conditioned reinforcers capable of maintaining self-administration behaviors in the absence of nicotine, and (3) a reinforcement enhancer that increases the incentive value of accompanying environmental stimuli. To state this in terms of the taxonomy above, nicotine serves as (1) an unconditioned reinforcer, (2) a UC that, via respondent conditioning, can establish neutral environmental stimuli as CSs that also serve as operant conditioned reinforcers, and (3) an EO that increases the reinforcing effectiveness of environmental stimuli associated with nicotine delivery. This multifunctional role of nicotine in the dual-reinforcement model may help explain why the abuse liability of cigarette smoke and intractability of tobacco use is so strong, despite nicotine's relatively weak unconditioned reinforcing effects compared to other drugs of abuse like major stimulants and opioids.

Other theories of tobacco use emphasize the role of antecedent stimuli in the control of tobacco use. For example, in a respondent conditioning model, nicotine as a US (or more specifically a UC in the present terms) is thought to establish antecedent stimuli predictive of nicotine delivery as CSs that can elicit CRs similar to the UR elicited by a nicotine US

(Eissenberg, 2004; Ferguson & Shiffman, 2009). Respondent conditioning theories stress that among the URs that can be elicited by nicotine are physiological responses that oppose nicotine's disruptive effects on normal internal regulatory processes. In other words, the URs compensate or defend against the dysregulation caused by nicotine to maintain homeostasis. When nicotine is absent after a history of nicotine exposure, the compensatory URs continue, internal dysregulation occurs, and a withdrawal syndrome manifests in a variety of signs (e.g., craving, urges, irritability, depressed mood). That is, the URs elicited by nicotine are the physiological responses that underlie withdrawal symptoms. As such, any stimulus that is predictive of nicotine administration, such as the sight/smell/taste of a cigarette or the context in which smoking occurs, can come to elicit a conditioned withdrawal CR, though weaker in magnitude than the UR.

Nicotine withdrawal symptoms, whether they are URs or CRs, are considered the primary source of motivation for smoking in respondent conditioning models (Eissenberg, 2004; Ferguson & Shiffman, 2009). From an operant perspective, their onset serves as an EO or conditioned EO that establishes their reduction or removal as a form of negative reinforcement (similar to onset of painful stimuli), which occurs with smoking or nicotine self-administration. As such, respondent conditioning models emphasize that smoking paired cues (CSs) play a significant role in provoking tobacco use, which manifests as lapses or relapse during a quit attempt (Eissenberg, 2004; Ferguson & Shiffman, 2009).

The reduction of CRs, such as cue-induced craving/urges, are a primary target in some smoking cessation interventions. For example, one form of "cue exposure" therapy emphasizes reducing the CR to smoking related CSs through respondent extinction. Treatment involves abstinent patients being repeatedly exposed to smoking related CSs without being able to smoke (US). Unfortunately, the evidence that this approach reduces cue-induced cravings or other CRs or smoking relapse is mixed (Ferguson & Shiffman, 2009; Niaura et al., 1999).

Other cue-exposure approaches that involve training behaviors that are incompatible with or redirect a person away from the CSs or smoking have been more successful (Ferguson & Shiffman, 2009). Consideration of the stimulus functions of nicotine points to several potential reasons for the limited efficacy of cue-exposure approaches. First, studies in nonhumans by Bevins and colleagues have shown that a nicotine CS can compete with environmental stimuli for control of a CR. That is, when nicotine and an environmental stimulus are both paired with a US (sucrose), nicotine becomes a stronger CS (i.e., elicits a stronger UR) than the environmental stimulus (i.e., nicotine overshadowing occurs, Murray, Wells, & Bevins, 2011). This suggests that cue-exposure therapy may target relatively weak CS-CR relations. Second, Bevins and colleagues have shown that extinction of a CS-CR relation can be context-specific (Bevins & Palmatier, 2004). Because cue-exposure therapy does not extinguish many of the CSs that can occur in the smoker's natural environment, those CSs remain capable of eliciting CRs (e.g., craving). Finally, cue exposure therapies and the respondent conditioning model on which they are based do not recognize that CSs could also serve an operant S^D function, because they are differentially correlated with the availability of nicotine. To the extent that smoking paired cues serve as S^Ds for smoking, reducing their control requires operant extinction, not respondent extinction. In this case, smoking behavior would have to be allowed to occur in the presence of the cues and not reinforced with nicotine. This could potentially be accomplished using denicotinized cigarettes or sham smoking an unlit cigarette. Therefore, the limited effects of respondent cue-exposure procedures may be due to targeting the wrong or weaker stimulus function of the cues.

4. Conclusion

The present chapter shows that nicotine exhibits many of the same stimulus functions as other drug and non-drug stimuli, and these functions play a key role in theories of tobacco use. It also shows that the behavioral effects of nicotine are malleable and cannot be predicted on the basis of its physical or pharmacological properties alone. For example, some stimulus functions can occur simultaneously and affect behavior in seemingly divergent ways. For example, the work of Goldberg and colleagues shows that the same dose of nicotine via the same route can serve as an unconditioned reinforcer, despite also serving as a US that elicits vomiting (a putative aversive effect, (Spealman & Goldberg, 1982). In addition, that same dose can punish or negatively reinforce operant behavior in a different context (Goldberg & Spealman, 1983; Spealman, 1983). These divergent stimulus functions have also been demonstrated in human laboratory studies (Harvey et al., 2004; Henningfield & Goldberg, 1983a), and generalize to some extent to clinical observations. For example, youth can become daily smokers and physically dependent on nicotine despite experiencing aversive US effects produced by the first cigarettes smoked (DiFranza et al., 2004; Pomerleau, Pomerleau, & Namenek, 1998). Taken together, an implication of these findings is that one cannot necessarily predict one stimulus function (e.g., reinforcer) from another (e.g., punisher) without considering the historical and current circumstances in which nicotine is administered. Moreover, the forgoing review shows that those functions can be strongly moderated by other environmental variables. Consideration of the multiple stimulus functions of nicotine and the environmental context within which those functions can manifest is necessary to gain a comprehensive understanding of tobacco use and develop the best interventions and public policies to reduce it.

Although many stimulus functions of nicotine have been demonstrated and factors modulating those functions have been elucidated, further research is needed to determine the full range of stimulus functions that nicotine can share with non-drug environmental stimuli. Preclinical studies are perhaps best suited for this task, as they can potentially provide more rigorous control of confounding variables. As noted above, some stimulus functions that have not yet been demonstrated include the respondent CC in higher-order conditioning, conditioned reinforcer, and conditioned punisher. Approaches to consider for demonstrating these functions were discussed above. Research on other stimulus functions has some limitations to address. For example, the goal tracking method to demonstrate a respondent CS function of nicotine is somewhat confounded by an inextricably intertwined operant contingency, suggesting that nicotine may also be serving an S^D function to some degree in that assay. Procedures involving clearer unconditioned reflexes would help clarify further this stimulus function of nicotine. The CS and conditioned reinforcer functions are an especially important focus, because they represent behavioral mechanisms through which nicotine could evoke tobacco use beyond its unconditioned reinforcing and EO functions in the dual-reinforcement model.

The taxonomy of stimulus functions applied here is an extension of that previously applied by behavioral pharmacologists (Thompson & Pickens, 1971) and appears useful for categorizing a wide range of nicotine's behavioral effects. The present chapter illustrates how a taxonomy of well-defined mutually-exclusive stimulus functions could help clarify the way nicotine's behavioral effects are conceptualized and guide research and theory accordingly (Zeiler, 1986). Continued research on the stimulus functions of nicotine could play a vital role in developing better clinical and regulatory approaches to preventing and reducing tobacco use and its harm to individual and public health.

Acknowledgments

The author thanks Andrew Harris and two anonymous reviewers for their helpful comments on earlier versions of the manuscript. Supported by grants R01-DA046318 and R01-DA048899, and a Career Development Award from the Hennepin Healthcare Research Institute.

Conflict of interest statement

The author has no conflicts of interest to declare.

References

Arbol, J. L., del Muñoz, J. R., Ojeda, L., Cascales, A. L., Irles, J. R., Miranda, M. T., et al. (2000). Plasma concentrations of beta-endorphin in smokers who consume different numbers of cigarettes per day. *Pharmacology Biochemistry and Behavior, 67*(1), 25–28.

Ator, N. A., & Griffiths, R. R. (1983). Nicotine self-administration in baboons. *Pharmacology Biochemistry and Behavior, 19*(6), 993–1003.

Bardo, M. T., & Bevins, R. A. (2000). Conditioned place preference: what does it add to our preclinical understanding of drug reward? *Psychopharmacology, 153*(1), 31–43.

Barrett, S. T., & Bevins, R. A. (2012). A quantitative analysis of the reward-enhancing effects of nicotine using reinforcer demand. *Behavioural Pharmacology, 23*(8), 781–789.

Benowitz, N. L. (2008). Clinical pharmacology of nicotine: implications for understanding, preventing, and treating tobacco addiction. *Clinical Pharmacology & Therapeutics, 83*(4), 531–541.

Benowitz, N. L., & Jacob, P. (1990). Intravenous nicotine replacement suppresses nicotine intake from cigarette smoking. *The Journal of Pharmacology and Experimental Therapeutics, 254*(3), 1000–1005.

Benwell, M. E. M., & Balfour, D. J. K. (1992). The effects of acute and repeated nicotine treatment on nucleus accumbens dopamine and locomotor activity. *British Journal of Pharmacology, 105*(4), 849–856.

Besheer, J., Palmatier, M. I., Metschke, D. M., & Bevins, R. A. (2004). Nicotine as a signal for the presence or absence of sucrose reward: a Pavlovian drug appetitive conditioning preparation in rats. *Psychopharmacology, 172*(1), 108–117.

Bevins, R. A., & Besheer, J. (2001). Individual differences in rat locomotor activity are diminished by nicotine through stimulation of central nicotinic acetylcholine receptors. *Physiology & Behavior, 72*(1–2), 237–244.

Bevins, R. A., Besheer, J., & Pickett, K. S. (2001). Nicotine-conditioned locomotor activity in rats: dopaminergic and GABAergic influences on conditioned expression. *Pharmacology Biochemistry and Behavior, 68*(1), 135–145.

Bevins, R. A., Eurek, S., & Besheer, J. (2005). Timing of conditioned responding in a nicotine locomotor conditioning preparation: manipulations of the temporal arrangement between context cues and drug administration. *Behavioural Brain Research, 159*(1), 135–143.

Bevins, R. A., & Palmatier, M. I. (2003). Nicotine-conditioned locomotor sensitization in rats: assessment of the US-preexposure effect. *Behavioural Brain Research, 143*(1), 65–74.

Bevins, R. A., & Palmatier, M. I. (2004). Extending the Role of Associative Learning Processes in Nicotine Addiction. *Behavioral and Cognitive Neuroscience Reviews, 3*(3), 143–158.

Branch, M. N. (1991). Behavioral Pharmacology. In I. H. Iversen, & K. A. Lattal (Eds.), *Experimental anaylsis of behavior, Part 2* (pp. 21–78). Elsevier.

Bunney, P. E., Burroughs, D., Hernandez, C., & LeSage, M. G. (2016). The effects of nicotine self-administration and withdrawal on concurrently available chow and sucrose intake in adult male rats. *Physiology & Behavior, 154*, 49–59.

Bunney, P. E., Hansen, M., & Lesage, M. (2018). Effects of isolated tobacco alkaloids and tobacco products on deprivation-induced food intake and meal patterns in rats. *Pharmacology, Biochemistry, and Behavior, 165*, 45–55.

Caggiula, A. R., Donny, E. C., Epstein, L. H., Sved, A. F., Knof, S., Rose, C., et al. (1998). The role of corticosteroids in nicotine's physiological and behavioral effects. *Psychoneuroendocrinology, 23*(2), 143–159.

Caggiula, A. R., Donny, E. C., Palmatier, M. I., Liu, X., Chaudhri, N., & Sved, A. F. (2009). The role of nicotine in smoking: a dual-reinforcement model. *Nebraska Symposium on Motivation Nebraska Symposium on Motivation, 55*, 91–109.

Caggiula, A. R., Donny, E. C., White, A. R., Chaudhri, N., Booth, S., Gharib, M. A., et al. (2001). Cue dependency of nicotine self-administration and smoking. *Pharmacology Biochemistry and Behavior, 70*(4), 515–530.

Caggiula, A. R., Donny, E. C., White, A. R., Chaudhri, N., Booth, S., Gharib, M. A., et al. (2002). Environmental stimuli promote the acquisition of nicotine self-administration in rats. *Psychopharmacology, 163*(2), 230–237.

Caggiula, A. R., Epstein, L. H., Antelman, S. M., Saylor, S. S., Perkins, K. A., Knopf, S., et al. (1991). Conditioned tolerance to the anorectic and corticosterone-elevating effects of nicotine. *Pharmacology Biochemistry and Behavior, 40*(1), 53–59.

Caine, S. B., Collins, G. T., Thomsen, M., Wright, C., Lanier, R. K., & Mello, N. K. (2014). Nicotine-like behavioral effects of the minor tobacco alkaloids nornicotine, anabasine, and anatabine in male rodents. *Experimental and Clinical Psychopharmacology, 22*(1), 9–22.

Catania, A. C. (1992). *Learning* (3rd ed.). Englewood Cliffs, NJ: Prentice-Hall, Inc.

Charntikov, S., Pittenger, S. T., Swalve, N., Barrett, S. T., & Bevins, R. A. (2020). Conditioned enhancement of the nicotine reinforcer. *Experimental and Clinical Psychopharmacology, 29*(4), 385–394.

Cherek, D. R., & Bennett, R. H. (1991). Effects of spirometric administration of tobacco smoke containing varying amounts of nicotine on human punished and non-punished operant responding. *Behavioural Pharmacology, 2*(1), 23–30.

Clarke, P. B. S., & Kumar, R. (1983). The effects of nicotine on locomotor activity in non-tolerant and tolerant rats. *British Journal of Pharmacology, 78*(2), 329–337.

Constantin, A., & Clarke, P. B. S. (2018). Reinforcement enhancement by nicotine in adult rats: behavioral selectivity and relation to mode of delivery and blood nicotine levels. *Psychopharmacology, 235*(3), 1–10.

Cornelius, M. E., Wang, T. W., Jamal, A., Loretan, C. G., & Neff, L. J. (2020). Tobacco Product Use Among Adults — United States, 2019. *Morbidity and Mortality Weekly Report, 69*(46), 1736–1742.

Corrigall, W. A., & Coen, K. M. (1989). Nicotine maintains robust self-administration in rats on a limited-access schedule. *Psychopharmacology, 99*(4), 473–478.

Craft, R. M., & Howard, J. L. (1988). Cue properties of oral and transdermal nicotine in the rat. *Psychopharmacology, 96*(3), 281–284.

DiFranza, J. R., Savageau, J. A., Fletcher, K., Ockene, J. K., Rigotti, N. A., McNeill, A. D., et al. (2004). Recollections and repercussions of the first inhaled cigarette. *Addictive Behaviors, 29*(2), 261–272.

Donny, E. C., Caggiula, A. R., Knopf, S., & Brown, C. (1995). Nicotine self-administration in rats. *Psychopharmacology, 122*(4), 390–394.

Donny, E. C., Caggiula, A. R., Mielke, M. M., Jacobs, K. S., Rose, C., & Sved, A. F. (1998). Acquisition of nicotine self-administration in rats: the effects of dose, feeding schedule, and drug contingency. *Psychopharmacology, 136*(1), 83–90.

Donny, E. C., Chaudhri, N., Caggiula, A. R., Evans-Martin, F. F., Booth, S., Gharib, M. A., et al. (2003). Operant responding for a visual reinforcer in rats is enhanced by noncontingent nicotine: implications for nicotine self-administration and reinforcement. *Psychopharmacology*, *169*(1), 68–76.

Donny, E. C., Denlinger, R. L., Tidey, J. W., Koopmeiners, J. S., Benowitz, N. L., Vandrey, R. G., et al. (2015). Randomized trial of reduced-nicotine standards for cigarettes. *The New England Journal of Medicine*, *373*(14), 1340–1349.

Donny, E. C., Houtsmuller, E., & Stitzer, M. L. (2007). Smoking in the absence of nicotine: behavioral, subjective and physiological effects over 11 days. *Addiction (Abingdon, England)*, *102*(2), 324–334.

Donny, E. C., Taylor, T. G., LeSage, M. G., Levin, M., Buffalari, D. M., Joel, D., et al. (2012). Impact of tobacco regulation on animal research: new perspectives and opportunities. *Nicotine & Tobacco Research*, *14*(11), 1319–1338.

Dougherty, J., Miller, D., Todd, G., & Kostenbauder, H. B. (1981). Reinforcing and other behavioral effects of nicotine. *Neuroscience and Biobehavioral Reviews*, *5*(4), 487–495.

Eikelboom, R., & Stewart, J. (1982). Conditioning of drug-induced physiological responses. *Psychological Review*, *89*(5), 507–528.

Eissenberg, T. (2004). Measuring the emergence of tobacco dependence: the contribution of negative reinforcement models. *Addiction*, *99*(s1), 5–29.

Ellson, D. G. (1941). Hallucinations produced by sensory conditioning. *Journal of Experimental Psychology*, *28*(1), 1–20.

Epstein, L. H., Bulik, C. M., Perkins, K. A., Caggiula, A. R., & Rodefer, J. (1991). Behavioral economic analysis of smoking: money and food as alternatives. *Pharmacology, Biochemistry, and Behavior*, *38*(4), 715–721.

Faulcon, L. M., Rudy, S., Limpert, J., Wang, B., & Murphy, I. (2020). Adverse experience reports of seizures in youth and young adult electronic nicotine delivery systems users. *Journal of Adolescent Health*, *66*(1), 15–17.

Ferguson, S. G., & Shiffman, S. (2009). The relevance and treatment of cue-induced cravings in tobacco dependence. *Journal of Substance Abuse Treatment*, *36*(3), 235–243.

Food and Drug Administration. (2017). *Assessment of abuse potential of drugs: Guidance for industry*. Silver Spring, MD: Center for Drug Evaluation Research.

Fudala, P. J., Teoh, K. W., & Iwamoto, E. T. (1985). Pharmacologic characterization of nicotine-induced conditioned place preference. *Pharmacology Biochemistry and Behavior*, *22*(2), 237–241.

Garcia, K. L. P., Lê, A. D., & Tyndale, R. F. (2014). Effect of food training and training dose on nicotine self-administration in rats. *Behavioural Brain Research*, *274*, 10–18.

Gasior, M., Shoaib, M., Yasar, S., Jaszyna, M., & Goldberg, S. R. (1999). Acquisition of nicotine discrimination and discriminative stimulus effects of nicotine in rats chronically exposed to caffeine. *The Journal of Pharmacology and Experimental Therapeutics*, *288*(3), 1053–1073.

Gentzke, A. S., Creamer, M., Cullen, K. A., Ambrose, B. K., Willis, G., Jamal, A., et al. (2019). Vital Signs: Tobacco Product Use Among Middle and High School Students — United States, 2011–2018. *Morbidity and Mortality Weekly Report*, *68*(6), 157–164.

Gentzke, A. S., Wang, T. W., Jamal, A., Park-Lee, E., Ren, C., Cullen, K. A., et al. (2020). Tobacco Product Use Among Middle and High School Students — United States, 2020. *MMWR. Morbidity and Mortality Weekly Report*, *69*(50), 1881–1888.

Glowa, J. R. (1986). Some effects of d-amphetamine, caffeine, nicotine and cocaine on schedule-controlled responding of the mouse. *Neuropharmacology*, *25*(10), 1127–1135.

Goldberg, S. R., & Spealman, R. D. (1983). Suppression of behavior by intravenous injections of nicotine or by electric shocks in squirrel monkeys: effects of chlordiazepoxide and mecamylamine. *The Journal of Pharmacology and Experimental Therapeutics*, *224*(2), 334–340.

Goldberg, S. R., Spealman, R. D., Risner, M. E., & Henningfield, J. E. (1983). Control of behavior by intravenous nicotine injections in laboratory animals. *Pharmacology, Biochemistry, and Behavior, 19*(6), 1011–1020.
Goldberg, S., & Spealman, R. (1982). Maintenance and suppression of behavior by intravenous nicotine injections in squirrel monkeys. *FASEB, 41*(2), 216–220.
Goldberg, S., Spealman, R., & Goldberg, D. (1981). Persistent behavior at high rates maintained by intravenous self-administration of nicotine. *Science, 214*(4520), 573–575.
Grebenstein, P., Burroughs, D., Hernandez, C., & LeSage, M. G. (2015). Increased weight gain and sucrose intake during extinction of nicotine self-administration in adult male rats. *Drug and Alcohol Dependence, 146*, e128.
Grebenstein, P. E., Burroughs, D., Roiko, S. A., Pentel, P. R., & LeSage, M. G. (2015). Predictors of the nicotine reinforcement threshold, compensation, and elasticity of demand in a rodent model of nicotine reduction policy. *Drug and Alcohol Dependence, 151*, 181–193.
Griffiths, R. R., & Henningfield, J. E. (1982). Experimental analysis of human cigarette smoking behavior. *Federation Proceedings, 41*(2), 234–240.
Grunberg, N. E. (1982). The effects of nicotine and cigarette smoking on food consumption and taste preferences. *Addictive Behaviors, 7*(4), 317–331.
Harris, A. C., Tally, L., Muelken, P., Banal, A., Schmidt, C. E., Cao, Q., et al. (2015). Effects of nicotine and minor tobacco alkaloids on intracranial-self-stimulation in rats. *Drug and Alcohol Dependence, 153*, 330–334.
Harrison, A. A., Gasparini, F., & Markou, A. (2002). Nicotine potentiation of brain stimulation reward reversed by DH beta E and SCH 23390, but not by eticlopride, LY 314582 or MPEP in rats. *Psychopharmacology, 160*(1), 56–66.
Harvey, D. M., Yasar, S., Heishman, S. J., Panlilio, L. V., Henningfield, J. E., & Goldberg, S. R. (2004). Nicotine serves as an effective reinforcer of intravenous drug-taking behavior in human cigarette smokers. *Psychopharmacology, 175*(2), 134–142.
Hatsukami, D., Mooney, M., Murphy, S., Lesage, M., Babb, D., & Hecht, S. (2007). Effects of high dose transdermal nicotine replacement in cigarette smokers. *Pharmacology, Biochemistry, and Behavior, 86*(1), 132–139.
Henningfield, J. E., Buchhalter, A. R., & Fant, R. V. (2016). Behavioral pharmacology contributions to regulation of drug and tobacco products by the Food and Drug Administration. *Behavior Analysis: Research and Practice, 16*(4), 179–189.
Henningfield, J. E., & Goldberg, S. R. (1983a). Control of behavior by intravenous nicotine injections in human subjects. *Pharmacology Biochemistry and Behavior, 19*(6), 1021–1026.
Henningfield, J. E., & Goldberg, S. R. (1983b). Nicotine as a reinforcer in human subjects and laboratory animals. *Pharmacology Biochemistry and Behavior, 19*(6), 989–992.
Henningfield, J. E., Smith, T. T., Kleykamp, B. A., Fant, R. V., & Donny, E. C. (2016). Nicotine self-administration research: the legacy of Steven R. Goldberg and implications for regulation, health policy, and research. *Psychopharmacology, 233*(23–24), 3829–3848.
Hirschhorn, I. D., & Rosecrans, J. A. (1974). Studies on the time course and the effect of cholinergic and adrenergic receptor blockers on the stimulus effect of nicotine. *Psychopharmacology, 40*(2), 109–120.
Holland, P. C. (1979). Differential effects of omission contingencies on various components of Pavlovian appetitive conditioned responding in rats. *Journal of Experimental Psychology: Animal Behavior Processes, 5*(2), 178–193.
Hukkanen, J., Jacob, P., & Benowitz, N. L. (2005). Metabolism and disposition kinetics of nicotine. *Pharmacological Reviews, 57*(1), 79–115.
Iwamoto, E. T., & Williamson, E. C. (1984). Nicotine-induced taste aversion: Characterization and preexposure effects in rats. *Pharmacology Biochemistry and Behavior, 21*(4), 527–532.

Jackson, K. J., Martin, B. R., Changeux, J. P., & Damaj, M. I. (2008). Differential role of nicotinic acetylcholine receptor subunits in physical and affective nicotine withdrawal signs. *The Journal of Pharmacology and Experimental Therapeutics*, *325*(1), 302–312.

Jorenby, D. E., Steinpreis, R. E., Sherman, J. E., & Baker, T. B. (1990). Aversion instead of preference learning indicated by nicotine place conditioning in rats. *Psychopharmacology*, *101*(4), 533–538.

Kenny, P. J., & Markou, A. (2005). Conditioned nicotine withdrawal profoundly decreases the activity of brain reward systems. *The Journal of Neuroscience*, *25*(26), 6208–6212.

Kirshenbaum, A., Green, J., Fay, M., Parks, A., Phillips, J., Stone, J., et al. (2015). Reinforcer devaluation as a consequence of acute nicotine exposure and withdrawal. *Psychopharmacology*, *232*(9), 1583–1594.

Koffarnus, M. N., & Winger, G. (2015). Individual differences in the reinforcing and punishing effects of nicotine in rhesus monkeys. *Psychopharmacology*, *232*(13), 2393–2403.

Koob, G. F., & Volkow, N. D. (2010). Neurocircuitry of addiction. *Neuropsychopharmacology: Official Publication of the American College of Neuropsychopharmacology*, *35*(1), 217–238.

Kunisawa, N., Iha, H. A., Nomura, Y., Onishi, M., Matsubara, N., Shimizu, S., et al. (2017). Serotonergic modulation of nicotine-induced kinetic tremor in mice. *Journal of Pharmacological Sciences*, *134*(2), 131–138.

Kunisawa, N., Iha, H. A., Shimizu, S., Tokudome, K., Mukai, T., Kinboshi, M., et al. (2016). Nicotine evokes kinetic tremor by activating the inferior olive via α7 nicotinic acetylcholine receptors. *Behavioural Brain Research*, *314*, 173–180.

Kunisawa, N., Shimizu, S., Kato, M., Iha, H. A., Iwai, C., Hashimura, M., et al. (2018). Pharmacological characterization of nicotine-induced tremor: Responses to anti-tremor and anti-epileptic agents. *Journal of Pharmacological Sciences*, *137*(2), 162–169.

Laraway, S., Snycerski, S., Michael, J., & Poling, A. (2003). Motivating operations and terms to describe them: some further refinements. *Journal of Applied Behavior Analysis*, *36*(3), 407–414.

Lazev, A. B., Herzog, T. A., & Brandon, T. H. (1999). Classical conditioning of environmental cues to cigarette smoking. *Experimental and Clinical Psychopharmacology*, 7(1), 56–63.

LeSage, M. G. (2009). Toward a nonhuman model of contingency management: effects of reinforcing abstinence from nicotine self-administration in rats with an alternative nondrug reinforcer. *Psychopharmacology*, *203*(1), 13–22.

LeSage, M. G., Keyler, D. E., Collins, G., & Pentel, P. R. (2003). Effects of continuous nicotine infusion on nicotine self-administration in rats: relationship between continuously infused and self-administered nicotine doses and serum concentrations. *Psychopharmacology*, *170*(3), 278–286.

LeSage, M. G., Keyler, D. E., Shoeman, D., Raphael, D., Collins, G., & Pentel, P. R. (2002). Continuous nicotine infusion reduces nicotine self-administration in rats with 23-h/day access to nicotine. *Pharmacology, Biochemistry, and Behavior*, *72*(1–2), 279–289.

LeSage, M. G., Shelley, D., Ross, J. T., Carroll, F. I., & Corrigall, W. A. (2009). Effects of the nicotinic receptor partial agonists varenicline and cytisine on the discriminative stimulus effects of nicotine in rats. *Pharmacology, Biochemistry, and Behavior*, *91*(3), 461–467.

LeSage, M. G., Smethells, J. R., & Harris, A. C. (2018). Status and future directions of preclinical behavioral pharmacology in tobacco regulatory science. *Behavior Analysis: Research and Practice*, *18*(3), 252–274.

Lobina, C., Carai, M. A. M., Froestl, W., Mugnaini, C., Pasquini, S., Corelli, F., et al. (2011). Activation of the GABAB receptor prevents nicotine-induced locomotor stimulation in mice. *Frontiers in Psychiatry*, *2*, 76.

Manzardo, A. M., Rio, J. A. D., Stein, L., & Belluzzi, J. D. (2001). Rats choose cocaine over dopamine agonists in a two-lever self-administration preference test. *Pharmacology, Biochemistry, and Behavior, 70*(2–3), 257–265.
Martin, C. D., Bool, H. M., George, A. M., Carr, K. A., Epstein, L. H., Hawk, L. W., et al. (2018). Social reinforcement as alternative to sucrose reinforcement is increased by nicotine and methylphenidate in male Fischer-344 rats. *Psychopharmacology, 235*(7), 1981–1985.
Matta, S. G., Balfour, D. J., Benowitz, N. L., Boyd, R. T., Buccafusco, J. J., Caggiula, A. R., et al. (2007). Guidelines on nicotine dose selection for in vivo research. *Psychopharmacology, 190*(3), 269–319.
Mazur, J. E. (1990). *Learning and behavior* (2nd ed.). Englewood Cliffs, NJ: Prentice-Hall, Inc.
McMahon, L. R. (2019). Green tobacco sickness: mecamylamine, varenicline, and nicotine vaccine as clinical research tools and potential therapeutics. *Expert Review of Clinical Pharmacology, 12*(3), 189–195.
Michael, J. (1993). Establishing operations. *The Behavior Analyst, 16*(2), 191–206.
Michael, J. (1995). What every student of behavior analysis ought to learn: a system for classifying the multiple effects of behavioral variables. *The Behavior Analyst, 18*(2), 273–284.
Michael, J. (2004). *Concepts and principles of behavior analysis*. Kalamazoo, MI: Association for Behavior Analysis.
Miech, R., Johnston, L., O'Malley, P. M., Bachman, J. G., & Patrick, M. E. (2019). Adolescent vaping and nicotine use in 2017–2018 — U.S. National Estimates. *New England Journal of Medicine*.
Miner, L. L., & Collins, A. C. (1989). Strain comparison of nicotine-induced seizure sensitivity and nicotinic receptors. *Pharmacology Biochemistry and Behavior, 33*(2), 469–475.
Moerke, M. J., Zhu, A. Z. X., Tyndale, R. F., Javors, M. A., & McMahon, L. R. (2017). The discriminative stimulus effects of i.v. nicotine in rhesus monkeys: Pharmacokinetics and apparent pA2 analysis with dihydro-β-erythroidine. *Neuropharmacology, 116*, 9–17.
Morrison, C. F. (1969). The effects of nicotine on punished behaviour. *Psychopharmacologia, 14*(3), 221–232.
Morrison, C. F., & Stephenson, J. A. (1969). Nicotine injections as the conditioned stimulus in discrimination learning. *Psychopharmacologia, 15*(5), 351–360.
Murray, J. E., Wells, N. R., & Bevins, R. A. (2011). Nicotine competes with a visual stimulus for control of conditioned responding. *Addiction Biology, 16*(1), 152–162.
Nemeth-Coslett, R., Henningfield, J. E., O'Keeffe, M. K., & Griffiths, R. R. (1987). Nicotine gum: dose-related effects on cigarette smoking and subjective ratings. *Psychopharmacology, 92*(4), 424–430.
Niaura, R., Abrams, D. B., Shadel, W. G., Rohsenow, D. J., Monti, P. M., & Sirota, A. D. (1999). Cue exposure treatment for smoking relapse prevention: a controlled clinical trial. *Addiction, 94*(5), 685–695.
NIDA. (2018). *Monitoring the future survey results show alarming rise in teen vaping*. https://www.drugabuse.gov/about-nida/noras-blog/2018/12/monitoring-future-survey-results-show-alarming-rise-in-teen-vaping.
Nishikawa, T., & Tsujimoto, A. (1975). Comparison of the cardiostimulatory effects of nicotine in dogs and monkeys. *Journal of Pharmacy and Pharmacology, 27*(9), 716–718.
O'Dell, L. E., Chen, S. A., Smith, R. T., Specio, S. E., Balster, R. L., Paterson, N. E., et al. (2007). Extended access to nicotine self-administration leads to dependence: Circadian measures, withdrawal measures, and extinction behavior in rats. *The Journal of Pharmacology and Experimental Therapeutics, 320*(1), 180–193.
O'Dell, L. E., & Koob, G. F. (2007). "Nicotine deprivation effect" in rats with intermittent 23-hour access to intravenous nicotine self-administration. *Pharmacology, Biochemistry, and Behavior, 86*(2), 346–353.

Olausson, P., Jentsch, J. D., & Taylor, J. R. (2004). Nicotine enhances responding with conditioned reinforcement. *Psychopharmacology*, *171*(2), 173–178.
Overton, D. A. (1991). A historical perspective on drug discrimination. *NIDA Research Monograph*, *116*, 5–24.
Palmatier, M. I., Liu, X., Matteson, G. L., Donny, E. C., Caggiula, A. R., & Sved, A. F. (2007). Conditioned reinforcement in rats established with self-administered nicotine and enhanced by noncontingent nicotine. *Psychopharmacology*, *195*(2), 235–243.
Palmatier, M. I., Matteson, G. L., Black, J. J., Liu, X., Caggiula, A. R., Craven, L., et al. (2007). The reinforcement enhancing effects of nicotine depend on the incentive value of non-drug reinforcers and increase with repeated drug injections. *Drug and Alcohol Dependence*, *89*(1), 52–59.
Palmatier, M. I., O'Brien, L. C., & Hall, M. J. (2012). The role of conditioning history and reinforcer strength in the reinforcement enhancing effects of nicotine in rats. *Psychopharmacology*, *219*(4), 1119–1131.
Perkins, K. A. (1992). Effects of tobacco smoking on caloric intake. *British Journal of Addiction*, *87*(2), 193–205.
Perkins, K. A., Epstein, L. H., Sexton, J. E., & Pastor, S. (1990). Effects of smoking cessation on consumption of alcohol and sweet, high-fat foods. *Journal of Substance Abuse*, *2*(3), 287–297.
Perkins, K. A., Epstein, L. H., Sexton, J. E., Solberg-Kassel, R., Stiller, R. L., & Jacob, R. G. (1992). Effects of nicotine on hunger and eating in male and female smokers. *Psychopharmacology*, *106*(1), 53–59.
Perkins, K. A., Grobe, J. E., Stiller, R. L., Fonte, C., & Goettler, J. E. (1992). Nasal spray nicotine replacement suppresses cigarette smoking desire and behavior. *Clinical Pharmacology & Therapeutics*, *52*(6), 627–634.
Perkins, K. A., Grobe, J. E., Weiss, D., Fonte, C., & Caggiula, A. (1996). Nicotine preference in smokers as a function of smoking abstinence. *Pharmacology Biochemistry and Behavior*, *55*(2), 257–263.
Pickens, R. (1977). Behavioral pharmacology: A brief history. In T. Thompson, & P. B. Dews (Eds.), *Vol. 1. Advances in behavioral pharmacology* (pp. 230–257).
Poling, A., & Byrne, T. (2000). *Behavioral pharmacology*. Reno, NV: Context Press.
Poling, A., Lotfizadeh, A., & Edwards, T. L. (2017). Predicting reinforcement: Utility of the motivating operations concept. *The Behavior Analyst*, *40*(1), 49–56.
Pomerleau, O. F., Pomerleau, C. S., & Namenek, R. J. (1998). Early experiences with tobacco among women smokers, ex-smokers, and never-smokers. *Addiction*, *93*(4), 595–599.
Powers, A. R., Mathys, C., & Corlett, P. R. (2017). Pavlovian conditioning–induced hallucinations result from overweighting of perceptual priors. *Science*, *357*(6351), 596–600.
Pratt, J. A., Stolerman, I. P., Garcha, H. S., Giardini, V., & Feyerabend, C. (1983). Discriminative stimulus properties of nicotine: further evidence for mediation at a cholinergic receptor. *Psychopharmacology*, *81*(1), 54–60.
Raiff, B. R., & Dallery, J. (2006). Effects of acute and chronic nicotine on responses maintained by primary and conditioned reinforcers in rats. *Experimental and Clinical Psychopharmacology*, *14*(3), 296–305.
Raiff, B. R., & Dallery, J. (2009). Responding maintained by primary reinforcing visual stimuli is increased by nicotine administration in rats. *Behavioural Processes*, *82*(1), 95–99.
Reid, M. S., Ho, L. B., & Berger, S. P. (1996). Effects of environmental conditioning on the development of nicotine sensitization: Behavioral and neurochemical analysis. *Psychopharmacology*, *126*(4), 301–310.
Revusky, S., Davey, V., & Zagorski, M. (1989). Heart rate conditioning with pentobarbital as a conditioned stimulus and amphetamine as an unconditioned stimulus. *Behavioral Neuroscience*, *103*(2), 296–307.

Rinker, J. A., Busse, G. D., & Riley, A. L. (2008). An assessment of sex differences in nicotine-induced conditioned taste aversions. *Pharmacology, Biochemistry, and Behavior, 88*(4), 427–431.

Risinger, F. O., & Oakes, R. A. (1995). Nicotine-induced conditioned place preference and conditioned place aversion in mice. *Pharmacology Biochemistry and Behavior, 51*(2–3), 457–461.

Risner, M. E., & Goldberg, S. R. (1983). A comparison of nicotine and cocaine self-administration in the dog: fixed-ratio and progressive-ratio schedules of intravenous drug infusion. *The Journal of Pharmacology and Experimental Therapeutics, 224*(2), 319–326.

Rose, J. E., & Corrigall, W. A. (1997). Nicotine self-administration in animals and humans: similarities and differences. *Psychopharmacology, 130*(1), 28–40.

Rose, J. E., Jarvik, M. E., & Ananda, S. (1984). Nicotine preference increases after cigarette deprivation. *Pharmacology Biochemistry and Behavior, 20*(1), 55–58.

Rush, M. L., & Lang, W. J. (1970). A comparison of conditional cardiovascular responses induced by centrally and peripherally acting drugs. *European Journal of Pharmacology, 11*(2), 130–138.

SAMHSA. (2020). *Key substance use and mental health indicators in the United States: Results from the 2019 National Survey on Drug Use and Health.* Rockville, MD: Center for Behavioral Health Statistics and Quality, Substance Abuse and Mental Health Services Administration.

Schindler, C. W., Panlilio, L. V., & Goldberg, S. R. (2002). Second-order schedules of drug self-administration in animals. *Psychopharmacology, 163*(3), 327–344.

Schlinger, H. D. (1993). Establishing operations: Another step toward a functional taxonomy of environmental events. *The Behavior Analyst, 16*(2), 207–209.

Schlinger, H. D., & Blakely, E. (1994). A descriptive taxonomy of environmental operations and its implications for behavior analysis. *The Behavior Analyst, 17*(1), 43–57.

Seyler, L. E., Pomerleau, O. F., Fertig, J. B., Hunt, D., & Parker, K. (1986). Pituitary hormone response to cigarette smoking. *Pharmacology Biochemistry and Behavior, 24*(1), 159–162.

Shiffman, S. M., Gritz, E. R., Maltese, J., Lee, M. A., Schneider, N. G., & Jarvik, M. E. (1983). Effects of cigarette smoking and oral nicotine on hand tremor. *Clinical Pharmacology & Therapeutics, 33*(6), 800–805.

Shoaib, M., Schindler, C. W., & Goldberg, S. R. (1997). Nicotine self-administration in rats: strain and nicotine pre-exposure effects on acquisition. *Psychopharmacology, 129*(1), 35–43.

Shoaib, M., Stolerman, I. P., & Kumar, R. C. (1994). Nicotine-induced place preferences following prior nicotine exposure in rats. *Psychopharmacology, 113*(3–4), 445–452.

Shoaib, M., & Perkins, K. A. (2020). Preclinical and clinical research on the discriminative stimulus effects of nicotine. *Neuropharmacology, 170,* 108063.

Singh, T., Kennedy, S., Marynak, K., Persoskie, A., Melstrom, P., & King, B. A. (2016). Characteristics of Electronic Cigarette Use Among Middle and High School Students — United States, 2015. *MMWR. Morbidity and Mortality Weekly Report, 65*(5051), 1425–1429.

Skinner, B. F. (1957). *Verbal behavior.* New York: Appleton-Century Crofts.

Smith, J. W., & Stolerman, I. P. (2009). Recognizing nicotine: the neurobiological basis of nicotine discrimination. *Handbook of Experimental Pharmacology, 192*(192), 295–333.

Sofuoglu, M., & LeSage, M. G. (2012). The reinforcement threshold for nicotine as a target for tobacco control. *Drug and Alcohol Dependence, 125*(1–2), 1–7.

Sorge, R., & Clarke, P. (2009). Rats self-administer intravenous nicotine delivered in a novel smoking-relevant procedure: effects of dopamine antagonists. *The Journal of Pharmacology and Experimental Therapeutics, 330*(2), 633–640.

Sorge, R., Pierre, V., & Clarke, P. (2009). Facilitation of intravenous nicotine self-administration in rats by a motivationally neutral sensory stimulus. *Psychopharmacology, 207*(2), 191–200.
Spealman, R. D. (1983). Maintenance of behavior by postponement of scheduled injections of nicotine in squirrel monkeys. *The Journal of Pharmacology and Experimental Therapeutics, 227*(1), 154–159.
Spealman, R. D., & Goldberg, S. R. (1982). Maintenance of schedule-controlled behavior by intravenous injections of nicotine in squirrel monkeys. *The Journal of Pharmacology and Experimental Therapeutics, 223*(2), 402–408.
Spring, B. (2003). Altered reward value of carbohydrate snacks for female smokers withdrawn from nicotine. *Pharmacology, Biochemistry, and Behavior, 76*(2), 351–360.
Spring, B., Wurtman, J., Gleason, R., Wurtman, R., & Kessler, K. (1991). Weight gain and withdrawal symptoms after smoking cessation: A preventive intervention using d-fenfluramine. *Health Psychology, 10*(3), 216–223.
Stolerman, I. P. (1989). Discriminative stimulus effects of nicotine in rats trained under different schedules of reinforcement. *Psychopharmacology, 97*(1), 131–138.
Stolerman, I. P., & Garcha, H. S. (1989). Temporal factors in drug discrimination: Experiments with nicotine. *Journal of Psychopharmacology, 3*(2), 88–97.
Stolerman, I. P., Garcha, H. S., & Mirza, N. R. (1995). Dissociations between the locomotor stimulant and depressant effects of nicotinic agonists in rats. *Psychopharmacology, 117*(4), 430–437.
Stolerman, I. P., Garcha, H. S., Pratt, J. A., & Kumar, R. (1984). Role of training dose in discrimination of nicotine and related compounds by rats. *Psychopharmacology, 84*(3), 413–419.
Stolerman, I. P., & Jarvis, M. J. (1995). The scientific case that nicotine is addictive. *Psychopharmacology, 117*(1), 2–10.
Stolerman, I. P., Naylor, C., Elmer, G. I., & Goldberg, S. R. (1999). Discrimination and self-administration of nicotine by inbred strains of mice. *Psychopharmacology, 141*(3), 297–306.
Stratton, K., Kwan, L. Y., & Eaton, D. L. (2018). *Public health consequences of E-cigarettes.* National Academies Press.
Suzuki, T., Ise, Y., Tsuda, M., Maeda, J., & Misawa, M. (1996). Mecamylamine-precipitated nicotine-withdrawal aversion in rats. *European Journal of Pharmacology, 314*(3), 281–284.
Takada, K., Barrett, J. E., Allen, M. S., Cook, J. M., & Katz, J. L. (1992). Punishment of schedule-controlled behavior with beta-carboline injections: antagonism and comparisons with other compounds. *The Journal of Pharmacology and Experimental Therapeutics, 261*(1), 138–145.
Takada, K., Hagen, T. J., Cook, J. M., Goldberg, S. R., & Katz, J. L. (1988). Discriminative stimulus effects of intravenous nicotine in squirrel monkeys. *Pharmacology Biochemistry and Behavior, 30*(1), 243–247.
Takada, K., Swedberg, M., Goldberg, S. R., & Katz, J. L. (1989). Discriminative stimulus effects of intravenous l-nicotine and nicotine analogs or metabolites in squirrel monkeys. *Psychopharmacology, 99*, 208–212.
Thompson, T., & Pickens, R. (1971). *Stimulus properties of drugs.* New York: Appleton-Century-Crofts.
Thompson, T., & Schuster, C. R. (1968). *Behavioral pharmacology*. Englewood Cliffs, NJ: Prentice-Hall.
Tsai, M., Byun, M. K., Shin, J., & Alexander, L. E. C. (2020). Effects of e-cigarettes and vaping devices on cardiac and pulmonary physiology. *The Journal of Physiology, 598*(22), 5039–5062.
Tunock, Y., Hieda, Y., Keyler, D. E., Brown, S., Ennifar, S., Fattom, A., et al. (2001). Inhibition of nicotine-induced seizures in rats by combining vaccination against nicotine with chronic nicotine infusion. *Experimental and Clinical Psychopharmacology, 9*(2), 228–254.

Tweed, J. O., Hsia, S. H., Lutfy, K., & Friedman, T. C. (2012). The endocrine effects of nicotine and cigarette smoke. *Trends in Endocrinology and Metabolism, 23*(7), 334–342.
USDHHS. (2010). *How tobacco smoke causes disease: The biology and behavioral basis for smoking-attributable disease: A Report of the surgeon general. Office on Smoking and Health: U.S. Department of Health and Human Services, Centers for Disease Control and Prevention.* National Center for Chronic Disease Prevention and Health Promotion.
USDHHS. (2014). The health consequences of smoking—50 years of progress: A report of the surgeon general. In *Office on Smoking and Health: U.S. Department of Health and Human Services, Centers for Disease Control and Prevention* National Center for Chronic Disease Prevention and Health Promotion.
Vastola, B. J., Douglas, L. A., Varlinskaya, E. I., & Spear, L. P. (2002). Nicotine-induced conditioned place preference in adolescent and adult rats. *Physiology & Behavior,* 77(1), 107–114.
Verendeev, A., & Riley, A. L. (2012). Conditioned taste aversion and drugs of abuse: History and interpretation. *Neuroscience & Biobehavioral Reviews, 36*(10), 2193–2205.
Walter, S., & Kuschinsky, K. (1989). Conditioning of nicotine effects on motility and behaviour in rats. *Naunyn-Schmiedeberg's Archives of Pharmacology, 339*(1–2), 208–213.
Wang, T. W., Gentzke, A. S., Neff, L. J., Glidden, E. V., Jamal, A., Park-Lee, E., et al. (2021). Characteristics of e-Cigarette use behaviors among US Youth, 2020. *JAMA Network Open, 4*(6), e2111336.
WHO. (2019). *Who report on the global tobacco epidemic 2019: Offer help to quit tobacco use.* World Health Organization.
Wing, V. C., & Shoaib, M. (2010a). A second-order schedule of food reinforcement in rats to examine the role of CB1 receptors in the reinforcement-enhancing effects of nicotine. *Addiction Biology, 15*(4), 380–392.
Wing, V. C., & Shoaib, M. (2010b). Second-order schedules of nicotine reinforcement in rats: effect of AM251. *Addiction Biology, 15*(4), 393–402.
Wing, V. C., & Shoaib, M. (2013). Effect of infusion rate on intravenous nicotine self-administration in rats. *Behavioural Pharmacology, 24*(5–6), 517–522.
Wright, J. M., Ren, S., Constantin, A., & Clarke, P. B. S. (2018). Enhancement of a visual reinforcer by d-amphetamine and nicotine in adult rats: relation to habituation and food restriction. *Psychopharmacology, 235*(3), 1–12.
Xu, X., Bishop, E. E., Kennedy, S. M., Simpson, S. A., & Pechacek, T. F. (2015). Annual healthcare spending attributable to cigarette smoking an update. *American Journal of Preventive Medicine, 48*(3), 326–333.
Xue, Y., Morris, M., Ni, L., Guthrie, S. K., Zubieta, J.-K., Gonzalez, K., et al. (2010). Venous plasma nicotine correlates of hormonal effects of tobacco smoking. *Pharmacology Biochemistry and Behavior, 95*(2), 209–215.
Young, R., & Glennon, R. A. (2002). Nicotine and bupropion share a similar discriminative stimulus effect. *European Journal of Pharmacology, 443*(1–3), 113–118.
Zacny, J. P., & Stitzer, M. L. (1985). Effects of smoke deprivation interval on puff topography. *Clinical Pharmacology & Therapeutics, 38*(1), 109–115.
Zeiler, M. D. (1986). Behavioral units: A historical introduction. In T. Thompson, & M. D. Zeiler (Eds.), *Analysis and integration of behavioral units* (pp. 1–12). Hillsdale, NJ: Erlbaum.

CHAPTER SIX

The incentive amplifying effects of nicotine: Roles in alcohol seeking and consumption

Christopher P. King[a,b] and Paul J. Meyer[a,*]
[a]Department of Psychology, State University of New York at Buffalo, Buffalo, NY, United States
[b]Clinical and Research Institute on Addictions, State University of New York at Buffalo, Buffalo, NY, United States
*Corresponding author: e-mail address: pmeyer@buffalo.edu

Contents

1. Introduction 172
2. Appetitive effects of nicotine 174
   2.1 Cues influence behavior by acquiring incentive value 175
   2.2 Nicotine imbues cues with incentive value via multiple mechanisms 175
   2.3 Nicotine amplifies motivation for alcohol by interacting with alcohol-associated cues 178
3. Consummatory effects of nicotine 183
   3.1 Nicotine's temporal factors regulating alcohol intake 184
   3.2 Behavioral models of co-use 185
4. Neurobiological underpinnings of nicotine's reinforcing and incentive amplifying effects 188
   4.1 Neurobiological substrates for nicotine and alcohol: Mesolimbic dopamine 189
   4.2 Neurobiological mechanisms of nicotine amplification of the incentive value of cues 193
   4.3 Neurobiological processes regulating intake: Interoception and the insular cortex 195
5. Conclusion 197
   5.1 Impact for treatment and cessation strategy 198
   5.2 Differences in drug histories on treatment outcome 199
   5.3 Final remarks 200
Acknowledgments 200
Conflict of interest 200
References 200

Abstract

Nicotine has a unique profile among drugs of abuse. To the noninitiated user, nicotine has powerful aversive effects and its relatively weak euphorigenic effects undergo rapid tolerance. Despite this, nicotine is commonly abused despite negative heath

Advances in Pharmacology, Volume 93
ISSN 1054-3589
https://doi.org/10.1016/bs.apha.2021.10.008

consequences, and nicotine users have enormous difficulty quitting. Further, nicotine is one of the most commonly co-abused substances, in that it is often taken in combination with other drugs. One explanation of this polydrug use is that nicotine has multiple appetitive and consummatory conditioning effects. For example, nicotine is a reinforcement enhancer in that it can potently increase the incentive value of other stimuli, including those surrounding drugs of abuse such as alcohol. In addition, nicotine also has a unique profile of neurobiological effects that alter regulation of alcohol intake and interoception. This review discusses the psychological and biological mechanisms surrounding nicotine's appetitive conditioning and consummatory effects, particularly its interactions with alcohol.

Abbreviations

aVTA anterior ventral tegmental area
CS conditioned stimulus
DLS dorsolateral quadrant of the neostriatum
GABA gamma aminobutyric acid
i.v. intravenous
IC insular cortex
DA dopamine
FR fixed ratio
mPFC medial prefrontal cortex
NAcc nucleus accumbens
NAccSh nucleus accumbens shell
NAchR nicotinic acetylcholine receptor
PR progressive-ratio
pVTA posterior ventral tegmental area
VTA ventral tegmental area
VP ventral pallidum
VS visual stimulus

1. Introduction

Nicotine is frequently taken in combination with other drugs, especially alcohol. Nicotine and alcohol use co-morbidity has been well established among human users (Weinberger, Funk, & Goodwin, 2016), with tobacco usage estimates as high as 90% among alcoholics (Batel, Pessione, Maitre, & Rueff, 1995; Burling & Ziff, 1988). Intensity of use between tobacco and alcohol are positively correlated (Istvan & Matarazzo, 1984), resulting in higher levels of individual intake. Further, attempts to quit smoking are more successful in individuals who are nonalcoholic, with at success rates as low as 7% of alcoholic smokers being able to successfully terminate use (DiFranza & Guerrera, 1990). In order to better characterize the relationship between alcohol and tobacco co-use, some lines of evidence have examined intake patterns during drinking episodes. For example, ecological studies have observed that smoking increases during episodes of drinking (Harrison, Hinson, & McKee, 2009). Subjective pleasure for drinking and smoking are positively correlated and are highest during peak intoxication (Piasecki et al., 2011; Piasecki, Wood, Shiffman, Sher, & Heath, 2012), suggesting that the intake of one substance may promote the use of the other when the two are concurrently available. However, tobacco and alcohol co-use research is currently in need of both human and animal research that better model the clinical condition, as well as how the two drugs interact (Van Skike et al., 2016).

Understanding nicotine's psychological and behavioral effects are necessary to explain the underpinnings of pathological polydrug use. First, although the direct effects of nicotine on the central nervous system certainly contribute to the maintenance of tobacco use, the psychological process underlying nicotine's appetitive effects are equally important, both in terms of nicotine's mediation of tobacco use and the enhancement drug use from other drug classes. For example, the sensorimotor stimuli (cues) associated with smoking are important for the maintenance of tobacco use because of the conditioned effects resulting from thousands of nicotine pairings with orosensory tobacco cues (Rose, Behm, & Levin, 1993; Rose, Behm, Westman, & Johnson, 2000; Rose & Levin, 1991). The motivational response to these cues that surround tobacco use are thought to be amplified by nicotine via "reinforcement enhancement" or "incentive amplification" (Bevins & Palmatier, 2004; Liu, Palmatier, Caggiula, Donny, & Sved, 2007; Palmatier et al., 2007), and in humans this reinforcement enhancement can extend to enhance the response other drug and nondrug rewards (Perkins & Karelitz, 2013; Perkins, Karelitz, & Boldry, 2017, 2019). As we will discuss in this chapter, in the case of alcohol, nicotine can alter the response to alcohol-paired cues and contexts, in addition to altering alcohol's reinforcing properties directly. These conditioning effects of nicotine first result in initiation of approach behaviors toward drug and nondrug cues and elicit conditioned motivational states, which can subsequently maintain both tobacco and alcohol use.

Second, intake of one substance appears to be directly linked to the other. Experimental studies in humans have sought to establish causal links using consummatory measures of intake and concepts of reward during tobacco and alcohol use. Under experimenter-controlled conditions, alcohol administration increases both the urge to smoke and subsequent smoking behavior (Epstein, Sher, Young, & King, 2007; King & Epstein, 2005; Mitchell, de Wit, & Zacny, 1995; Rose et al., 2004), suggesting alcohol potentiates both tobacco-directed appetitive and consummatory behaviors. The reciprocal has also been demonstrated under laboratory conditions, where subjects who smoked nicotinized cigarettes report increased alcohol-induced pleasure derived relative to those who smoked de-nicotinized cigarettes (Barrett, Tichauer, Leyton, & Pihl, 2006; Kouri, McCarthy, Faust, & Lukas, 2004). Thus, alcohol and tobacco are both taken together, show positively correlated usage, and appear to increase the craving and intake of each other bidirectionally (for review see Verplaetse & McKee, 2017).

This review will discuss two major domains of nicotine's effects on drug-taking, with special attention to its interactions with alcohol. Here, we separate these domains into being defined as affecting either the (1) appetitive (conditioning, seeking, motivational, and approach) or (2) consummatory (intake and reward) components of alcohol-directed behavior. In this regard, preclinical animal models are widely employed given their utility in characterizing precise neurobiological processes, drug–drug interactions, and long-term changes that are involved across nicotine's various actions (Koob, Kenneth Lloyd, & Mason, 2009).

2. Appetitive effects of nicotine

Although smoked tobacco has been referred to as one of the most addictive and harmful drugs (Nutt, King, Saulsbury, & Blakemore, 2007), the evidence indicating that nicotine is reinforcing in the absence of tobacco smoke or other stimuli is scant and debated (Dar & Frenk, 2004; Henningfield & Goldberg, 1983; Henningfield, Miyasato, & Jasinski, 1983; Perkins, Grobe, Caggiula, Wilson, & Stiller, 1997) (Perkins, 2004; Perkins et al., 2017; Rose, Behm, Westman, Bates, & Salley, 2003; Rose & Corrigall, 1997). Notably, studies demonstrating intravenous nicotine self-administration in human smokers have required the presence of auditory, visual, or olfactory smoke cues coincident with nicotine infusion (Harvey et al., 2004; Rose, Behm, Westman, & Bates, 2003). As noted throughout this chapter, these external cues are critical for nicotine's reinforcing properties.

2.1 Cues influence behavior by acquiring incentive value

Reward-associated stimuli (cues) strongly influence may forms of motivated behavior. In most situations, cues are inherent to the rewards they are associated with (e.g., the smell of a freshly baked brownie, the taste of alcohol). However, in modern environments, and in laboratory preparations, cues can be spatially and temporally separated from their rewards (e.g., a neon alcohol advertisement, a deck of cards at a casino, an empty cigarette box). In these examples, cues have properties that fall into two categories: they predict the availability of rewards, and they can incentivize several behavioral responses. What is the incentive value of a cue and how is it determined? Generally, a cue that has acquired incentive value promotes some form of motivated response. Specifically, in the laboratory, cues can be said to have acquired incentive value if (1) it becomes attractive and individuals will approach it (e.g., during a Pavlovian conditioned approach paradigm), (2) an individual will work for it (e.g., during a conditioned reinforcement test), or (3) it energizes an ongoing instrumental action (e.g., during drug self-administration or Pavlovian to instrumental transfer Milton & Everitt, 2010; Robinson, Yager, Cogan, & Saunders, 2014). In using these measures, several laboratories have demonstrated that the incentive value of cues are experimentally dissociable from their predictive value (Robinson et al., 2014; Robinson & Flagel, 2009) and subserved by different neurobiological mechanisms (Flagel et al., 2011; Flagel, Watson, Robinson, & Akil, 2007; Saunders & Robinson, 2012). Further, there is substantial individual variability in the attribution of incentive value to reward cues (Meyer et al., 2012), which may be a vulnerability trait for addiction-related traits (Meyer, Ma, & Robinson, 2012; Saunders & Robinson, 2010, 2011).

2.2 Nicotine imbues cues with incentive value via multiple mechanisms

2.2.1 Evidence from Pavlovian paradigms

Nicotine increases the incentive value of cues by each of these three measures, albeit via different biopsychological mechanisms. For example, our laboratory has shown that nicotine-paired cues are attractive in a Pavlovian paradigm (Fig. 1). To demonstrate this, rats were equipped with an intravenous (i.v.) catheter and were then presented with a cue (an 8-s presentation of a lever), that predicted the subsequent delivery of 0.03 mg/kg intravenous nicotine infusions (Fig. 1A). These rats learned to

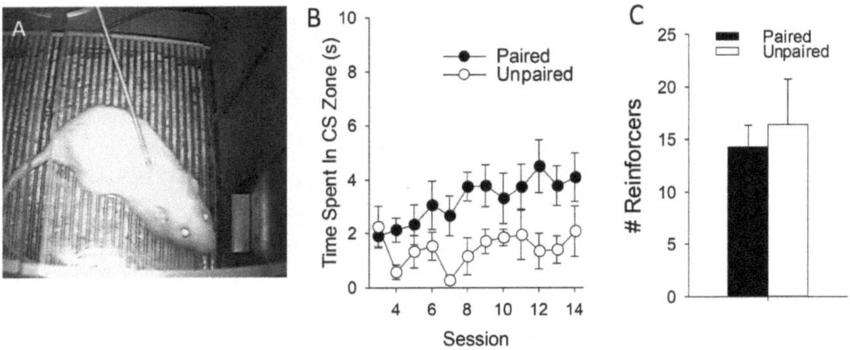

Fig. 1 A nicotine-predictive cue elicits approach in a Pavlovian conditioning paradigm. (A) Rats were equipped with an intravenous catheter and trained to associate an 8-s presentation of a retractable lever with a 0.03 mg/kg infusion of nicotine over eight trials on a VI-15 m schedule for 14 days. (B) Rats approached the nicotine-paired cue to a greater degree than animals presented with the lever and nicotine in an unpaired fashion. (C) On a subsequent test for conditioned reinforcement, rats nose-poked for 3-s presentations of the conditioned stimulus in the absence of nicotine during a 40-min test, but there were no differences in paired and unpaired groups.

approach the lever cue, compared to rats that received unpaired cue/nicotine presentations (Fig. 1B). This demonstration of approach behavior shows that nicotine can imbue its associated cues with incentive value through Pavlovian mechanisms. However, paired rats did not show differences from unpaired rats when working for the cue itself via conditioned reinforcement (Fig. 1C), although a similar study demonstrated that a cue paired with nicotine did acquire this additional reinforcing value (Yager & Robinson, 2015). Thus, within strictly associative Pavlovian conditioning paradigms, nicotine-paired cues can acquire incentive value. As discussed later, the incentive value acquired through these associative processes also plays an important role in nicotine self-administration in animal models as well as smoking behavior in humans.

2.2.2 Evidence from operant paradigms

The incentive properties of cues are particularly important in the study of addiction because they strongly enhance the maintenance of drug-taking and relapse into drug addiction. For example, in a seminal study by Caggiula (Caggiula et al., 2001), rats were trained to press a lever at high rates to obtain i.v. infusions of nicotine that were paired with visual cues. When the cues were removed, the number of acquired nicotine infusions was immediately and substantially reduced, despite nicotine still being freely available. Reintroduction of the cues immediately restored responding for nicotine. Nicotine cues are therefore critical for motivating drug-taking behavior during ongoing nicotine self-administration and is another example of the cues controlling behavior via their incentive properties. Similarly, nicotine-associated cues enhance nicotine-directed behavior by increasing the motivation to obtain the drug (Chaudhri et al., 2007), slow the extinction of operant responding for nicotine when nicotine is no longer available, and reinstate nicotine seeking after extinction (Feltenstein, Ghee, & See, 2012; LeSage, Burroughs, Dufek, Keyler, & Pentel, 2004; Versaggi, King, & Meyer, 2016).

In a series of follow-up studies on Caggiula's initial study, Palmatier et al. demonstrated that cues need not be directly associated with nicotine to produce these effects. In a particularly elegant experiment (Palmatier et al., 2006), four groups of rats were trained to respond for nicotine and/or a visual cue. One group lever-pressed for a visual stimulus (VS), one group pressed only for 0.03 mg/kg nicotine, and a third group pressed for VS-nicotine combination on a single lever. Crucially, the fourth group could concurrently press for the VS and nicotine on separate levers. The nicotine-only group responded the least, with responding lower than the VS-only group. The VS/nicotine single lever group responded at high levels, as had been shown many times. However, the separate nicotine-VS lever group responded for nicotine at similarly low levels as the nicotine group, but responded at high levels for the VS, in fact as high as the VS/nicotine single-lever group. This demonstrates a crucial finding: nicotine self-administration is primarily driven not by its own reinforcing effects, but by its ability to enhance the incentive value of other reinforcers. Subsequent studies further characterized this phenomenon, having very important implications regarding nicotine's effects on cues. For example, nicotine enhances the reinforcing value of a stimulus even when nicotine is given noncontingently at the beginning of the session (Chaudhri et al., 2006; Chaudhri et al., 2006; Chaudhri et al., 2007; Liu et al., 2007; Palmatier et al., 2007; Perkins et al., 2019; Versaggi et al., 2016). Also, the incentive amplification induced by nicotine depends on the initial reinforcing value of the stimulus (Palmatier et al., 2007). In addition, nicotine can enhance the incentive value of stimuli in Pavlovian and operant paradigms (Palmatier et al., 2013; Stringfield, Boettiger, & Robinson, 2018; Versaggi et al., 2016). Thus, nicotine enhances the incentive and reinforcing properties of stimuli across a variety of reward conditioning protocols, consequently imbuing those stimuli with the enhanced capacity to instigate motivated behavior or maintain responding.

In humans, nicotine-paired cues clearly instigate motivated behavior as well. Nicotine cues can induce nicotine craving (Carter & Tiffany, 1999), evoke conditioned physiological responses (Carter & Tiffany, 1999; Erblich, Bovbjerg, & Sloan, 2011; Winkler et al., 2011) maintain smoking behavior independently of nicotine intake (Donny, Houtsmuller, & Stitzer, 2007), and are necessary for the subjective positive experiences induced by nicotine (Alia-Klein et al., 2007; Rose et al., 2000). Thus, smoking, nicotine self-administration, and other smoking-associated behaviors are principally controlled by nicotine's interactions with reward-associated cues. This incentive amplification may explain why the initiation and maintenance of smoking behavior is often highest in the presence of other rewarding situations, such as social interaction (Nguyen & Zhu, 2009). However, the isolation of the nicotine's incentive amplifying effects have been only measured directly in a few studies, with mixed results (Addicott, Oliver, & Joseph McClernon, 2017; Barr, Pizzagalli, Culhane, Goff, & Evins, 2008; Perkins, Grottenthaler, & Wilson, 2009; Wignall & de Wit, 2011). Specifically, one study (Barr et al., 2008); found that nicotine, delivered via transdermal patch to non-smokers, biased responding toward reward stimuli, while another (Perkins et al., 2009), found that intranasal nicotine or smoking had no effect on an operant task in which nondependent smokers responded for various nondrug rewards on an escalating fixed-ratio (FR) (FR11, FR12, etc.) schedule of responding. However, expended effort is only one measure of a reward's incentive value, and as described above, nicotine may amplify the incentive properties of other reward (including alcohol) through multiple mechanisms (Robinson et al., 2014).

2.3 Nicotine amplifies motivation for alcohol by interacting with alcohol-associated cues

As described above, nicotine's conditioned effects are not limited to nicotine cues, because nicotine similarly increases responding for cues associated with other reinforcers (Caggiula et al., 2009), including alcohol (Le, Wang, Harding, Juzytsch, & Shaham, 2003). Thus, one mechanism for the comorbidity of alcohol and nicotine use (Weinberger et al., 2016; Weinberger, Platt, Jiang, & Goodwin, 2015) is that nicotine enhances the reinforcing properties of alcohol-associated cues separately from the pharmacological interactions between these drugs. Consistent with this, rodent studies show that nicotine produces a high-approach, low-avoidance alcohol phenotype

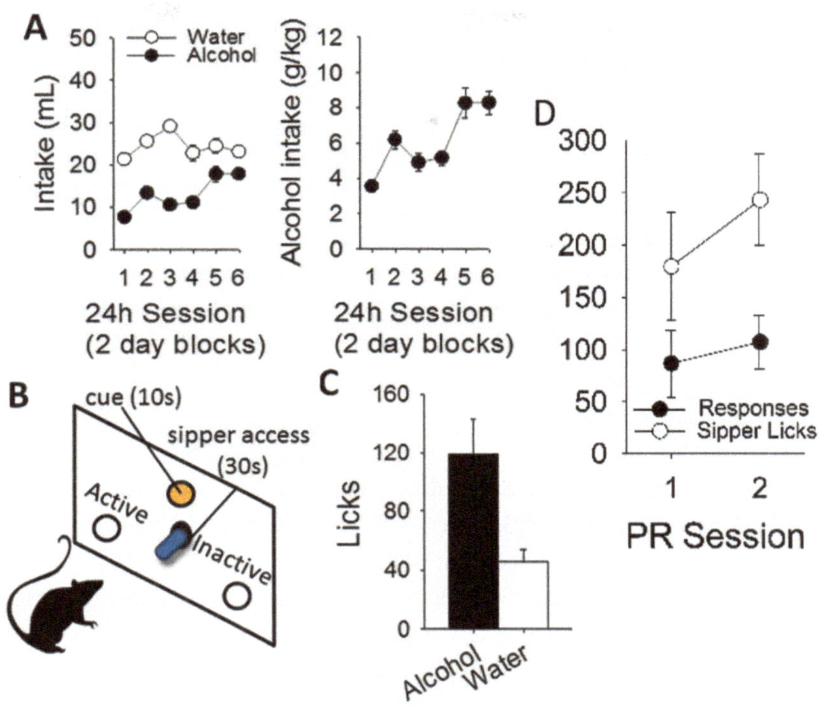

Fig. 2 Home-cage ethanol exposure promotes operant ethanol self-administration. (A) 20% alcohol *v/v* is given every other day in the home-cage for 4 weeks, resulting in escalated intake and increased preference. Then, (B) rats are trained to operantly respond for alcohol by nosepoking for 30 s presentations of an alcohol sipper. During self-administration, consummatory behavior is measured using contact lickometers to measure (C) alcohol intake, and also (D) appetitive nosepoking behavior during tests such as progressive ratio.

in response to alcohol associated cues. For example, nicotine enhances the approach response evoked by an alcohol-predictive cue in Pavlovian paradigms (Angelyn, Loney, & Meyer, 2021; Loney, Angelyn, Cleary, & Meyer, 2019; Maddux & Chaudhri, 2017; Srey, Maddux, & Chaudhri, 2015). We have shown nicotine enhanced the response to a cue that predicted access to a retractable sipper bottle containing ethanol, without affecting the response to a similar, nonpredictive stimulus. In other experiments, nicotine reduced the conditioned taste (but not place) aversion induced by ethanol (Loney et al., 2019; Loney, Pautassi, Kapadia, & Meyer, 2018), indicating that nicotine alters the motivational effects of alcohol-associated cues in some, but not all, Pavlovian paradigms.

2.3.1 *Alcohol self-administration models assess the effects of motivation and intake*

Alcohol self-administration involves both the preparatory responding and motivation to gain access to alcohol, as well as the subsequent consumption of alcohol following its delivery. In our laboratory, we use a procedure in which the appetitive and consummatory phases of ethanol self-administration can be dissociated [Figs. 2 and 3; see also Schier, Dilly, & Gonzales, 2013; Simms, Bito-Onon, Chatterjee, & Bartlett, 2010]. First, rats are given 24-h access to 20% ethanol or water, three times a week for 4 weeks. This produces escalation in ethanol intake (Fig. 2A). Then, rats make responses that are reinforced with a 30-s presentation of a bottle containing 20% ethanol (Fig. 2B). A cue-light is illuminated with the bottle presentation. Using contact lickometers, we can dissociate the appetitive (nose-poking or lever-pressing) and consummatory (licking and consumption) aspects of ethanol drinking (Fig. 2C). In addition, the motivational properties of ethanol reinforcement can be assessed using a progressive ratio (PR) test, in which work requirement to access alcohol sipper becomes increasingly difficult. The PR test is used as a standard measure of ethanol reinforcement with minimal influence of post-ingestive factors. A shown in Fig. 2, the alcohol exposure provided in the home cage produces increases in both the appetitive (Fig. 2D) and consummatory measures (Fig. 2C) of alcohol-directed behavior. Using this design, it is therefore possible to specifically observe nicotine's effects on appetitive alcohol-directed behavior, separately from its effects on regulating intake.

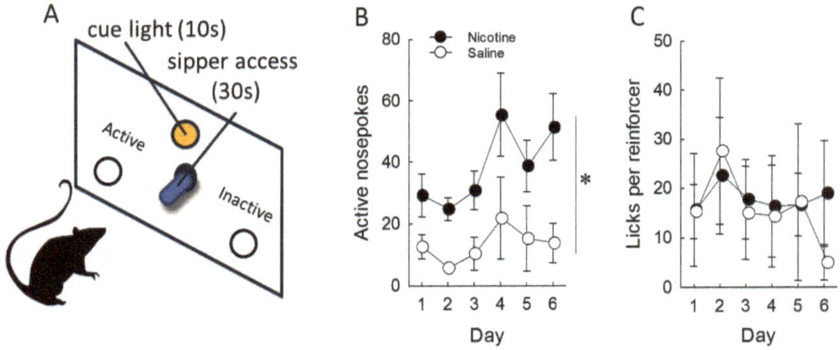

Fig. 3 Nicotine enhanced operant responding for alcohol. (A) Rats were tested for both alcohol-directed responding and intake in daily 1-h sessions under saline or 0.4 mg/kg injections of nicotine. (B) Nicotine enhances responding for alcohol in the presence of cues relative to saline treated rats, however (C) this did not result in heightened intake.

2.3.2 Nicotine enhances responding for alcohol in the presence of cues

Being able to distinguish between the appetitive and consummatory consequences of nicotine is important, particularly in order to dissociate the mechanisms by which nicotine modifies behavior. Factors regulating intake will be discussed in detail below, however generally speaking, nicotine reduces alcohol intake when it is given acutely, immediately prior to testing (Le, Corrigall, Harding, Juzytsch, & Li, 2000; Sharpe & Samson, 2002). In contrast, chronic nicotine also increases responding for alcohol in the presence of cues (Le et al., 2003), even when delivered continuously over a 24-h period via osmotic pump (Clark, Lindgren, Brooks, Watson, & Little, 2001). Using our method of alcohol self-administration to identify appetitive-specific effects of nicotine (Fig. 3A), we have found that nicotine enhances responding for presentations of an alcohol sipper (Fig. 3B) in the presence of alcohol-paired cues without affecting subsequent intake (Fig. 3C). These data fit with the general body of work suggesting nicotine can enhance responding for other reward-paired stimuli, crucially those paired with alcohol. These alcohol cues presented alongside the alcohol reinforcement can acquire incentive value, as measured by their ability to cause the reinstatement of an extinguished response (Lamparelli & Meyer, 2018). Nicotine enhances this effect and may be one reason why alcohol abstinence is hard to maintain in smokers (Smith et al., 2020).

2.3.3 Occasion-setters and discriminative stimuli

In the experimental designs described in this chapter, cue presentation was contingent on the rats' response. However, cues can be presented independent of the subject's response, for example acting as "occasion-setters" to signal drug-availability or acting as a discriminative stimulus (S^d). Nicotine itself can serve as a S^d to occasion motivated responding (Randall, Cannady, & Besheer, 2016; Troisi 2nd, Dooley 2nd, & Craig, 2013; Wooters, Bevins, & Bardo, 2009), and nicotine can also alter the response to other S^d presentations. In an example using rats, we tested the effect of nicotine injections in a discriminative stimulus (S^d)-modulated alcohol self-administration and reinstatement procedure. Here, rats nose-poked for presentations of an alcohol bottle in the presence of an "alcohol-available" S^d (illumination of a houselight; Fig. 4A). We found that this S^d effectively modulated alcohol self-administration compared to a separate alcohol "nonavailable" DS (S^{delta}), and that nicotine specifically enhanced appetitive responding only in the presence of the S^d during self-administration (Fig. 4B). Further, the enhancement was also observed during a reinstatement test when

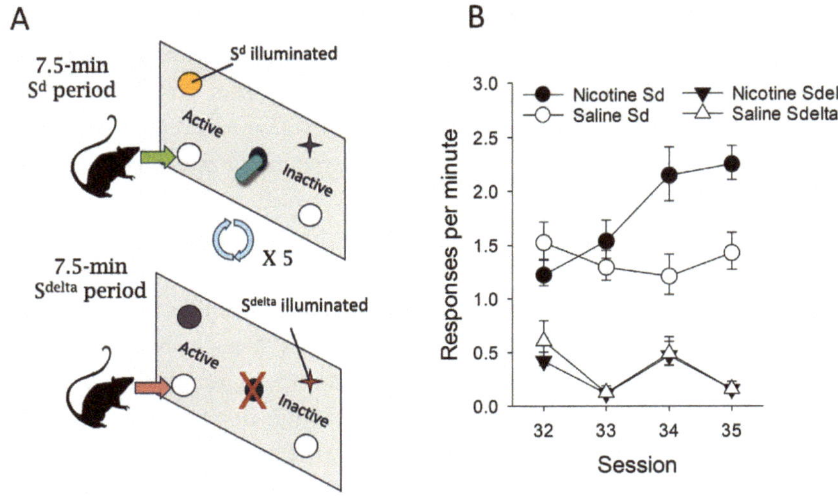

Fig. 4 Nicotine enhances responding for alcohol in the presence of a discriminative stimulus signaling alcohol availability. (A) Rats were trained to respond for alcohol in 7.5 min "alcohol-available" (S^d) periods, where active nose-pokes resulted in presentation of an alcohol sipper solution. Each 7.5 min Sd period was followed by a 7.5 min "alcohol nonavailable" period signaled by a separate "S^{delta}" stimulus. (B) Rats specifically responded for alcohol during the Sd period, and Sd-induced responding specifically was enhanced by nicotine.

the alcohol bottle and its associated cues were removed (Angelyn & Meyer, 2019). Since these cues were not response contingent, the term "reinforcement enhancement" in reference to nicotine's effects is insufficient. Instead, because nicotine's immediate effects on regulating appetitive behavior through cues therefore also extend to other salient stimuli that signal reward availability such as occasion setters and discriminative stimuli, nicotine is better described as acting more generally as an amplifier of the incentive value of cues (Bevins and Palmatier, 2004), including alcohol cues. Further, this incentive amplification can apply to complex contextual stimuli, which have powerful control over not only nicotine seeking (Conklin, 2006; McClernon et al., 2016), but alcohol seeking as well (Zipori et al., 2017).

Collectively, these findings indicate that nicotine promotes appetitive alcohol responding by amplifying the incentive value of alcohol-associated cues. This is consistent with Cagiulla's ideas regarding nicotine's effects on reinforcement (Caggiula et al., 2009), with the modification that nicotine amplifies the incentive value of cues generally, whether they are response-contingent or not. However, one aspect of alcohol and nicotine co-use that may be unique to the combination of these drugs is the effect of nicotine on alcohol taste cues. While oral cues can instigate alcohol seeking (Knight et al., 2016), higher doses of alcohol can condition an aversion to alcohol-associated tastes (e.g., Anderson, Varlinskaya, & Spear, 2010). Nicotine interferes with this conditioned taste aversion to alcohol-associated flavors (Bienkowski, Piasecki, Koros, Stefanski, & Kostowski, 1998; Kunin, Smith, & Amit, 1999; Loney et al., 2018; Loney et al., 2019; Loney & Meyer, 2019; Rinker et al., 2011), which is likely due to an alteration of the interoceptive properties of alcohol by nicotine (discussed more later), and not to a general effect of nicotine on learning, because nicotine does not alter a taste aversion induced by the nausea-producing drug lithium chloride. In this manner, in addition to increasing the incentive value of environmental alcohol cues, nicotine may also facilitate alcohol seeking by altering the aversive interoceptive effects of higher doses of alcohol.

3. Consummatory effects of nicotine

Thus far we have discussed data showing that nicotine enhances the incentive salience of drug paired cues, instigates seeking and approach behavior, and enhances reinforcement for alcohol in the presence of cues (Le et al., 2003). During ongoing drug self-administration, in addition to the presence of discrete alcohol and nicotine cues, drug-directed behavior is also influenced by lifetime experience with both substances, as well as the individual's own ability to titrate their alcohol and nicotine intake. As discussed, nicotine's profile of effects envelopes both appetitive and consummatory processes, including nicotine's enhancement of responding for alcohol during self-administration and reinstatement (Le et al., 2003), its promotion of intake in a time-dependent manner (Le et al., 2000), and its effects when given chronically at higher doses (Bito-Onon, Simms, Chatterjee, Holgate, & Bartlett, 2011). However, the relationship between intake and responding is not always straightforward. In one study using rats (Le et al., 2010), alcohol and nicotine were made available together in one group, while other groups self-administered only one drug. Alcohol self-administration occurred at the expense of nicotine, but later the extinction of responding for alcohol was delayed in rats that had nicotine concurrently available, indicating separable intake and operant response consequences of nicotine. Priming with either nicotine or alcohol during a subsequent reinstatement test increased responding for both drugs.

Thus, this study showed that self-administered nicotine, although itself decreased by alcohol, increased responding for self-administered alcohol. Thus, segregation of the appetitive and consequential intake effects of nicotine is crucial to fully understand the interaction between drugs.

Several studies have used responding for alcohol and alcohol intake interchangeably as endpoints for nicotine's effects on alcohol-directed behavior. Importantly however, the effects of nicotine are highly dependent on when it is given, for how long, and the exact behaviors being measured and when. Our studies show that although nicotine increases alcohol's appetitive effects in standard self-administration paradigms, it either does not change or reduces alcohol intake acutely. Instead, nicotine-induced changes related to the ingestive, consummatory aspects of alcohol and are likely due to nicotine's chronic effects, which is discussed in this section.

3.1 Nicotine's temporal factors regulating alcohol intake

3.1.1 Acute effects on intake

Alcohol intake involves the reinforcing properties of alcohol during and following drinking, as well as processes involving of fluid intake and regulation (Samson, Slawecki, Sharpe, & Chappell, 1998). Naturally, given its high face validity, quantified alcohol intake is the one of the most frequently reported methods for operationalizing alcohol-directed behavior. However, the timing, dosing, and experience with nicotine may differentially alter alcohol intake, and thus with the wealth of methods to measure alcohol-directed behavior under nicotine, each measure and experimental design may target different psychological processes.

Perhaps the simplest way to model the interaction between nicotine and alcohol in rodents is to look at how consumption of one substance changes while under the influence of the other. The simplicity of this design is likely one of the reasons why this approach has historically been one of the most widely employed. For example, a number of early studies from Samson and colleagues have demonstrated that alcohol intake in rats is acutely suppressed when measured following subcutaneous injections of nicotine (Hendrickson, Zhao-Shea, Pang, Gardner, & Tapper, 2010; Nadal & Samson, 1999; Sharpe & Samson, 2002). Nicotine is anorexigenic (Jo, Talmage, & Role, 2002), which likely suppresses alcohol intake during early phases of nicotine exposure. Home-cage alcohol intake is suppressed specifically via nicotinic acetylcholine receptors (Dyr, Koros, Bienkowski, & Kostowski, 1999) including the α4 subtype (Hendrickson et al., 2010).

Importantly, these studies occurred in the absence of a dedicated testing environment and alcohol-paired CSs, thus more directly reflecting the consummatory phase of alcohol intake.

3.1.2 Protracted effects on intake

In humans, experience and history with nicotine undoubtably contributes to the longer-term behavioral and neurobiological changes, with age of smoking onset predicting alcohol use problems later (Chen et al., 2002; Grant, 1998; Jensen et al., 2003). Thus, in the laboratory, intake-specific effects of nicotine are similarly influenced by an individual's history and timing of exposure, particularly when experienced outside the testing environment. For example, alcohol-experienced rats show a suppression of intake when nicotine is given immediately prior to a relapse to alcohol intake test, but instead showed heightened intake when nicotine is was given during a withdrawal period on the days prior (Alen, Gomez, Gonzalez-Cuevas, Navarro, & Lopez-Moreno, 2009; Doyon et al., 2013). Indeed, other designs have similarly demonstrated nicotine can later enhance alcohol intake when it is first given in the absence of alcohol (Hauser et al., 2012; Lopez-Moreno et al., 2004), and during adolescence (Kemppainen, Hyytia, & Kiianmaa, 2009). Importantly, these data suggest that longer-term intake-specific effects may be divorced from the other more immediate effects, where intake is heightened when it is temporally separated from the drinking event (Alen et al., 2009). Thus, procedures that generally employ longer nicotine exposure periods across days better facilitate alcohol intake in the home cage (Blomqvist, Ericson, Johnson, Engel, & Soderpalm, 1996; Olausson, Ericson, Lof, Engel, & Soderpalm, 2001; Smith, Horan, Gaskin, & Amit, 1999). Taken together, it is likely that the intake specific processes surrounding nicotine are a result longer-term exposure periods, which eventually come to interact with the various appetitive and conditioning properties in various drug-taking settings. Indeed, nicotine delivered continuously by osmotic minipump can also promote the acquisition and maintenance of alcohol self-administration (Clark et al., 2001); perhaps, better reflecting the chronic nature of tobacco use.

3.2 Behavioral models of co-use

A brief summary of these data suggests that, at least acutely, experimenter-delivered nicotine has suppressive effects on both alcohol intake and seeking when it is given in close temporal proximity but can enhance it when given chronically or separately from the testing session.

Despite the great utility of studies that utilize noncontingent injections, controlled site-specific infusions, and other highly experimentally controlled methods, individuals can titrate their own tobacco and alcohol use under normal conditions. It stands to reason rodent studies employing dual self-administration protocols may model key components of voluntary human usage, although very few groups have tried this. Marshall and colleagues originally reported that, when nicotine and alcohol solutions were presented together, there were no changes in consumption relative to when they were presented alone (Marshall, Dadmarz, Hofford, Gottheil, & Vogel, 2003). Other attempts to model co-use using operant conditioning instead of free intake were later attempted, but either nicotine self-administration decreased in the presence of alcohol (Le et al., 2010), or the concurrent availability of both decreased the intake of both (Funk, Lo, Coen, & Le, 2016).

It is likely that the specific parameters surrounding drug-availability, timing, training, and presence of cues are important for these models. Other variations to this procedure have been deployed, but with mixed results. Orally self-administering rats demonstrate preference for an alcohol only solution over alcohol and nicotine (Hauser et al., 2012), but show heightened intake for a cocktail of intravenous nicotine and alcohol over either by itself (Karatayev et al., 2015), likely reflecting factors surrounding relative aversion and reward due to route of administration. As discussed previously, nicotine has been shown to enhance intake when taken sufficiently in advance of alcohol, and in one instance during daily alternating access to alcohol and nicotine, nicotine enhanced alcohol intake when nicotine was taken earlier in the day (Le, Funk, Lo, & Coen, 2014), suggesting that that timing of drug-taking is important both under experimenter controlled and voluntary conditions.

Because nicotine enhances appetitive responding for alcohol in the presence of cues (see Fig. 3), we assessed the immediate effect of nicotine availability on free-alcohol consumption in the absence of cues using a procedure in which rats were allowed to freely self-administer nicotine in the presence of an alcohol sipper (Fig. 5) that required no appetitive responding. In contrast to Le and colleagues, we found that i.v. nicotine was readily self-administered (Fig. 5A), but at the expense of alcohol responding (Fig. 5B), crucially in rats that had an established history of home cage drinking (adapted from: (Simms et al., 2008; Simms et al., 2010)). Upon nicotine removal, responding for nicotine rapidly decreased (Fig. 5C), and alcohol consumption increased to saline levels (Fig. 5D). Recently, Chandler and

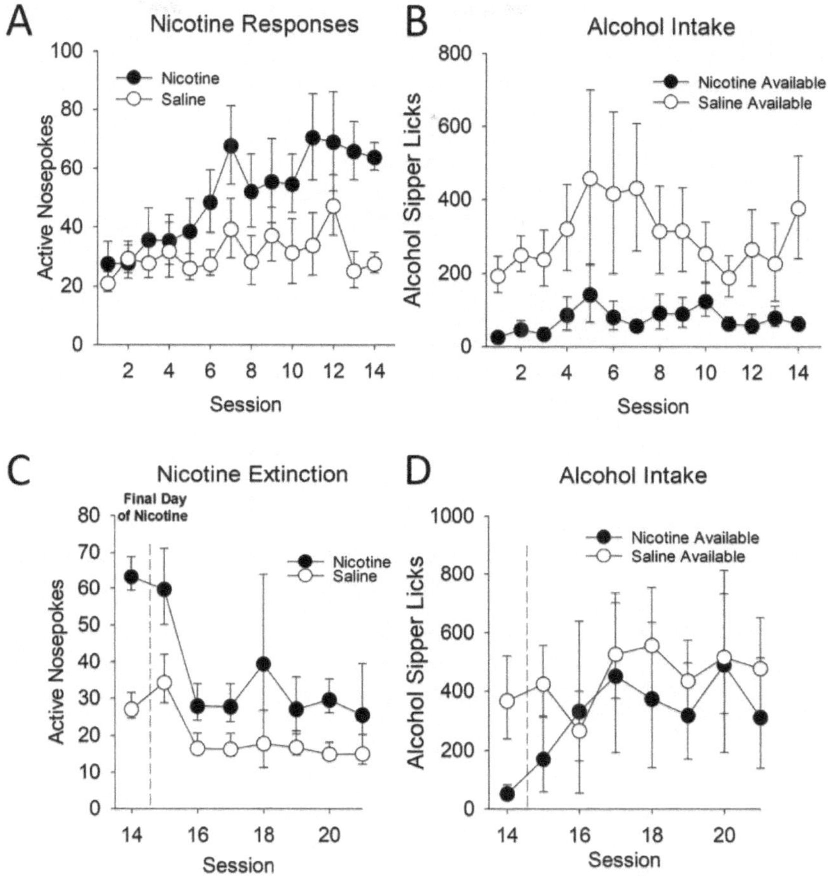

Fig. 5 Alcohol and nicotine continuous access. Rats were trained to lever press for nicotine or saline in the presence of a continuously available 20% alcohol sipper. Nicotine responses are shown on the left panels, and alcohol intake is shown in the right panels. (A) Rats lever pressed for nicotine more than saline controls. However, (B) rats with nicotine available consumed less alcohol. When nicotine was removed, (C) responding on the nicotine lever decreased, and (D) alcohol intake increased quickly to control levels.

colleagues have sought to optimize i.v. nicotine and alcohol intakes under co-use conditions, with the primary goal of evaluating pharmacological manipulations (naltrexone and varenicline) directed at reducing intake of one or both substances. Specifically, they demonstrated that alcohol consumption escalated during nicotine availability, but only when the fixed-ratio response requirement was sufficiently high (Chandler, Maggio, Peng, Nixon, & Bardo, 2020).

These data together suggest that (1) alcohol and nicotine can both be readily self-administered, but only when (2) either the response requirement for nicotine is sufficiently high to discourage high levels of intake, or (3) nicotine-availability is sufficiently separated from alcohol to avoid the immediate alcohol suppressing effects. Further, separation of both the motivational and intake-specific effects of nicotine are especially crucial, given the differential effect of nicotine on both under various conditions.

The future utility of validating co-use models may provide important insights into the unique neuroadaptive changes surrounding motivation and regulation of intake when the subject can regulate their own consumption of both nicotine and alcohol. This may be especially useful because pharmacological treatments differ in efficacy among individuals with both tobacco and alcohol use histories, and the use of well-designed animal models of co-use may help reconcile currently existing disparities with behavioral outcomes and treatment mechanisms between sets of models, making them more generalizable (Motschman et al., 2016). Future models of co-use will thus likely be most successful when they are able to exploit the availability of cues, the long-term potentiating effects of nicotine, and dissociate both the appetitive/motivational components of drug-seeking from intake.

4. Neurobiological underpinnings of nicotine's reinforcing and incentive amplifying effects

As discussed, nicotine produces a range of appetitive and consummatory effects on alcohol. The neurobiological processes underling tobacco and alcohol co-use are complicated and involve drug actions across a range of neurotransmitter systems and brain areas. Each of these systems may engage different psychological and behavioral processes, producing an ensemble of changes working in concert to modify alcohol and nicotine directed behavior across the lifetime of the individual. It is therefore difficult to disentangle the direct effects of nicotine on alcohol-directed behavior from the synergistic effect of both taken in conjunction, although some lines of evidence have been useful in dissociating the various drug- and neuroanatomical specific effects involved in co-use.

4.1 Neurobiological substrates for nicotine and alcohol: Mesolimbic dopamine

The involvement of the mesolimbic dopamine system in drug reinforcement and learning has been well documented and is probably the most widely examined neural system to date in the development of drug addiction across a variety of compounds. In addition to its involvement in the response to drug cues, the reinforcing properties of most drugs of abuse depend on the activity of the limbic system (Everitt & Robbins, 2005, 2013; Nestler, 2005; Robinson & Berridge, 1993, 2000, 2008), and are necessary for the maintenance of drug-taking across different drug-classes such as the psychomotor stimulants, opioids, nicotine, and alcohol. It is thus reasonable to predict that the reinforcing and motivational properties of alcohol and its associated cues are directly modified by nicotine through convergent neuroadaptations in dopaminergic circuitry.

Functionally, as a key structure in the mesolimbic dopamine system, the ventral tegmental area (VTA) has been characterized for its role encoding the motivational value of rewards and their associated cues (D'Ardenne, McClure, Nystrom, & Cohen, 2008; Schultz, 1997, 1998, 2015), principally through phasic bursts of firing (Tsai et al., 2009) which can instigate reward seeking behavior (Adamantidis et al., 2011). The firing of dopamine-containing cell bodies in the VTA results in dopaminergic overflow in downstream forebrain regions such as the nucleus accumbens (NAcc) (Sombers, Beyene, Carelli, & Wightman, 2009) that contrast tonic single-spike firing (Hyland, Reynolds, Hay, Perk, & Miller, 2002). Thus, these transient increases in NAcc dopamine release become linked to reward cues and initiation of reward seeing behavior (Owesson-White, Cheer, Beyene, Carelli, & Wightman, 2008; Roitman, Stuber, Phillips, Wightman, & Carelli, 2004). These actions likely underlie the conditioned, appetitive effects of drugs such as nicotine following drug-use.

The direct, immediate actions of addictive drugs within the mesolimbic dopamine system therefore result in abnormal motivational learning when compared to conventional reinforcers (Di Chiara, 1998; Di Chiara et al., 1999; Pierce & Kumaresan, 2006). Like many drugs of abuse, nicotine and alcohol involve actions on mesolimbic dopamine, principally by increasingly dopamine release in the NAcc through various mechanisms. Although here we discuss convergent nicotine and alcohol reinforcement mechanisms, an exhaustive review of the complex cellular and neurobiological mechanisms of alcohol and nicotine reinforcement is beyond the scope of this review. These systems have recently been reviewed in excellent detail elsewhere (e.g., for a recent review see Morel, Montgomery, & Han, 2019).

4.1.1 Mechanisms of nicotine reinforcement

Nicotine binds to the various subtypes of the nicotinic acetylcholine receptor (NAchR) that are neuroanatomically distributed (Gotti et al., 2009), and for example can stimulate dopamine release via VTA and NAcc actions (Ferrari, Le Novere, Picciotto, Changeux, & Zoli, 2002). In addition to being expressed at multiple nodes in the midbrain, dorsal, and ventral striatum, it is further expressed in the habenular-peduncular pathway, amygdala, hippocampus, and cortical areas (Tuesta, Fowler, & Kenny, 2011). Furthermore, nicotinic receptor subtype distribution varies anatomically as well (for a full review, see: (Fowler, Arends, & Kenny, 2008), although the α4, α7, and β2 have received a great deal of addition given their location in the VTA (Charpantier, Barneoud, Moser, Besnard, & Sgard, 1998), involvement in nicotine self-administration (Brunzell & McIntosh, 2012; Laviolette & van der Kooy, 2003), and involvement in reinforcement within in the VTA (Pons et al., 2008). Furthermore, β2-containing nicotinic receptors stimulate dopamine release from the VTA (Mameli-Engvall et al., 2006), and systemic antagonism of α4β2 reduces the conditioned reinforcing properties of nicotine (Liu et al., 2007; Liu, Zhao-Shea, McIntosh, Gardner, & Tapper, 2012). The appraisal of the β2-containing nicotinic receptor in drug-related behaviors, and its proximity to the VTA-NAcc pathway have made this an attractive target for nicotine actions on reinforcement.

4.1.2 Mechanisms of alcohol reinforcement

Alcohol-elicited dopamine release is a key process in reinforcement (Gonzales, Job, & Doyon, 2004), and alcohol is largely been identified as reinforcing in the VTA (Gatto, McBride, Murphy, Lumeng, & Li, 1994; Rodd et al., 2004), stimulating VTA dopamine neurons directly (Appel, Liu, McElvain, & Brodie, 2003; Brodie, Pesold, & Appel, 1999) resulting in downstream DA release in areas including the NAcc (Di Chiara & Imperato, 1985) to promote self-administration (Rassnick, Pulvirenti, & Koob, 1992). However, the VTA is a relatively large and heterogeneous structure, with separate neuroanatomical regions distinguished by various afferent targets (Swanson, 1982; Walsh & Han, 2014) and cytoarchitectural distinctions (Sanchez-Catalan, Kaufling, Georges, Veinante, & Barrot, 2014). The multiple projections of the VTA innervate the forebrain

(Swanson, 1982) including areas crucial for drug reinforcement such as the NAcc. The various regions of the VTA have been simplified into dimensions based on neuroanatomical location, for example, as either anterior (aVTA) or posterior (pVTA), both of which are differentially sensitive to different drugs of reinforcement (Sanchez-Catalan et al., 2014). Alcohol-stimulated dopamine release, particularly in the pVTA, innervates a variety of forebrain regions including the ventral pallidum (VP), medial prefrontal cortex (mPFC), NAcc core (Ding, Ingraham, Rodd, & McBride, 2015), and NAcc (Boileau et al., 2003; Rassnick et al., 1992; Weiss, Lorang, Bloom, & Koob, 1993) which are understood to drive the reinforcing effects of alcohol. At least in the pVTA, repeated exposure to alcohol via microinjections appears to sensitize the release of NAcc shell (NAccSh) DA (Ding, Rodd, Engleman, & McBride, 2009).

4.1.3 Mechanisms of nicotine-alcohol interactions

Nicotine and alcohol are thought to produce complex interactions on reinforcement through their direct actions on each other within the mesolimbic system, which have also been previously discussed in several other excellent reviews (Doyon, Thomas, Ostroumov, Dong, & Dani, 2013; Hendrickson, Guildford, & Tapper, 2013). Passive administration of nicotine and alcohol together produces an additive effect of dopamine release in the NAcc (Tizabi, Bai, Copeland Jr., & Taylor, 2007) which likely involves interactions within the VTA (Tizabi, Copeland, Louis, & Taylor, 2002). Specifically, the reinforcing value of lower doses of nicotine and alcohol together are enhanced in the pVTA (Truitt et al., 2015), as both taken at subthreshold doses together intracranially, resulting in robust brain-derived neurotrophic factor (BDNF) upregulation and drug-elicited dopamine and glutamate release in the NAccSh (Waeiss, Knight, Engleman, Hauser, & Rodd, 2020). The alcohol-enhanced firing rate of VTA neurons is further exacerbated by nicotine (Clark & Little, 2004) but is concentration-dependent. Regardless, at least locally, nicotine appears to sensitize local dopamine release in the NAccSh to the subsequent effects of alcohol (Ding et al., 2012). These studies together would support an enhancement of the reinforcing and motivational properties of combined nicotine and alcohol, although they largely model acute effects, rather than neuroadaptations following prolonged consumption and drug history. Further, these studies largely focus on localized effects under intracranial manipulations.

4.1.4 Protracted changes in nicotine–alcohol interactions

As discussed previously, nicotine appears to better enhance voluntary alcohol intake when it is given in exposure windows either developmentally or temporally dissociated from the period of alcohol consumption. In contrast to the previously described studies, subchronic nicotine can actually blunt alcohol-induced DA release in the NAccSh (Lopez-Moreno et al., 2008). The effect of nicotine pre-exposure can persist long after it is metabolized, attenuating the alcohol-induced release of NAcc DA and VTA firing, while producing concurrent increases in alcohol consumption (Doyon, Dong, et al., 2013). In addition, although nicotine can acutely increase VTA firing, NAchRs are rapidly desensitized, producing acute tolerance to nicotine's effects (Pidoplichko, DeBiasi, Williams, & Dani, 1997). The repeated combination of desensitization (Grady, Wageman, Patzlaff, & Marks, 2012) and NAchR upregulation (Fasoli et al., 2016; Staley et al., 2006) specifically on VTA gamma aminobutyric acid (GABA) inhibitory interneurons (Nashmi et al., 2007) may result in acceleration of DA-ergic blunting. These pre-exposures specifically in development appear to amplify inhibitory synaptic GABA mechanisms (Thomas et al., 2018) resulting in increased alcohol consumption.

Paradoxically, despite chronically induced decreases in alcohol induced DA release following nicotine, intake is amplified. Indeed, blunted DA function has thought to be a consequence of alcohol dependence (Martinez et al., 2005; Volkow et al., 1996). Interestingly, phasic firing appears to be a crucial feature surrounding the response to rewards and associated cues, as tonic stimulation of the VTA blunts alcohol intake (Bass et al., 2013). In light of this, it is likely that other mechanisms other than simply DA surges in the NAcc, such as changes in inhibitory GABA function (Chester & Cunningham, 2002) that can regulate consumption (Nie, Rewal, Gill, Ron, & Janak, 2011) may underlie persistent changes following nicotine histories. There is some evidence to suggest that the GABA-alcohol interaction may be especially important, given GABAergic inhibitory currents in the cerebellum are related to variation in alcohol consumption (Kaplan, Mohr, & Rossi, 2013; Richardson & Rossi, 2017).

Additional work separating cue and intake-specific effects under different drug histories will be important in elucidating the specific neuroadaptations following concurrent nicotine and alcohol use. It is, however, likely that the varieties of effects produced by nicotine in the mesolimbic system underlie features that alter cue conditioning and intake, and likely do so differently following prolonged experience with the drug. Further, nicotine-driven escalations in alcohol intake may involve other non-mesolimbic actions of nicotine.

4.2 Neurobiological mechanisms of nicotine amplification of the incentive value of cues

Because nicotine has weak reinforcing properties when administered alone, most studies examining nicotine reinforcement either present nicotine in combination with cues or measure the response to the cues themselves. Human studies using fMRI have indicated the appetitive activation (i.e., craving) activated by nicotine cues (typically presented on a video screen) is associated with activation of limbic brain areas described in reinforcement, including the NAcc (ventral striatum), amygdala, and areas of the cortex, including the prefrontal, cingulate, insular, and orbitofrontal cortices (Brody et al., 2002; McClernon, Hiott, Huettel, & Rose, 2005; Seungdamrong & Yasunaga, 1975; Smolka et al., 2006; Wilson, Sayette, Delgado, & Fiez, 2005). In one study, smokers were presented cues after smoking cigarettes, thus minimizing the effects of nicotine withdrawal. Not only was robust cue-induced craving observed, but robust activation of the ventral striatum, amygdala, orbitofrontal cortex, hippocampus, medial thalamus, and left insula were observed as well (Franklin et al., 2007). However, no non-nicotine sessions were included in the design, so it is unclear whether the neural cue responsivity was due to the acquired incentive properties of the cues (through Pavlovian mechanisms), or whether the brain activation was due to more generalized noncontingent incentive amplifying properties of nicotine. Another study measured the neural response to money-predictive (or neutral) cues after oral nicotine or placebo, and on some trials the outcome was unexpected (Addicott et al., 2017). Nicotine amplified the neural response to all cues in this task, including money-predictive cues, neutral cues, and those that preceded unexpected outcomes, particularly in the anterior insula/inferior frontal gyrus. This was also associated with a decrease in cue-induced activity in the dorsal striatum. Together, these data suggest a key role for the insular cortex (discussed in detail below) in nicotine's ability to amplify the incentive value of cues.

Several studies, especially those in rodent models, indicate that nicotine self-administration is dependent on the mesolimbic dopamine system (Corrigall, Coen, & Adamson, 1994), which is likely regulated by brainstem areas that can influence the rewarding and aversive properties of nicotine (Laviolette, Alexson, & van der Kooy, 2002). However, in most of these investigations, nicotine is presented in combination with an associated cue, and thus the primary reinforcing effects of nicotine cannot be dissociated from its incentive amplifying effects. However, one study used a Pavlovian conditioned approach paradigm to demonstrate that dopamine receptors are required for the enhancement of the sign-tracking response by nicotine (Palmatier, Kellicut, Brianna Sheppard, Brown, & Robinson, 2014). This finding, in combination with others showing that sign-tracking requires dopamine neurotransmission (Danna & Elmer, 2010; Flagel et al., 2011), indicates that nicotine likely amplifies the incentive value of reward-associated stimuli via dopaminergic neurotransmission. Also, several studies have measured the role dopamine and related brain areas during cue-induced reinstatement, which largely support a role for the mesocorticolimbic circuity described above (Caggiula et al., 2001). In addition, transition to nicotine self-administration is accompanied by a reduction in the aversive properties of nicotine (and alcohol), which is associated with changes in the lateral habenula and peduncular nuclei (Baldwin, Alanis, & Salas, 2011; Fowler & Kenny, 2012; Glover, McDougle, Siegel, Jhou, & Chandler, 2016; Pang et al., 2016; Wolfman et al., 2018; Zhao-Shea et al., 2015).

At least some of the appetitive effects of nicotine are similar to other drug categories, and may be explained by actions within the mesocorticolimbic dopamine system which is important in coupling incentive salience to reward-paired cues (Berridge, 2012). In humans, DA-stimulating drugs such as d-amphetamine can enhance the positive response to stimuli independently of its euphorigenic effects (Wardle & de Wit, 2012). Amphetamine likely shares mechanistic overlap with nicotine, for example by enhancing the conditioned reinforcing value of CSs via its DA-promoting actions in the NAcc (Parkinson, Olmstead, Burns, Robbins, & Everitt, 1999; Taylor & Robbins, 1984, 1986; Wyvell & Berridge, 2000) and enhancing sign-tracking in the dorsolateral quadrant of the neostriatum (DLS) (DiFeliceantonio & Berridge, 2016). It is likely that these various pharmacological actions may converge simultaneously, as nicotine and amphetamine given in conjunction can further enhance VS responding (McNealy, Ramsay, Barrett, & Bevins, 2021), perhaps via their combined DA actions in the NAcc which is involved in conditioned reinforcement (Wolterink et al., 1993) and sign-tracking (Fraser & Janak, 2017). Besides the psychomotor stimulants, other drug categories including intra-NAcc agonists targeting opioid receptors can also enhance incentive salience measures such as pavlovian instrumental transfer (Peciña & Berridge, 2013) and conditioned reinforcement (Phillips, Robbins, & Everitt, 1994). Thus, it seems highly likely that there are DA-modulated actions on both reinforcement and incentive salience in the mesolimbic forebrain that can be recapitulated by different drug classes.

The neurobiological basis for the effects of nicotine on alcohol cue responsivity, however, is less well-studied and may reflect unique drug-drug interactions. The combination of these drugs can serve as a complex discriminative stimulus (Ford, Davis, McCracken, & Grant, 2013; Ford, McCracken, Davis, Ryabinin, & Grant, 2012; Randall et al., 2016; Troisi 2nd et al., 2013) that involves the NAcc and prefrontal cortex, (Chatterjee & Bartlett, 2010; Randall, McElligott, & Besheer, 2020), and alcohol cues activate similar circuitry. One study (King, McNamara, Angstadt, & Phan, 2010) showed that the neural response to smoking cues in the NAcc is enhanced by alcohol. The converse study has not been done, but one study found similar activation in the insular and cingulate cortices during separately presented alcohol and nicotine cues in co-users of these drugs (Liu, Claus, Calhoun, & Hutchison, 2014). A role for the insular cortex in nicotine's interoceptive effects has been implicated in humans as well (Naqvi & Bechara, 2009, 2010), and in animals the insular cortex has been implicated in nicotine and alcohol self-administration (Forget, Pushparaj, & Le Foll, 2010; Jaramillo et al., 2018; Jaramillo, Van Voorhies, Randall, & Besheer, 2018), as well as the enhancement of opioid self-administration by nicotine. Together, these data from humans and animals suggest that, whereas the reinforcing effects of nicotine, alcohol, and their associated cues are dependent on the activation of mesocorticolimbic circuitry, the incentive amplification properties of nicotine, and thereby its effects on alcohol-associated cues, are largely due to its actions within the insular cortex.

4.3 Neurobiological processes regulating intake: Interoception and the insular cortex

Although initiation and regulation of alcohol intake is likely driven by concepts of reinforcement and conditioned motivation, quantity of intake is also likely to driven by postingestive feedback, including relative interoceptive state of intoxication, and the postingestive rewarding effects of alcohol. Interoception refers to perception of internal state (Craig, 2010), which can refer to both internal processes antecedent to drug-taking (Paulus & Stewart, 2014), as well perception of state when the drug is onboard. Nicotine can alter interoception, for example, by blunting the subjective effects of other drugs. In humans, for example, transdermal nicotine patches reduce subjective intoxication for alcohol (McKee, O'Malley, Shi, Mase, & Krishnan-Sarin, 2008) and cocaine (Kouri, Stull, & Lukas, 2001), and both nicotine and alcohol produce tolerance to the somatic effects of alcohol (Collins, Wilkins, Slobe, Cao, & Bullock, 1996). In rodents, experience with nicotine in periadolescence and adulthood can also reduce the subsequent aversive properties of alcohol (Rinker et al., 2011), as well as interfere with the conditioned taste aversion induced by ethanol, cocaine, and morphine in adult rats (Loney & Meyer, 2019) which is largely dependent on the interoceptive aversive properties of these drugs.

4.3.1 Insular cortex

The insular cortex (IC) has received a great deal of attention for its role in interoception, and integration of limbic and sensory information (Gogolla, 2017), including properties surrounding drug conditioning (Arguello et al., 2017; Thompson, Bevins, & Murray, 2019) which likely explains its involvement in response to nicotine and alcohol cues. The interoceptive subjective effect of drugs is also important for regulation of intake and dose control, and loss of IC function can both enhance or reduce intake in rodents (Rotge et al., 2017) depending on whether the loss of function occurs prior to or following drug-experience. Nicotine and the IC have been of special interest, especially following several lines of evidence indicating damage following stroke in smokers can interrupt smoking (Naqvi, Rudrauf, Damasio, & Bechara, 2007), reduce perception of withdrawal (Abdolahi et al., 2015), and predict continued cessation of tobacco use following stroke (Gaznick, Tranel, McNutt, & Bechara, 2014; Suner-Soler et al., 2012).

The IC contains NAchRs available to nicotine, that normally receive input from the basal forebrain (Toyoda, 2019), specifically including β2-NAchRs that depress pyramidal neurons in layer V, likely via GABAergic action (Sato, Kawano, Yin, Kato, & Toyoda, 2017; Toyoda, 2018). Thus, convergent evidence for the IC in integration of interoceptive status via the nicotinic system appears likely. Crucially, both systemic nicotine and intra-IC nicotine produce rightward shifts in morphine conditioned place preference and aversion (Loney, King, & Meyer, 2021), suggesting that dose perception is blunted via the IC for both the rewarding and aversive properties of the drug under nicotine. While other studies have shown the importance of the IC specifically in drug-conditioning (Geddes, Han, Baldwin, Norgren, & Grigson, 2008; Li, Zhu, Meng, Li, & Sui, 2013), very few have demonstrated disruptions specifically as rightward dose-response shifts, such that perception of dose is less sensitive under both appetitive and aversive conditioning. This raises the interesting possibility that escalation of alcohol intake under nicotine may also be driven by interoceptive factors surrounding the perception of intoxication, in addition to changes in motivational strength involving neuroadaptive changes in mesolimbic dopamine. To date however, escalation of drug-intake under control of IC NAchRs has yet to be established but raises an interesting possibility for dysregulated intake control.

5. Conclusion

In the current review, we discuss the various nicotine effects on drug-seeking and drug-taking behavior, ranging from the antecedent "appetitive" drug-seeking and approach behaviors, to the actual consummatory intake of drug and the resulting internal consequences. For alcohol in particular, the complex characterization of appetitive and consummatory processes have come a long way since early separation of the terms (Freedland, Sharpe, Samson, & Porrino, 2001; Samson, Czachowski, Chappell, & Legg, 2003; Sharpe & Samson, 2001) to include a robust ensemble of conditioning and reinforcing effects. Here, we argue that the behavioral effects of nicotine can be conceptualized as domains that influence appetitive conditioning (cues, context, and motivation), as well as consummatory behavior (intake and interoception), summarized in Fig. 6. By increasing the incentive value of both nicotine and alcohol paired stimuli, facilitating approach behaviors and resulting in activation of conditioned motivational states, nicotine can lead to behaviors that increase the likelihood of alcohol consumption. Then, nicotine can alter the reinforcing and intake properties of alcohol directly by both interfacing with the mesolimbic dopamine system and blunting at least some of the interoceptive properties of alcohol to promote consumption. Relatively few studies have directly tried to dissociate the primary vs reinforcement enhancing effects of nicotine, which highlight the need for additional work that directly assesses modulation alcohol seeking in the presence of cues separately from the reinforcing properties of alcohol consumption directly.

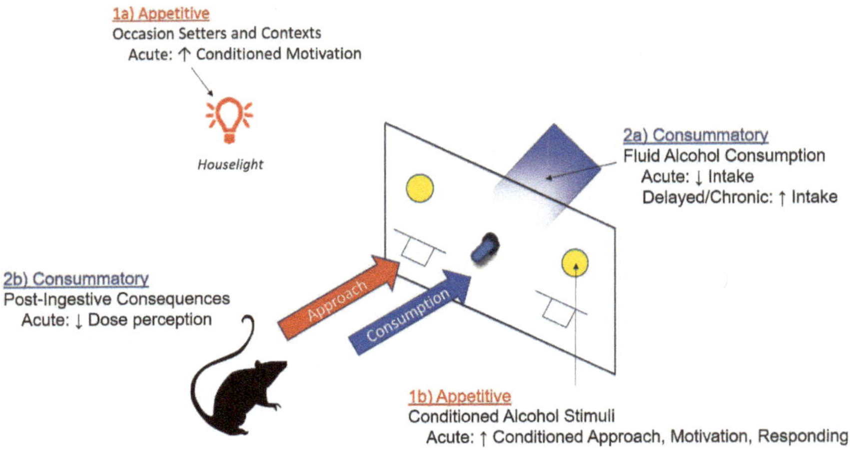

Fig. 6 Schematic of how nicotine's effects on the appetitive and consummatory processes of alcohol. Nicotine can enhance appetitive responding and approach toward alcohol in the presence of (1a) alcohol-paired occasions setters and contexts and (1b) discrete alcohol paired conditioned stimuli. Following approach and initiation of alcohol consumption, nicotine also can (2a) increase alcohol consumption following chronic treatment, although acute nicotine and decrease intake in some situations. Finally, (2b) nicotine is suggested to further enhance alcohol intake by blunting the postingestive consequences of alcohol, for example, by blocking the perception of dose and intoxication.

5.1 Impact for treatment and cessation strategy

Development and validation of pharmacotherapies used for nicotine, alcohol, and codependence often involves using well validated rodent models with an understanding of the behavior concepts described in this review. Preclinical and clinical research do not always directly map onto each other. For example, although varenicline is used in treating alcohol and nicotine dependence (Bold et al., 2019; Erwin & Slaton, 2014; Hurt et al., 2018; McKee et al., 2009), preclinical data suggest that varenicline shows difficulty in reducing combined alcohol and nicotine intake (Funk et al., 2016; Maggio et al., 2018; Waeiss et al., 2019). Naltrexone has also been thought to be more effective in heavy drinkers that smoke (Fucito et al., 2012; King, Cao, Vanier, & Wilcox, 2009), although rodent models have had difficulty demonstrating reduced nicotine intake (Le et al., 2014; Maggio et al., 2018).

Importantly, this pattern of results show that it worth considering the behavioral model and outcome measure being used. For example, preclinical pharmacotheraputics often focus on drugs that reduce intake. Given what we know about the appetitive and motivational conditioning effects, however, consideration of measures that reflect likelihood of initiating drug-use and motivation to work for drug, rather than expression free intake, may make better sense from a prevention perspective. Medications, mechanisms, and the generalization of varenicline's effects even in clinical data may also complicate the general pattern of findings (Motschman et al., 2016). As clinical models continue to improve the characterization of data in individuals and research groups (Gorelick & McPherson, 2015), and as animal models continue to refine observations to the various processes surrounding drug actions, well-defined behavioral measures will hopefully yield more convergent mechanistic data.

5.2 Differences in drug histories on treatment outcome

Considering the multitude of biobehavioral effects of nicotine, clinical outcomes and research may benefit by prioritizing the treatment of tobacco use disorder, an approach that has not directly been examined using preclinical modeling. Indeed, smoking is negatively related to treatment and clinical outcome for quitting drinking (Chiappetta, Garcia-Rodriguez, Jin, Secades-Villa, & Blanco, 2014; Weinberger et al., 2015). Instead, a "multimorbid" treatment approach that addresses both nicotine and other comorbid drug use may yield better outcomes (MacLean, Sofuoglu, & Rosenheck, 2018). In individuals undergoing treatment for alcohol use, smoking cessation does not appear to interfere with success maintaining alcohol abstinence (Gulliver, Kamholz, & Helstrom, 2006), which may be crucial maximizing treatment outcomes (Yokoyama et al., 2014) particularly in maximizing long-term success rates (Tsoh, Chi, Mertens, & Weisner, 2011). Approaches to encourage smoking cessation using contingency management may benefit from providing intermittent alternate reinforcement (Chudzynski, Roll, McPherson, Cameron, & Howell, 2015; Packer, Howell, McPherson, & Roll, 2012). Use of urinalysis to verify abstinence may be better predictor of substance use outcome (McPherson, Packer, Cameron, Howell, & Roll, 2014), and some recent evidence suggests that contingency management for both treatment of alcohol and tobacco use together can improve urinalysis outcomes for both (Orr et al., 2018). Preclinical models may eventually benefit from co-use models that examine behavioral outcomes following nicotine removal, or examining alternative reinforcement (Venniro et al., 2018).

5.3 Final remarks

The variety of approaches to studying drug-directed behavior under nicotine is remarkable, with the design of each study assessing different behavioral consequences of the drug. While these behavioral effects involve dissociable processes and multiple biological substrates, we suggest that it is useful to dissociate the various properties of nicotine into these various components of drug-directed behavior, specifically because it helps prevent the conflation of processes leading to, and resulting from, bouts of drug use.

Acknowledgments

We would like to acknowledge the work of Alexander Lamparelli, Hailley Angelyn, Cassandra Whalen (née Versaggi), and Laketta Jackson for collecting and analyzing the data presented in this chapter. Research reported in this publication was supported by grants from the Office of the Director, National Institutes of Health (NIH), the National Institute on Alcohol Abuse and Alcoholism (AA024112 and AA007583), and the National Institute on Drug Abuse (P50 DA037844). The content is solely the responsibility of the authors and does not necessarily represent the official views of the NIH.

Conflict of interest

The authors C.P.K. and P.J.M. have no conflicts of interest to declare.

References

Abdolahi, A., Williams, G. C., Benesch, C. G., Wang, H. Z., Spitzer, E. M., Scott, B. E., et al. (2015). Damage to the insula leads to decreased nicotine withdrawal during abstinence. *Addiction, 110*(12), 1994–2003. https://doi.org/10.1111/add.13061.

Adamantidis, A. R., Tsai, H. C., Boutrel, B., Zhang, F., Stuber, G. D., Budygin, E. A., et al. (2011). Optogenetic interrogation of dopaminergic modulation of the multiple phases of reward-seeking behavior. *The Journal of Neuroscience, 31*(30), 10829–10835. https://doi.org/10.1523/JNEUROSCI.2246-11.2011.

Addicott, M. A., Oliver, J. A., & Joseph McClernon, F. (2017). Nicotine increases anterior insula activation to expected and unexpected outcomes among nonsmokers. *Psychopharmacology, 234*(7), 1145–1154. https://doi.org/10.1007/s00213-017-4550-8.

Alen, F., Gomez, R., Gonzalez-Cuevas, G., Navarro, M., & Lopez-Moreno, J. A. (2009). Nicotine causes opposite effects on alcohol intake: Evidence in an animal experimental model of abstinence and relapse from alcohol. *Nicotine & Tobacco Research, 11*(11), 1304–1311. https://doi.org/10.1093/ntr/ntp139.

Alia-Klein, N., Goldstein, R. Z., Tomasi, D., Zhang, L., Fagin-Jones, S., Telang, F., et al. (2007). What is in a word? No versus yes differentially engage the lateral orbitofrontal cortex. *Emotion, 7*(3), 649–659. https://doi.org/10.1037/1528-3542.7.3.649.

Anderson, R. I., Varlinskaya, E. I., & Spear, L. P. (2010). Ethanol-induced conditioned taste aversion in male Sprague-dawley rats: Impact of age and stress. *Alcoholism, Clinical and Experimental Research, 34*(12), 2106–2115. https://doi.org/10.1111/j.1530-0277.2010.01307.x.

Angelyn, H., Loney, G. C., & Meyer, P. J. (2021). Nicotine enhances goal-tracking in ethanol and food Pavlovian conditioned approach paradigms. *Frontiers in Neuroscience, 15*, 561766. https://doi.org/10.3389/fnins.2021.561766.

Angelyn, H., & Meyer, P. (2019). *Nicotine enhances reinstatement elicited by a discriminative stimulus that predicts alcohol availability.* (Paper presented at the Alcoholism-Clinical and Experimental Research).

Appel, S. B., Liu, Z., McElvain, M. A., & Brodie, M. S. (2003). Ethanol excitation of dopaminergic ventral tegmental area neurons is blocked by quinidine. *The Journal of Pharmacology and Experimental Therapeutics, 306*(2), 437–446. https://doi.org/10.1124/jpet.103.050963.

Arguello, A. A., Wang, R., Lyons, C. M., Higginbotham, J. A., Hodges, M. A., & Fuchs, R. A. (2017). Role of the agranular insular cortex in contextual control over cocaine-seeking behavior in rats. *Psychopharmacology, 234*(16), 2431–2441. https://doi.org/10.1007/s00213-017-4632-7.

Baldwin, P. R., Alanis, R., & Salas, R. (2011). The Role of the Habenula in nicotine addiction. *Journal of Addiction Research & Therapy, S1*(2), 002. https://doi.org/10.4172/2155-6105.S1-002.

Barr, R. S., Pizzagalli, D. A., Culhane, M. A., Goff, D. C., & Evins, A. E. (2008). A single dose of nicotine enhances reward responsiveness in nonsmokers: Implications for development of dependence. *Biological Psychiatry, 63*(11), 1061–1065. https://doi.org/10.1016/j.biopsych.2007.09.015.

Barrett, S. P., Tichauer, M., Leyton, M., & Pihl, R. O. (2006). Nicotine increases alcohol self-administration in non-dependent male smokers. *Drug and Alcohol Dependence, 81*(2), 197–204. https://doi.org/10.1016/j.drugalcdep.2005.06.009.

Bass, C. E., Grinevich, V. P., Gioia, D., Day-Brown, J. D., Bonin, K. D., Stuber, G. D., et al. (2013). Optogenetic stimulation of VTA dopamine neurons reveals that tonic but not phasic patterns of dopamine transmission reduce ethanol self-administration. *Frontiers in Behavioral Neuroscience*, 7, 173. https://doi.org/10.3389/fnbeh.2013.00173.

Batel, P., Pessione, F., Maitre, C., & Rueff, B. (1995). Relationship between alcohol and tobacco dependencies among alcoholics who smoke. *Addiction, 90*(7), 977–980. https://doi.org/10.1046/j.1360-0443.1995.90797711.x.

Berridge, K. C. (2012). From prediction error to incentive salience: Mesolimbic computation of reward motivation. *The European Journal of Neuroscience, 35*(7), 1124–1143. https://doi.org/10.1111/j.1460-9568.2012.07990.x.

Bevins, R. A., & Palmatier, M. I. (2004). Extending the role of associative learning processes in nicotine addiction. *Behavioral and Cognitive Neuroscience Reviews, 3*(3), 143–158. https://doi.org/10.1177/1534582304272005.

Bienkowski, P., Piasecki, J., Koros, E., Stefanski, R., & Kostowski, W. (1998). Studies on the role of nicotinic acetylcholine receptors in the discriminative and aversive stimulus properties of ethanol in the rat. *European Neuropsychopharmacology, 8*(2), 79–87. https://doi.org/10.1016/s0924-977x(97)00052-7.

Bito-Onon, J. J., Simms, J. A., Chatterjee, S., Holgate, J., & Bartlett, S. E. (2011). Varenicline, a partial agonist at neuronal nicotinic acetylcholine receptors, reduces nicotine-induced increases in 20% ethanol operant self-administration in Sprague-Dawley rats. *Addiction Biology, 16*(3), 440–449. https://doi.org/10.1111/j.1369-1600.2010.00309.x.

Blomqvist, O., Ericson, M., Johnson, D. H., Engel, J. A., & Soderpalm, B. (1996). Voluntary ethanol intake in the rat: Effects of nicotinic acetylcholine receptor blockade or subchronic nicotine treatment. *European Journal of Pharmacology, 314*(3), 257–267. https://doi.org/10.1016/s0014-2999(96)00583-3.

Boileau, I., Assaad, J. M., Pihl, R. O., Benkelfat, C., Leyton, M., Diksic, M., et al. (2003). Alcohol promotes dopamine release in the human nucleus accumbens. *Synapse, 49*(4), 226–231. https://doi.org/10.1002/syn.10226.

Bold, K. W., Zweben, A., Fucito, L. M., Piepmeier, M. E., Muvvala, S., Wu, R., et al. (2019). Longitudinal findings from a randomized clinical trial of Varenicline for alcohol use disorder with comorbid cigarette smoking. *Alcoholism, Clinical and Experimental Research*, *43*(5), 937–944. https://doi.org/10.1111/acer.13994.

Brodie, M. S., Pesold, C., & Appel, S. B. (1999). Ethanol directly excites dopaminergic ventral tegmental area reward neurons. *Alcoholism, Clinical and Experimental Research*, *23*(11), 1848–1852. https://doi.org/10.1111/j.1530-0277.1999.tb04082.x.

Brody, A. L., Mandelkern, M. A., London, E. D., Childress, A. R., Lee, G. S., Bota, R. G., et al. (2002). Brain metabolic changes during cigarette craving. *Archives of General Psychiatry*, *59*(12), 1162–1172. https://doi.org/10.1001/archpsyc.59.12.1162.

Brunzell, D. H., & McIntosh, J. M. (2012). Alpha7 nicotinic acetylcholine receptors modulate motivation to self-administer nicotine: Implications for smoking and schizophrenia. *Neuropsychopharmacology*, *37*(5), 1134–1143.

Burling, T. A., & Ziff, D. C. (1988). Tobacco smoking: A comparison between alcohol and drug abuse inpatients. *Addictive Behaviors*, *13*(2), 185–190. https://doi.org/10.1016/0306-4603(88)90010-x.

Caggiula, A. R., Donny, E. C., Palmatier, M. I., Liu, X., Chaudhri, N., & Sved, A. F. (2009). The role of nicotine in smoking: A dual-reinforcement model. *Nebraska Symposium on Motivation*, *55*, 91–109. https://doi.org/10.1007/978-0-387-78748-0_6.

Caggiula, A. R., Donny, E. C., White, A. R., Chaudhri, N., Booth, S., Gharib, M. A., et al. (2001). Cue dependency of nicotine self-administration and smoking. *Pharmacology, Biochemistry, and Behavior*, *70*(4), 515–530. https://doi.org/10.1016/s0091-3057(01)00676-1.

Carter, B. L., & Tiffany, S. T. (1999). Meta-analysis of cue-reactivity in addiction research. *Addiction*, *94*(3), 327–340.

Chandler, C. M., Maggio, S. E., Peng, H., Nixon, K., & Bardo, M. T. (2020). Effects of ethanol, naltrexone, nicotine and varenicline in an ethanol and nicotine co-use model in Sprague-Dawley rats. *Drug and Alcohol Dependence*, *212*, 107988. https://doi.org/10.1016/j.drugalcdep.2020.107988.

Charpantier, E., Barneoud, P., Moser, P., Besnard, F., & Sgard, F. (1998). Nicotinic acetylcholine subunit mRNA expression in dopaminergic neurons of the rat substantia nigra and ventral tegmental area. *Neuroreport*, *9*(13), 3097–3101. https://doi.org/10.1097/00001756-199809140-00033.

Chatterjee, S., & Bartlett, S. E. (2010). Neuronal nicotinic acetylcholine receptors as pharmacotherapeutic targets for the treatment of alcohol use disorders. *CNS & Neurological Disorders Drug Targets*, *9*(1), 60–76. https://doi.org/10.2174/187152710790966597.

Chaudhri, N., Caggiula, A. R., Donny, E. C., Booth, S., Gharib, M., Craven, L., et al. (2006). Operant responding for conditioned and unconditioned reinforcers in rats is differentially enhanced by the primary reinforcing and reinforcement-enhancing effects of nicotine. *Psychopharmacology*, *189*(1), 27–36. https://doi.org/10.1007/s00213-006-0522-0.

Chaudhri, N., Caggiula, A. R., Donny, E. C., Booth, S., Gharib, M., Craven, L., et al. (2007). Self-administered and noncontingent nicotine enhance reinforced operant responding in rats: Impact of nicotine dose and reinforcement schedule. *Psychopharmacology*, *190*(3), 353–362. https://doi.org/10.1007/s00213-006-0454-8.

Chaudhri, N., Caggiula, A. R., Donny, E. C., Palmatier, M. I., Liu, X., & Sved, A. F. (2006). Complex interactions between nicotine and nonpharmacological stimuli reveal multiple roles for nicotine in reinforcement. *Psychopharmacology*, *184*(3–4), 353–366. https://doi.org/10.1007/s00213-005-0178-1.

Chen, X., Unger, J. B., Palmer, P., Weiner, M. D., Johnson, C. A., Wong, M. M., et al. (2002). Prior cigarette smoking initiation predicting current alcohol use. *Addictive Behaviors*, *27*(5), 799–817. https://doi.org/10.1016/s0306-4603(01)00211-8.

Chester, J. A., & Cunningham, C. L. (2002). GABAA receptor modulation of the rewarding and aversive effects of ethanol. *Alcohol, 26*(3), 131–143. https://doi.org/10.1016/s0741-8329(02)00199-4.

Chiappetta, V., Garcia-Rodriguez, O., Jin, C. J., Secades-Villa, R., & Blanco, C. (2014). Predictors of quit attempts and successful quit attempts among individuals with alcohol use disorders in a nationally representative sample. *Drug and Alcohol Dependence, 141*, 138–144. https://doi.org/10.1016/j.drugalcdep.2014.05.019.

Chudzynski, J., Roll, J. M., McPherson, S., Cameron, J. M., & Howell, D. N. (2015). Reinforcement schedule effects on Long-term behavior change. *Psychological Record, 65*(2), 347–353. https://doi.org/10.1007/s40732-014-0110-3.

Clark, A., Lindgren, S., Brooks, S. P., Watson, W. P., & Little, H. J. (2001). Chronic infusion of nicotine can increase operant self-administration of alcohol. *Neuropharmacology, 41*(1), 108–117.

Clark, A., & Little, H. J. (2004). Interactions between low concentrations of ethanol and nicotine on firing rate of ventral tegmental dopamine neurones. *Drug and Alcohol Dependence, 75*(2), 199–206. https://doi.org/10.1016/j.drugalcdep.2004.03.001.

Collins, A. C., Wilkins, L. H., Slobe, B. S., Cao, J. Z., & Bullock, A. E. (1996). Long-term ethanol and nicotine treatment elicit tolerance to ethanol. *Alcoholism, Clinical and Experimental Research, 20*(6), 990–999. https://doi.org/10.1111/j.1530-0277.1996.tb01936.x.

Conklin, C. A. (2006). Environments as cues to smoke: Implications for human extinction-based research and treatment. *Experimental and Clinical Psychopharmacology, 14*(1), 12–19. https://doi.org/10.1037/1064-1297.14.1.12.

Corrigall, W. A., Coen, K. M., & Adamson, K. L. (1994). Self-administered nicotine activates the mesolimbic dopamine system through the ventral tegmental area. *Brain Research, 653*(1–2), 278–284. https://doi.org/10.1016/0006-8993(94)90401-4.

Craig, A. D. (2010). The sentient self. *Brain Structure & Function, 214*(5–6), 563–577. https://doi.org/10.1007/s00429-010-0248-y.

Danna, C. L., & Elmer, G. I. (2010). Disruption of conditioned reward association by typical and atypical antipsychotics. *Pharmacology, Biochemistry, and Behavior, 96*(1), 40–47. https://doi.org/10.1016/j.pbb.2010.04.004.

Dar, R., & Frenk, H. (2004). Do smokers self-administer pure nicotine? A review of the evidence. *Psychopharmacology, 173*(1–2), 18–26. https://doi.org/10.1007/s00213-004-1781-2.

D'Ardenne, K., McClure, S. M., Nystrom, L. E., & Cohen, J. D. (2008). BOLD responses reflecting dopaminergic signals in the human ventral tegmental area. *Science, 319*(5867), 1264–1267. https://doi.org/10.1126/science.1150605.

Di Chiara, G. (1998). A motivational learning hypothesis of the role of mesolimbic dopamine in compulsive drug use. *Journal of Psychopharmacology, 12*(1), 54–67. https://doi.org/10.1177/026988119801200108.

Di Chiara, G., & Imperato, A. (1985). Ethanol preferentially stimulates dopamine release in the nucleus accumbens of freely moving rats. *European Journal of Pharmacology, 115*(1), 131–132. https://doi.org/10.1016/0014-2999(85)90598-9.

Di Chiara, G., Tanda, G., Bassareo, V., Pontieri, F., Acquas, E., Fenu, S., et al. (1999). Drug addiction as a disorder of associative learning. Role of nucleus accumbens shell/extended amygdala dopamine. *Annals of the New York Academy of Sciences, 877*(1 ADVANCING FRO), 461–485. https://doi.org/10.1111/j.1749-6632.1999.tb09283.x.

DiFeliceantonio, A. G., & Berridge, K. C. (2016). Dorsolateral neostriatum contribution to incentive salience: Opioid or dopamine stimulation makes one reward cue more motivationally attractive than another. *The European Journal of Neuroscience, 43*(9), 1203–1218. https://doi.org/10.1111/ejn.13220.

DiFranza, J. R., & Guerrera, M. P. (1990). Alcoholism and smoking. *Journal of Studies on Alcohol*, *51*(2), 130–135. https://doi.org/10.15288/jsa.1990.51.130.

Ding, Z. M., Ingraham, C. M., Rodd, Z. A., & McBride, W. J. (2015). The reinforcing effects of ethanol within the posterior ventral tegmental area depend on dopamine neurotransmission to forebrain cortico-limbic systems. *Addiction Biology*, *20*(3), 458–468. https://doi.org/10.1111/adb.12138.

Ding, Z. M., Katner, S. N., Rodd, Z. A., Truitt, W., Hauser, S. R., Deehan, G. A., Jr., et al. (2012). Repeated exposure of the posterior ventral tegmental area to nicotine increases the sensitivity of local dopamine neurons to the stimulating effects of ethanol. *Alcohol*, *46*(3), 217–223. https://doi.org/10.1016/j.alcohol.2011.11.007.

Ding, Z. M., Rodd, Z. A., Engleman, E. A., & McBride, W. J. (2009). Sensitization of ventral tegmental area dopamine neurons to the stimulating effects of ethanol. *Alcoholism, Clinical and Experimental Research*, *33*(9), 1571–1581. https://doi.org/10.1111/j.1530-0277.2009.00985.x.

Donny, E. C., Houtsmuller, E., & Stitzer, M. L. (2007). Smoking in the absence of nicotine: Behavioral, subjective and physiological effects over 11 days. *Addiction*, *102*(2), 324–334. https://doi.org/10.1111/j.1360-0443.2006.01670.x.

Doyon, W. M., Dong, Y., Ostroumov, A., Thomas, A. M., Zhang, T. A., & Dani, J. A. (2013). Nicotine decreases ethanol-induced dopamine signaling and increases self-administration via stress hormones. *Neuron*, *79*(3), 530–540.

Doyon, W. M., Thomas, A. M., Ostroumov, A., Dong, Y., & Dani, J. A. (2013). Potential substrates for nicotine and alcohol interactions: A focus on the mesocorticolimbic dopamine system. *Biochemical Pharmacology*, *86*(8), 1181–1193. https://doi.org/10.1016/j.bcp.2013.07.007.

Dyr, W., Koros, E., Bienkowski, P., & Kostowski, W. (1999). Involvement of nicotinic acetylcholine receptors in the regulation of alcohol drinking in Wistar rats. *Alcohol and Alcoholism*, *34*(1), 43–47. https://doi.org/10.1093/alcalc/34.1.43.

Epstein, A. M., Sher, T. G., Young, M. A., & King, A. C. (2007). Tobacco chippers show robust increases in smoking urge after alcohol consumption. *Psychopharmacology*, *190*(3), 321–329. https://doi.org/10.1007/s00213-006-0438-8.

Erblich, J., Bovbjerg, D. H., & Sloan, R. P. (2011). Exposure to smoking cues: Cardiovascular and autonomic effects. *Addictive Behaviors*, *36*(7), 737–742. https://doi.org/10.1016/j.addbeh.2011.02.011.

Erwin, B. L., & Slaton, R. M. (2014). Varenicline in the treatment of alcohol use disorders. *The Annals of Pharmacotherapy*, *48*(11), 1445–1455. https://doi.org/10.1177/1060028014545806.

Everitt, B. J., & Robbins, T. W. (2005). Neural systems of reinforcement for drug addiction: From actions to habits to compulsion. *Nature Neuroscience*, *8*(11), 1481–1489. https://doi.org/10.1038/nn1579.

Everitt, B. J., & Robbins, T. W. (2013). From the ventral to the dorsal striatum: Devolving views of their roles in drug addiction. *Neuroscience and Biobehavioral Reviews*, *37*(9 Pt A), 1946–1954. https://doi.org/10.1016/j.neubiorev.2013.02.010.

Fasoli, F., Moretti, M., Zoli, M., Pistillo, F., Crespi, A., Clementi, F., et al. (2016). In vivo chronic nicotine exposure differentially and reversibly affects upregulation and stoichiometry of alpha4beta2 nicotinic receptors in cortex and thalamus. *Neuropharmacology*, *108*, 324–331. https://doi.org/10.1016/j.neuropharm.2016.04.048.

Feltenstein, M. W., Ghee, S. M., & See, R. E. (2012). Nicotine self-administration and reinstatement of nicotine-seeking in male and female rats. *Drug and Alcohol Dependence*, *121*(3), 240–246. https://doi.org/10.1016/j.drugalcdep.2011.09.001.

Ferrari, R., Le Novere, N., Picciotto, M. R., Changeux, J. P., & Zoli, M. (2002). Acute and long-term changes in the mesolimbic dopamine pathway after systemic or local single nicotine injections. *The European Journal of Neuroscience*, *15*(11), 1810–1818. https://doi.org/10.1046/j.1460-9568.2001.02009.x.

Flagel, S. B., Clark, J. J., Robinson, T. E., Mayo, L., Czuj, A., Willuhn, I., et al. (2011). A selective role for dopamine in stimulus-reward learning. *Nature, 469*(7328), 53–57. https://doi.org/10.1038/nature09588.

Flagel, S. B., Watson, S. J., Robinson, T. E., & Akil, H. (2007). Individual differences in the propensity to approach signals vs goals promote different adaptations in the dopamine system of rats. *Psychopharmacology, 191*(3), 599–607. https://doi.org/10.1007/s00213-006-0535-8.

Ford, M. M., Davis, N. L., McCracken, A. D., & Grant, K. A. (2013). Contribution of NMDA glutamate and nicotinic acetylcholine receptor mechanisms in the discrimination of ethanol-nicotine mixtures. *Behavioural Pharmacology, 24*(7), 617–622. https://doi.org/10.1097/FBP.0b013e3283654216.

Ford, M. M., McCracken, A. D., Davis, N. L., Ryabinin, A. E., & Grant, K. A. (2012). Discrimination of ethanol-nicotine drug mixtures in mice: Dual interactive mechanisms of overshadowing and potentiation. *Psychopharmacology, 224*(4), 537–548. https://doi.org/10.1007/s00213-012-2781-2.

Forget, B., Pushparaj, A., & Le Foll, B. (2010). Granular insular cortex inactivation as a novel therapeutic strategy for nicotine addiction. *Biological Psychiatry, 68*(3), 265–271. https://doi.org/10.1016/j.biopsych.2010.01.029.

Fowler, C. D., Arends, M. A., & Kenny, P. J. (2008). Subtypes of nicotinic acetylcholine receptors in nicotine reward, dependence, and withdrawal: Evidence from genetically modified mice. *Behavioural Pharmacology, 19*(5–6), 461–484. https://doi.org/10.1097/FBP.0b013e32830c360e.

Fowler, C. D., & Kenny, P. J. (2012). Habenular signaling in nicotine reinforcement. *Neuropsychopharmacology, 37*(1), 306–307. https://doi.org/10.1038/npp.2011.197.

Franklin, T. R., Wang, Z., Wang, J., Sciortino, N., Harper, D., Li, Y., et al. (2007). Limbic activation to cigarette smoking cues independent of nicotine withdrawal: A perfusion fMRI study. *Neuropsychopharmacology, 32*(11), 2301–2309. https://doi.org/10.1038/sj.npp.1301371.

Fraser, K. M., & Janak, P. H. (2017). Long-lasting contribution of dopamine in the nucleus Accumbens Core, but not dorsal lateral striatum, TO sign-tracking. *bioRxiv.*. https://doi.org/10.1101/132977.

Freedland, C. S., Sharpe, A. L., Samson, H. H., & Porrino, L. J. (2001). Effects of SR141716A on ethanol and sucrose self-administration. *Alcoholism, Clinical and Experimental Research, 25*(2), 277–282. https://doi.org/10.1111/j.1530-0277.2001.tb02209.x.

Fucito, L. M., Park, A., Gulliver, S. B., Mattson, M. E., Gueorguieva, R. V., & O'Malley, S. S. (2012). Cigarette smoking predicts differential benefit from naltrexone for alcohol dependence. *Biological Psychiatry, 72*(10), 832–838. https://doi.org/10.1016/j.biopsych.2012.03.023.

Funk, D., Lo, S., Coen, K., & Le, A. D. (2016). Effects of varenicline on operant self-administration of alcohol and/or nicotine in a rat model of co-abuse. *Behavioural Brain Research, 296*, 157–162. https://doi.org/10.1016/j.bbr.2015.09.009.

Gatto, G. J., McBride, W. J., Murphy, J. M., Lumeng, L., & Li, T. K. (1994). Ethanol self-infusion into the ventral tegmental area by alcohol-preferring rats. *Alcohol, 11*(6), 557–564. https://doi.org/10.1016/0741-8329(94)90083-3.

Gaznick, N., Tranel, D., McNutt, A., & Bechara, A. (2014). Basal ganglia plus insula damage yields stronger disruption of smoking addiction than basal ganglia damage alone. *Nicotine & Tobacco Research, 16*(4), 445–453. https://doi.org/10.1093/ntr/ntt172.

Geddes, R. I., Han, L., Baldwin, A. E., Norgren, R., & Grigson, P. S. (2008). Gustatory insular cortex lesions disrupt drug-induced, but not lithium chloride-induced, suppression of conditioned stimulus intake. *Behavioral Neuroscience, 122*(5), 1038–1050. https://doi.org/10.1037/a0012748.

Glover, E. J., McDougle, M. J., Siegel, G. S., Jhou, T. C., & Chandler, L. J. (2016). Role for the Rostromedial tegmental nucleus in signaling the aversive properties of alcohol. *Alcoholism, Clinical and Experimental Research, 40*(8), 1651–1661. https://doi.org/10.1111/acer.13140.

Gogolla, N. (2017). The insular cortex. *Current Biology, 27*(12), R580–R586. https://doi.org/10.1016/j.cub.2017.05.010.

Gonzales, R. A., Job, M. O., & Doyon, W. M. (2004). The role of mesolimbic dopamine in the development and maintenance of ethanol reinforcement. *Pharmacology & Therapeutics, 103*(2), 121–146. https://doi.org/10.1016/j.pharmthera.2004.06.002.

Gorelick, D. A., & McPherson, S. (2015). Improving the analysis and modeling of substance use. *The American Journal of Drug and Alcohol Abuse, 41*(6), 475–478. https://doi.org/10.3109/00952990.2015.1085264.

Gotti, C., Clementi, F., Fornari, A., Gaimarri, A., Guiducci, S., Manfredi, I., et al. (2009). Structural and functional diversity of native brain neuronal nicotinic receptors. *Biochemical Pharmacology, 78*(7), 703–711. https://doi.org/10.1016/j.bcp.2009.05.024.

Grady, S. R., Wageman, C. R., Patzlaff, N. E., & Marks, M. J. (2012). Low concentrations of nicotine differentially desensitize nicotinic acetylcholine receptors that include α5 or α6 subunits and that mediate synaptosomal neurotransmitter release. *Neuropharmacology, 62*(5–6), 1935–1943.

Grant, B. F. (1998). Age at smoking onset and its association with alcohol consumption and DSM-IV alcohol abuse and dependence: Results from the national longitudinal alcohol epidemiologic survey. *Journal of Substance Abuse, 10*(1), 59–73. https://doi.org/10.1016/s0899-3289(99)80141-2.

Gulliver, S. B., Kamholz, B. W., & Helstrom, A. W. (2006). Smoking cessation and alcohol abstinence: What do the data tell us? *Alcohol Research & Health: The Journal of the National Institute on Alcohol Abuse and Alcoholism, 29*(3), 208–212.

Harrison, E. L., Hinson, R. E., & McKee, S. A. (2009). Experimenting and daily smokers: Episodic patterns of alcohol and cigarette use. *Addictive Behaviors, 34*(5), 484–486. https://doi.org/10.1016/j.addbeh.2008.12.013.

Harvey, D. M., Yasar, S., Heishman, S. J., Panlilio, L. V., Henningfield, J. E., & Goldberg, S. R. (2004). Nicotine serves as an effective reinforcer of intravenous drug-taking behavior in human cigarette smokers. *Psychopharmacology, 175*(2), 134–142. https://doi.org/10.1007/s00213-004-1818-6.

Hauser, S. R., Getachew, B., Oster, S. M., Dhaher, R., Ding, Z. M., Bell, R. L., et al. (2012). Nicotine modulates alcohol-seeking and relapse by alcohol-preferring (P) rats in a time-dependent manner. *Alcoholism, Clinical and Experimental Research, 36*(1), 43–54. https://doi.org/10.1111/j.1530-0277.2011.01579.x.

Hauser, S. R., Katner, S. N., Deehan, G. A., Jr., Ding, Z. M., Toalston, J. E., Scott, B. J., et al. (2012). Development of an oral operant nicotine/ethanol co-use model in alcohol-preferring (p) rats. *Alcoholism, Clinical and Experimental Research, 36*(11), 1963–1972. https://doi.org/10.1111/j.1530-0277.2012.01800.x.

Hendrickson, L. M., Guildford, M. J., & Tapper, A. R. (2013). Neuronal nicotinic acetylcholine receptors: Common molecular substrates of nicotine and alcohol dependence. *Frontiers in Psychiatry, 4*, 29. https://doi.org/10.3389/fpsyt.2013.00029.

Hendrickson, L. M., Zhao-Shea, R., Pang, X., Gardner, P. D., & Tapper, A. R. (2010). Activation of alpha4* nAChRs is necessary and sufficient for varenicline-induced reduction of alcohol consumption. *The Journal of Neuroscience, 30*(30), 10169–10176. https://doi.org/10.1523/JNEUROSCI.2601-10.2010.

Henningfield, J. E., & Goldberg, S. R. (1983). Nicotine as a reinforcer in human subjects and laboratory animals. *Pharmacology, Biochemistry, and Behavior, 19*(6), 989–992. https://doi.org/10.1016/0091-3057(83)90405-7.

Henningfield, J. E., Miyasato, K., & Jasinski, D. R. (1983). Cigarette smokers self-administer intravenous nicotine. *Pharmacology, Biochemistry, and Behavior, 19*(5), 887–890. https://doi.org/10.1016/0091-3057(83)90099-0.

Hurt, R. T., Ebbert, J. O., Croghan, I. T., Schroeder, D. R., Hurt, R. D., & Hays, J. T. (2018). Varenicline for tobacco-dependence treatment in alcohol-dependent smokers: A randomized controlled trial. *Drug and Alcohol Dependence, 184*, 12–17. https://doi.org/10.1016/j.drugalcdep.2017.11.017.

Hyland, B. I., Reynolds, J. N., Hay, J., Perk, C. G., & Miller, R. (2002). Firing modes of midbrain dopamine cells in the freely moving rat. *Neuroscience, 114*(2), 475–492. https://doi.org/10.1016/s0306-4522(02)00267-1.

Istvan, J., & Matarazzo, J. D. (1984). Tobacco, alcohol, and caffeine use: A review of their interrelationships. *Psychological Bulletin, 95*(2), 301–326. https://doi.org/10.1037/0033-2909.95.2.301.

Jaramillo, A. A., Randall, P. A., Stewart, S., Fortino, B., Van Voorhies, K., & Besheer, J. (2018). Functional role for cortical-striatal circuitry in modulating alcohol self-administration. *Neuropharmacology, 130*, 42–53. https://doi.org/10.1016/j.neuropharm.2017.11.035.

Jaramillo, A. A., Van Voorhies, K., Randall, P. A., & Besheer, J. (2018). Silencing the insular-striatal circuit decreases alcohol self-administration and increases sensitivity to alcohol. *Behavioural Brain Research, 348*, 74–81. https://doi.org/10.1016/j.bbr.2018.04.007.

Jensen, M. K., Sorensen, T. I., Andersen, A. T., Thorsen, T., Tolstrup, J. S., Godtfredsen, N. S., et al. (2003). A prospective study of the association between smoking and later alcohol drinking in the general population. *Addiction, 98*(3), 355–363. https://doi.org/10.1046/j.1360-0443.2003.00304.x.

Jo, Y. H., Talmage, D. A., & Role, L. W. (2002). Nicotinic receptor-mediated effects on appetite and food intake. *Journal of Neurobiology, 53*(4), 618–632. https://doi.org/10.1002/neu.10147.

Kaplan, J. S., Mohr, C., & Rossi, D. J. (2013). Opposite actions of alcohol on tonic GABA(a) receptor currents mediated by nNOS and PKC activity. *Nature Neuroscience, 16*(12), 1783–1793. https://doi.org/10.1038/nn.3559.

Karatayev, O., Lukatskaya, O., Moon, S. H., Guo, W. R., Chen, D., Algava, D., et al. (2015). Nicotine and ethanol co-use in Long-Evans rats: Stimulatory effects of perinatal exposure to a fat-rich diet. *Alcohol, 49*(5), 479–489. https://doi.org/10.1016/j.alcohol.2015.03.002.

Kemppainen, H., Hyytia, P., & Kiianmaa, K. (2009). Behavioral consequences of repeated nicotine during adolescence in alcohol-preferring AA and alcohol-avoiding ANA rats. *Alcoholism, Clinical and Experimental Research, 33*(2), 340–349. https://doi.org/10.1111/j.1530-0277.2008.00838.x.

King, A., Cao, D., Vanier, C., & Wilcox, T. (2009). Naltrexone decreases heavy drinking rates in smoking cessation treatment: An exploratory study. *Alcoholism, Clinical and Experimental Research, 33*(6), 1044–1050. https://doi.org/10.1111/j.1530-0277.2009.00925.x.

King, A. C., & Epstein, A. M. (2005). Alcohol dose-dependent increases in smoking urge in light smokers. *Alcoholism, Clinical and Experimental Research, 29*(4), 547–552. https://doi.org/10.1097/01.alc.0000158839.65251.fe.

King, A., McNamara, P., Angstadt, M., & Phan, K. L. (2010). Neural substrates of alcohol-induced smoking urge in heavy drinking nondaily smokers. *Neuropsychopharmacology, 35*(3), 692–701. https://doi.org/10.1038/npp.2009.177.

Knight, C. P., Hauser, S. R., Deehan, G. A., Jr., Toalston, J. E., McBride, W. J., & Rodd, Z. A. (2016). Oral conditioned cues can enhance or inhibit ethanol (EtOH)-seeking and EtOH-relapse drinking by alcohol-preferring (P) rats. *Alcoholism, Clinical and Experimental Research, 40*(4), 906–915. https://doi.org/10.1111/acer.13027.

Koob, G. F., Kenneth Lloyd, G., & Mason, B. J. (2009). Development of pharmacotherapies for drug addiction: A Rosetta stone approach. *Nature Reviews Drug Discovery*, *8*(6), 500–515. https://doi.org/10.1038/nrd2828.

Kouri, E. M., McCarthy, E. M., Faust, A. H., & Lukas, S. E. (2004). Pretreatment with transdermal nicotine enhances some of ethanol's acute effects in men. *Drug and Alcohol Dependence*, *75*(1), 55–65. https://doi.org/10.1016/j.drugalcdep.2004.01.011.

Kouri, E. M., Stull, M., & Lukas, S. E. (2001). Nicotine alters some of cocaine's subjective effects in the absence of physiological or pharmacokinetic changes. *Pharmacology Biochemistry and Behavior*, *69*(1–2), 209–217. https://doi.org/10.1016/s0091-3057(01)00529-9.

Kunin, D., Smith, B. R., & Amit, Z. (1999). Nicotine and ethanol interaction on conditioned taste aversions induced by both drugs. *Pharmacology, Biochemistry, and Behavior*, *62*(2), 215–221.

Lamparelli, A., & Meyer, P. (2018). *Nicotine differentially enhances alcohol self-administration in two schedules of reinforcement*. (Paper presented at the Alcoholism-Clinical and Experimental Research).

Laviolette, S. R., Alexson, T. O., & van der Kooy, D. (2002). Lesions of the tegmental pedunculopontine nucleus block the rewarding effects and reveal the aversive effects of nicotine in the ventral tegmental area. *The Journal of Neuroscience*, *22*(19), 8653–8660. https://doi.org/10.1523/jneurosci.22-19-08653.2002.

Laviolette, S. R., & van der Kooy, D. (2003). The motivational valence of nicotine in the rat ventral tegmental area is switched from rewarding to aversive following blockade of the alpha7-subunit-containing nicotinic acetylcholine receptor. *Psychopharmacology*, *166*(3), 306–313. https://doi.org/10.1007/s00213-002-1317-6.

Le, A. D., Corrigall, W. A., Harding, J. W., Juzytsch, W., & Li, T. K. (2000). Involvement of nicotinic receptors in alcohol self-administration. *Alcoholism, Clinical and Experimental Research*, *24*(2), 155–163. https://doi.org/10.1111/j.1530-0277.2000.tb04585.x.

Le, A. D., Funk, D., Lo, S., & Coen, K. (2014). Operant self-administration of alcohol and nicotine in a preclinical model of co-abuse. *Psychopharmacology*, *231*(20), 4019–4029. https://doi.org/10.1007/s00213-014-3541-2.

Le, A. D., Lo, S., Harding, S., Juzytsch, W., Marinelli, P. W., & Funk, D. (2010). Coadministration of intravenous nicotine and oral alcohol in rats. *Psychopharmacology*, *208*(3), 475–486. https://doi.org/10.1007/s00213-009-1746-6.

Le, A. D., Wang, A., Harding, S., Juzytsch, W., & Shaham, Y. (2003). Nicotine increases alcohol self-administration and reinstates alcohol seeking in rats. *Psychopharmacology*, *168*(1–2), 216–221. https://doi.org/10.1007/s00213-002-1330-9.

LeSage, M. G., Burroughs, D., Dufek, M., Keyler, D. E., & Pentel, P. R. (2004). Reinstatement of nicotine self-administration in rats by presentation of nicotine-paired stimuli, but not nicotine priming. *Pharmacology, Biochemistry, and Behavior*, *79*(3), 507–513. https://doi.org/10.1016/j.pbb.2004.09.002.

Li, C. L., Zhu, N., Meng, X. L., Li, Y. H., & Sui, N. (2013). Effects of inactivating the agranular or granular insular cortex on the acquisition of the morphine-induced conditioned place preference and naloxone-precipitated conditioned place aversion in rats. *Journal of Psychopharmacology*, *27*(9), 837–844. https://doi.org/10.1177/0269881113492028.

Liu, J., Claus, E. D., Calhoun, V. D., & Hutchison, K. E. (2014). Brain regions affected by impaired control modulate responses to alcohol and smoking cues. *Journal of Studies on Alcohol and Drugs*, *75*(5), 808–816. https://doi.org/10.15288/jsad.2014.75.808.

Liu, X., Palmatier, M. I., Caggiula, A. R., Donny, E. C., & Sved, A. F. (2007). Reinforcement enhancing effect of nicotine and its attenuation by nicotinic antagonists in rats. *Psychopharmacology*, *194*(4), 463–473. https://doi.org/10.1007/s00213-007-0863-3.

Liu, L., Zhao-Shea, R., McIntosh, J. M., Gardner, P. D., & Tapper, A. R. (2012). Nicotine persistently activates ventral tegmental area dopaminergic neurons via nicotinic acetylcholine receptors containing alpha4 and alpha6 subunits. *Molecular Pharmacology*, *81*(4), 541–548. https://doi.org/10.1124/mol.111.076661.

Loney, G. C., Angelyn, H., Cleary, L. M., & Meyer, P. J. (2019). Nicotine produces a high-approach, low-avoidance phenotype in response to alcohol-associated cues in male rats. *Alcoholism, Clinical and Experimental Research*, *43*(6), 1284–1295. https://doi.org/10.1111/acer.14043.

Loney, G. C., King, C. P., & Meyer, P. J. (2021). Systemic nicotine enhances opioid self-administration and modulates the formation of opioid-associated memories partly through actions within the insular cortex. *Scientific Reports*, *11*(1), 3321. https://doi.org/10.1038/s41598-021-81955-5.

Loney, G. C., & Meyer, P. J. (2019). Nicotine pre-treatment reduces sensitivity to the interoceptive stimulus effects of commonly abused drugs as assessed with taste conditioning paradigms. *Drug and Alcohol Dependence*, *194*, 341–350. https://doi.org/10.1016/j.drugalcdep.2018.07.048.

Loney, G. C., Pautassi, R. M., Kapadia, D., & Meyer, P. J. (2018). Nicotine affects ethanol-conditioned taste, but not place, aversion in a simultaneous conditioning procedure. *Alcohol*, *71*, 47–55. https://doi.org/10.1016/j.alcohol.2018.02.005.

Lopez-Moreno, J. A., Scherma, M., Rodriguez de Fonseca, F., Gonzalez-Cuevas, G., Fratta, W., & Navarro, M. (2008). Changed accumbal responsiveness to alcohol in rats pre-treated with nicotine or the cannabinoid receptor agonist WIN 55,212-2. *Neuroscience Letters*, *433*(1), 1–5. https://doi.org/10.1016/j.neulet.2007.11.074.

Lopez-Moreno, J. A., Trigo-Diaz, J. M., Rodriguez de Fonseca, F., Gonzalez Cuevas, G., Gomez de Heras, R., Crespo Galan, I., et al. (2004). Nicotine in alcohol deprivation increases alcohol operant self-administration during reinstatement. *Neuropharmacology*, *47*(7), 1036–1044. https://doi.org/10.1016/j.neuropharm.2004.08.002.

MacLean, R. R., Sofuoglu, M., & Rosenheck, R. (2018). Tobacco and alcohol use disorders: Evaluating multimorbidity. *Addictive Behaviors*, *78*, 59–66. https://doi.org/10.1016/j.addbeh.2017.11.006.

Maddux, J. N., & Chaudhri, N. (2017). Nicotine-induced enhancement of Pavlovian alcohol-seeking behavior in rats. *Psychopharmacology*, *234*(4), 727–738. https://doi.org/10.1007/s00213-016-4508-2.

Maggio, S. E., Saunders, M. A., Baxter, T. A., Nixon, K., Prendergast, M. A., Zheng, G., et al. (2018). Effects of the nicotinic agonist varenicline, nicotinic antagonist r-bPiDI, and DAT inhibitor (R)-modafinil on co-use of ethanol and nicotine in female P rats. *Psychopharmacology*, *235*(5), 1439–1453. https://doi.org/10.1007/s00213-018-4853-4.

Mameli-Engvall, M., Evrard, A., Pons, S., Maskos, U., Svensson, T. H., Changeux, J. P., et al. (2006). Hierarchical control of dopamine neuron-firing patterns by nicotinic receptors. *Neuron*, *50*(6), 911–921. https://doi.org/10.1016/j.neuron.2006.05.007.

Marshall, C. E., Dadmarz, M., Hofford, J. M., Gottheil, E., & Vogel, W. H. (2003). Self-administration of both ethanol and nicotine in rats. *Pharmacology*, *67*(3), 143–149. https://doi.org/10.1159/000067801.

Martinez, D., Gil, R., Slifstein, M., Hwang, D. R., Huang, Y., Perez, A., et al. (2005). Alcohol dependence is associated with blunted dopamine transmission in the ventral striatum. *Biological Psychiatry*, *58*(10), 779–786. https://doi.org/10.1016/j.biopsych.2005.04.044.

McClernon, F. J., Conklin, C. A., Kozink, R. V., Adcock, R. A., Sweitzer, M. M., Addicott, M. A., et al. (2016). Hippocampal and insular response to smoking-related environments: Neuroimaging evidence for drug-context effects in nicotine dependence. *Neuropsychopharmacology*, *41*(3), 877–885. https://doi.org/10.1038/npp.2015.214.

McClernon, F. J., Hiott, F. B., Huettel, S. A., & Rose, J. E. (2005). Abstinence-induced changes in self-report craving correlate with event-related FMRI responses to smoking cues. *Neuropsychopharmacology, 30*(10), 1940–1947. https://doi.org/10.1038/sj.npp.1300780.

McKee, S. A., Harrison, E. L., O'Malley, S. S., Krishnan-Sarin, S., Shi, J., Tetrault, J. M., et al. (2009). Varenicline reduces alcohol self-administration in heavy-drinking smokers. *Biological Psychiatry, 66*(2), 185–190. https://doi.org/10.1016/j.biopsych.2009.01.029.

McKee, S. A., O'Malley, S. S., Shi, J., Mase, T., & Krishnan-Sarin, S. (2008). Effect of transdermal nicotine replacement on alcohol responses and alcohol self-administration. *Psychopharmacology, 196*(2), 189–200. https://doi.org/10.1007/s00213-007-0952-3.

McNealy, K. R., Ramsay, M. E., Barrett, S. T., & Bevins, R. A. (2021). Reward-enhancing effects of d-amphetamine and its interactions with nicotine were greater in female rats and persisted across schedules of reinforcement. *Behavioural Pharmacology, 32*(5).

McPherson, S., Packer, R. R., Cameron, J. M., Howell, D. N., & Roll, J. M. (2014). Biochemical marker of use is a better predictor of outcomes than self-report metrics in a contingency management smoking cessation analog study. *The American Journal on Addictions, 23*(1), 15–20. https://doi.org/10.1111/j.1521-0391.2013.12059.x.

Meyer, P. J., Lovic, V., Saunders, B. T., Yager, L. M., Flagel, S. B., Morrow, J. D., et al. (2012). Quantifying individual variation in the propensity to attribute incentive salience to reward cues. *PLoS One, 7*(6). https://doi.org/10.1371/journal.pone.0038987, e38987.

Meyer, P. J., Ma, S. T., & Robinson, T. E. (2012). A cocaine cue is more preferred and evokes more frequency-modulated 50-kHz ultrasonic vocalizations in rats prone to attribute incentive salience to a food cue. *Psychopharmacology, 219*(4), 999–1009. https://doi.org/10.1007/s00213-011-2429-7.

Milton, A. L., & Everitt, B. J. (2010). The psychological and neurochemical mechanisms of drug memory reconsolidation: Implications for the treatment of addiction. *The European Journal of Neuroscience, 31*(12), 2308–2319. https://doi.org/10.1111/j.1460-9568.2010.07249.x.

Mitchell, S. H., de Wit, H., & Zacny, J. P. (1995). Effects of varying ethanol dose on cigarette consumption in healthy normal volunteers. *Behavioural Pharmacology, 6*(4), 359–365. https://doi.org/10.1097/00008877-199506000-00006.

Morel, C., Montgomery, S., & Han, M. H. (2019). Nicotine and alcohol: The role of midbrain dopaminergic neurons in drug reinforcement. *The European Journal of Neuroscience, 50*(3), 2180–2200. https://doi.org/10.1111/ejn.14160.

Motschman, C. A., Gass, J. C., Wray, J. M., Germeroth, L. J., Schlienz, N. J., Munoz, D. A., et al. (2016). Selection criteria limit generalizability of smoking pharmacotherapy studies differentially across clinical trials and laboratory studies: A systematic review on varenicline. *Drug and Alcohol Dependence, 169*, 180–189. https://doi.org/10.1016/j.drugalcdep.2016.10.018.

Nadal, R., & Samson, H. H. (1999). Operant ethanol self-administration after nicotine treatment and withdrawal. *Alcohol, 17*(2), 139–147. https://doi.org/10.1016/s0741-8329(98)00045-7.

Naqvi, N. H., & Bechara, A. (2009). The hidden island of addiction: The insula. *Trends in Neurosciences, 32*(1), 56–67. https://doi.org/10.1016/j.tins.2008.09.009.

Naqvi, N. H., & Bechara, A. (2010). The insula and drug addiction: An interoceptive view of pleasure, urges, and decision-making. *Brain Structure & Function, 214*(5–6), 435–450. https://doi.org/10.1007/s00429-010-0268-7.

Naqvi, N. H., Rudrauf, D., Damasio, H., & Bechara, A. (2007). Damage to the insula disrupts addiction to cigarette smoking. *Science, 315*(5811), 531–534. https://doi.org/10.1126/science.1135926.

Nashmi, R., Xiao, C., Deshpande, P., McKinney, S., Grady, S. R., Whiteaker, P., et al. (2007). Chronic nicotine cell specifically upregulates functional alpha 4* nicotinic receptors: Basis for both tolerance in midbrain and enhanced long-term potentiation in perforant path. *The Journal of Neuroscience*, *27*(31), 8202–8218. https://doi.org/10.1523/JNEUROSCI.2199-07.2007.

Nestler, E. J. (2005). Is there a common molecular pathway for addiction? *Nature Neuroscience*, *8*(11), 1445–1449. https://doi.org/10.1038/nn1578.

Nguyen, Q. B., & Zhu, S. H. (2009). Intermittent smokers who used to smoke daily: A preliminary study on smoking situations. *Nicotine & Tobacco Research*, *11*(2), 164–170. https://doi.org/10.1093/ntr/ntp012.

Nie, H., Rewal, M., Gill, T. M., Ron, D., & Janak, P. H. (2011). Extrasynaptic delta-containing GABAA receptors in the nucleus accumbens dorsomedial shell contribute to alcohol intake. *Proceedings of the National Academy of Sciences of the United States of America*, *108*(11), 4459–4464. https://doi.org/10.1073/pnas.1016156108.

Nutt, D., King, L. A., Saulsbury, W., & Blakemore, C. (2007). Development of a rational scale to assess the harm of drugs of potential misuse. *Lancet*, *369*(9566), 1047–1053. https://doi.org/10.1016/S0140-6736(07)60464-4.

Olausson, P., Ericson, M., Lof, E., Engel, J. A., & Soderpalm, B. (2001). Nicotine-induced behavioral disinhibition and ethanol preference correlate after repeated nicotine treatment. *European Journal of Pharmacology*, *417*(1–2), 117–123. https://doi.org/10.1016/s0014-2999(01)00903-7.

Orr, M. F., Lederhos Smith, C., Finlay, M., Martin, S. C., Brooks, O., Oluwoye, O. A., et al. (2018). Pilot investigation: Randomized-controlled analog trial for alcohol and tobacco smoking co-addiction using contingency management. *Behavioural Pharmacology*, *29*(5), 462–468. https://doi.org/10.1097/FBP.0000000000000379.

Owesson-White, C. A., Cheer, J. F., Beyene, M., Carelli, R. M., & Wightman, R. M. (2008). Dynamic changes in accumbens dopamine correlate with learning during intracranial self-stimulation. *Proceedings of the National Academy of Sciences of the United States of America*, *105*(33), 11957–11962. https://doi.org/10.1073/pnas.0803896105.

Packer, R. R., Howell, D. N., McPherson, S., & Roll, J. M. (2012). Investigating reinforcer magnitude and reinforcer delay: A contingency management analog study. *Experimental and Clinical Psychopharmacology*, *20*(4), 287–292. https://doi.org/10.1037/a0027802.

Palmatier, M. I., Evans-Martin, F. F., Hoffman, A., Caggiula, A. R., Chaudhri, N., Donny, E. C., et al. (2006). Dissociating the primary reinforcing and reinforcement-enhancing effects of nicotine using a rat self-administration paradigm with concurrently available drug and environmental reinforcers. *Psychopharmacology*, *184*(3–4), 391–400. https://doi.org/10.1007/s00213-005-0183-4.

Palmatier, M. I., Kellicut, M. R., Brianna Sheppard, A., Brown, R. W., & Robinson, D. L. (2014). The incentive amplifying effects of nicotine are reduced by selective and non-selective dopamine antagonists in rats. *Pharmacology, Biochemistry, and Behavior*, *126*, 50–62. https://doi.org/10.1016/j.pbb.2014.08.012.

Palmatier, M. I., Marks, K. R., Jones, S. A., Freeman, K. S., Wissman, K. M., & Sheppard, A. B. (2013). The effect of nicotine on sign-tracking and goal-tracking in a Pavlovian conditioned approach paradigm in rats. *Psychopharmacology*, *226*(2), 247–259. https://doi.org/10.1007/s00213-012-2892-9.

Palmatier, M. I., Matteson, G. L., Black, J. J., Liu, X., Caggiula, A. R., Craven, L., et al. (2007). The reinforcement enhancing effects of nicotine depend on the incentive value of non-drug reinforcers and increase with repeated drug injections. *Drug and Alcohol Dependence*, *89*(1), 52–59. https://doi.org/10.1016/j.drugalcdep.2006.11.020.

Pang, X., Liu, L., Ngolab, J., Zhao-Shea, R., McIntosh, J. M., Gardner, P. D., et al. (2016). Habenula cholinergic neurons regulate anxiety during nicotine withdrawal via nicotinic acetylcholine receptors. *Neuropharmacology*, *107*, 294–304. https://doi.org/10.1016/j.neuropharm.2016.03.039.

Parkinson, J. A., Olmstead, M. C., Burns, L. H., Robbins, T. W., & Everitt, B. J. (1999). Dissociation in effects of lesions of the nucleus Accumbens Core and Shell on appetitive Pavlovian approach behavior and the potentiation of conditioned reinforcement and locomotor activity byd-amphetamine. *The Journal of Neuroscience, 19*(6), 2401–2411. https://doi.org/10.1523/jneurosci.19-06-02401.1999.

Paulus, M. P., & Stewart, J. L. (2014). Interoception and drug addiction. *Neuropharmacology, 76*(Pt B), 342–350. https://doi.org/10.1016/j.neuropharm.2013.07.002.

Peciña, S., & Berridge, K. C. (2013). Dopamine or opioid stimulation of nucleus accumbens similarly amplify cue-triggered 'wanting' for reward: Entire core and medial shell mapped as substrates for PIT enhancement. *European Journal of Neuroscience, 37*(9), 1529–1540. https://doi.org/10.1111/ejn.12174.

Perkins, K. A. (2004). Response to Dar and Frenk (2004), "do smokers self-administer pure nicotine? A review of the evidence". *Psychopharmacology, 175*(2), 256–258. author reply 259-261 https://doi.org/10.1007/s00213-004-1930-7.

Perkins, K. A., Grobe, J. E., Caggiula, A., Wilson, A. S., & Stiller, R. L. (1997). Acute reinforcing effects of low-dose nicotine nasal spray in humans. *Pharmacology, Biochemistry, and Behavior, 56*(2), 235–241. https://doi.org/10.1016/s0091-3057(96)00216-x.

Perkins, K. A., Grottenthaler, A., & Wilson, A. S. (2009). Lack of reinforcement enhancing effects of nicotine in non-dependent smokers. *Psychopharmacology, 205*(4), 635–645. https://doi.org/10.1007/s00213-009-1574-8.

Perkins, K. A., & Karelitz, J. L. (2013). Reinforcement enhancing effects of nicotine via smoking. *Psychopharmacology, 228*(3), 479–486. https://doi.org/10.1007/s00213-013-3054-4.

Perkins, K. A., Karelitz, J. L., & Boldry, M. C. (2017). Nicotine acutely enhances reinforcement from non-drug rewards in humans. *Frontiers in Psychiatry, 8*(65), 65. https://doi.org/10.3389/fpsyt.2017.00065.

Perkins, K. A., Karelitz, J. L., & Boldry, M. C. (2019). Reinforcement enhancing effects of nicotine via patch and nasal spray. *Nicotine & Tobacco Research, 21*(6), 778–783. https://doi.org/10.1093/ntr/nty038.

Phillips, G. D., Robbins, T. W., & Everitt, B. J. (1994). Mesoaccumbens dopamine-opiate interactions in the control over behaviour by a conditioned reinforcer. *Psychopharmacology, 114*(2), 345–359. https://doi.org/10.1007/BF02244858.

Piasecki, T. M., Jahng, S., Wood, P. K., Robertson, B. M., Epler, A. J., Cronk, N. J., et al. (2011). The subjective effects of alcohol-tobacco co-use: An ecological momentary assessment investigation. *Journal of Abnormal Psychology, 120*(3), 557–571. https://doi.org/10.1037/a0023033.

Piasecki, T. M., Wood, P. K., Shiffman, S., Sher, K. J., & Heath, A. C. (2012). Responses to alcohol and cigarette use during ecologically assessed drinking episodes. *Psychopharmacology, 223*(3), 331–344. https://doi.org/10.1007/s00213-012-2721-1.

Pidoplichko, V. I., DeBiasi, M., Williams, J. T., & Dani, J. A. (1997). Nicotine activates and desensitizes midbrain dopamine neurons. *Nature, 390*(6658), 401–404. https://doi.org/10.1038/37120.

Pierce, R. C., & Kumaresan, V. (2006). The mesolimbic dopamine system: The final common pathway for the reinforcing effect of drugs of abuse? *Neuroscience and Biobehavioral Reviews, 30*(2), 215–238. https://doi.org/10.1016/j.neubiorev.2005.04.016.

Pons, S., Fattore, L., Cossu, G., Tolu, S., Porcu, E., McIntosh, J. M., et al. (2008). Crucial role of alpha4 and alpha6 nicotinic acetylcholine receptor subunits from ventral tegmental area in systemic nicotine self-administration. *The Journal of Neuroscience, 28*(47), 12318–12327. https://doi.org/10.1523/JNEUROSCI.3918-08.2008.

Randall, P. A., Cannady, R., & Besheer, J. (2016). The nicotine + alcohol interoceptive drug state: Contribution of the components and effects of varenicline in rats. *Psychopharmacology, 233*(15–16), 3061–3074. https://doi.org/10.1007/s00213-016-4354-2.

Randall, P. A., McElligott, Z. A., & Besheer, J. (2020). Role of mPFC and nucleus accumbens circuitry in modulation of a nicotine plus alcohol compound drug state. *Addiction Biology*, *25*(4). https://doi.org/10.1111/adb.12782, e12782.

Rassnick, S., Pulvirenti, L., & Koob, G. F. (1992). Oral ethanol self-administration in rats is reduced by the administration of dopamine and glutamate receptor antagonists into the nucleus accumbens. *Psychopharmacology*, *109*(1), 92–98.

Richardson, B. D., & Rossi, D. J. (2017). Recreational concentrations of alcohol enhance synaptic inhibition of cerebellar unipolar brush cells via pre- and postsynaptic mechanisms. *Journal of Neurophysiology*, *118*(1), 267–279. https://doi.org/10.1152/jn.00963.2016.

Rinker, J. A., Hutchison, M. A., Chen, S. A., Thorsell, A., Heilig, M., & Riley, A. L. (2011). Exposure to nicotine during periadolescence or early adulthood alters aversive and physiological effects induced by ethanol. *Pharmacology, Biochemistry, and Behavior*, *99*(1), 7–16. https://doi.org/10.1016/j.pbb.2011.03.009.

Robinson, T. E., & Berridge, K. C. (1993). The neural basis of drug craving: An incentive-sensitization theory of addiction. *Brain Research. Brain Research Reviews*, *18*(3), 247–291. https://doi.org/10.1016/0165-0173(93)90013-p.

Robinson, T. E., & Berridge, K. C. (2000). The psychology and neurobiology of addiction: An incentive-sensitization view. *Addiction*, *95*(Suppl 2), S91–117. https://doi.org/10.1080/09652140050111681.

Robinson, T. E., & Berridge, K. C. (2008). Review. In *The incentive sensitization theory of addiction: Some current issues*. Philosophical: Transactions of the Royal Society of London.

Robinson, T. E., & Flagel, S. B. (2009). Dissociating the predictive and incentive motivational properties of reward-related cues through the study of individual differences. *Biological Psychiatry*, *65*(10), 869–873. https://doi.org/10.1016/j.biopsych.2008.09.006.

Robinson, T. E., Yager, L. M., Cogan, E. S., & Saunders, B. T. (2014). On the motivational properties of reward cues: Individual differences. *Neuropharmacology*, *76*(*Part B*(0)), 450–459. https://doi.org/10.1016/j.neuropharm.2013.05.040.

Rodd, Z. A., Bell, R. L., Melendez, R. I., Kuc, K. A., Lumeng, L., Li, T. K., et al. (2004). Comparison of intracranial self-administration of ethanol within the posterior ventral tegmental area between alcohol-preferring and Wistar rats. *Alcoholism, Clinical and Experimental Research*, *28*(8), 1212–1219. https://doi.org/10.1097/01.alc.0000134401.30394.7f.

Roitman, M. F., Stuber, G. D., Phillips, P. E., Wightman, R. M., & Carelli, R. M. (2004). Dopamine operates as a subsecond modulator of food seeking. *The Journal of Neuroscience*, *24*(6), 1265–1271. https://doi.org/10.1523/JNEUROSCI.3823-03.2004.

Rose, J. E., Behm, F. M., & Levin, E. D. (1993). Role of nicotine dose and sensory cues in the regulation of smoke intake. *Pharmacology, Biochemistry, and Behavior*, *44*(4), 891–900. https://doi.org/10.1016/0091-3057(93)90021-k.

Rose, J. E., Behm, F. M., Westman, E. C., & Bates, J. E. (2003). Mecamylamine acutely increases human intravenous nicotine self-administration. *Pharmacology, Biochemistry, and Behavior*, *76*(2), 307–313. https://doi.org/10.1016/j.pbb.2003.08.011.

Rose, J. E., Behm, F. M., Westman, E. C., Bates, J. E., & Salley, A. (2003). Pharmacologic and sensorimotor components of satiation in cigarette smoking. *Pharmacology, Biochemistry, and Behavior*, *76*(2), 243–250. https://doi.org/10.1016/j.pbb.2003.07.002.

Rose, J. E., Behm, F. M., Westman, E. C., & Johnson, M. (2000). Dissociating nicotine and nonnicotine components of cigarette smoking. *Pharmacology, Biochemistry, and Behavior*, *67*(1), 71–81. https://doi.org/10.1016/s0091-3057(00)00301-4.

Rose, J. E., Brauer, L. H., Behm, F. M., Cramblett, M., Calkins, K., & Lawhon, D. (2004). Psychopharmacological interactions between nicotine and ethanol. *Nicotine & Tobacco Research*, *6*(1), 133–144. https://doi.org/10.1080/14622200310001656957.

Rose, J. E., & Corrigall, W. A. (1997). Nicotine self-administration in animals and humans: Similarities and differences. *Psychopharmacology, 130*(1), 28–40. https://doi.org/10.1007/s002130050209.

Rose, J. E., & Levin, E. D. (1991). Inter-relationships between conditioned and primary reinforcement in the maintenance of cigarette smoking. *British Journal of Addiction, 86*(5), 605–609. https://doi.org/10.1111/j.1360-0443.1991.tb01816.x.

Rotge, J. Y., Cocker, P. J., Daniel, M. L., Belin-Rauscent, A., Everitt, B. J., & Belin, D. (2017). Bidirectional regulation over the development and expression of loss of control over cocaine intake by the anterior insula. *Psychopharmacology, 234*(9–10), 1623–1631. https://doi.org/10.1007/s00213-017-4593-x.

Samson, H. H., Czachowski, C. L., Chappell, A., & Legg, B. (2003). Measuring the appetitive strength of ethanol: Use of an extinction trial procedure. *Alcohol, 31*(1–2), 77–86. https://doi.org/10.1016/j.alcohol.2003.09.002.

Samson, H. H., Slawecki, C. J., Sharpe, A. L., & Chappell, A. (1998). Appetitive and consummatory behaviors in the control of ethanol consumption: A measure of ethanol seeking behavior. *Alcoholism, Clinical and Experimental Research, 22*(8), 1783–1787. https://doi.org/10.1111/j.1530-0277.1998.tb03980.x.

Sanchez-Catalan, M. J., Kaufling, J., Georges, F., Veinante, P., & Barrot, M. (2014). The antero-posterior heterogeneity of the ventral tegmental area. *Neuroscience, 282*, 198–216. https://doi.org/10.1016/j.neuroscience.2014.09.025.

Sato, H., Kawano, T., Yin, D. X., Kato, T., & Toyoda, H. (2017). Nicotinic activity depresses synaptic potentiation in layer V pyramidal neurons of mouse insular cortex. *Neuroscience, 358*, 13–27. https://doi.org/10.1016/j.neuroscience.2017.06.031.

Saunders, B. T., & Robinson, T. E. (2010). A cocaine cue acts as an incentive stimulus in some but not others: Implications for addiction. *Biological Psychiatry, 67*(8), 730–736. https://doi.org/10.1016/j.biopsych.2009.11.015.

Saunders, B. T., & Robinson, T. E. (2011). Individual variation in the motivational properties of cocaine. *Neuropsychopharmacology, 36*(8), 1668–1676. https://doi.org/10.1038/npp.2011.48.

Saunders, B. T., & Robinson, T. E. (2012). The role of dopamine in the accumbens core in the expression of Pavlovian-conditioned responses. *The European Journal of Neuroscience, 36*(4), 2521–2532. https://doi.org/10.1111/j.1460-9568.2012.08217.x.

Schier, C. J., Dilly, G. A., & Gonzales, R. A. (2013). Intravenous ethanol increases extracellular dopamine in the medial prefrontal cortex of the Long-Evans rat. *Alcoholism, Clinical and Experimental Research, 37*(5), 740–747. https://doi.org/10.1111/acer.12042.

Schultz, W. (1997). Dopamine neurons and their role in reward mechanisms. *Current Opinion in Neurobiology*, 7(2), 191–197. https://doi.org/10.1016/s0959-4388(97)80007-4.

Schultz, W. (1998). Predictive reward signal of dopamine neurons. *Journal of Neurophysiology, 80*(1), 1–27. https://doi.org/10.1152/jn.1998.80.1.1.

Schultz, W. (2015). Neuronal reward and decision signals: From theories to data. *Physiological Reviews, 95*(3), 853–951. https://doi.org/10.1152/physrev.00023.2014.

Seungdamrong, S., & Yasunaga, S. (1975). Relative severity of hemolysis in the subtypes of ABO incompatible hemolytic disease. *IMJ. Illinois Medical Journal, 148*(5), 526–527 (530).

Sharpe, A. L., & Samson, H. H. (2001). Effect of naloxone on appetitive and consummatory phases of ethanol self-administration. *Alcoholism, Clinical and Experimental Research, 25*(7), 1006–1011. https://doi.org/10.1111/j.1530-0277.2001.tb02309.x.

Sharpe, A. L., & Samson, H. H. (2002). Repeated nicotine injections decrease operant ethanol self-administration. *Alcohol, 28*(1), 1–7. https://doi.org/10.1016/s0741-8329(02)00238-0.

Simms, J. A., Bito-Onon, J. J., Chatterjee, S., & Bartlett, S. E. (2010). Long-Evans rats acquire operant self-administration of 20% ethanol without sucrose fading. *Neuropsychopharmacology, 35*(7), 1453–1463. https://doi.org/10.1038/npp.2010.15.

Simms, J. A., Steensland, P., Medina, B., Abernathy, K. E., Chandler, L. J., Wise, R., et al. (2008). Intermittent access to 20% ethanol induces high ethanol consumption in Long-Evans and Wistar rats. *Alcoholism, Clinical and Experimental Research, 32*(10), 1816–1823. https://doi.org/10.1111/j.1530-0277.2008.00753.x.

Smith, B. R., Horan, J. T., Gaskin, S., & Amit, Z. (1999). Exposure to nicotine enhances acquisition of ethanol drinking by laboratory rats in a limited access paradigm. *Psychopharmacology, 142*(4), 408–412. https://doi.org/10.1007/s002130050906.

Smith, C. L., Jenkins, G., Burduli, E., Tham, P., Miguel, A., Roll, J., et al. (2020). Crossover associations of alcohol and smoking, craving and biochemically verified alcohol and nicotine use in heavy drinking smokers. *Behavioural Pharmacology, 31*(7), 702–705. https://doi.org/10.1097/FBP.0000000000000568.

Smolka, M. N., Buhler, M., Klein, S., Zimmermann, U., Mann, K., Heinz, A., et al. (2006). Severity of nicotine dependence modulates cue-induced brain activity in regions involved in motor preparation and imagery. *Psychopharmacology, 184*(3–4), 577–588. https://doi.org/10.1007/s00213-005-0080-x.

Sombers, L. A., Beyene, M., Carelli, R. M., & Wightman, R. M. (2009). Synaptic overflow of dopamine in the nucleus accumbens arises from neuronal activity in the ventral tegmental area. *The Journal of Neuroscience, 29*(6), 1735–1742. https://doi.org/10.1523/JNEUROSCI.5562-08.2009.

Srey, C. S., Maddux, J. M., & Chaudhri, N. (2015). The attribution of incentive salience to Pavlovian alcohol cues: A shift from goal-tracking to sign-tracking. *Frontiers in Behavioral Neuroscience, 9*, 54. https://doi.org/10.3389/fnbeh.2015.00054.

Staley, J. K., Krishnan-Sarin, S., Cosgrove, K. P., Krantzler, E., Frohlich, E., Perry, E., et al. (2006). Human tobacco smokers in early abstinence have higher levels of β2* nicotinic acetylcholine receptors than nonsmokers. *Journal of Neuroscience, 26*(34), 8707–8714.

Stringfield, S. J., Boettiger, C. A., & Robinson, D. L. (2018). Nicotine-enhanced Pavlovian conditioned approach is resistant to omission of expected outcome. *Behavioural Brain Research, 343*, 16–20. https://doi.org/10.1016/j.bbr.2018.01.023.

Suner-Soler, R., Grau, A., Gras, M. E., Font-Mayolas, S., Silva, Y., Davalos, A., et al. (2012). Smoking cessation 1 year poststroke and damage to the insular cortex. *Stroke, 43*(1), 131–136. https://doi.org/10.1161/STROKEAHA.111.630004.

Swanson, L. W. (1982). The projections of the ventral tegmental area and adjacent regions: A combined fluorescent retrograde tracer and immunofluorescence study in the rat. *Brain Research Bulletin, 9*(1–6), 321–353. https://doi.org/10.1016/0361-9230(82)90145-9.

Taylor, J. R., & Robbins, T. W. (1984). Enhanced behavioural control by conditioned reinforcers following microinjections of d-amphetamine into the nucleus accumbens. *Psychopharmacology, 84*(3), 405–412. https://doi.org/10.1007/BF00555222.

Taylor, J. R., & Robbins, T. W. (1986). 6-Hydroxydopamine lesions of the nucleus accumbens, but not of the caudate nucleus, attenuate enhanced responding with reward-related stimuli produced by intra-accumbens d-amphetamine. *Psychopharmacology, 90*(3), 390–397. https://doi.org/10.1007/bf00179197.

Thomas, A. M., Ostroumov, A., Kimmey, B. A., Taormina, M. B., Holden, W. M., Kim, K., et al. (2018). Adolescent nicotine exposure alters GABAA receptor signaling in the ventral tegmental area and increases adult ethanol self-administration. *Cell Reports, 23*(1), 68–77. https://doi.org/10.1016/j.celrep.2018.03.030.

Thompson, B. M., Bevins, R. A., & Murray, J. E. (2019). Interoceptive Stimulus Effects of Drugs of Abuse. In *Neural Mechanisms of Addiction* (pp. 89–101). Elsevier.

Tizabi, Y., Bai, L., Copeland, R. L., Jr., & Taylor, R. E. (2007). Combined effects of systemic alcohol and nicotine on dopamine release in the nucleus accumbens shell. *Alcohol and Alcoholism, 42*(5), 413–416. https://doi.org/10.1093/alcalc/agm057.

Tizabi, Y., Copeland, R. L., Louis, V. A., & Taylor, R. E. (2002). Effects of combined systemic alcohol and central nicotine administration into ventral tegmental area on dopamine release in the nucleus Accumbens. *Alcoholism: Clinical and Experimental Research*, *26*(3), 394–399. https://doi.org/10.1111/j.1530-0277.2002.tb02551.x.

Toyoda, H. (2018). Nicotine facilitates synaptic depression in layer V pyramidal neurons of the mouse insular cortex. *Neuroscience Letters*, *672*, 78–83. https://doi.org/10.1016/j.neulet.2018.02.046.

Toyoda, H. (2019). Role of nicotinic acetylcholine receptors for modulation of microcircuits in the agranular insular cortex. *Journal of Oral Biosciences*, *61*(1), 5–11. https://doi.org/10.1016/j.job.2018.12.001.

Troisi, J. R., 2nd, Dooley, T. F., 2nd, & Craig, E. M. (2013). The discriminative stimulus effects of a nicotine-ethanol compound in rats: Extinction with the parts differs from the whole. *Behavioral Neuroscience*, *127*(6), 899–912. https://doi.org/10.1037/a0034824.

Truitt, W. A., Hauser, S. R., Deehan, G. A., Jr., Toalston, J. E., Wilden, J. A., Bell, R. L., et al. (2015). Ethanol and nicotine interaction within the posterior ventral tegmental area in male and female alcohol-preferring rats: Evidence of synergy and differential gene activation in the nucleus accumbens shell. *Psychopharmacology*, *232*(3), 639–649. https://doi.org/10.1007/s00213-014-3702-3.

Tsai, H. C., Zhang, F., Adamantidis, A., Stuber, G. D., Bonci, A., de Lecea, L., et al. (2009). Phasic firing in dopaminergic neurons is sufficient for behavioral conditioning. *Science*, *324*(5930), 1080–1084. https://doi.org/10.1126/science.1168878.

Tsoh, J. Y., Chi, F. W., Mertens, J. R., & Weisner, C. M. (2011). Stopping smoking during first year of substance use treatment predicted 9-year alcohol and drug treatment outcomes. *Drug and Alcohol Dependence*, *114*(2–3), 110–118. https://doi.org/10.1016/j.drugalcdep.2010.09.008.

Tuesta, L. M., Fowler, C. D., & Kenny, P. J. (2011). Recent advances in understanding nicotinic receptor signaling mechanisms that regulate drug self-administration behavior. *Biochemical Pharmacology*, *82*(8), 984–995. https://doi.org/10.1016/j.bcp.2011.06.026.

Van Skike, C. E., Maggio, S. E., Reynolds, A. R., Casey, E. M., Bardo, M. T., Dwoskin, L. P., et al. (2016). Critical needs in drug discovery for cessation of alcohol and nicotine polysubstance abuse. *Progress in Neuro-Psychopharmacology & Biological Psychiatry*, *65*, 269–287. https://doi.org/10.1016/j.pnpbp.2015.11.004.

Venniro, M., Zhang, M., Caprioli, D., Hoots, J. K., Golden, S. A., Heins, C., et al. (2018). Volitional social interaction prevents drug addiction in rat models. *Nature Neuroscience*, *21*(11), 1520–1529. https://doi.org/10.1038/s41593-018-0246-6.

Verplaetse, T. L., & McKee, S. A. (2017). An overview of alcohol and tobacco/nicotine interactions in the human laboratory. *The American Journal of Drug and Alcohol Abuse*, *43*(2), 186–196. https://doi.org/10.1080/00952990.2016.1189927.

Versaggi, C. L., King, C. P., & Meyer, P. J. (2016). The tendency to sign-track predicts cue-induced reinstatement during nicotine self-administration, and is enhanced by nicotine but not ethanol. *Psychopharmacology*, *233*(15–16), 2985–2997. https://doi.org/10.1007/s00213-016-4341-7.

Volkow, N. D., Wang, G. J., Fowler, J. S., Logan, J., Hitzemann, R., Ding, Y. S., et al. (1996). Decreases in dopamine receptors but not in dopamine transporters in alcoholics. *Alcoholism, Clinical and Experimental Research*, *20*(9), 1594–1598. https://doi.org/10.1111/j.1530-0277.1996.tb05936.x.

Waeiss, R. A., Knight, C. P., Engleman, E. A., Hauser, S. R., & Rodd, Z. A. (2020). Co-administration of ethanol and nicotine heightens sensitivity to ethanol reward within the nucleus accumbens (NAc) shell and increasing NAc shell BDNF is sufficient to enhance ethanol reward in naive Wistar rats. *Journal of Neurochemistry*, *152*(5), 556–569. https://doi.org/10.1111/jnc.14914.

Waeiss, R. A., Knight, C. P., Hauser, S. R., Pratt, L. A., McBride, W. J., & Rodd, Z. A. (2019). Therapeutic challenges for concurrent ethanol and nicotine consumption: Naltrexone and varenicline fail to alter simultaneous ethanol and nicotine intake by female alcohol-preferring (P) rats. *Psychopharmacology*, *236*(6), 1887–1900. https://doi.org/10.1007/s00213-019-5174-y.

Walsh, J. J., & Han, M. H. (2014). The heterogeneity of ventral tegmental area neurons: Projection functions in a mood-related context. *Neuroscience*, *282*, 101–108. https://doi.org/10.1016/j.neuroscience.2014.06.006.

Wardle, M. C., & de Wit, H. (2012). Effects of amphetamine on reactivity to emotional stimuli. *Psychopharmacology*, *220*(1), 143–153. https://doi.org/10.1007/s00213-011-2498-7.

Weinberger, A. H., Funk, A. P., & Goodwin, R. D. (2016). A review of epidemiologic research on smoking behavior among persons with alcohol and illicit substance use disorders. *Preventive Medicine*, *92*, 148–159. https://doi.org/10.1016/j.ypmed.2016.05.011.

Weinberger, A. H., Platt, J., Jiang, B., & Goodwin, R. D. (2015). Cigarette smoking and risk of alcohol use relapse among adults in recovery from alcohol use disorders. *Alcoholism, Clinical and Experimental Research*, *39*(10), 1989–1996. https://doi.org/10.1111/acer.12840.

Weiss, F., Lorang, M. T., Bloom, F. E., & Koob, G. F. (1993). Oral alcohol self-administration stimulates dopamine release in the rat nucleus accumbens: Genetic and motivational determinants. *The Journal of Pharmacology and Experimental Therapeutics*, *267*(1), 250–258.

Wignall, N. D., & de Wit, H. (2011). Effects of nicotine on attention and inhibitory control in healthy nonsmokers. *Experimental and Clinical Psychopharmacology*, *19*(3), 183–191. https://doi.org/10.1037/a0023292.

Wilson, S. J., Sayette, M. A., Delgado, M. R., & Fiez, J. A. (2005). Instructed smoking expectancy modulates cue-elicited neural activity: A preliminary study. *Nicotine & Tobacco Research*, 7(4), 637–645. https://doi.org/10.1080/14622200500185520.

Winkler, M. H., Weyers, P., Mucha, R. F., Stippekohl, B., Stark, R., & Pauli, P. (2011). Conditioned cues for smoking elicit preparatory responses in healthy smokers. *Psychopharmacology*, *213*(4), 781–789. https://doi.org/10.1007/s00213-010-2033-2.

Wolfman, S. L., Gill, D. F., Bogdanic, F., Long, K., Al-Hasani, R., McCall, J. G., et al. (2018). Nicotine aversion is mediated by GABAergic interpeduncular nucleus inputs to laterodorsal tegmentum. *Nature Communications*, *9*(1), 2710. https://doi.org/10.1038/s41467-018-04654-2.

Wolterink, G., Phillips, G., Cador, M., Donselaar-Wolterink, I., Robbins, T. W., & Everitt, B. J. (1993). Relative roles of ventral striatal D1 and D2 dopamine receptors in responding with conditioned reinforcement. *Psychopharmacology*, *110*(3), 355–364. https://doi.org/10.1007/BF02251293.

Wooters, T. E., Bevins, R. A., & Bardo, M. T. (2009). Neuropharmacology of the interoceptive stimulus properties of nicotine. *Current Drug Abuse Reviews*, *2*(3), 243–255. https://doi.org/10.2174/1874473710902030243.

Wyvell, C. L., & Berridge, K. C. (2000). Intra-Accumbens amphetamine increases the conditioned incentive salience of sucrose reward: Enhancement of reward "wanting" without enhanced "liking" or response reinforcement. *The Journal of Neuroscience*, *20*(21), 8122–8130. https://doi.org/10.1523/jneurosci.20-21-08122.2000.

Yager, L. M., & Robinson, T. E. (2015). Individual variation in the motivational properties of a nicotine cue: Sign-trackers vs. goal-trackers. *Psychopharmacology*, *232*(17), 3149–3160. https://doi.org/10.1007/s00213-015-3962-6.

Yokoyama, A., Mizukami, T., Nakayama, H., Takimura, T., Sakuma, H., Yoshimura, A., et al. (2014). Concurrent inpatient smoking cessation and alcohol abstinence programs for alcoholics and their outcomes. *Nihon Arukoru Yakubutsu Igakkai zasshi = Japanese Journal of Alcohol Studies & Drug Dependence*, *49*(6), 381–390.

Zhao-Shea, R., DeGroot, S. R., Liu, L., Vallaster, M., Pang, X., Su, Q., et al. (2015). Increased CRF signalling in a ventral tegmental area-interpeduncular nucleus-medial habenula circuit induces anxiety during nicotine withdrawal. *Nature Communications*, *6*, 6770. https://doi.org/10.1038/ncomms7770.

Zipori, D., Sadot-Sogrin, Y., Goltseker, K., Even-Chen, O., Rahamim, N., Shaham, O., et al. (2017). Re-exposure to nicotine-associated context from adolescence enhances alcohol intake in adulthood. *Scientific Reports*, 7(1), 2479. https://doi.org/10.1038/s41598-017-02177-2.

CHAPTER SEVEN

Environmental influence on the preclinical evaluation of substance use disorder therapeutics

Matthew L. Banks*
Department of Pharmacology and Toxicology, Virginia Commonwealth University School of Medicine, Richmond, VA, United States
*Corresponding author: e-mail address: mbanks7@vcu.edu

Contents

1. Introduction 220
2. Drug dependence and withdrawal on candidate medication effectiveness 223
3. Schedule-related variables on candidate medication effectiveness 225
4. Subject housing variables on candidate medication effectiveness 230
5. Subject variables on candidate medication effectiveness 231
6. Conclusion 232
Acknowledgments 233
Conflicts of interest 233
References 234

Abstract

Substance use disorders (SUD) develop as a result of complex interactions between the environment, the subject, and the drug of abuse. Preclinical basic research investigating each of these tripartite components of SUD individually has resulted in advancements in our fundamental knowledge regarding the progression from drug abuse to SUD and severe drug addiction and the underlying behavioral and neurobiological mechanisms. How these complex interactions between the environment, the subject, and the drug of abuse impact the effectiveness of candidate or clinically used medications for SUD has not been as extensively investigated. The focus of this chapter will address the current state of our knowledge how these environmental, subject, and pharmacological variables have been shown to impact candidate or clinical SUD medication evaluation in preclinical research using drug self-administration procedures as the primary dependent measure. The results discussed in this chapter highlight the importance of considering environmental variables such as the schedule of reinforcement, concurrent availability of alternative nondrug reinforcers, and experimental housing conditions in the context of SUD therapeutic evaluation. The thesis of this chapter is that improved

Advances in Pharmacology, Volume 93
ISSN 1054-3589
https://doi.org/10.1016/bs.apha.2021.10.004

understanding of environmental variables in the context of SUD research will facilitate the utility of preclinical drug self-administration studies in the evaluation and development of candidate SUD therapeutics.

Abbreviations

SUD substance use disorder
OUD opioid use disorder
NAc nucleus accumbens

1. Introduction

"Thoroughly conscious ignorance is the prelude to every real advance in science."
James Clerk Maxwell

Substance use disorders (SUD) are categorized under the broader umbrella of mental health disorders (American Psychiatric Association, 2013) and characterized by the misallocation of behavior towards to the procurement and use of abused substance(s) at the expense of adaptive behaviors maintained by nondrug alternative reinforcers (e.g., social interaction with family or friends, employment, heath, etc.) (Ahmed, 2010; Banks & Negus, 2012; Heyman, 2009). The progression from initial drug experimentation to SUD diagnosis and severe SUD or addiction occurs insidiously over some time frame that could range weeks to years and is the result of complex interactions between three main factors: the subject, the abused substance, and the environment (Heilig et al., 2021; Leshner, 1997). Despite our limited understanding of these complex interactions, there are some basic tenets of SUD. First, both the subject and the abused substance have to occupy the same environment in the same way that a ligand and its receptor must be present in the same environment in any basic pharmacology experiment. Although a subject and an abused substance occupying the same environment is necessary for SUD, this condition is insufficient for the development of SUD. Second, the subject must also emit some type of behavior leading to the consumption of the abused substance so that the substance can activate reinforcement-dependent signally pathways that lead to more abuse substance consumption. Just like the presence of ligand in an environment where the receptor is located is insufficient to activate the receptor and associated signaling pathways. The ligand must also interact with and activate that receptor to a sufficient degree to initiate the associated signaling pathways.

As one thought experiment highlighting the complex interactions between these three factors, consider two different environmental contexts. In context A, a person lives in an environment where not a single substance of abuse is available for consumption. In this context, the development of a SUD would be impossible because the subject never has access to and consumes the abused substance. The abused substance must be present in the environment and be consumed by the subject to reach its target. An example of this context in the preclinical research setting would be a rat housed in the vivarium with ad libitum access to food, water, and social interaction. Context A serves as an anchor point along an environmental continuum of abused substance access. In context B, a person lives in an environment where only a single substance of abuse is available for consumption and there are no nondrug alternative reinforcers in the environment. In this latter dystopian context, the development of a SUD would also be impossible based on the criteria defined in the Diagnostic and Statistical Manual version 5 criteria for SUD (American Psychiatric Association, 2013) and teleological theories of addiction (Rachlin, 1997). Consumption of the abused substance in this context may certainly have health consequences for the individual, but would not occur at the expense of more adaptive behaviors maintained by nondrug alternative reinforcers because there are none. An example of this context is the conventional preclinical research setting where a rat implanted with an indwelling venous catheter is placed in an operant chamber with a single response lever. Response-contingent methamphetamine infusions would be available every time the lever was pressed without availability of any other consequent stimuli that could function as reinforcers. Thus, Context B serves as a second anchor point along this environmental continuum of abuse substance access at the other extreme of Context A. The natural environment that we as humans live and behave within falls somewhere between Contexts A and B. The position of any individual person along this continuum at any given time in the individual's lifespan depends upon numerous other circumstances that are beyond the scope of this manuscript. If the environmental context is an important component of the development of a SUD, then this manuscript proposes that the environmental context may also be an important in the preclinical evaluation of candidate therapeutics for SUD and clinical effectiveness of current SUD therapeutics.

One of the primary goals of preclinical research is the development of therapeutics for the treatment of both human and nonhuman diseases and disorders such as SUD consistent with the mission statements of most national research funding agencies. For example, the mission of the National Institutes of Health is "to seek fundamental knowledge about the nature and behavior of living systems and the application of that knowledge to enhance health, lengthen life, and reduce illness and disability" (https://www.nih.gov/about-nih/what-we-do/mission-goals). This goal can be achieved through two major research pathways. One pathway is the advancement of our fundamental knowledge regarding the nature and behavior of humans and nonhumans. Improvements in our knowledge base is hypothesized to lead to the identification of biological targets that could be accessed by subsequent development of candidate therapeutics directed at those biological targets through the applied research pathway mentioned next. The second other pathway is the direct evaluation of these candidate therapeutics on preclinical endpoints such as drug self-administration that have been shown to be both *sensitive* and *selective* (for review, see (Banks, Townsend, & Negus, 2019; Comer et al., 2008; Haney & Spealman, 2008; Mello & Negus, 1996)). This later applied research pathway will be the focus of this chapter.

In this manuscript, *sensitivity* refers to the degree to which the preclinical endpoint or dependent measure is altered by a clinically therapeutic in a manner and direction consistent with the clinical use of that therapeutic. For example, the mu-opioid receptor partial agonist buprenorphine is clinically used for the treatment of opioid use disorder (OUD) and chronic buprenorphine treatment decreases opioid self-administration in humans (Greenwald, Comer, & Fiellin, 2014), rhesus monkeys (Mello, Bree, & Mendelson, 1983; Negus, 2006), and rats (Bossert et al., 2020; Townsend et al., 2021). Using this framework, preclinical opioid self-administration would be categorized as a *sensitive* preclinical endpoint for the evaluation of candidate therapeutics for OUD consistent with the extant literature (Haney & Spealman, 2008; Mello & Negus, 1996; Townsend, Negus, & Banks, 2020).

Selectivity in this manuscript refers to the degree to which a candidate or clinically utilized therapeutic results in an effect only (i.e., selectively) on the primary preclinical endpoint of interest and does not produce an effect that would result in a false-positive outcome. As one example, kappa-opioid receptor agonists were developed and evaluated as candidate therapeutics for SUD and shown to decrease preclinical drug self-administration endpoints with some degree of behavioral selectivity for drug self-administration under single operant schedules of reinforcement compared to food-maintained responding (for review, see (Banks et al., 2019)). However, these kappa-opioid agonists treatment effects on preclinical drug self-administration endpoints were insufficiently *selective* for behavior maintained by the drug of abuser relative to behavior maintained by other nondrug reinforcers such as food in the context of a drug-vs-food choice procedure in monkeys (Negus, 2004). Furthermore, these preclinical results were consistent with kappa agonist effects on drug-vs-money "choice" self-administration studies in humans (Walsh, Geter-Douglas, Strain, & Bigelow, 2001). Thus, drug self-administration endpoints under single operant schedules of reinforcement were *sensitive* to buprenorphine, but were not *selective* for kappa-opioid agonists. The literature contains numerous examples like the kappa-opioid agonist results described above (see (Czoty, Stoops, & Rush, 2016; Venniro, Banks, Heilig, Epstein, & Shaham, 2020)). The issue of failed translation and selectivity would be expected in any area of scientific research. However, we need to openly acknowledge these failures and to identify and test possible hypotheses regarding the causes of these failures. This manuscript will focus on our current scientific knowledge regarding the influence of environmental factors in the context of preclinical evaluation of candidate medications for SUD and discuss opportunities for future research directions.

2. Drug dependence and withdrawal on candidate medication effectiveness

One classic example how the environmental/pharmacological context matters with regards to medication effectiveness for SUD is opioid dependence and withdrawal. Methadone is a high-efficacy mu-opioid receptor agonist that is clinically approved worldwide for the treatment of opioid use disorder (Livingston, Mahoney, Manglik, Sunahara, & Traynor, 2018; Mattick, Breen, Kimber, & Davoli, 2009). Notably, methadone is probably the most effective medication clinically available for the treatment of any SUD (Epstein, Heilig, & Shaham, 2018; Klimas et al., 2019; Kreek, Reed, & Butelman, 2019; Noble & Marie, 2019). High-efficacy agonist medications like methadone are used almost exclusively in patients with a high degree of opioid dependence (SAMHSA, 2018). In agreement with this contextual use of agonist medications in dependent patients but not in non-dependent patients, high-efficacy agonist medications have little effect on opioid self-administration in non-dependent laboratory animals (for review, see (Townsend, Negus, & Banks, 2020)). For example, in non-dependent subjects, repeated methadone treatment has failed to decrease opioid self-administration in dogs (Jones & Prada, 1977), rhesus monkeys (Mello et al., 1983; Negus, 2006), and rats (unpublished observations by our laboratory); however, see (Hiranita et al., 2014) for evidence that acute methadone treatment decreased opioid self-administration in non-dependent rats.

However, once opioid dependence is established by a history of either opioid self-administration (Gipson, Dunn, Bull, Ulangkaya, & Hossain, 2020; Griffiths, Wurster, & Brady, 1975; Lenoir, Cantin, Vanhille, Serre, & Ahmed, 2013; Negus, 2006; Negus & Rice, 2009; Townsend et al., 2021) or repeated opioid administration (Mavrikaki, Lintz, Constantino, Page, & Chartoff, 2021; Seaman & Collins, 2021; Spragg, 1940), termination of opioid exposure elicits somatic withdrawal signs including withdrawal-associated increases in opioid self-administration (Cooper, Truong, Shi, & Woods, 2008; Griffiths et al., 1975; Jones & Prada, 1977; Negus, 2006; Spragg, 1940; Townsend et al., 2019). Under these experimental conditions, methadone treatment consistently decreased opioid self-administration in both monkeys (Griffiths et al., 1975; Negus, 2006) and rats (Townsend, Kim, et al., 2021) in subjects that have been rendered opioid dependent and undergoing withdrawal. These results have been interpreted to suggest that the clinical effectiveness of high-efficacy opioid agonists like methadone to attenuate withdrawal-associated increases in opioid self-administration contributes to their effectiveness as medications for OUD in opioid-dependent patients. Overall, the therapeutic effectiveness of clinically available OUD medications appears to best achieved by matching the continuum of medications that progress from the opioid antagonist naltrexone in non-dependent/post-dependent subjects to the intermediate-efficacy agonist buprenorphine in modestly dependent subjects to the high-efficacy agonist methadone in highly dependent subjects. Moreover, even though there are Food and Drug Administration-approved pharmacotherapies for OUD that fall along this opioid dependence continuum, there are still research and therapeutic opportunities for new medications particularly at the highly opioid-dependent end of the continuum where methadone falls.

In contrast to the rich literature on OUD medications as a function of opioid dependence and withdrawal, much less is known regarding the influence of dependence and withdrawal on the effectiveness of either candidate or clinically available medications for other substances use disorders. For other drugs of abuse such as cocaine, there is much weaker evidence for cocaine dependence and withdrawal enhancing the reinforcing effects of cocaine. For example, increased breakpoints for cocaine under a progressive-ratio procedure have been reported after some periods of cocaine exposure and abstinence in rats (Morgan et al., 2002; Morgan,

Smith, & Roberts, 2005; Orio, Edwards, George, Parsons, & Koob, 2009; Paterson & Markou, 2003; Wee, Mandyam, Lekic, & Koob, 2008). However, numerous other studies determining effects of cocaine exposure and withdrawal have failed to observe increased cocaine-maintained breakpoints in both rats and nonhuman primates, and in some cases, breakpoints for cocaine decreased during periods of cocaine abstinence (Banks & Negus, 2010; Czoty, Martelle, & Nader, 2006; Li, Depoortere, & Emmett-Oglesby, 1994; Liu, Roberts, & Morgan, 2005; Morgan & Roberts, 2004; Yanagita, 1975, 1979). Collectively, these results have been interpreted to suggest that cocaine dependence and withdrawal do not robustly enhance cocaine reinforcement. Whether cocaine dependence and withdrawal might alter either the sensitivity or selectivity of candidate medications to decrease cocaine self-administration remains to be empirically evaluated. Furthermore, even less is known about the effects of drug dependence and withdrawal on drug self-administration endpoints for other drugs of abuse such as methamphetamine or nicotine. The role of drug dependence and withdrawal in the medication development process therefore represents a rich opportunity for future preclinical and clinical research across all classes of abuse drugs.

3. Schedule-related variables on candidate medication effectiveness

A schedule of reinforcement is the operational parameters established by the investigator in the laboratory that define the components of the three-term contingency $S^D \rightarrow R \rightarrow S^C$ as promulgated by Skinner (Skinner, 1938). Under these conditions, the S^D designates a *discriminative stimulus*, R designates a *response* on the part of the organism, and S^C designates a *consequent stimulus*. For example, in a typical nonhuman drug self-administration study, a monkey implanted with a chronic indwelling venous catheter would be placed in an experimental chamber that contains a stimulus light and a response lever and connected to an infusion pump containing a dose of an abused drug. The investigator can then program contingencies such that when the stimulus light is illuminated (the discriminative stimulus), then depression of the response lever (the response) will result in delivery of a drug infusion (the consequent stimulus). Conversely, when the stimulus light is not illuminated, then responding fails to result in a drug infusion. Consequent stimuli that increase responding leading to their delivery are operationally defined as *reinforcers* (S^R), whereas consequent stimuli that decrease responding leading to their delivery are defined as *punishers* (S^P) (Ferster & Skinner, 1957).

Numerous different schedules of reinforcement in drug self-administration studies have been and continue to be utilized in the evaluation of candidate medications for SUD. One example of a candidate medication that has decreased drug self-administration across a broad range of schedules of reinforcement is the monoamine transporter substrate amphetamine (Czoty et al., 2016; Negus & Henningfield, 2015). Amphetamine maintenance (i.e., repeated administration by continuous intravenous infusion, oral, or osmotic pump for at least three days) decreases cocaine self-administration in rats, monkeys, and humans under fixed-ratio schedules (Allain et al., 2020; Siciliano et al., 2018), second-order schedules (Negus & Mello, 2003a), progressive-ratio schedules (Chiodo, Läck, & Roberts, 2008; Czoty, Gould, Martelle, & Nader, 2011; Hamilton, Czoty, Gage, & Nader, 2010; Negus & Mello, 2003b; Rush, Stoops, Sevak, & Hays, 2010; Zimmer, Chiodo, & Roberts, 2014), and concurrent "choice" schedules (Banks, Blough, & Negus, 2013a, 2013b; Lile et al., 2020; Negus, 2003). Furthermore, these nonhuman and human laboratory studies are consistent with amphetamine maintenance treatment effectiveness for reducing cocaine use in clinical trials (Castells, Cunill, Pérez-Mañá, Vidal, & Capellà, 2016; Grabowski et al., 2001; Levin et al., 2015; Levin et al., 2020; Mariani et al., 2012). Although amphetamine maintenance has consistently decreased cocaine self-administration across these numerous schedules of reinforcement, differences in effectiveness have been observed. For example, under both second-order, fixed-ratio, and progressive-ratio schedules of reinforcement, amphetamine maintenance robustly decreased cocaine self-administration in both monkeys and rats (Allain et al., 2020; Chiodo et al., 2008; Czoty et al., 2011; Hamilton et al., 2010; Negus & Mello, 2003a; Negus & Mello, 2003b). However, under a concurrent "choice" schedule of cocaine and food availability, amphetamine maintenance attenuated, but did not eliminate, cocaine-vs-food choice in monkeys and rats (Banks et al., 2013a, 2013b; Negus, 2003; Thomsen, Barrett, Negus, & Caine, 2013). This dichotomy of amphetamine maintenance effectiveness on different cocaine self-administration endpoints has also been reported within the same subjects (Hutsell, Negus, & Banks, 2016). Although amphetamine maintenance decreased cocaine self-administration across these different schedules of reinforcement, there also appears to be differences in amphetamine effectiveness across these different experimental (i.e., environmental) contexts that might have clinical implications in the deployment of amphetamine as a therapeutic for cocaine use disorder.

In contrast to the nuanced effects of amphetamine maintenance on cocaine self-administration discussed above, there are several more striking preclinical examples of candidate medication effectiveness depending upon the schedule of reinforcement and two will be discussed. The first example involves kappa-opioid agonists such as U69,593 or enadoline maintenance effects on cocaine self-administration. Kappa opioid receptors are $G_{i/o}$-protein coupled receptors that are ubiquitously expressed in the central and peripheral nervous system and hypothesized to be involved in SUD (for review, see (Chavkin & Koob, 2015; Crowley & Kash, 2015; Tejeda & Bonci, 2019; Wee & Koob, 2010)). Activation of kappa receptors results either by endogenous release of the dynorphin peptide (Chavkin, James, & Goldstein, 1982; Oka et al., 1982) or synthetic kappa agonist administration results in inhibition of neuronal function. For example, administration of synthetic kappa agonists (e.g., U59,593, U50,488, or salvinorin A) decrease extracellular nucleus accumbens (NAc) dopamine levels (Carlezon et al., 2006; Di Chiara & Imperato, 1988; Leitl et al., 2014). On the basis of this preclinical evidence, kappa agonists were hypothesized to attenuate cocaine-induced increases in NAc dopamine levels and thus reduce drug self-administration and be effective SUD medications. Maintenance (i.e., repeated drug administration for at least 3 days) treatments with ethylketocyclazine, U50,488, enadoline, spiradoline, PD117302, bremazocine, and cyclazocine all produced sustained decreases in cocaine self-administration under fixed-ratio and second-order schedules of reinforcement in rhesus monkeys (Cosgrove & Carroll, 2002; Mello & Negus, 1998; Negus, Mello, Portoghese, & Lin, 1997). However, kappa agonist doses that decreased cocaine self-administration under these rate-based schedules of reinforcement failed to demonstrate a robust degree of behavioral selectivity when compared to kappa agonist maintenance treatment effects on food-maintained responding. Moreover, when U50,488 maintenance effects were examined on cocaine self-administration under a concurrent "choice" schedule of cocaine and food pellet availability in rhesus monkeys, U50,488 maintenance increased, not decreased, cocaine choice (Negus, 2004). Consistent with these cocaine choice results in monkeys, enadoline maintenance failed to attenuate cocaine-vs.-money choice in humans and there was a trend for increased cocaine choice at the largest enadoline dose examined (Walsh et al., 2001). Thus, kappa agonist maintenance effects on cocaine self-administration depended upon the schedule of reinforcement. Furthermore, consistent with these cocaine self-administration studies, similar differences in kappa agonist effects on opioid self-administration between rate-based schedules of reinforcement such as progressive-ratio procedures and drug-food choice procedures have also been reported (Townsend, 2021; Townsend et al., 2017).

A second and more recent example of candidate medication effectiveness depending upon the schedule of reinforcement is the 5-HT_{2C} agonist lorcaserin. 5-HT_{2C} receptors are G_q/G_{11}-coupled receptors located primarily on GABAergic neurons (Hannon & Hoyer, 2008). As a result, 5-HT_{2C} receptor activation excites GABA neurons, subsequently inhibiting dopamine neurons resulting in an attenuation of the abuse-related effects of cocaine. For example, acute pretreatment with the 5-HT_{2C} agonist RO 60–0175 attenuated cocaine-induced extracellular NAc dopamine increases in both rats (Cathala et al., 2015; Navailles, Moison, Cunningham, & Spampinato, 2008) and monkeys (Manvich, Kimmel, & Howell, 2012). Because of the neuroanatomical distribution within the mesolimbic pathway, these receptors have emerged as pharmacological targets for substance use disorder treatments (Collins & France, 2018; Higgins, Fletcher, & Shanahan, 2020; Howell & Cunningham, 2015). Maintenance treatments with the 5-HT_{2C} agonist lorcaserin have produced sustained and behaviorally selective decreases in cocaine self-administration under fixed-ratio schedules of reinforcement in rhesus monkeys (Collins, Gerak, Javors, & France, 2016; Gerak, Collins, & France, 2016). However, when lorcaserin maintenance was evaluated under a concurrent "choice" schedule of cocaine and food pellet availability, lorcaserin failed to attenuate cocaine choice in rhesus monkeys (Banks & Negus, 2017b) and cocaine-vs-money choice in humans (Pirtle et al., 2019). Lorcaserin maintenance has also been reported to be ineffective in decreasing cocaine use in a double-blind clinical trial (Negus & Banks, 2020). Furthermore, similar results regarding the failure of lorcaserin maintenance to decrease opioid choice in both monkeys and humans has been reported (Brandt et al., 2020; Townsend, Negus, Poklis, & Banks, 2020). Because of the consistency between preclinical and human laboratory studies using concurrent "choice" schedules to evaluate candidate SUD medications, we have proposed that preclinical choice procedures might have particular utility in the evaluation of candidate SUD therapeutics because preclinical choice procedures appear to have a higher degree of *selectivity* than conventional single-operant drug self-administration procedures (Banks et al., 2019; Banks & Negus, 2017a).

Behavioral strategies for SUD, such as contingency management or the therapeutic workplace, share the common goal of decreasing abused drug consumption by increasing the relative cost (i.e., response requirement) for the abused drug relative to other nondrug commodities (Bigelow, Stitzer, Griffiths, & Liebson, 1981; Budney, Higgins, Delaney, Kent, & Bickel, 1991; Silverman, Holtyn, & Toegel, 2019; Vocci & Montoya, 2009). This type of behavioral strategy can be modeled in preclinical studies by manipulating the response requirement for one of the consequent stimuli under a concurrent schedule of reinforcement. For example, preclinical research in both monkeys (Maguire, Gerak, & France, 2013; Nader & Woolverton, 1992; Negus, 2003) and rats (Cantin et al., 2010; Chow & Beckmann, 2020; Thomsen et al., 2013; Venniro et al., 2018) demonstrate that manipulation of the response requirement can significantly alter behavioral allocation between concurrently available drug and nondrug reinforcers such that lower response requirements for the alternative nondrug reinforcer or higher response requirements for the drug reinforcer both decrease behavior directed towards the drug resulting in a decrease in overall drug choice. Conversely, higher response requirements for the alternative nondrug reinforcer or lower response requirements for the drug reinforcer both increase behavior directed towards the drug resulting in increased overall drug choice. Furthermore, these preclinical studies are congruent with human laboratory drug self-administration studies (Hart, Haney, Foltin, & Fischman, 2000; Lile et al., 2016; Stoops, Lile, Glaser, Hays, & Rush, 2012).

There is a paucity of studies that have examined interactions between behavioral manipulations such as response requirement and the effectiveness of candidate medications to decrease drug self-administration. In one study, cocaine choice in male rhesus monkeys was reported to be most sensitive to continuous treatment with the monoamine transporter substrate phenmetrazine under conditions where the response requirement for cocaine was low, the cocaine choice dose-effect function was shifted leftward, and cocaine-vs-food choice was maintained by small cocaine doses (Banks et al., 2013a, 2013b). Conversely, cocaine choice was relatively insensitive to phenmetrazine maintenance when the relative response requirement for cocaine was high, the cocaine choice dose-effect function was shifted rightward, and cocaine-vs-food choice was maintained by large cocaine doses (Banks et al., 2013a, 2013b). These results were consistent with a previous cocaine self-administration study under a single-operant drug self-administration procedure demonstrating that smaller unit cocaine doses were more vulnerable to pharmacological treatments than larger unit cocaine doses (Collins et al., 2016; Glowa et al., 1995). These preclinical results were interpretated to suggest that candidate medication effectiveness may be influenced by the relative contingencies of drug and nondrug reinforcer availability. However, this interpretation has not been rigorously tested across different classes of abused drugs and represents an opportunity for future preclinical and clinical research.

4. Subject housing variables on candidate medication effectiveness

Subject housing variables are a category of independent variables for which there is a tremendous amount of research on the how these variables impact the progression from initial drug use to SUD and addiction, but a paucity of research on how these variables impact candidate medication effectiveness. For instance, both nonhumans and humans are social animals that are sensitive to manipulations in their social environment. Studies in nonhuman primates and rodents have established that social housing conditions can influence drug self-administration (Czoty, McCabe, & Nader, 2005; Morgan et al., 2002; Nader et al., 2012; Smith, 2012). For example, subordinate male monkeys acquired cocaine self-administration at lower doses than dominate males (Morgan et al., 2002) and subordinates also displayed a leftward shift in the cocaine-vs-food choice dose-effect function compared to dominates (Czoty et al., 2005). In contrast, dominant female monkeys acquired cocaine self-administration at lower doses than subordinate females (Nader et al., 2012). Introduction of social interaction as a consequent stimulus in rats decreased both heroin and methamphetamine self-administration (Venniro et al., 2018; Venniro, Russell, Zhang, & Shaham, 2019). Furthermore, social housing conditions have shown to influence acquisition and maintenance of cocaine self-administration in rats (Lacy, Strickland, Feinstein, Robinson, & Smith, 2016; Robinson, Lacy, Strickland, Magee, & Smith, 2016; Smith, 2012; Smith & Pitts, 2014). Overall, this literature supports the interpretation that environmental variables, such as housing conditions, can influence drug self-administration endpoints and potential vulnerability to drugs of abuse.

In contrast to the literature cited above, there has only been one candidate medication that has been evaluated to decrease cocaine self-administration under the same schedule of reinforcement, but under different social housing conditions. Buspirone is a mixed serotonin agonist and dopamine D2-like D3/D4 antagonist that is clinically used in the treatment of anxiety-related mental health disorders (Bergman et al., 2013; Boess &

Martin, 1994; Tallman et al., 1997). Repeated buspirone treatment failed to decrease cocaine self-administration in a cocaine-food choice procedure in male rhesus monkeys that were singly housed (John, Banala, Newman, & Nader, 2015). In contrast, acute buspirone administered either intravenously or orally decreased cocaine choice and increased food choice in dominant male cynomolgus monkeys that were socially housed (Czoty & Nader, 2015). Buspirone had either no effect or slightly increased cocaine choice in subordinate cynomolgus monkeys (Czoty & Nader, 2015). Acknowledging potential interpretative limitations including different species of monkeys and different buspirone dosing regimens (i.e., acute vs. repeated) were used between these two studies, these results highlight the potential unexplored research opportunities for determining how subject housing variables such as social housing and other subject housing variables such as limited nesting and bedding (to model an impoverished environment) impact candidate medication effectiveness on preclinical drug self-administration endpoints in the development of SUD therapeutics.

5. Subject variables on candidate medication effectiveness

Just like subject housing-related independent variables above, subject variables are another category of rich independent variables for which there is a tremendous amount of research focused on the transition from initial drug use to SUD and addiction, but only a paucity of research focused on how these subject variables (e.g., genetics, age, life history, or comorbidities) impact candidate medication effectiveness. In 2015, the National Institutes of Health published a notice regarding the consideration and implementation of sex as a biological variable (SABV) with the expectation that SABV be factored into research designs, analyses, and reporting in vertebrate animal and human studies (Clayton, 2016). Numerous commentaries and reviews have been written regarding the scientific premise and practice for inclusion of SABV in biomedical nonhuman research (Becker & Koob, 2016; Mauvais-Jarvis et al., 2021; Shansky, 2019). The role of SABV in the preclinical evaluation of any clinically approved and used medication for any SUD has not been systematically examined to the best of this author's knowledge and represents an opportunity for both future preclinical and clinical research. A recent preclinical study determining the effectiveness of the novel mu-opioid receptor agonist oliceridine (i.e., TRV130) to decrease oxycodone self-administration suggested nuanced sex differences (Bossert et al., 2020).

For example, oliceridine maintenance decreased extinction responding and reacquisition of oxycodone self-administration in male rats; however, oliceridine maintenance only decreased extinction responding in female rats. These results were interpreted to suggest that the clinical effectiveness of oliceridine as a candidate medication for OUD relapse might include potential sex differences. Moreover, these results highlight the potential of SABV in future research in the development of candidate medications for SUD and improve the success rate of translating positive preclinical results into positive clinical outcomes by taking a personalized medicine approach (Nader, 2016).

6. Conclusion

The diagnosis of SUD results from a subject's behavior being misallocated towards the procurement, use, and recovery from the abused substance at the expense of behaviors directed towards more adaptative nondrug reinforcers (e.g., job, family, or health). The environmental context is an important component of complex interactions between the subject and the abused substance because the abused substance resides outside the subject's body and the subject must emit some behavior in the environment where the abused substance is located and consume the substance. Pharmacological variables such as dependence and withdrawal are well-established as important determinants of medication effectiveness for some drug classes such as opioids, but are less well defined for most other drug classes including monoamine transporter ligands, nicotinic agonists, and ethanol. The available literature discussed in this chapter provides preliminary and supporting evidence for environmental variables such as the schedule of reinforcement and subject housing conditions to influence the effectiveness of candidate medications to attenuate drug self-administration. Subject-related variables such as SABV have only recently been examined in the context of SUD medication development and represent a potential mechanism towards a more personalized medicine approach to SUD treatment. Overall, the role of environmental and subject-related variables in the preclinical evaluation of candidate SUD therapeutics represents multiple new avenues for research opportunities.

One potential future direction would be the inclusion of other nondrug reinforcers than food in preclinical drug choice procedures. Food as the nondrug alternative reinforcer has been exclusively used in the context of preclinical drug-choice self-administration procedures for presumably a number of reasons including ease of use and ability to readily manipulate reinforcer magnitude. Furthermore, food-maintained responding has also been the primary nondrug reinforcer as the comparator for behavioral selectivity of candidate medication effectiveness to interpret whether the candidate medication produced a selective decrease drug self-administration versus a more generalized decrease in positively-reinforced operant behavior. However, food is one of many numerous nondrug reinforcers in our natural environment and the degree to which candidate medications or clinically available SUD medications promote a reallocation of behavior away from drugs and towards different nondrug reinforcers in humans or nonhumans has not been systematically examined. As one example, social interaction as a reinforcer has been utilized in preclinical studies including both monkeys and rats (Corwin & Schuster, 1993; Venniro et al., 2018). The working hypothesis would be that medications that both decrease preclinical drug self-administration and promote behavioral reallocation to several different nondrug reinforcers might have greater clinical utility than medications that promote behavioral reallocation to a more limited range of nondrug reinforcers.

Another potential future direction for subject-related variables is the role of age in the effectiveness of candidate or clinically used medications for SUD. For example, dopamine D2 receptor availability decreases as a function of increasing age as measured using positron emission tomography (Volkow et al., 1998). Whether mu-opioid receptor availability also changes as a function of age has not been empirically determined to the best of the authors knowledge. Moreover, how these age-related changes in receptor expression and age-related changes in receptor function impact SUD medication effectiveness across these different age groups remain unexplored scientific research areas.

Acknowledgments

The author is supported by National Institutes of Health Grants UG3DA050311, P30DA033934, and R21DA053820. The National Institute on Drug Abuse had no role in study design, collection, analysis, or interpretation of the data, or in the writing or decision to submit the manuscript for publication. The manuscript content is solely the responsibility of the author and does not necessarily reflect the official views of the National Institutes of Health.

Conflicts of interest

The author declares there are no competing financial interests or potential conflicts of interest in relation to the research described.

References

Ahmed, S. H. (2010). Validation crisis in animal models of drug addiction: Beyond non-disordered drug use toward drug addiction. *Neuroscience and Biobehavioral Reviews*, *35*(2), 172–184. https://doi.org/10.1016/j.neubiorev.2010.04.005.

Allain, F., Delignat-Lavaud, B., Beaudoin, M.-P., Jacquemet, V., Robinson, T. E., Trudeau, L.-E., et al. (2020). Amphetamine maintenance therapy during intermittent cocaine self-administration in rats attenuates psychomotor and dopamine sensitization and reduces addiction-like behavior. *Neuropsychopharmacology*. https://doi.org/10.1038/s41386-020-0773-1.

American Psychiatric Association. (2013). *Diagnositc and statistical manual of mental disorders* (5th ed.). Arlington, VA: American Psychiatric Association.

Banks, M. L., Blough, B. E., & Negus, S. S. (2013a). Effects of 14-day treatment with the schedule III anorectic phendimetrazine on choice between cocaine and food in rhesus monkeys (vol 131, pg 204, 2013). *Drug and Alcohol Dependence*, *133*(2), 794. https://doi.org/10.1016/j.drugalcdep.2013.08.005.

Banks, M. L., Blough, B. E., & Negus, S. S. (2013b). Interaction between behavioral and pharmacological treatment strategies to decrease cocaine choice in Rhesus monkeys. *Neuropsychopharmacology*, *38*(3), 395–404. http://www.nature.com/npp/journal/v38/n3/suppinfo/npp2012193s1.html.

Banks, M. L., & Negus, S. S. (2010). Effects of extended cocaine access and cocaine withdrawal on choice between cocaine and food in rhesus monkeys. *Neuropsychopharmacology*, *35*(2), 493–504. https://doi.org/10.1038/npp.2009.154.

Banks, M. L., & Negus, S. S. (2012). Preclinical determinants of drug choice under concurrent schedules of drug self-administration. *Advances in Pharmacological Sciences*, *2012*, 281768. https://doi.org/10.1155/2012/281768.

Banks, M. L., & Negus, S. S. (2017a). Insights from preclinical choice models on treating drug addiction. *Trends in Pharmacological Sciences*, *38*, 181–194. https://doi.org/10.1016/j.tips.2016.11.002.

Banks, M. L., & Negus, S. S. (2017b). Repeated 7-day treatment with the 5-HT2C agonist Lorcaserin or the 5-HT2A antagonist Pimavanserin alone or in combination fails to reduce cocaine vs food choice in male Rhesus monkeys. *Neuropsychopharmacology*, *42*, 1082–1092. https://doi.org/10.1038/npp.2016.259.

Banks, M. L., Townsend, E. A., & Negus, S. S. (2019). Testing the 10 most wanted: A preclinical algorithm to screen candidate opioid use disorder medications. *Neuropsychopharmacology*. https://doi.org/10.1038/s41386-019-0336-5.

Becker, J. B., & Koob, G. F. (2016). Sex differences in animal models: Focus on addiction. *Pharmacological Reviews*, *68*(2), 242–263. https://doi.org/10.1124/pr.115.011163.

Bergman, J., Roof, R. A., Furman, C. A., Conroy, J. L., Mello, N. K., Sibley, D. R., et al. (2013). Modification of cocaine self-administration by buspirone (buspar®): Potential involvement of D3 and D4 dopamine receptors. *The International Journal of Neuropsychopharmacology*, *16*(2), 445–458. https://doi.org/10.1017/s1461145712000661.

Bigelow, G. E., Stitzer, M. L., Griffiths, R. R., & Liebson, I. A. (1981). Contingency management approaches to drug self-administration and drug abuse: Efficacy and limitations. *Addictive Behaviors*, *6*(3), 241–252. https://doi.org/10.1016/0306-4603(81)90022-8.

Boess, F. G., & Martin, I. L. (1994). Molecular biology of 5-HT receptors. *Neuropharmacology*, *33*(3–4), 275–317. https://doi.org/10.1016/0028-3908(94)90059-0.

Bossert, J. M., Kiyatkin, E. A., Korah, H., Hoots, J. K., Afzal, A., Perekopskiy, D., et al. (2020). In a rat model of opioid maintenance, the G protein–biased mu opioid receptor agonist TRV130 decreases relapse to oxycodone seeking and taking and prevents oxycodone-induced brain hypoxia. *Biological Psychiatry*. https://doi.org/10.1016/j.biopsych.2020.02.014.

Brandt, L., Jones, J. D., Martinez, S., Manubay, J. M., Mogali, S., Ramey, T., et al. (2020). Effects of lorcaserin on oxycodone self-administration and subjective responses in participants with opioid use disorder. *Drug and Alcohol Dependence, 107859*. https://doi.org/10.1016/j.drugalcdep.2020.107859.

Budney, A. J., Higgins, S. T., Delaney, D. D., Kent, L., & Bickel, W. K. (1991). Contingent reinforcement of abstinence with individuals abusing cocaine and marijuana. *Journal of Applied Behavior Analysis, 24*(4), 657–665. https://doi.org/10.1901/jaba.1991.24-657.

Cantin, L., Lenoir, M., Augier, E., Vanhille, N., Dubreucq, S., Serre, F., et al. (2010). Cocaine is low on the value ladder of rats: Possible evidence for resilience to addiction. *PLoS One, 5*(7), e11592. https://doi.org/10.1371/journal.pone.0011592.

Carlezon, W. A., Béguin, C., DiNieri, J. A., Baumann, M. H., Richards, M. R., Todtenkopf, M. S., et al. (2006). Depressive-like effects of the κ-opioid receptor agonist Salvinorin a on behavior and neurochemistry in rats. *The Journal of Pharmacology and Experimental Therapeutics, 316*(1), 440–447. https://doi.org/10.1124/jpet.105.092304.

Castells, X., Cunill, R., Pérez-Mañá, C., Vidal, X., & Capellà, D. (2016). Psychostimulant drugs for cocaine dependence. *Cochrane Database of Systematic Reviews, 9*. https://doi.org/10.1002/14651858.CD007380.pub4.

Cathala, A., Devroye, C., Maitre, M., Piazza, P. V., Abrous, D. N., Revest, J.-M., et al. (2015). Serotonin2C receptors modulate dopamine transmission in the nucleus accumbens independently of dopamine release: Behavioral, neurochemical and molecular studies with cocaine. *Addiction Biology, 20*(3), 445–457. https://doi.org/10.1111/adb.12137.

Chavkin, C., James, I., & Goldstein, A. (1982). Dynorphin is a specific endogenous ligand of the kappa opioid receptor. *Science, 215*(4531), 413–415. https://doi.org/10.1126/science.6120570.

Chavkin, C., & Koob, G. F. (2015). Dynorphin, dysphoria, and dependence: The stress of addiction. *Neuropsychopharmacology, 41*, 373. https://doi.org/10.1038/npp.2015.258.

Chiodo, K. A., Läck, C. M., & Roberts, D. C. S. (2008). Cocaine self-administration reinforced on a progressive ratio schedule decreases with continuous d-amphetamine treatment in rats. *Psychopharmacology, 200*(4), 465–473. https://doi.org/10.1007/s00213-008-1222-8.

Chow, J. J., & Beckmann, J. S. (2020). Remifentanil-food choice follows predictions of relative subjective value. *Drug and Alcohol Dependence, 108369*. https://doi.org/10.1016/j.drugalcdep.2020.108369.

Clayton, J. A. (2016). Studying both sexes: A guiding principle for biomedicine. *The FASEB Journal, 30*(2), 519–524. https://doi.org/10.1096/fj.15-279554.

Collins, G. T., & France, C. P. (2018). Effects of lorcaserin and buspirone, administered alone and as a mixture, on cocaine self-administration in male and female rhesus monkeys. *Experimental and Clinical Psychopharmacology, 26*(5), 488–496. https://doi.org/10.1037/pha0000209.

Collins, G. T., Gerak, L. R., Javors, M. A., & France, C. P. (2016). Lorcaserin reduces the discriminative stimulus and reinforcing effects of cocaine in Rhesus monkeys. *The Journal of Pharmacology and Experimental Therapeutics, 356*(1), 85–95. https://doi.org/10.1124/jpet.115.228833.

Comer, S. D., Ashworth, J. B., Foltin, R. W., Johanson, C. E., Zacny, J. P., & Walsh, S. L. (2008). The role of human drug self-administration procedures in the development of medications. *Drug and Alcohol Dependence, 96*(1–2), 1–15. https://doi.org/10.1016/j.drugalcdep.2008.03.001.

Cooper, Z. D., Truong, Y. N.-T., Shi, Y.-G., & Woods, J. H. (2008). Morphine deprivation increases self-administration of the Fast- and Short-Acting μ-opioid receptor agonist remifentanil in the rat. *The Journal of Pharmacology and Experimental Therapeutics, 326*(3), 920–929. https://doi.org/10.1124/jpet.108.139196.

Corwin, R. L., & Schuster, C. R. (1993). Anorectic specificity as measured in a choice paradigm in rhesus monkeys. *Pharmacology, Biochemistry, and Behavior, 45*(1), 131–141. https://doi.org/10.1016/0091-3057(93)90096-C.

Cosgrove, K. P., & Carroll, M. E. (2002). Effects of Bremazocine on self-administration of smoked cocaine base and orally delivered ethanol, phencyclidine, saccharin, and food in Rhesus monkeys: A behavioral economic analysis. *The Journal of Pharmacology and Experimental Therapeutics, 301*(3), 993–1002. https://doi.org/10.1124/jpet.301.3.993.

Crowley, N. A., & Kash, T. L. (2015). Kappa opioid receptor signaling in the brain: Circuitry and implications for treatment. *Progress in Neuro-Psychopharmacology & Biological Psychiatry, 62*, 51–60. https://doi.org/10.1016/j.pnpbp.2015.01.001.

Czoty, P. W., Gould, R. W., Martelle, J. L., & Nader, M. A. (2011). Prolonged attenuation of the reinforcing strength of cocaine by chronic d-Amphetamine in Rhesus monkeys. *Neuropsychopharmacology, 36*(2), 539–547. https://doi.org/10.1038/npp.2010.185.

Czoty, P. W., Martelle, J. L., & Nader, M. A. (2006). Influence of abstinence and conditions of cocaine access on the reinforcing strength of cocaine in nonhuman primates. *Drug and Alcohol Dependence, 85*(3), 213–220. https://doi.org/10.1016/j.drugalcdep.2006.04.009.

Czoty, P. W., McCabe, C., & Nader, M. A. (2005). Assessment of the relative reinforcing strength of cocaine in socially housed monkeys using a choice procedure. *The Journal of Pharmacology and Experimental Therapeutics, 312*(1), 96–102. https://doi.org/10.1124/jpet.104.073411.

Czoty, P. W., & Nader, M. A. (2015). Effects of oral and intravenous administration of Buspirone on food-cocaine choice in socially housed male Cynomolgus monkeys. *Neuropsychopharmacology, 40*(5), 1072–1083. https://doi.org/10.1038/npp.2014.300.

Czoty, P. W., Stoops, W. W., & Rush, C. R. (2016). Evaluation of the "pipeline" for development of medications for cocaine use disorder: A review of translational preclinical, human laboratory, and clinical trial research. *Pharmacological Reviews, 68*(3), 533–562. https://doi.org/10.1124/pr.115.011668.

Di Chiara, G., & Imperato, A. (1988). Drugs abused by humans preferentially increase synaptic dopamine concentrations in the mesolimbic system of freely moving rats. *Proceedings of the National Academy of Sciences of the United States of America, 85*(14), 5274–5278. Retrieved from http://www.pnas.org/content/85/14/5274.abstract.

Epstein, D. H., Heilig, M., & Shaham, Y. (2018). Science-based actions can help address the opioid crisis. *Trends in Pharmacological Sciences, 39*(11), 911–916. https://doi.org/10.1016/j.tips.2018.06.002.

Ferster, C. B., & Skinner, B. F. (1957). *Schedules of reinforcement*. East Norwalk, CT, US: Appleton-Century-Crofts.

Gerak, L. R., Collins, G. T., & France, C. P. (2016). Effects of lorcaserin on cocaine and methamphetamine self-administration and reinstatement of extinguished responding in rhesus monkeys. *The Journal of Pharmacology and Experimental Therapeutics, 359*(3), 383–391. https://doi.org/10.1124/jpet.116.236307.

Gipson, C. D., Dunn, K. E., Bull, A., Ulangkaya, H., & Hossain, A. (2020). Establishing preclinical withdrawal syndrome symptomatology following heroin self-administration in male and female rats. *Experimental and Clinical Psychopharmacology*. https://doi.org/10.1037/pha0000375.

Glowa, J. R., Wojnicki, F. H. E., Matecka, D., Bacher, J. D., Mansbach, R. S., Balster, R. L., et al. (1995). Effects of dopamine reuptake inhibitors on food- and cocaine-maintained responding: I. dependence on unit dose of cocaine. *Experimental and Clinical Psychopharmacology, 3*(3), 219–231. https://doi.org/10.1037/1064-1297.3.3.219.

Grabowski, J., Rhoades, H., Schmitz, J., Stotts, A., Daruzska, L. A., Creson, D., et al. (2001). Dextroamphetamine for cocaine-dependence treatment: A double-blind randomized clinical trial. *Journal of Clinical Psychopharmacology, 21*(5), 522–526.

Greenwald, M. K., Comer, S. D., & Fiellin, D. A. (2014). Buprenorphine maintenance and mu-opioid receptor availability in the treatment of opioid use disorder: Implications for clinical use and policy. *Drug and Alcohol Dependence, 144*, 1–11. https://doi.org/10.1016/j.drugalcdep.2014.07.035.

Griffiths, R. R., Wurster, R. M., & Brady, J. V. (1975). Discrete-trial choice procedure: Effects of naloxone and methadone on choice between food and heroin. *Pharmacological Reviews, 27*(3), 357–365.

Hamilton, L. R., Czoty, P. W., Gage, H. D., & Nader, M. A. (2010). Characterization of the dopamine receptor system in adult rhesus monkeys exposed to cocaine throughout gestation. *Psychopharmacology, 210*(4), 481–488. https://doi.org/10.1007/s00213-010-1847-2.

Haney, M., & Spealman, R. (2008). Controversies in translational research: Drug self-administration. *Psychopharmacology, 199*(3), 403–419. https://doi.org/10.1007/s00213-008-1079-x.

Hannon, J., & Hoyer, D. (2008). Molecular biology of 5-HT receptors. *Behavioural Brain Research, 195*(1), 198–213. https://doi.org/10.1016/j.bbr.2008.03.020.

Hart, C. L., Haney, M., Foltin, R. W., & Fischman, M. W. (2000). Alternative reinforcers differentially modify cocaine self-administration by humans. *Behavioural Pharmacology, 11*(1), 87–91.

Heilig, M., MacKillop, J., Martinez, D., Rehm, J., Leggio, L., & Vanderschuren, L. (2021). Addiction as a brain disease revised: Why it still matters, and the need for consilience. *Neuropsychopharmacology*. https://doi.org/10.1038/s41386-020-00950-y.

Heyman, G. H. (2009). *Addiction: A disorder of choice*. Cambridge: Harvard University Press.

Higgins, G. A., Fletcher, P. J., & Shanahan, W. R. (2020). Lorcaserin: A review of its preclinical and clinical pharmacology and therapeutic potential. *Pharmacology & Therapeutics, 205*, 107417. https://doi.org/10.1016/j.pharmthera.2019.107417.

Hiranita, T., Kohut, S. J., Soto, P. L., Tanda, G., Kopajtic, T. A., & Katz, J. L. (2014). Preclinical efficacy of N-substituted Benztropine analogs as antagonists of methamphetamine self-administration in rats. *The Journal of Pharmacology and Experimental Therapeutics, 348*(1), 174–191. https://doi.org/10.1124/jpet.113.208264.

Howell, L. L., & Cunningham, K. A. (2015). Serotonin 5-HT2 receptor interactions with dopamine function: Implications for therapeutics in cocaine use disorder. *Pharmacological Reviews, 67*(1), 176–197. https://doi.org/10.1124/pr.114.009514.

Hutsell, B. A., Negus, S. S., & Banks, M. L. (2016). Effects of 21-day d-amphetamine and risperidone treatment on cocaine vs food choice and extended-access cocaine intake in male rhesus monkeys. *Drug and Alcohol Dependence, 168*, 36–44. https://doi.org/10.1016/j.drugalcdep.2016.08.637.

John, W. S., Banala, A. K., Newman, A. H., & Nader, M. A. (2015). Effects of buspirone and the dopamine D3 receptor compound PG619 on cocaine and methamphetamine self-administration in rhesus monkeys using a food-drug choice paradigm. *Psychopharmacology, 232*(7), 1279–1289. https://doi.org/10.1007/s00213-014-3760-6.

Jones, B. E., & Prada, J. A. (1977). Effects of methadone and morphine maintenance on drug-seeking behavior in the dog. *Psychopharmacology, 54*(2), 109–112. https://doi.org/10.1007/BF00426764.

Klimas, J., Gorfinkel, L., Giacomuzzi, S. M., Ruckes, C., Socías, M. E., Fairbairn, N., et al. (2019). Slow release oral morphine versus methadone for the treatment of opioid use disorder. *BMJ Open, 9*(4), e025799. https://doi.org/10.1136/bmjopen-2018-025799.

Kreek, M. J., Reed, B., & Butelman, E. R. (2019). Current status of opioid addiction treatment and related preclinical research. *Science Advances, 5*(10), eaax9140. https://doi.org/10.1126/sciadv.aax9140.

Lacy, R. T., Strickland, J. C., Feinstein, M. A., Robinson, A. M., & Smith, M. A. (2016). The effects of sex, estrous cycle, and social contact on cocaine and heroin self-administration in rats. *Psychopharmacology, 233*(17), 3201–3210. https://doi.org/10.1007/s00213-016-4368-9.

Leitl, M. D., Onvani, S., Bowers, M. S., Cheng, K., Rice, K. C., Carlezon, W. A., Jr., et al. (2014). Pain-related depression of the mesolimbic dopamine system in rats: Expression, blockade by analgesics, and role of endogenous kappa-opioids. *Neuropsychopharmacology, 39*(3), 614–624. https://doi.org/10.1038/npp.2013.236.

Lenoir, M., Cantin, L., Vanhille, N., Serre, F., & Ahmed, S. H. (2013). Extended heroin access increases heroin choices over a potent nondrug alternative. *Neuropsychopharmacology, 38*(7), 1209–1220. https://doi.org/10.1038/npp.2013.17.

Leshner, A. I. (1997). Addiction is a brain disease, and it matters. *Science, 278*(5335), 45–47. https://doi.org/10.1126/science.278.5335.45.

Levin, F. R., Mariani, J. J., Pavlicova, M., Choi, C. J., Mahony, A. L., Brooks, D. J., et al. (2020). Extended release mixed amphetamine salts and topiramate for cocaine dependence: A randomized clinical replication trial with frequent users. *Drug and Alcohol Dependence, 206*, 107700. https://doi.org/10.1016/j.drugalcdep.2019.107700.

Levin, F. R., Mariani, J. J., Specker, S., Mooney, M., Mahony, A., Brooks, D. J., et al. (2015). Extended-release mixed amphetamine salts vs placebo for comorbid adult attention-deficit/hyperactivity disorder and cocaine use disorder: A randomized clinical trial. *JAMA Psychiatry, 72*(6), 593–602. https://doi.org/10.1001/jamapsychiatry.2015.41.

Li, D. H., Depoortere, R. Y., & Emmett-Oglesby, M. W. (1994). Tolerance to the reinforcing effects of cocaine in a progressive ratio paradigm. *Psychopharmacology, 116*(3), 326–332. https://doi.org/10.1007/BF02245336.

Lile, J. A., Johnson, A. R., Banks, M. L., Hatton, K. W., Hays, L. R., Nicholson, K. L., et al. (2020). Pharmacological validation of a translational model of cocaine use disorder: Effects of d-amphetamine maintenance on choice between intravenous cocaine and a nondrug alternative in humans and rhesus monkeys. *Experimental and Clinical Psychopharmacology, 28*(2), 169–180. https://doi.org/10.1037/pha0000302.

Lile, J. A., Stoops, W. W., Rush, C. R., Negus, S. S., Glaser, P. E. A., Hatton, K. W., et al. (2016). Development of a translational model to screen medications for cocaine use disorder II: Choice between intravenous cocaine and money in humans. *Drug and Alcohol Dependence*. https://doi.org/10.1016/j.drugalcdep.2016.05.022.

Liu, Y., Roberts, D. C. S., & Morgan, D. (2005). Effects of extended-access self-administration and deprivation on breakpoints maintained by cocaine in rats. *Psychopharmacology, 179*(3), 644–651. https://doi.org/10.1007/s00213-004-2089-y.

Livingston, K. E., Mahoney, J. P., Manglik, A., Sunahara, R. K., & Traynor, J. R. (2018). Measuring ligand efficacy at the mu-opioid receptor using a conformational biosensor. *eLife*, 7, e32499. https://doi.org/10.7554/eLife.32499.

Maguire, D. R., Gerak, L. R., & France, C. P. (2013). Delay discounting of food and remifentanil in rhesus monkeys. *Psychopharmacology, 229*(2), 323–330. https://doi.org/10.1007/s00213-013-3121-x.

Manvich, D. F., Kimmel, H. L., & Howell, L. L. (2012). Effects of serotonin 2C receptor agonists on the behavioral and neurochemical effects of cocaine in squirrel monkeys. *The Journal of Pharmacology and Experimental Therapeutics, 341*(2), 424–434. https://doi.org/10.1124/jpet.111.186981.

Mariani, J. J., Pavlicova, M., Bisaga, A., Nunes, E. V., Brooks, D. J., & Levin, F. R. (2012). Extended-release mixed amphetamine salts and Topiramate for cocaine dependence: A randomized controlled trial. *Biological Psychiatry, 72*(11), 950–956. https://doi.org/10.1016/j.biopsych.2012.05.032.

Mattick, R. P., Breen, C., Kimber, J., & Davoli, M. (2009). Methadone maintenance therapy versus no opioid replacement therapy for opioid dependence. *Cochrane Database of Systematic Reviews, 3*. https://doi.org/10.1002/14651858.CD002209.pub2.

Mauvais-Jarvis, F., Berthold, H. K., Campesi, I., Carrero, J.-J., Dhakal, S., Franconi, F., et al. (2021). Sex- and gender-based pharmacological response to drugs. *Pharmacological Reviews*, *73*(2), 730–762. https://doi.org/10.1124/pharmrev.120.000206.

Mavrikaki, M., Lintz, T., Constantino, N., Page, S., & Chartoff, E. (2021). Chronic opioid exposure differentially modulates oxycodone self-administration in male and female rats. *Addiction Biology*, *26*(3), e12973. https://doi.org/10.1111/adb.12973.

Mello, N. K., Bree, M. P., & Mendelson, J. H. (1983). Comparison of buprenorphine and methadone effects on opiate self-administration in primates. *The Journal of Pharmacology and Experimental Therapeutics*, *225*(2), 378–386.

Mello, N. K., & Negus, S. S. (1996). Preclinical evaluation of pharmacotherapies for treatment of cocaine and opioid abuse using drug self-administration procedures. *Neuropsychopharmacology*, *14*(6), 375–424.

Mello, N. K., & Negus, S. S. (1998). Effects of kappa opioid agonists on cocaine- and food-maintained responding by Rhesus monkeys. *The Journal of Pharmacology and Experimental Therapeutics*, *286*(2), 812–824.

Morgan, D., Grant, K. A., Gage, H. D., Mach, R. H., Kaplan, J. R., Prioleau, O., et al. (2002). Social dominance in monkeys: Dopamine D2 receptors and cocaine self-administration. *Nature Neuroscience*, *5*(2), 169–174. Retrieved from https://doi.org/10.1038/nn798.

Morgan, D., & Roberts, D. C. S. (2004). Sensitization to the reinforcing effects of cocaine following binge-abstinent self-administration. *Neuroscience and Biobehavioral Reviews*, *27*(8), 803–812. https://doi.org/10.1016/j.neubiorev.2003.11.004.

Morgan, D., Smith, M. A., & Roberts, D. C. S. (2005). Binge self-administration and deprivation produces sensitization to the reinforcing effects of cocaine in rats. *Psychopharmacology*, *178*(2), 309–316. https://doi.org/10.1007/s00213-004-1992-6.

Nader, M. A. (2016). Chapter 1–Animal models for addiction medicine: From vulnerable phenotypes to addicted individuals. In E. Hamed, & P. P. Martin (Eds.), *Vol. 224. Prog Brain Res* (pp. 3–24). Elsevier.

Nader, M. A., Nader, S. H., Czoty, P. W., Riddick, N. V., Gage, H. D., Gould, R. W., et al. (2012). Social dominance in female monkeys: Dopamine receptor function and cocaine reinforcement. *Biological Psychiatry*, *72*(5), 414–421. https://doi.org/10.1016/j.biopsych.2012.03.002.

Nader, M. A., & Woolverton, W. L. (1992). Effects of increasing response requirement on choice between cocaine and food in rhesus monkeys. *Psychopharmacology*, *108*(3), 295–300.

Navailles, S., Moison, D., Cunningham, K. A., & Spampinato, U. (2008). Differential regulation of the Mesoaccumbens dopamine circuit by Serotonin2C receptors in the ventral tegmental area and the nucleus Accumbens: An in vivo microdialysis study with cocaine. *Neuropsychopharmacology*, *33*(2), 237–246.

Negus, S. S. (2003). Rapid assessment of choice between cocaine and food in Rhesus monkeys: Effects of environmental manipulations and treatment with d-amphetamine and Flupenthixol. *Neuropsychopharmacology*, *28*(5), 919–931.

Negus, S. S. (2004). Effects of the kappa opioid agonist U50,488 and the kappa opioid antagonist nor-binaltorphimine on choice between cocaine and food in rhesus monkeys. *Psychopharmacology*, *176*(2), 204–213.

Negus, S. S. (2006). Choice between heroin and food in nondependent and heroin-dependent Rhesus monkeys: Effects of naloxone, buprenorphine, and methadone. *The Journal of Pharmacology and Experimental Therapeutics*, *317*(2), 711–723. https://doi.org/10.1124/jpet.105.095380.

Negus, S. S., & Banks, M. L. (2020). Learning from lorcaserin: Lessons from the negative clinical trial of lorcaserin to treat cocaine use disorder. *Neuropsychopharmacology*, *45*(12), 1967–1973. https://doi.org/10.1038/s41386-020-00815-4.

Negus, S. S., & Henningfield, J. (2015). Agonist medications for the treatment of cocaine use disorder. *Neuropsychopharmacology*, *40*(8), 1815–1825. https://doi.org/10.1038/npp.2014.322.

Negus, S. S., & Mello, N. K. (2003a). Effects of chronic d-amphetamine treatment on cocaine- and food-maintained responding under a second-order schedule in rhesus monkeys. *Drug and Alcohol Dependence*, *70*(1), 39–52. Doi: S0376871602003393.

Negus, S. S., & Mello, N. K. (2003b). Effects of chronic d-amphetamine treatment on cocaine- and food-maintained responding under a progressive-ratio schedule in rhesus monkeys. *Psychopharmacology*, *167*(3), 324–332.

Negus, S. S., Mello, N. K., Portoghese, P. S., & Lin, C.-E. (1997). Effects of kappa opioids on cocaine self-administration by Rhesus monkeys. *The Journal of Pharmacology and Experimental Therapeutics*, *282*(1), 44–55.

Negus, S. S., & Rice, K. C. (2009). Mechanisms of withdrawal-associated increases in heroin self-administration: Pharmacologic modulation of heroin vs food choice in heroin-dependent Rhesus monkeys. *Neuropsychopharmacology*, *34*(4), 899–911. Retrieved from https://doi.org/10.1038/npp.2008.127.

Noble, F., & Marie, N. (2019). Management of opioid addiction with opioid substitution treatments: Beyond methadone and buprenorphine. *Frontiers in Psychiatry*, *9*(742). https://doi.org/10.3389/fpsyt.2018.00742.

Oka, T., Negishi, K., Suda, M., Sawa, A., Fujino, M., & Wakimasu, M. (1982). Evidence that dynorphin-$(1-13)$ acts as an agonist on opioid κ-receptors. *European Journal of Pharmacology*, 77(2), 137–141. https://doi.org/10.1016/0014-2999(82)90008-5.

Orio, L., Edwards, S., George, O., Parsons, L. H., & Koob, G. F. (2009). A role for the endocannabinoid system in the increased motivation for cocaine in extended-access conditions. *The Journal of Neuroscience*, *29*(15), 4846–4857. https://doi.org/10.1523/jneurosci.0563-09.2009.

Paterson, N. E., & Markou, A. (2003). Increased motivation for self-administered cocaine after escalated cocaine intake. *Neuroreport*, *14*(17), 2229–2232. https://doi.org/10.1097/00001756-200312020-00019.

Pirtle, J. L., Hickman, M. D., Boinpelly, V. C., Surineni, K., Thakur, H. K., & Grasing, K. W. (2019). The serotonin-2C agonist Lorcaserin delays intravenous choice and modifies the subjective and cardiovascular effects of cocaine: A randomized, controlled human laboratory study. *Pharmacology, Biochemistry, and Behavior*, *180*, 52–59. https://doi.org/10.1016/j.pbb.2019.02.010.

Rachlin, H. (1997). Four teleological theories of addiction. *Psychonomic Bulletin & Review*, *4*(4), 462–473. https://doi.org/10.3758/BF03214335.

Robinson, A. M., Lacy, R. T., Strickland, J. C., Magee, C. P., & Smith, M. A. (2016). The effects of social contact on cocaine intake under extended-access conditions in male rats. *Experimental and Clinical Psychopharmacology*, *24*(4), 285–296. https://doi.org/10.1037/pha0000078.

Rush, C. R., Stoops, W. W., Sevak, R. J., & Hays, L. R. (2010). Cocaine choice in humans during D-amphetamine maintenance. *Journal of Clinical Psychopharmacology*, *30*(2), 152–159. https://doi.org/10.1097/JCP.0b013e3181d21967.

SAMHSA. (2018). Medications for opioid use disorder. *Greatment improvement protocol (TIP) series 63, full document. HHS publication no. (SMA) 19-5063FULLDOC*. Rockville, MD.

Seaman, R. W., Jr., & Collins, G. T. (2021). Impact of morphine dependence and withdrawal on the reinforcing effectiveness of fentanyl, cocaine, and methamphetamine in rats. *Frontiers in Pharmacology*, *12*, 691700. https://doi.org/10.3389/fphar.2021.691700.

Shansky, R. M. (2019). Are hormones a "female problem" for animal research? *Science*, *364*(6443), 825–826. https://doi.org/10.1126/science.aaw7570.

Siciliano, C. A., Saha, K., Calipari, E. S., Fordahl, S. C., Chen, R., Khoshbouei, H., et al. (2018). Amphetamine reverses escalated cocaine intake via restoration of dopamine

transporter conformation. *The Journal of Neuroscience, 38*(2), 484–497. https://doi.org/10.1523/jneurosci.2604-17.2017.
Silverman, K., Holtyn, A. F., & Toegel, F. (2019). The utility of operant conditioning to address poverty and drug addiction. *Perspectives on Behavior Science, 42*(3), 525–546. https://doi.org/10.1007/s40614-019-00203-4.
Skinner, B. (1938). *The behavior of organisms*. New York, NY, USA: Appleton-Century-Crofts.
Smith, M. A. (2012). Peer influences on drug self-administration: Social facilitation and social inhibition of cocaine intake in male rats. *Psychopharmacology, 224*(1), 81–90. https://doi.org/10.1007/s00213-012-2737-6.
Smith, M. A., & Pitts, E. G. (2014). Social preference and drug self-administration: A preclinical model of social choice within peer groups. *Drug and Alcohol Dependence, 135*, 140–145. https://doi.org/10.1016/j.drugalcdep.2013.12.001.
Spragg, S. D. S. (1940). Morphine addiction in chimpanzees. In *Comparative psychology monographs: Vol. 79* (pp. 1–132). Baltimore, MD: The John Hopkins Press.
Stoops, W. W., Lile, J. A., Glaser, P. E., Hays, L. R., & Rush, C. R. (2012). Alternative reinforcer response cost impacts cocaine choice in humans. *Progress in Neuro-Psychopharmacology & Biological Psychiatry, 36*(1), 189–193. Doi:S0278-5846(11)00286-7 [pii] https://doi.org/10.1016/j.pnpbp.2011.10.003.
Tallman, J. F., Primus, R. J., Brodbeck, R., Cornfield, L., Meade, R., Woodruff, K., et al. (1997). I. NGD 94–1: Identification of a novel, high-affinity antagonist at the human dopamine D^4 receptor. *The Journal of Pharmacology and Experimental Therapeutics, 282*(2), 1011–1019.
Tejeda, H. A., & Bonci, A. (2019). Dynorphin/kappa-opioid receptor control of dopamine dynamics: Implications for negative affective states and psychiatric disorders. *Brain Research, 1713*, 91–101. https://doi.org/10.1016/j.brainres.2018.09.023.
Thomsen, M., Barrett, A. C., Negus, S. S., & Caine, S. B. (2013). Cocaine versus food choice procedure in rats: Environmental manipulations and effects of amphetamine. *Journal of the Experimental Analysis of Behavior, 99*(2), 211–233. https://doi.org/10.1002/jeab.15.
Townsend, E. A. (2021). Effects of kappa opioid receptor agonists on fentanyl vs. food choice in male and female rats: Contingent vs. non-contingent administration. *Psychopharmacology, 238*(4), 1017–1028. https://doi.org/10.1007/s00213-020-05749-9.
Townsend, E. A., Blake, S., Faunce, K. E., Hwang, C. S., Natori, Y., Zhou, B., et al. (2019). Conjugate vaccine produces long-lasting attenuation of fentanyl vs. food choice and blocks expression of opioid withdrawal-induced increases in fentanyl choice in rats. *Neuropsychopharmacology*. https://doi.org/10.1038/s41386-019-0385-9.
Townsend, E. A., Bremer, P. T., Jacob, N. T., Negus, S. S., Janda, K. D., & Banks, M. L. (2021). A synthetic opioid vaccine attenuates fentanyl-vs-food choice in male and female rhesus monkeys. *Drug and Alcohol Dependence, 218*, 108348. https://doi.org/10.1016/j.drugalcdep.2020.108348.
Townsend, E. A., Kim, R. K., Robinson, H. L., Marsh, S. A., Banks, M. L., & Hamilton, P. J. (2021). Opioid withdrawal produces sex-specific effects on fentanyl-vs.-food choice and mesolimbic transcription. *Biological Psychiatry Global Open Science*. https://doi.org/10.1016/j.bpsgos.2021.04.009.
Townsend, E. A., Naylor, J. E., Negus, S. S., Edwards, S. R., Qureshi, H. N., McLendon, H. W., et al. (2017). Effects of nalfurafine on the reinforcing, thermal antinociceptive, and respiratory-depressant effects of oxycodone: Modeling an abuse-deterrent opioid analgesic in rats. *Psychopharmacology, 234*(17), 2597–2605. https://doi.org/10.1007/s00213-017-4652-3.
Townsend, E. A., Negus, S. S., & Banks, M. L. (2020). Medications development for treatment of opioid use disorder. *Cold Spring Harbor Perspectives in Medicine*. https://doi.org/10.1101/cshperspect.a039263.

Townsend, E. A., Negus, S. S., Poklis, J. L., & Banks, M. L. (2020). Lorcaserin maintenance fails to attenuate heroin vs. food choice in rhesus monkeys. *Drug and Alcohol Dependence*, 107848. https://doi.org/10.1016/j.drugalcdep.2020.107848.

Venniro, M., Banks, M. L., Heilig, M., Epstein, D. H., & Shaham, Y. (2020). Improving translation of animal models of addiction and relapse by reverse translation. *Nature Reviews. Neuroscience*. https://doi.org/10.1038/s41583-020-0378-z.

Venniro, M., Russell, T. I., Zhang, M., & Shaham, Y. (2019). Operant social reward decreases incubation of heroin craving in male and female rats. *Biological Psychiatry*. https://doi.org/10.1016/j.biopsych.2019.05.018.

Venniro, M., Zhang, M., Caprioli, D., Hoots, J. K., Golden, S. A., Heins, C., et al. (2018). Volitional social interaction prevents drug addiction in rat models. *Nature Neuroscience*, *21*(11), 1520–1529. https://doi.org/10.1038/s41593-018-0246-6.

Vocci, F. J., & Montoya, I. D. (2009). Psychological treatments for stimulant misuse, comparing and contrasting those for amphetamine dependence and those for cocaine dependence. *Current Opinion in Psychiatry*, *22*(3), 263–268. https://doi.org/10.1097/YCO.0b013e32832a3b44.

Volkow, N., Gur, R., Wang, G.-J., Folwer, J., Modberg, P., Ding, Y.-S., et al. (1998). Association between decline in brain dopamine activity with age and cognitive and motor impairment in healthy individuals. *The American Journal of Psychiatry*, *155*(3), 344–349. https://doi.org/10.1176/ajp.155.3.344.

Walsh, S. L., Geter-Douglas, B., Strain, E. C., & Bigelow, G. E. (2001). Enadoline and Butorphanol: Evaluation of κ-agonists on cocaine pharmacodynamics and cocaine self-administration in humans. *The Journal of Pharmacology and Experimental Therapeutics*, *299*(1), 147–158.

Wee, S., & Koob, G. F. (2010). The role of the dynorphin–κ opioid system in the reinforcing effects of drugs of abuse. *Psychopharmacology*, *210*(2), 121–135. https://doi.org/10.1007/s00213-010-1825-8.

Wee, S., Mandyam, C. D., Lekic, D. M., & Koob, G. F. (2008). α1-Noradrenergic system role in increased motivation for cocaine intake in rats with prolonged access. *European Neuropsychopharmacology*, *18*(4), 303–311. https://doi.org/10.1016/j.euroneuro.2007.08.003.

Yanagita, T. (1975). Some methodological problems in assessing dependence-producing properties of drugs in animals. *Pharmacological Reviews*, *27*(4), 503–509.

Yanagita, T. (1979). Self-administration studies on psychological dependence. *Trends in Pharmacological Sciences*, *1*(1), 161–164. https://doi.org/10.1016/0165-6147(79)90057-9.

Zimmer, B., Chiodo, K., & Roberts, D. S. (2014). Reduction of the reinforcing effectiveness of cocaine by continuous d-amphetamine treatment in rats: Importance of active self-administration during treatment period. *Psychopharmacology*, *231*(5), 949–954. https://doi.org/10.1007/s00213-013-3305-4.

CHAPTER EIGHT

Examining the effects of psychoactive drugs on complex behavioral processes in laboratory animals

Brian D. Kangas*
[a]Behavioral Biology Program, McLean Hospital, Belmont, MA, United States
[b]Department of Psychiatry, Harvard Medical School, Boston, MA, United States
*Corresponding author: e-mail address: bkangas@mclean.harvard.edu

Contents

1. Introduction 244
2. Cognitive tasks in pharmacology 245
   2.1 Learning 246
   2.2 Cognitive flexibility 249
   2.3 Memory 252
   2.4 Attention 255
   2.5 Motivation 257
   2.6 Impulsivity 259
3. Caveats and considerations 262
4. On terms coda 263
5. Conclusion 264
Acknowledgments 265
Conflict of interest statement 265
References 265

Abstract

Behavioral pharmacology has been aided significantly by the development of innovative cognitive tasks designed to examine complex behavioral processes in laboratory animals. Performance outcomes under these conditions have provided key metrics of drug action which serve to supplement traditional in vivo assays of physiologic and behavioral effects of psychoactive drugs. This chapter provides a primer of cognitive tasks designed to assay different aspects of complex behavior, including learning, cognitive flexibility, memory, attention, motivation, and impulsivity. Both capstone studies and recent publications are highlighted throughout to illustrate task value for two distinct but often interconnected translational strategies. First, task performance in laboratory animals can be utilized to elucidate how *drugs of abuse* affect complex behavioral processes. Here, the expectation is that adverse effects on such processes

Advances in Pharmacology, Volume 93
ISSN 1054-3589
https://doi.org/10.1016/bs.apha.2021.09.001

will have predictive relevance to consequences that will be experienced by humans. Second, these same task outcomes can be used to evaluate *candidate therapeutics*. In this case, the extent to which drug doses with medicinal value perturb task performance can contribute critical information for a more complete safety profile appraisal and advance the process of medications development. Methodological and theoretical considerations are discussed and include an emphasis on determining selectivity in drug action on complex behavioral processes.

1. Introduction

Psychoactive drugs can have profound effects on complex behavioral processes. The intersection between behavioral science and pharmacology offers an approach to better understand these interactions and, like many endeavors in biomedical science, can be aided in significant ways by translational research in laboratory animals. Indeed, the last 65 years of research in behavioral pharmacology using rodents, birds, and nonhuman primates have produced substantial increases in our understanding of drug effects on behavioral processes. During the last few decades, advances in the development and empirical validation of cognitive tasks for laboratory animals have served as important complements to efforts elucidating drug action using other behavioral methodologies, including schedule-controlled responding, drug discrimination, and self-administration.

The reasons for studying the effects of psychoactive drugs in cognitive tasks can be divided into two general categories. The first involves deriving detailed characterizations of the effects *drugs of abuse* have on complex behavioral processes. Here, the expectation is that either brief or long-term perturbations in task performance following either acute or chronic drug treatment will be predictive of consequences experienced by humans. That is, understanding how commonly used and abused drugs adversely affect different aspects of complex behavioral processes allows for an enhanced appraisal of inherent risks which can be levied against perceived recreational benefits.

A second reason for studying the effects of psychoactive drugs on cognitive task performance in laboratory animals is to evaluate *candidate therapeutics* on complex behavioral processes. In this case, determining the effects of a novel pharmacotherapeutic on task performance at doses known to have medicinal value can contribute to a preclinical appraisal of the drug's safety. Indeed, establishing a *therapeutic index* that quantifies the distance between doses that produce desirable treatment outcomes and those that adversely affect task performance can complement traditional toxicological measures (Weiss & Laties, 1975) and indices of abuse liability (Ator & Griffiths, 2003) for appraising a candidate medication's clinical viability and side-effect profile. In some cases, an established pharmacotherapeutic may have adverse effects on cognition that are targeted for reduction or elimination in a novel candidate medication. Thus, a preclinical approach that defines the existing therapeutic as a *standard* to improve upon, via retention of medicinal effects with fewer unwanted behaviorally disruptive effects, can serve to advance drug development.

Importantly, although the two approaches described above can be conducted independently, it is increasingly common for these pursuits to progress in a highly interconnected manner. For example, many endeavors in the development of psychoactive therapeutics focus on improving the safety profile of existing medications. Often, these existing medications, though efficacious for their intended purposes, are also drugs of abuse in certain populations. Indeed, abuse liability is a common undesirable feature of several categories of commonly prescribed pharmacotherapies, including opioid analgesics for pain management (Wightman, Perrone, Portelli, & Nelson, 2012), psychomotor stimulants for attention deficit disorders (Romach, Schoedel, & Sellers, 2014), and benzodiazepines for anxiety (Ator, 2005). Having the existing medication serve as the standard to be improved upon allows for systematic comparisons of candidate therapeutics designed to have lower abuse liability while simultaneously evaluating potential for accompanying side-effects on complex behavioral processes. This strategy can provide a more complete preclinical safety profile of both existing and candidate medications and, at the same time, reveal potentially hazardous consequences for those who might consume it illicitly.

2. Cognitive tasks in pharmacology

This section is designed to serve as a primer of commonly used cognitive tasks in laboratory animals for the pursuits in behavioral pharmacology and medications development defined above. It is important to note that this is not intended to serve as an exhaustive list. In fact, novel methods are continually being developed to examine behavioral phenotypes that emerge from clinical observations and laboratory discoveries. Rather, the diverse tasks highlighted in this chapter are examples of those associated with long-standing contributions to an enhanced understanding of drug action on complex behavioral processes. Finally, it is important to note that every task discussed below can be understood from a neuropharmacological perspective that seeks to explicate their neurobiological and pharmacological mechanisms of action; however, the scope of this chapter expressly prioritizes the behavioral level of analysis. Nevertheless, many of the references cited below were selected to guide the interested reader to the relevant neural and receptor pharmacology literature as well.

2.1 Learning

The extent to which a drug perturbs learning can provide a foundational assessment of its actions on complex behavioral processes. In particular, discrimination learning has provided a vital approach to the study of both abused drugs and candidate medications. Studying the rate at which a subject acquires a new discrimination allows for measurement of the magnitude of a drug's adverse consequences and the extent to which tolerance develops to those effects. Discriminative behavior can also be used as a means to determine a subject's sensitivity to the reinforcement contingencies that maintain such performance and how a drug might modify those complex processes.

2.1.1 Repeated acquisition

The ***repeated acquisition task*** is an assay commonly used to examine fundamental aspects of *discrimination learning* and how it develops over time. In its typical arrangement, a subject is presented with two concurrently-available stimuli: one arbitrarily designated as S^+ (responses to it result in reinforcement) and the other as S^- (responses to it result in a timeout period). Following sufficient experience with the contingencies, subjects eventually acquire the discrimination, indicated by exclusive responding to the S^+ stimulus. Following mastery of a given discrimination, the subject is exposed to a novel S^+/S^- pair until mastery is again observed. This is repeated with numerous S^+/S^- stimulus pairs across sessions to allow for measurement of acquisition rate across successive discriminations. Although it had been known for some time that laboratory animals can acquire multiple distinct discriminations, seminal work by Harlow (1949) using this paradigm in monkeys illustrated a profound effect and fundamental principle of learning: the rate at which a subject acquires such discriminations increases systematically as a function of the number of previously mastered discriminations until very few trials are required to learn new discriminations. He called this phenomenon a *learning set*. The importance of this finding lies not simply in the characterization of the subject's ever-expanding discriminative repertoire but, for the present purposes, a method to examine acute drug treatment on the ability to learn new things and how chronic drug treatment might impact the ability to develop a learning set (i.e., *learn-to-learn*). Although early capstone studies manually presented three-dimensional S^+/S^- objects to subjects (Warren, 1965), subsequent studies in behavioral pharmacology used automated procedures in operant conditioning chambers to examine drug effects on novel discrimination learning by repeatedly training unique chained response sequences across multiple operanda (Thompson, 1973). For example, a subject responding in a chamber with two levers might need to press the left, then right, then right again, then left lever to obtain reward. These 3–5 step sequences allowed for some of the first systematic studies characterizing the deleterious effects of Δ^9-tetrahydrocannabinol (Δ^9-THC) and other cannabinoid agonists in rats and monkeys (Branch, Dearing, & Lee, 1980; Thompson & Winsauer, 1985; Winsauer, Lambert, & Moerschbaecher, 1999) and subsequent tolerance (Delatte, Winsauer, & Moerschbaecher, 2002), as well as adverse stimulant and opioid effects (Evans & Wenger, 1992; Moerschbaecher, Thompson, & Winsauer, 1983; Winsauer, Silvester, Moerschbaecher, & France, 2000). More recently, advances in modern touch-sensitive technology for rodents and nonhuman primates (Bussey et al., 2008; Dumont, Salewski, & Beraldo, 2021; Kangas & Bergman, 2012, 2017) have provided an ability to train a near-infinite number of distinct visual discriminations using unique photographic stimuli (Kangas & Bergman, 2014) to examine the effects of psychoactive drugs on acquisition rates to master novel discriminations and, as well, the development of learning-to-learn repertoires. In addition to systematic replication of Δ^9-THC's adverse effects on discrimination learning (Withey et al., 2021), repeated acquisition studies have detailed comparisons of Δ^9-THC and ligands designed to elevate levels of endogenous cannabinoids to examine the prospect that endocannabinoids may have similar medicinal value with fewer unwanted side-effects than Δ^9-THC (Di Marzo, 2018). This advantage was indeed documented in learning (Kangas et al., 2016) and antiemesis (Wooldridge et al., 2020) endpoints, thus representing an instance of the important interplay between studying drugs of abuse and therapeutic potential discussed above. In addition to studies of experimenter-administered drugs, touchscreen-based repeated acquisition tasks have also been used to characterize the effects of self-administered drugs, such as methamphetamine (Kangas & Bergman, 2016) and cocaine (Kangas, Doyle, Kohut, Bergman, & Kaufman, 2019). These studies revealed that, although significant adverse effects on the rate of acquisition were associated with high daily drug intake, tolerance to the disruptive effects on learning was reliably produced following remedial training, even during chronic conditions. Interestingly, matched studies of other self-administered drugs of abuse, for example, the prescription opioid oxycodone (Kibaly et al., 2021), have documented no deleterious effects on the development of this behavioral repertoire, even during conditions of high daily intake (Withey, Doyle, Porter, Bergman, & Kangas, 2020), providing evidence that the abuse liability of a drug does not necessarily predict its adverse effects on discrimination learning.

2.1.2 Probabilistic reward task

The ***probabilistic reward task*** is designed to examine a subject's *sensitivity to reward*. It also utilizes discrimination methodology; however, in this paradigm, rather than examining the development of discrimination learning, the same two stimuli are presented across numerous trials with asymmetric probabilistic contingencies that reward correct responses in the presence of one stimulus (rich) more often than correct responses in the presence of the other stimulus (lean). This provides a quantitative means to identify reward learning deficits that are prominent in anhedonic populations and for which no approved medications exist. For example, in the human variant of the probabilistic reward task (Pizzagalli, Jahn, & O'Shea, 2005), subjects are instructed to distinguish between two lines that vary slightly in length. Unbeknownst to the subjects, 3:1 asymmetrical probabilistic contingencies are arranged such that 60% of correct responses to one of the stimuli are rewarded (e.g., long line: rich stimulus) and 20% of correct responses to the other are rewarded (e.g., short line: lean stimulus). As predicted by signal detection theory (Luc, Pizzagalli, & Kangas, 2021; McCarthy & Davison, 1979), healthy subjects reliably exhibit a response bias toward the more richly rewarded stimulus. However, subjects with anhedonia display a blunted response bias that has been repeatedly documented to correlate with current and future anhedonia across diverse clinical populations (Vrieze et al., 2013). Anhedonia, or the loss of pleasure or lack of reactivity to previously rewarding stimuli, is most closely associated with major depressive disorders (Whitton, Treadway, & Pizzagalli, 2015), but is also prominent in other neuropsychiatric conditions, including bipolar disorder (Hasler, Drevets, Gould, Gottesman, & Manji, 2006), schizophrenia (Horan, Kring, & Blanchard, 2006), post-traumatic stress disorder (Nawijn et al., 2015), and substance use disorder (Markou, Kosten, & Koob, 1998). Given the transdiagnostic prevalence of anhedonic phenotypes across neuropsychiatric disorders, the probabilistic reward task has been *reverse-translated* for use in rodents and nonhuman primates to help bridge the preclinical gap between therapeutic discovery and treatment. For example, in an auditory-based variant, rats were trained to discriminate between two tone durations that, following acquisition, were programmed with a 3:1 rich:lean probabilistic contingency (Der-Avakian, D'Souza, Pizzagalli, & Markou, 2013). Expected response biases toward the more richly rewarded stimulus were observed as was pharmacological blunting of response bias following administration of low doses of the direct dopamine D_2-family agonist pramipexole as seen previously in humans (Pizzagalli et al., 2008). In addition, chronic social defeat stress blunted response biases relative to non-stressed controls (Der-Avakian et al., 2017) and, in turn, revealed a role of dopaminergic and glucocorticoid systems in aspects of reward responsiveness (Lamontagne, Melendez, & Olmstead, 2018). To align formal similarity with the human task, touchscreen-based variants also have been developed using visual line-length discriminations under probabilistic contingencies designed for rats (Kangas, Wooldridge, Luc, Bergman, & Pizzagalli, 2020) and marmosets (Wooldridge, Bergman, Pizzagalli, & Kangas, 2021). Expected response biases were observed in both species and subsequent studies confirmed pharmacological sensitivity by showing that drugs known to enhance hedonic tone, such as amphetamine (McIntyre et al., 2017), scopolamine (Jaffe, Novakovic, & Peselow, 2013), and ketamine (Coyle & Laws, 2015), dose-dependently enhanced reward responsiveness in these reverse-translated animal tasks. Coordinated pursuits of this sort leverage human and laboratory animal behavior under discrimination learning tasks as quantitative metrics to advance medications development for disorders in which anhedonic phenotypes are prominent.

2.2 Cognitive flexibility

Although the development of discrimination learning repertoires can be viewed as fundamental adaptive behavior, so too is the ability to modify response allocation in the face of changing contingencies. The capacity to efficiently inhibit a previously reinforced response in a shifting environment has obvious survival value and, as such, the extent to which a drug perturbs these complex behavioral processes has been a ripe source of investigation in behavioral pharmacology and medications development.

2.2.1 Discrimination reversal

The ***discrimination reversal task*** is commonly used to probe *cognitive flexibility*, that is, a subject's ability to inhibit a response that was previously associated with reward delivery and respond effectively in accord with the new contingencies. The first phase of the discrimination reversal task often mirrors that of the repeated acquisition task in which a novel S^+/S^- stimulus discrimination is mastered. At some point following discrimination mastery, in an otherwise unsignaled manner, responses to the stimulus that was previously S^+ produces the consequences associated with the stimulus that was previously S^-, and vice versa. Because this reversal in contingencies is not signaled to the subject, responses to the stimulus that was previously S^+ (now S^-) persist for a period of time. Following sufficient exposure to these updated conditions, the subject will inhibit this response and instead respond with increased probability to the stimulus that was previously S^- (now S^+). The rate at which this shift in response allocation occurs serves as a primary dependent variable related to the construct of cognitive flexibility/response inhibition and, like acquisition rate of the initial discrimination, is a highly useful behavioral endpoint to examine the effects of psychoactive drugs, especially those with high abuse liability (Izquierdo & Jentsch, 2012). One prominent example of its use in behavioral pharmacology is in studies of psychomotor stimulants. Compulsive phenotypes defined, in part, by deficits in inhibitory control have been long associated with substance use disorders involving this drug class (London, Kohno, Morales, & Ballard, 2015). Studies examining nonhuman primate performance during a discrimination reversal task have discovered, for example, that chronic methamphetamine-induced performance deficits were significantly more pronounced during discrimination reversal, relative to initial acquisition, but also included individual differences that revealed a correlation between the magnitude of impaired cognitive flexibility and changes in dopaminergic transmission, specifically via reduced dopamine D_2-like receptors and dopamine transporter availability (Groman et al., 2012). Assessments of individual differences in reversal learning and inhibitory control also uncovered a relationship between the magnitude of task deficits and structural alterations of increased gray matter density in the putamen (Groman, Morales, Lee, London, & Jentsch, 2013), in line with previous neuroimaging observations in humans (Chang et al., 2005). Increases in gray matter density, among other structural changes, were also recently shown to correlate with deficits in reversal learning following chronic self-administered cocaine, even after extended periods of abstinence (Jedema et al., 2021). These studies and others demonstrate the value of examining reversal learning and response inhibition metrics that comprise the construct of cognitive flexibility and, as well, how interrogating individual differences in task performance can reveal mechanistic order when determining behavior, drug, and brain interactions.

2.2.2 Probabilistic reversal learning

The ***probabilistic reversal learning task*** shares several features with the discrimination reversal task described above to assay *cognitive flexibility* but with asymmetric probabilistic contingencies programmed. Specifically, subjects are presented with a concurrent choice between two options: responding on one results in reward more often (e.g., 80% of the time), whereas responding on the other option results in reward less often (e.g., 20% of the time). After the subject is exclusively responding on the rich alternative for some predefined number of trials, the probabilities programmed on each response alternative switch in an otherwise unsignaled manner. This task is often comprised of numerous trials allowing for multiple reversals in a daily session and the number of completed reversals serves as a primary dependent measure. Like the discrimination reversal task, the shift in response allocation in the face of changing contingencies is thought to assay cognitive flexibility and, in turn, can serve as a useful construct to examine underlying neural mechanism and pharmacological modulation. In addition, as with several of the tasks highlighted in this chapter, variants designed for human subjects that are commonly used for similar ends permit coordinated studies of cross-species continuity (Fellows & Farah, 2003; Lawrence, Sahakian, Rogers, Hodge, & Robbins, 1999). Moreover, the use of probabilistic schedules of reinforcement lend themselves well to innovative computational analyses of expected and unexpected reinforcement/punishment outcomes in laboratory animals that are similar to those used in human studies (Costa, Tran, Turchi, & Averbeck, 2015; Kanen, Ersche, Fineberg, Robbins, & Cardinal, 2019). The probabilistic reversal learning task has revealed deficits in cognitive flexibility during nicotine withdrawal (Jackson, Silk, Buhidma, & Shoaib, 2017) and following chronic administration of abused drugs such as methamphetamine (Groman, Rich, Smith, Lee, & Taylor, 2018) and cocaine (Groman et al., 2020) but not alcohol (Aguirre et al., 2020). It has also been used to provide preclinical indications of performance enhancement, for example, following oxytocin treatment (Roberts et al., 2019). Recent work also has employed this task with aims to develop improved medications for mood disorders, given the fact that deficits in reversal learning have been associated with depression (Mukherjee, Filipowicz, Vo, Satterthwaite, & Kable, 2020). To date, probabilistic reversal learning studies in rats have yielded encouraging, though mixed, findings. For example, during systematic studies examining serotonergic mechanisms in sensitivity to reward and negative feedback, Bari et al. (2010) documented the ability of acute and sub-chronic treatment with a high but not low dose of citalopram to enhance reversal learning. Studies of other antidepressants have documented that agomelatine and mirtazapine, but not escitalopram, clomipramine, and venlafaxine, improved certain aspects of reversal learning (Drozd, Rychlik, Fijalkowska, & Rygula, 2019), whereas Wilkinson, Grogan, Mellor, and Robinson (2020) also observed enhancement effects with citalopram, but not reboxetine, venlafaxine, or the fast-acting antidepressants ketamine and scopolamine (however, see Rychlik, Bollen, & Rygula, 2017, for positive ketamine findings). Rigorous testing across numerous drugs designed for the same indication serves as an important example of how to use performance outcomes under the same task to provide preclinical ranking of candidate therapeutics.

2.3 Memory

A preponderance of animal research on the behavioral pharmacology of memorial processes involves examining the effects of psychoactive drugs on delayed stimulus control. This is typically arranged by training a conditional discrimination between a stimulus (e.g., visual, auditory, or spatial cue) and a response. After the conditional discrimination has been mastered, a delay is introduced between stimulus presentation and the opportunity to respond. This procedural variable is called a *retention interval* and its duration is negatively correlated with performance accuracy. That is, as the retention interval increases, stimulus control decreases. Evaluation of a variety of retention intervals across trials allows for characterization of a *forgetting function*, usually described by a negative exponential curve which has been repeatedly documented to be sensitive to, and modified by, drug treatment.

2.3.1 Delayed matching-to-sample

The ***delayed matching-to-sample task*** is used to examine *short-term recognition memory* (Blough, 1959; Kangas, Berry, & Branch, 2011; White, 1985). In its most common iteration, a subject is presented with one of two sample stimuli (e.g., a red or green light centered in between a left and right response lever). After completion of an observing response in the presence of that stimulus, it is extinguished for a period of time, followed by simultaneous illumination of two comparison stimuli (a red and green light, one presented above the left and the other presented above the right lever). A correct response is defined by responding on the lever associated with the comparison stimulus that matched the physical characteristics of the previously presented sample stimulus and is reinforced, whereas selection of the non-matching stimulus will terminate the trial without reward. A range of species-relevant retention intervals are examined across trials in a mixed manner to derive a forgetting function. Alternatively, procedural variants have been developed in which the retention interval increases following correct matches and decreases following incorrect matches and these titration contingences allow for precise determinations of memorial capacities under the conditions arranged (Cumming & Berryman, 1965; Kangas, Vaidya, & Branch, 2010). In another task variant, the ***delayed matching-to-position task*** is designed to assay *short-term spatial memory* (Dunnett, 1985). Instead of probing the ability to recognize a previously presented stimulus following a retention interval, a stimulus is presented in a location within the experimental chamber, for example, a light presented above one of two levers. After an observing response is made on the illuminated lever, another response is required on a different side of the chamber and, thereafter, the levers are protracted after the retention interval elapses. A response to the previously illuminated lever will be reinforced, whereas responses to other levers will terminate the trial without reward. A long-standing research domain using these tasks has detailed the adverse effects on short-term memory of diverse drugs of abuse, including alcohol (Mello, 1971), cannabinoids (Kangas et al., 2016), psychomotor stimulants (Branch & Dearing, 1982; Harper, Wisnewski, Hunt, & Schenk, 2005; Jedema et al., 2021; LeSage, Clark, & Poling, 1993) and, in the latter drug class, how pretreatment with other drugs might mitigate such undesirable effects on memory (Harper, 2013; Macaskill, Harrow, & Harper, 2015). Studies examining the effects of ongoing *chronic* drug treatment on delayed matching-to-sample performance are less common but have documented evidence of tolerance to the memory disruptive effects of illicit drugs, such as cocaine (Kangas & Branch, 2012). Forgetting functions derived from delayed matching-to-sample procedures can also be assessed for the ability of drug administration to improve short-term memory. Although the laudable goal of developing so-called cognitive enhancers has been elusive, there have been promising findings. For example, a compelling line of research examining administration of nicotinic and other pharmacologically-similar cholinergic ligands have revealed upward shifts in portions of the forgetting function (Buccafusco, Letchworth, Bencherif, & Lippiello, 2005; Elrod, Buccafusco, & Jackson, 1988); however, interpretive caution is required (Soto, Dallery, Ator, & Katz, 2013). Finally, the delayed matching-to-sample task has been effectively used in medications development to offer preclinical appraisals of candidate therapeutics with the goal of developing drugs that do not perturb short-term memory at doses that have medicinal value. Recent positive examples in nonhuman primates across diverse areas of study include trace amine-associated receptor 1 agonists for narcolepsy treatment (Goonawardena et al., 2019), kynurenic acid for use in cannabis use disorder pharmacotherapies (Justinova et al., 2013), and the pseudoirreversible mu opioid receptor antagonist methocinnamox for conditions of opioid abuse and overdose (Minervini, Disney, Husbands, & France, 2020).

2.3.2 Self-ordered spatial search

The ***self-ordered spatial search task***, like delayed matching-to-position, examines *short-term spatial memory* via the ability of a subject to remember spatial dimensions of stimuli presented. This task is based on the Hamilton search task (Hamilton, 1911) and the radial arm maze task (Levin, 1988), which was later adapted for use in human neuropsychological assessments (Owen, Downes, Sahakian, Polkey, & Robbins, 1990) and nonhuman primates using standard operant conditioning chambers (Levin & Bowman, 1986) and touchscreen-equipped chambers (Weed et al., 1999). In the prototypical touchscreen-based task variant, a subject is presented with a variable number of simultaneously available response boxes in different locations on the touchscreen. If the subject touches each of the response boxes once, and only once, reinforcement is delivered. Responding on a box that had already been touched in that trial terminates that trial without reward and leads to a timeout. Memorial processes are tested by introducing a variable delay (retention interval) after each box touch where all boxes disappear and then reappear in the same position, thus, requiring the subject to remember which have and have not been touched. Like delayed matching-to-sample and -position tasks, difficulty in the self-ordered spatial search task can be adjusted depending on subject performance by increasing the retention interval following each response and/or number of boxes presented in each trial. This task, often used as one component of a larger battery, has demonstrated value by elucidating deficits in spatial working memory following central nervous system dysfunction caused by simian immunodeficiency virus infection (Weed et al., 2004) or acute treatment with a variety of psychoactive drugs, including scopolamine (Levin & Bowman, 1986; Taffe, Weed, & Gold, 1999), ketamine (Taffe, Davis, Gutierrez, & Gold, 2002), dopamine antagonists (Von Huben et al., 2006), and Δ^9-THC (Wright, Vandewater, & Taffe, 2013). Other studies in monkeys conducted over a year after a short-course but high dose MDMA treatment regimen exhibited substantial and lasting serotonergic depletion in several cortical regions without producing persistent deficits on several cognitive tasks, including in the self-ordered spatial search task (Taffe et al., 2002).

Interestingly, however, subsequent challenges with the mixed $5HT_{2A/2C}$ antagonist ketanserin, the $5HT_{2C}$ agonist 1-(3-Chlo-rophenyl)piperazine dihydrochloride, and the $5HT_{1A}$ agonist (±)8-hydroxy-DPAT hydrobromide significantly worsened five-choice serial reaction time (Section 2.4.2) and progressive ratio (Section 2.5.1) performance without perturbing self-ordered spatial search. This provides evidence that previous history with a drug associated with abuse liability and long-lasting neurochemical alterations will not necessarily have enduring deleterious effects on complex behavior, despite task-selective vulnerabilities to receptor-mediated physiologic challenges.

2.4 Attention

Systematic evaluation of a drug's ability to enhance or impair attentional processes can serve as a metric of potential medicinal value in the case of the former or unwanted side-effects in the case of the latter. Although the discovery of pharmacologic enhancers of learning and memory has been elusive and often produce only ephemeral outcomes, the ability of a drug to extend sustained attention to task engagement has been repeatedly detected in animal models. This has been observed primarily with psychomotor stimulant drugs which, indicative of translational relevance, are employed successfully in the clinical management of attention deficit disorders. Like learning and memory tasks, animal models of attention also serve as valuable assessments of the extent to which a drug adversely affects the subject's ability to maintain effective and efficient task performance. An understanding of which drugs (at which doses) can enhance or perturb performance that requires sustained vigilant responding can contribute to a comprehensive appraisal of their medicinal value.

2.4.1 Psychomotor vigilance

The ***psychomotor vigilance task***, like all tasks highlighted in this chapter, has several procedural variants to assay *sustained attention*. However, many of the task elements can be traced back to studies from the 1940s, in which World War II service members were performing extended signal detection tasks, often tracking the movements of a clock (Mackworth, 1948) or blips on a radar screen (Anderson & Lindsley, 1944) which proved to have high translational relevance to mission success. Indeed, both Nazi Germany and the Allied Powers began experimenting with amphetamines and other psychomotor stimulants to extend battle-ready attentional processes and sustained vigilance during combat (Rasmussen, 2011). In a standard variant of the psychomotor vigilance task, responses are reinforced following detection of a visual stimulus on a computer screen. The precise location, intensity, and duration of stimulus presentation can vary depending on the species, response, and experimental goals. However, reaction time thresholds are typically a primary dependent measure, which usually degrade following extended exposure to the task or environmental stressors such as sleep deprivation (Deurveilher, Bush, Rusak, Eskes, & Semba, 2015; Dinges et al., 1997). In the context of interconnected approaches designed to understand both drugs of abuse and candidate therapeutics, animal variants of the psychomotor vigilance task are devised to reveal the extent to which a drug can either worsen attentional processes, improve them via slowing its time-dependent degradation, or enhance wakefulness following conditions of sleep deprivation (McCarthy et al., 2017). Not surprisingly, administration of drugs such as Δ^9-THC in monkeys produced dose-related decrements on sustained vigilance (Kangas et al., 2016); however, studies with relatively low doses of the psychomotor stimulants caffeine, nicotine, cocaine, and amphetamine in rats documented systematic improvements in task metrics (Davis, Roma, & Hienz, 2016; Evenden, Turpin, Oliver, & Jennings, 1993) similar to findings observed in human studies (Silber, Croft, Papafotiou, & Stough, 2006).

2.4.2 Five-choice serial reaction time

The ***five-choice serial reaction time task*** shares several characteristics with the psychomotor vigilance task but also has distinct features to assay *attentional processes*. Rather than responding to stimuli on a computer screen, the five-choice serial reaction time task is typically conducted in specialized chambers designed for rats and mice and include five transilluminated nose-poke apertures. In its typical arrangement, one of the five nose-poke apertures is illuminated for an interval that can vary in difficulty by its duration or brightness and by requiring a response within a very limited duration for reward. Task performance can be evaluated by analyzing session-wide hits, misses, premature responses, and response omissions. Although sometimes used to probe impulse control (see Section 2.6), the development of this task originally stemmed from studies examining attentional processes related to attention deficit disorders via lesion and drug studies in rats (Carli, Robbins, Evenden, & Everitt, 1983; Robbins, 2002). Subsequent use of this task has highlighted its value across drug classes, including documenting adverse effects on attentional processes following treatment with amphetamine (Cole & Robbins, 1987), scopolamine (Jones & Higgins, 1995; Shannon & Eberle, 2006), to a lesser extent morphine (Maguire, Henson, & France, 2016; Pattij, Schetters, Janssen, Wiskerke, & Schoffelmeer, 2009), and during both cocaine and heroin withdrawal (Dalley et al., 2005). Consistent with their attention-enhancing profile, low doses of nicotine, caffeine, and amphetamine have been shown to enhance accuracy and other performance metrics in this task (Bizarro, Patel, Murtagh, & Stolerman, 2004; Grottick & Higgins, 2002; Stolerman, Mirza, Hahn, & Shoaib, 2000). Finally, this task has also served an innovative role in medications development, for example, in studies examining the ability of orexin/hypocretin antagonists to reduce cocaine-induced premature responding as a behavioral marker of drug-induced deficits in executive functioning (Gentile et al., 2018).

2.5 Motivation

It is well known that motivation can be increased or decreased by psychoactive drugs. One common approach to studying drug effects on motivational processes in laboratory animals is to examine how pharmacological treatment modifies responding for an appetitive consequence, for example, a palatable food reward. After establishing stable baseline consumption, subsequent drug administration can probe whether the rate of operant responding increases, decreases, or is unaffected, with the assumption that dose-related changes in responding reflect pharmacological mediation of reward value. Another common approach to studying motivation is to examine the conditions under which a subject will respond for the drug itself. In this case, self-administration procedures can be arranged to derive the relationship between response output and unit dose, which can serve as an index of motivational limits for procurement of a given drug dose.

2.5.1 Progressive ratio

The ***progressive ratio task*** has been used for decades to examine *motivational processes* via how much a laboratory animal will respond for a given reinforcer (Hodos, 1961). In its standard arrangement, a subject will respond on a lever or other operandum under a ratio schedule of reinforcement with a small response requirement for the first reward. The response requirement subsequently increases following each reward delivery until the subject ceases to respond for some pre-determined period of time. The largest response requirement completed defines the *break point* and this value serves as a primary dependent measure. As with all behavioral assays, parameters in the progressive ratio task (e.g., ratio step-size, break-point criteria, reinforcer magnitude) can influence outcomes and should be carefully selected and, preferably, accompanied with control studies using varied procedural parameters to increase interpretive confidence in the data's predictive relevance to constructs of motivation (Bradshaw & Killeen, 2012; Stafford & Branch, 1998). Caveats aside, the progressive ratio task has been used in numerous studies to examine how drugs modify response output for palatable food rewards (Higgins et al., 2021; Kangas et al., 2016; Slezak, Desai, & Katz, 2017) and to determine the relative reinforcing effectiveness for administration of drug rewards across diverse classes, including the exploration of $GABA_A$ receptor subtypes in the reinforcing effects of benzodiazepines (Berro & Rowlett, 2020), the mitigating factors of exercise in the abuse potential of speedballs (Lacy, Strickland, Brophy, Witte, & Smith, 2014), and sex differences in addiction-like behavioral phenotypes during cocaine withdrawal (Towers, Bakhti-Suroosh, & Lynch, 2021). In addition, progressive ratio tasks have been used to appraise candidate therapeutics in innovative ways. For example, atypical dopamine uptake inhibitors have been studied with respect to anergia in rat progressive ratio performance with an aim to develop novel treatments for motivational dysfunction (Rotolo et al., 2019). In addition, chronic treatment of bupropion-like dopamine reuptake inhibitors have been examined as candidate nicotine-replacement agents designed to aid in nicotine cessation via the reduction of progressive ratio break points in nicotine self-administration (Coen, Adamson, & Corrigall, 2009).

2.5.2 Economic demand

The ***economic demand task*** and associated quantitative metrics are designed to capture similar features of *motivation for reward* as those assayed under the progressive ratio task. However, in economic demand tasks, a given response requirement for reward is typically varied across sessions or, in within-session task variants, across fixed-time components. Motivation is quantified by examining the number of rewards earned under a variety of response requirement conditions using equations derived from behavioral economics. In its most popular iteration, Hursh and Silberberg (2008) promulgated the following exponential demand equation that has been employed by a considerable number of empirical investigations:

$$\log Q = \log Q_0 + k\left(e^{-aQ_0C} - 1\right)$$

where Q is quantity consumed, Q_0 is consumption as price approaches 0 (baseline consumption), k is a constant representing the range of consumption in log units, α is the rate of change in consumption as price goes up (elasticity), and C is cost (response requirement). In addition to avoiding certain shortcomings of the progressive ratio task, for example, response requirement sequence effects (Maguire, Minervini, Dodda, & France, 2020), this quantitative framework allows for interrogation of different aspects of motivation for reward. For example, the equation can distinguish between a subject's response output for reward when costs are near-zero (Q_0) and the extent to which a subject will defend its levels of reward consumption as costs increases (elasticity or α). Importantly, task and equation variants continue to be developed to better model economic demand data (Koffarnus, Franck, Stein, & Bickel, 2015). Nevertheless, a close conceptual correspondence already has been successfully demonstrated for this quantitative framework in research with laboratory animals and humans (Strickland & Lacy, 2020) to examine motivation to respond for, and associated reinforcing effectiveness of, a variety of commonly abused drugs, including cocaine (O'Connor, Aston-Jones, & James, 2021), ethanol (Kim & Kearns, 2019), fentanyl (McConnell et al., 2021), and nicotine (Powell, Beckmann, Marusich, & Gipson, 2020), to name just a few recent examples.

2.6 Impulsivity

Impulsivity as a construct has been well-associated with drug use and abuse (Jentsch et al., 2014; Perry & Carroll, 2008). A highly active and provocative debate continues as to whether individuals with substance use disorders are more impulsive than healthy controls (trait theory) or if drug exposure itself can decrease levels of self-control (state theory). Although the nuances of this debate are beyond the scope of the present chapter and are offered elsewhere (de Wit, 2009; Odum, 2011), there are several diverse tasks that can assist in contributing to this important topic. In addition to the tasks highlighted below, it should be noted that the discrimination reversal task (Section 2.2.1) and five-choice serial reaction time task (Section 2.4.2), which were described above in the context of their ability to probe cognitive flexibility and attention, respectively, are also highly relevant to impulsivity insomuch as deficits in response inhibition have been associated with indices of impulsive behavior and drug addiction (Izquierdo & Jentsch, 2012; Smith, Mattick, Jamadar, & Iredale, 2014).

2.6.1 Stop signal task

The ***stop signal task*** is another paradigm originally developed in the human laboratory (Logan & Cowan, 1984), subsequently used in the clinic to characterize impulse control disorders (Aron & Poldrack, 2005), and reverse-translated for rats (Eagle & Robbins, 2003) and monkeys (Liu, Heitz, & Bradberry, 2009) to yield effective coordinated and bi-directional cross-species methods in medications development (Robbins, 2017). The stop signal task, also known as the ***go/no-go task***, assays *motoric impulsivity* by measuring the amount of time to respond in the presence of a "go" stimulus or, alternatively, inhibit a response after it has been initiated (i.e., the ability to stop) following subsequent presentation of a "stop" stimulus. For example, a trial-initiating response is required first, followed by presentation of a "go" stimulus (e.g., a green light) after a variable delay. Responding quickly within a narrowly defined window of time (limited hold) results in reward. However, in a minority of trials, a "stop" stimulus (e.g., a tone) is presented after the "go" stimulus, which signals that inhibition of the prepotent response is required to obtain reward. Following sufficient training, a negative correlation is observed between the stop signal delay and performance accuracy, with a zero-delay producing high levels of response inhibition and longer delays producing lower stop accuracies. Impulsivity in this context is defined by a subject requiring extended training, relative to normative outcomes under the conditions arranged, to successfully inhibit responding following stop signals. Impulsivity is also associated with an increase in reaction time on trials following stop signal trials (i.e., post-stop trial slowing). In addition to the rich literature using this task to characterize the neurobiology of response inhibition (Bari & Robbins, 2013) and attention deficit disorders (Alderson, Rapport, & Kofler, 2007), other studies have used this task to examine drugs of abuse. For example, findings in monkeys with an extensive history of cocaine intake, but during forced-abstinence conditions, revealed longer stop signal reaction times and lower post-stop trial slowing (Liu et al., 2009). This impulsive phenotype is highly consistent with studies of impulsivity deficits in chronic cocaine users (Fillmore & Rush, 2002). Other studies using the stop signal task have documented that amphetamine and methylphenidate increase both premature responding and responses after the stop signal, whereas atomoxetine produced small performance enhancements on stop signal accuracy and reduced premature responding in rats (Maguire & France, 2019), consistent with its medicinal profile as an effective treatment for attention deficit disorders in humans.

2.6.2 Delay discounting

The ***delay discounting task*** is designed to assay another distinct aspect of impulsivity, namely, *impulsive choice*, and represents yet another task that includes tailored variants for both humans and laboratory animals to foster coordinated and bi-directional research aimed at understanding how psychoactive drugs, among numerous other variables, modulate this fundamental behavioral process (Madden & Bickel, 2010). This paradigm has in recent years generated substantial interest and numerous procedural variants. However, at its core, a delay discounting task assays the rate at which a given reward is devalued as a function of time, with the rate of decay serving as a primary dependent variable. This can be measured by arranging conditions that allow the subject to repeatedly choose between smaller magnitude rewards delivered sooner and larger magnitude rewards delivered later. Protocols that titrate the delay but hold reward magnitudes constant (Mazur, 1987) or titrate the reward magnitude but hold delays constant (Richards, Mitchell, de Wit, & Seiden, 1997) are aimed at defining *indifference points*, which can be compiled across a parametric space to derive a subject's discounting function. Discussions regarding how best to fit these functions, for example, exponential vs hyperbolic curves (Madden, Bickel, & Jacobs, 1999; McKerchar et al., 2009), provide important insights into the nature of the behavioral process. Notwithstanding these debates, subjects that reliably demonstrate preference for smaller-sooner rewards over larger-later rewards are deemed more impulsive relative to subjects that reliably choose larger-later rewards over smaller-sooner rewards and are deemed self-controlled (Ainslie, 1974). In the context of this chapter, two fundamental uses of this task are to better understand how drug exposure can modify discounting processes for other rewards and, as well, how drugs as the rewards themselves are discounted (Heyman, 2009; Lamb, Maguire, Ginsburg, Pinkston, & France, 2016; Setlow, Mendez, Mitchell, & Simon, 2009). Indeed, highly robust observations of steeper discounting functions have been associated with substance use disorders in humans across multiple drug classes (Bickel et al., 2020). In addition, delay discounting studies in laboratory animals have revealed functional similarities in heightened impulsivity metrics following exposure to alcohol (Poulos, Le, & Parker, 1995), cocaine (Perry, Nelson, & Carroll, 2008), D-amphetamine (Cardinal, Robbins, & Everitt, 2000), and nicotine (Dallery & Locey, 2005). Effects of opioid treatment on delay discounting tasks in rats, however, have produced mixed findings with some studies documenting the inability of chronic heroin intake to modulate discounting functions for a food reward (Harty, Whaley, Halperin, & Ranaldi, 2011). Whereas other studies have shown that morphine-dependent rats had increased measures of impulsivity for a food reward, relative to drug-free control subjects, that subsequently subsided following abstinence (Harvey-Lewis, Perdrizet, & Franklin, 2012). In nonhuman primates, both acute and daily morphine administration were associated with individual differences in their capacity to increase impulsive choice for a food reward (Maguire, Gerak, & France, 2016). It may be fruitful to consider viewing these inconsistencies and individual differences in sensitivity to the effects of opioids on delay discounting in the context of a potential preclinical indicator of vulnerability for drug abuse, given functional similarity to this phenomenon observed in humans (Madden, Petry, Badger, & Bickel, 1997).

3. Caveats and considerations

It is worth remembering that the enterprise of behavioral pharmacology was largely founded on systematic evaluations of drug effects on scheduled-controlled operant behavior (Dews, 1955; Kelleher & Morse, 1968). Although it is common to describe cognitive tasks as *complex*, each task highlighted in this chapter can be distilled to chained operant arrangements, with schedules of reinforcement serving as their backbone. As such, each link in the chain can itself have complex control over behavior. Indeed, even *simple* schedules of reinforcement are only simple insomuch as they are easy to describe; however, their effects on behavior and as determinants of drug action can nevertheless be exceedingly complex (Ferster & Skinner, 1957; McKearney & Barrett, 1978).

In addition, every psychoactive drug by its categorical nature will produce *non-specific* effects on behavior at some dose. Therefore, when examining drug action on these and other cognitive tasks, it is worthwhile to interrogate each link in the chain and attend carefully to how a drug *selectively* (or *non-selectively*) modifies each procedural variable that comprises the assay. An example from the repeated acquisition literature is instructive. For the reasons discussed in Section 2.1.1, one might arrange the conditions for a laboratory animal to learn new visual discriminations daily. Following stability in acquisition rate, if pre-session drug treatment dose-dependently increases the number of trials required to master a novel discrimination, an obvious conclusion is that the drug adversely affected learning processes. However, a skeptic might wonder whether the drug impaired the ability of the subject to learn something new *or* if the drug had non-specific behavioral effects that hindered the ability of the subject to engage in the task and demonstrate whether it was able to learn something new. This distinction is subtle but nonetheless crucial. One solution is to test this competing hypothesis by modifying the repeated acquisition task to include probe trials that are intermittently programmed throughout the daily session, for example, every 10 trials, in which the subject is presented with the same S^+/S^- stimuli they have a long and accurate history discriminating. Then, task performance during sessions following drug treatment can be juxtaposed using accuracies during probe trials with accuracies during trials using novel stimuli. If a drug adversely affects discriminative performance during trials with novel stimuli but not during probe trials, one may conclude the dose *selectively* impaired the subject's ability to *learn* a new discrimination but not necessarily its ability to discriminate. This particular approach already has been shown to successfully appraise selectivity in discrimination learning studies with MDMA, methamphetamine, and methylphenidate in rats (Galizio, McKinney, Cerutti, & Pitts, 2009) and cannabinoid agonists in monkeys (Kangas et al., 2016).

Another tactic to help elucidate selectivity in drug action on complex behavioral processes is to examine a drug under a *battery* of diverse cognitive tasks. As discussed in detail elsewhere (Bussey et al., 2008; Dumont et al., 2021; Kangas & Bergman, 2017), the flexibility inherent in touch-sensitive apparatus allows for the ability to expose laboratory animals to a variety of tasks, including all of those highlighted in the present chapter. However, whether using touchscreen-based or traditional operant conditioning chambers, examination of the same drugs at the same doses across diverse tasks allows for measurement of selectivity in a drug's ability to produce desirable or undesirable effects on various behavioral endpoints. The extent to which relevant drug doses impact certain task performances but not others provide critical verification of selective impact on some but not all behavioral outcomes, thereby affirming the drug is not simply decreasing the probability, rate, or accuracy of all responding. This approach also provides an important way to rank drugs designed for the same medicinal target.

4. On terms coda

Although discussing cognitive tasks in regard to their ability to assay so-called *cognitive function* may serve descriptive ends, it is nevertheless important to maintain focus on precision in operational definitions. And while it is linguistically convenient to have task types (nouns) to categorize task performance (verbs), one should not fall into the trap of confusing the contingencies arranged and dependent measures studied with their associated hypothetical constructs that should serve only as shorthand.

Perhaps the most cogent warning was offered 100 years ago in one of the first psychology textbooks:

> *Instead of "memory" we should say "remembering"; instead of "thought" we should say "thinking"; instead of "sensation" we should say "seeing, hearing," etc. But, like other learned branches, psychology is prone to transform its verbs into nouns. Then what happens? We forget that our nouns are merely substitutes for verbs, and go hunting for the* things *denoted by the nouns; but there are no such things, there are only the activities that we started with, seeing, remembering, and so on. Intelligence, consciousness, the unconscious, are by rights not nouns, nor even adjectives or verbs; they are adverbs. The real facts are that the individual acts intelligently—more or less so—acts consciously or unconsciously, as he may also act skillfully, persistently, excitedly. It is a safe rule, then, on encountering any menacing psychological noun, to strip off its linguistic mask, and see what manner of activity lies behind.*
> *Woodworth (1921, p. 5–6)*

Here, Woodworth presents the hazards of reification when discussing cognition and we encounter a thorny affair when studying behavior. Our constrained linguistic structure presents limitations in talking about process and activity. The structure of Western languages, including English, necessitates segmenting the world around us into categories of verbs that *require* their organization around nouns. These arbitrary segmentations that imply discrete, unidirectional actions across time, instead of ongoing, multiply determined *processes,* likely contribute to obfuscation of the dynamics of behavioral processes. To be sure, as behavioral pharmacology continues to progress, we will need categorical terms to help elucidate the complicated, multifaceted, and fluid nature of drug/behavior interactions. And some of those words will necessarily have to be nouns. It is commonplace and, under some circumstances, useful shorthand to specify drugs that might, for example, impair memory, improve attention, or foster cognitive flexibility. However, as this early comment by Woodworth emphasizes, a fastidious focus on *activity* will help avoid confusing our subject matter with the words we must use to describe it.

5. Conclusion

As the numerous and diverse tasks highlighted in this chapter show, empirically validated methods have been developed for laboratory animals that include tailored variants for the species, drug class, and experimental questions required to illuminate the many intricacies of drug action on complex behavioral processes. These tools have proven effective in advancing our understanding of both abused drugs and candidate therapeutics. Moreover, considerable value has been added via coordinated bi-directional translational research with functionally similar tasks in human subjects. These extant tasks, along with the continued development of innovative paradigms stemming from clinical observations and laboratory discoveries, will be needed to both minimize existing knowledge gaps regarding drug abuse sequela and improve pharmacotherapeutic treatment options for various medical conditions.

Acknowledgments

Preparation of this chapter was supported in part by R01-DA047575 from the National Institute on Drug Abuse.

Conflict of interest statement

The author has no conflicts of interest to declare.

References

Aguirre, C. G., Stolyarova, A., Das, K., Kolli, S., Marty, V., Ray, L., et al. (2020). Sex-dependent effects of chronic intermittent voluntary alcohol consumption on attentional, not motivational, measures during probabilistic learning and reversal. *PLoS One*, *15*, e0234729.

Ainslie, G. (1974). Impulse control in pigeons. *Journal of the Experimental Analysis of Behavior*, *21*, 485–489.

Alderson, R. M., Rapport, M. D., & Kofler, M. J. (2007). Attention-deficit/hyperactivity disorder and behavioral inhibition: A meta-analytic review of the stop-signal paradigm. *Journal of Abnormal Child Psychology*, *35*, 745–758.

Anderson, J. H., & Lindsley, D. B. (1944). *Radar operator fatigue: The effects of length and repetition of operating periods on efficiency of performance*. Office of Scientific Research and Development Report No. O. S. R. D. 33334.

Aron, A. R., & Poldrack, R. A. (2005). The cognitive neuroscience of response inhibition: Relevance for genetic research in attention-deficit/hyperactivity disorder. *Biological Psychiatry*, *57*, 1285–1292.

Ator, N. A. (2005). Contributions of GABAA receptor subtype selectivity to abuse liability and dependence potential of pharmacological treatments for anxiety and sleep disorders. *CNS Spectrums*, *10*, 31–39.

Ator, N. A., & Griffiths, R. R. (2003). Principles of drug abuse liability assessment in laboratory animals. *Drug and Alcohol Dependence*, *70*, S55–S72.

Bari, A., & Robbins, T. W. (2013). Inhibition and impulsivity: Behavioral and neural basis of response control. *Progress in Neurobiology*, *108*, 44–79.

Bari, A., Theobald, D. E., Caprioli, D., Mar, A. C., Aidoo-Micah, A., Dalley, J. W., et al. (2010). Serotonin modulates sensitivity to reward and negative feedback in a probabilistic reversal learning task in rats. *Neuropsychopharmacology*, *35*, 1290–1301.

Berro, L. F., & Rowlett, J. K. (2020). GABAA receptor subtypes and the reinforcing effects of benzodiazepines in remifentanil-experienced rhesus monkeys. *Drug and Alcohol Dependence*, *213*, 108076.

Bickel, W. K., Athamneh, L. N., Snider, S. E., Craft, W. H., DeHart, W. B., Kaplan, B. A., et al. (2020). Reinforcer pathology: Implications for substance abuse intervention. *Current Topics in Behavioral Neurosciences*, *47*, 139–162.

Bizarro, L., Patel, S., Murtagh, C., & Stolerman, I. P. (2004). Differential effects of psychomotor stimulants on attentional performance in rats: Nicotine, amphetamine, caffeine and methylphenidate. *Behavioural Pharmacology*, *15*, 195–206.

Blough, D. S. (1959). Delayed matching in the pigeon. *Journal of the Experimental Analysis of Behavior*, *2*, 151–160.

Bradshaw, C. M., & Killeen, P. R. (2012). A theory of behaviour on progressive ratio schedules, with applications in behavioural pharmacology. *Psychopharmacology*, *222*, 549–564.

Branch, M. N., & Dearing, M. E. (1982). Effects of acute and daily cocaine administration on performance under a delayed-matching-to-sample procedure. *Pharmacology, Biochemistry, and Behavior*, *16*, 713–718.

Branch, M. N., Dearing, M. E., & Lee, D. M. (1980). Acute and chronic effects of delta 9-tetrahydrocannabinol on complex behavior of squirrel monkeys. *Psychopharmacology*, *71*, 247–256.

Buccafusco, J. J., Letchworth, S. R., Bencherif, M., & Lippiello, P. M. (2005). Long-lasting cognitive improvement with nicotinic receptor agonists: Mechanisms of pharmacokinetic-pharmacodynamic discordance. *Trends in Pharmacological Sciences*, *26*, 352–360.

Bussey, T. J., Padain, T. L., Skillings, E. A., Winters, B. D., Morton, A. J., & Saksida, L. M. (2008). The touchscreen cognitive testing method for rodents: How to get the best out of your rat. *Learning & Memory*, *15*, 516–523.

Cardinal, R. N., Robbins, T. W., & Everitt, B. J. (2000). The effects of d-amphetamine, chlordiazepoxide, alpha-flupenthixol and behavioural manipulations on choice of signalled and unsignalled delayed reinforcement in rats. *Psychopharmacology*, *152*, 362–375.

Carli, M., Robbins, T. W., Evenden, J. L., & Everitt, B. J. (1983). Effects of lesions to ascending noradrenergic neurones on performance of a 5-choice serial reaction task in rats; implications for theories of dorsal noradrenergic bundle function based on selective attention and arousal. *Behavioural Brain Research*, *9*, 361–380.

Chang, L., Cloak, C., Patterson, K., Grob, C., Miller, E. N., & Ernst, T. (2005). Enlarged striatum in abstinent methamphetamine abusers: A possible compensatory response. *Biological Psychiatry*, *57*, 967–974.

Coen, K. M., Adamson, K. L., & Corrigall, W. A. (2009). Medication-related pharmacological manipulations of nicotine self-administration in the rat maintained on fixed- and progressive-ratio schedules of reinforcement. *Psychopharmacology*, *201*, 557–568.

Cole, B. J., & Robbins, T. W. (1987). Amphetamine impairs the discriminative performance of rats with dorsal noradrenergic bundle lesions on a 5-choice serial reaction time task: New evidence for central dopaminergic-noradrenergic interactions. *Psychopharmacology*, *91*, 458–466.

Costa, V. D., Tran, V. L., Turchi, J., & Averbeck, B. B. (2015). Reversal learning and dopamine: A bayesian perspective. *Journal of Neuroscience*, *35*, 2407–2416.

Coyle, C. M., & Laws, K. R. (2015). The use of ketamine as an antidepressant: A systematic review and meta-analysis. *Human Psychopharmacology: Clinical and Experimental*, *30*, 152–163.

Cumming, W. W., & Berryman, R. (1965). The complex discriminated operant: Studies of matching-to-sample and related problems. In D. I. Mostofsky (Ed.), *Stimulus generalization* (pp. 284–330). Stanford, CA: Stanford University Press.

Dallery, J., & Locey, M. L. (2005). Effects of acute and chronic nicotine on impulsive choice in rats. *Behavioural Pharmacology*, *16*, 15–23.

Dalley, J. W., Lääne, K., Pena, Y., Theobald, D. E., Everitt, B. J., & Robbins, T. W. (2005). Attentional and motivational deficits in rats withdrawn from intravenous self-administration of cocaine or heroin. *Psychopharmacology*, *182*, 579–587.

Davis, C. M., Roma, P. G., & Hienz, R. D. (2016). A rodent model of the human psychomotor vigilance test: Performance comparisons. *Journal of Neuroscience Methods, 259*, 57–71.

de Wit, H. (2009). Impulsivity as a determinant and consequence of drug use: A review of underlying processes. *Addiction Biology, 14*, 22–31.

Delatte, M. S., Winsauer, P. J., & Moerschbaecher, J. M. (2002). Tolerance to the disruptive effects of Delta(9)-THC on learning in rats. *Pharmacology, Biochemistry, and Behavior, 74*, 129–140.

Der-Avakian, A., D'Souza, M. S., Potter, D. N., Chartoff, E. H., Carlezon, W. A., Pizzagalli, D. A., et al. (2017). Social defeat disrupts reward learning and potentiates striatal nociceptin/orphanin FQ mRNA in rats. *Psychopharmacology, 234*, 1603–1614.

Der-Avakian, A., D'Souza, M. S., Pizzagalli, D. A., & Markou, A. (2013). Assessment of reward responsiveness in the response bias probabilistic reward task in rats: Implications for cross-species translational research. *Translational Psychiatry, 3*, e297.

Deurveilher, S., Bush, J. E., Rusak, B., Eskes, G. A., & Semba, K. (2015). Psychomotor vigilance task performance during and following chronic sleep restriction in rats. *Sleep, 38*, 515–528.

Dews, P. B. (1955). Studies on behavior. I. Differential sensitivity to pentobarbital of pecking performance in pigeons depending on the schedule of reward. *Journal of Pharmacology and Experimental Therapeutics, 138*, 393–401.

Di Marzo, V. (2018). New approaches and challenges to targeting the endocannabinoid system. *Nature Reviews. Drug Discovery, 17*, 623–639.

Dinges, D. F., Pack, F., Williams, K., Gillen, K. A., Powell, J. W., Ott, G. E., et al. (1997). Cumulative sleepiness, mood disturbance, and psychomotor vigilance performance decrements during a week of sleep restricted to 4-5 hours per night. *Sleep, 20*, 267–277.

Drozd, R., Rychlik, M., Fijalkowska, A., & Rygula, R. (2019). Effects of cognitive judgement bias and acute antidepressant treatment on sensitivity to feedback and cognitive flexibility in the rat version of the probabilistic reversal-learning test. *Behavioural Brain Research, 359*, 619–629.

Dumont, J. R., Salewski, R., & Beraldo, F. (2021). Critical mass: The rise of a touchscreen technology community for rodent cognitive testing. *Genes, Brain, and Behavior, 20*, e12650.

Dunnett, S. B. (1985). Comparative effects of cholinergic drugs and lesions of nucleus basalis or fimbria-fornix on delayed matching in rats. *Psychopharmacology, 87*, 357–363.

Eagle, D. M., & Robbins, T. W. (2003). Inhibitory control in rats performing a stop-signal reaction-time task: Effects of lesions of the medial striatum and d-amphetamine. *Behavioral Neuroscience, 117*, 1302–1317.

Elrod, K., Buccafusco, J. J., & Jackson, W. J. (1988). Nicotine enhances delayed matching-to-sample performance by primates. *Life Sciences, 43*, 277–287.

Evans, E. B., & Wenger, G. R. (1992). Effects of drugs of abuse on acquisition of behavioral chains in squirrel monkeys. *Psychopharmacology, 107*, 55–60.

Evenden, J. L., Turpin, M., Oliver, L., & Jennings, C. (1993). Caffeine and nicotine improve visual tracking by rats: A comparison with amphetamine, cocaine and apomorphine. *Psychopharmacology, 110*, 169–176.

Fellows, L. K., & Farah, M. J. (2003). Ventromedial frontal cortex mediates affective shifting in humans: Evidence from a reversal learning paradigm. *Brain, 126*, 1830–1837.

Ferster, C. B., & Skinner, B. F. (1957). *Schedules of reinforcement*. East Norwalk, CT, US: Appleton-Century-Crofts.

Fillmore, M. T., & Rush, C. R. (2002). Impaired inhibitory control of behavior in chronic cocaine users. *Drug and Alcohol Dependence, 66*, 265–273.

Galizio, M., McKinney, P., Cerutti, D. T., & Pitts, R. C. (2009). Effects of MDMA, methamphetamine and methylphenidate on repeated acquisition and performance in rats. *Pharmacology, Biochemistry, and Behavior, 94*, 305–311.

Gentile, T. A., Simmons, S. J., Watson, M. N., Connelly, K. L., Brailoiu, E., Zhang, Y., et al. (2018). Effects of suvorexant, a dual orexin/hypocretin receptor antagonist, on impulsive behavior associated with cocaine. *Neuropsychopharmacology*, *43*, 1001–1009.

Goonawardena, A. V., Morairty, S. R., Dell, R., Orellana, G. A., Hoener, M. C., Wallace, T. L., et al. (2019). Trace amine-associated receptor 1 agonism promotes wakefulness without impairment of cognition in Cynomolgus macaques. *Neuropsychopharmacology*, *44*, 1485–1493.

Groman, S. M., Hillmer, A. T., Liu, H., Fowles, K., Holden, D., Morris, E. D., et al. (2020). Dysregulation of decision making related to metabotropic glutamate 5, but not midbrain D3, receptor availability following cocaine self-administration in rats. *Biological Psychiatry*, *88*, 777–787.

Groman, S. M., Lee, B., Seu, E., James, A. S., Feiler, K., Mandelkern, M. A., et al. (2012). Dysregulation of D_2-mediated dopamine transmission in monkeys after chronic escalating methamphetamine exposure. *Journal of Neuroscience*, *32*, 5843–5852.

Groman, S. M., Morales, A. M., Lee, B., London, E. D., & Jentsch, J. D. (2013). Methamphetamine-induced increases in putamen gray matter associate with inhibitory control. *Psychopharmacology*, *229*, 527–538.

Groman, S. M., Rich, K. M., Smith, N. J., Lee, D., & Taylor, J. R. (2018). Chronic exposure to methamphetamine disrupts reinforcement-based decision making in rats. *Neuropsychopharmacology*, *43*, 770–780.

Grottick, A. J., & Higgins, G. A. (2002). Assessing a vigilance decrement in aged rats: Effects of pre-feeding, task manipulation, and psychostimulants. *Psychopharmacology*, *164*, 33–41.

Hamilton, G. V. (1911). A study of trial and error reactions in mammals. *Journal of Animal Behavior*, *1*, 33–66.

Harlow, H. F. (1949). The formation of learning sets. *Psychological Review*, *56*, 51–65.

Harper, D. N. (2013). Attenuation of the disruptive effects of (+/−)3,4-methylenedioxymethamphetamine and cocaine on delayed matching-to-sample performance with D1 versus D2 antagonists. *Addiction Biology*, *18*, 912–920.

Harper, D. N., Wisnewski, R., Hunt, M., & Schenk, S. (2005). (+/−)3,4-methylenedioxymethamphetamine, d-amphetamine, and cocaine impair delayed matching-to-sample performance by an increase in susceptibility to proactive interference. *Behavioral Neuroscience*, *119*, 455–463.

Harty, S. C., Whaley, J. E., Halperin, J. M., & Ranaldi, R. (2011). Impulsive choice, as measured in a delay discounting paradigm, remains stable after chronic heroin administration. *Pharmacology, Biochemistry, and Behavior*, *98*, 337–340.

Harvey-Lewis, C., Perdrizet, J., & Franklin, K. B. (2012). The effect of morphine dependence on impulsive choice in rats. *Psychopharmacology*, *223*, 477–487.

Hasler, G., Drevets, W. C., Gould, T. D., Gottesman, I. I., & Manji, H. K. (2006). Toward constructing an endophenotype strategy for bipolar disorders. *Biological Psychiatry*, *60*, 93–105.

Heyman, G. M. (2009). *Addiction: A disorder of choice*. Cambridge, MA: Harvard University Press.

Higgins, G. A., Carroll, N. K., Brown, M., MacMillan, C., Silenieks, L. B., Thevarkunnel, S., et al. (2021). Low doses of psilocybin and ketamine enhance motivation and attention in poor performing rats: Evidence for an antidepressant property. *Frontiers in Pharmacology*, *12*, 640241.

Hodos, W. (1961). Progressive ratio as a measure of reward strength. *Science*, *134*, 943–944.

Horan, W. P., Kring, A. M., & Blanchard, J. J. (2006). Anhedonia in schizophrenia: A review of assessment strategies. *Schizophrenia Bulletin*, *32*, 259–273.

Hursh, S. R., & Silberberg, A. (2008). Economic demand and essential value. *Psychological Review*, *115*, 186–198.

Izquierdo, A., & Jentsch, J. D. (2012). Reversal learning as a measure of impulsive and compulsive behavior in addictions. *Psychopharmacology, 219*, 607–620.
Jackson, A., Silk, S., Buhidma, Y., & Shoaib, M. (2017). Varenicline, the clinically effective smoking cessation agent, restores probabilistic response reversal performance during withdrawal from nicotine. *Addiction Biology, 22*, 1316–1328.
Jaffe, R. J., Novakovic, V., & Peselow, E. D. (2013). Scopolamine as an antidepressant: A systematic review. *Clinical Neuropharmacology, 36*, 24–26.
Jedema, H. P., Song, X., Aizenstein, H. J., Bonner, A. R., Stein, E. A., Yang, Y., et al. (2021). Long-term cocaine self-administration produces structural brain changes that correlate with altered cognition. *Biological Psychiatry, 89*, 376–385.
Jentsch, J. D., Ashenhurst, J. R., Cervantes, M. C., Groman, S. M., James, A. S., & Pennington, Z. T. (2014). Dissecting impulsivity and its relationships to drug addictions. *Annals of the New York Academy of Sciences, 1327*, 1–26.
Jones, D. N., & Higgins, G. A. (1995). Effect of scopolamine on visual attention in rats. *Psychopharmacology, 120*, 142–149.
Justinova, Z., Mascia, P., Wu, H. Q., Secci, M. E., Redhi, G. H., Panlilio, L. V., et al. (2013). Reducing cannabinoid abuse and preventing relapse by enhancing endogenous brain levels of kynurenic acid. *Nature Neuroscience, 16*, 1652–1661.
Kanen, J. W., Ersche, K. D., Fineberg, N. A., Robbins, T. W., & Cardinal, R. N. (2019). Computational modelling reveals contrasting effects on reinforcement learning and cognitive flexibility in stimulant use disorder and obsessive-compulsive disorder: Remediating effects of dopaminergic D2/3 receptor agents. *Psychopharmacology, 236*, 2337–2358.
Kangas, B. D., & Bergman, J. (2012). A novel touch-sensitive apparatus for behavioral studies in unrestrained squirrel monkeys. *Journal of Neuroscience Methods, 209*, 331–336.
Kangas, B. D., & Bergman, J. (2014). Repeated acquisition and discrimination reversal in the squirrel monkey (Saimiri sciureus). *Animal Cognition, 17*, 221–228.
Kangas, B. D., & Bergman, J. (2016). Effects of self-administered methamphetamine on discrimination learning and reversal in nonhuman primates. *Psychopharmacology, 233*, 373–380.
Kangas, B. D., & Bergman, J. (2017). Touchscreen technology in the study of cognition-related behavior. *Behavioural Pharmacology, 28*, 623–629.
Kangas, B. D., Berry, M. S., & Branch, M. N. (2011). On the development and mechanics of delayed matching-to-sample performance. *Journal of the Experimental Analysis of Behavior, 95*, 221–236.
Kangas, B. D., & Branch, M. N. (2012). Effects of acute and chronic cocaine administration on titrating-delay matching-to-sample performance. *Journal of the Experimental Analysis of Behavior, 97*, 151–161.
Kangas, B. D., Doyle, R. J., Kohut, S. J., Bergman, J., & Kaufman, M. J. (2019). Effects of chronic cocaine self-administration and N-acetylcysteine on learning, cognitive flexibility, and reinstatement in nonhuman primates. *Psychopharmacology, 236*, 2143–2153.
Kangas, B. D., Leonard, M. Z., Shukla, V. G., Alapafuja, S. O., Nikas, S. P., Makriyannis, A., et al. (2016). Comparisons of Δ9-tetrahydrocannabinol and anandamide on a battery of cognition-related behavior in nonhuman primates. *Journal of Pharmacology and Experimental Therapeutics, 357*, 125–133.
Kangas, B. D., Vaidya, M., & Branch, M. N. (2010). Titrating-delay matching-to-sample in the pigeon. *Journal of the Experimental Analysis of Behavior, 94*, 69–81.
Kangas, B. D., Wooldridge, L. M., Luc, O. T., Bergman, J., & Pizzagalli, D. A. (2020). Empirical validation of a touchscreen probabilistic reward task in rats. *Translational Psychiatry, 10*, 285.

Kelleher, R. T., & Morse, W. H. (1968). Determinants of the specificity of behavioral effects of drugs. *Ergebnisse der Physiologie Biologischen Chemieund Experinmentellen Pharmakologie*, *60*, 1–56.

Kibaly, C., Alderete, J. A., Liu, S. H., Nasef, H. S., Law, P. Y., Evans, C. J., et al. (2021). Oxycodone in the opioid epidemic: High 'liking', 'wanting', and abuse liability. *Cellular and Molecular Neurobiology*, *41*, 899–926.

Kim, J. S., & Kearns, D. N. (2019). Reduced ethanol self-administration in rats produced by the introduction of a high value non-drug alternative reinforcer. *Pharmacology, Biochemistry, and Behavior*, *184*, 172744.

Koffarnus, M. N., Franck, C. T., Stein, J. S., & Bickel, W. K. (2015). A modified exponential behavioral economic demand model to better describe consumption data. *Experimental and Clinical Psychopharmacology*, *23*, 504–512.

Lacy, R. T., Strickland, J. C., Brophy, M. K., Witte, M. A., & Smith, M. A. (2014). Exercise decreases speedball self-administration. *Life Sciences*, *114*, 86–92.

Lamb, R. J., Maguire, D. R., Ginsburg, B. C., Pinkston, J. W., & France, C. P. (2016). Determinants of choice, and vulnerability and recovery in addiction. *Behavioural Processes*, *127*, 35–42.

Lamontagne, S. J., Melendez, S. I., & Olmstead, M. C. (2018). Investigating dopamine and glucocorticoid systems as underlying mechanisms of anhedonia. *Psychopharmacology*, *235*, 3103–3113.

Lawrence, A. D., Sahakian, B. J., Rogers, R. D., Hodge, J. R., & Robbins, T. W. (1999). Discrimination, reversal, and shift learning in Huntington's disease: Mechanisms of impaired response selection. *Neuropsychologia*, *37*, 1359–1374.

LeSage, M., Clark, R., & Poling, A. (1993). MDMA and memory: The acute and chronic effects of MDMA in pigeons performing under a delayed-matching-to-sample procedure. *Psychopharmacology*, *110*, 327–332.

Levin, E. D. (1988). Psychopharmacological effects in the radial-arm maze. *Neuroscience and Biobehavioral Reviews*, *12*, 169–175.

Levin, E. D., & Bowman, R. E. (1986). Scopolamine effects on Hamilton search task performance in monkeys. *Pharmacology, Biochemistry, and Behavior*, *24*, 819–821.

Liu, S., Heitz, R. P., & Bradberry, C. W. (2009). A touch screen based stop signal response task in rhesus monkeys for studying impulsivity associated with chronic cocaine self-administration. *Journal of Neuroscience Methods*, *177*, 67–72.

Logan, G. D., & Cowan, W. B. (1984). On the ability to inhibit thought and action: A theory of an act of control. *Psychological Review*, *91*, 295–327.

London, E. D., Kohno, M., Morales, A. M., & Ballard, M. E. (2015). Chronic methamphetamine abuse and corticostriatal deficits revealed by neuroimaging. *Brain Research*, *1628*, 174–185.

Luc, O. T., Pizzagalli, D. A., & Kangas, B. D. (2021). Toward a quantification of anhedonia: Unified matching law and signal detection for clinical assessment and drug development. *Perspectives on Behavior Science*. Advance online publication https://doi.org/10.1007/s40614-021-00288-w.

Macaskill, A. C., Harrow, C. C., & Harper, D. N. (2015). The disruptive effects of methamphetamine on delayed-matching-to-sample performance reflect proactive interference and are reduced by SCH23390. *Pharmacology, Biochemistry, and Behavior*, *128*, 62–67.

Mackworth, N. H. (1948). The breakdown of vigilance during prolonged visual search. *Quarterly Journal of Experimental Psychology*, *1*, 6–21.

Madden, G. J., & Bickel, W. K. (2010). *Impulsivity: The behavioral and neurological science of discounting*. Washington, DC: American Psychological Association.

Madden, G. J., Bickel, W. K., & Jacobs, E. A. (1999). Discounting of delayed rewards in opioid-dependent outpatients: Exponential or hyperbolic discounting functions? *Experimental and Clinical Psychopharmacology*, 7, 284–293.

Madden, G. J., Petry, N. M., Badger, G. J., & Bickel, W. K. (1997). Impulsive and self-control choices in opioid-dependent patients and non-drug-using control participants: Drug and monetary rewards. *Experimental and Clinical Psychopharmacology, 5*, 256–262.

Maguire, D. R., & France, C. P. (2019). Effects of amphetamine, methylphenidate, atomoxetine, and morphine in rats responding under an adjusting stop signal reaction time task. *Psychopharmacology, 236*, 1959–1972.

Maguire, D. R., Gerak, L. R., & France, C. P. (2016). Effect of daily morphine administration and its discontinuation on delay discounting of food in rhesus monkeys. *Behavioural Pharmacology, 27*, 155–164.

Maguire, D. R., Henson, C., & France, C. P. (2016). Daily morphine administration increases impulsivity in rats responding under a 5-choice serial reaction time task. *British Journal of Pharmacology, 173*, 1350–1362.

Maguire, D. R., Minervini, V., Dodda, V., & France, C. P. (2020). Impact of order of fixed-ratio presentation on demand for self-administered remifentanil in male rats. *Behavioural Pharmacology, 31*, 216–220.

Markou, A., Kosten, T. R., & Koob, G. F. (1998). Neurobiological similarities in depression and drug dependence: A self-medication hypothesis. *Neuropsychopharmacology, 18*, 135–174.

Mazur, J. E. (1987). An adjusting procedure for studying delayed reinforcement. In M. L. Commons, J. E. Mazur, J. A. Nevin, & H. Rachlin (Eds.), *The effect of delay and of intervening events of reinforcement value: Vol. 5. Quantitative analysis of behavior* (pp. 55–73). Hillsdale, NJ: Erlbaum.

McCarthy, D., & Davison, M. (1979). Signal probability, reinforcement, and signal detection. *Journal of the Experimental Analysis of Behavior, 32*, 373–382.

McCarthy, A., Loomis, S., Eastwood, B., Wafford, K. A., Winsky-Sommerer, R., & Gilmour, G. (2017). Modelling maintenance of wakefulness in rats: Comparing potential non-invasive sleep-restriction methods and their effects on sleep and attentional performance. *Journal of Sleep Research, 26*, 179–187.

McConnell, S. A., Brandner, A. J., Blank, B. A., Kearns, D. N., Koob, G. F., Vendruscolo, L. F., et al. (2021). Demand for fentanyl becomes inelastic following extended access to fentanyl vapor self-administration. *Neuropharmacology, 182*, 108355.

McIntyre, R. S., Lee, Y., Zhou, A. J., Rosenblat, J. D., Peters, E. M., Lam, R. W., et al. (2017). The efficacy of psychostimulants in major depressive episodes: A systematic review and meta-analysis. *Journal of Clinical Psychopharmacology, 37*, 412–418.

McKearney, J. W., & Barrett, J. E. (1978). Schedule-controlled behavior and the effects of drugs. In D. E. Blackman, & D. J. Sanger (Eds.), *Contemporary research in behavioral pharmacology* (pp. 1–68). New York: Plenum Press.

McKerchar, T. L., Green, L., Myerson, J., Pickford, T. S., Hill, J. C., & Stout, S. C. (2009). A comparison of four models of delay discounting in humans. *Behavioural Processes, 81*, 256–259.

Mello, N. K. (1971). Alcohol effects on delayed matching to sample performance by rhesus monkey. *Physiology & Behavior, 7*, 77–101.

Minervini, V., Disney, A., Husbands, S. M., & France, C. P. (2020). Methocinnamox (MCAM) antagonizes the behavioral suppressant effects of morphine without impairing delayed matching-to-sample accuracy in rhesus monkeys. *Psychopharmacology, 237*, 3057–3065.

Moerschbaecher, J. M., Thompson, D. M., & Winsauer, P. J. (1983). Effects of heroin, methadone, LAAM and cyclazocine on acquisition and performance of response sequences in monkeys. *Pharmacology, Biochemistry, and Behavior, 19*, 701–710.

Mukherjee, D., Filipowicz, A., Vo, K., Satterthwaite, T. D., & Kable, J. W. (2020). Reward and punishment reversal-learning in major depressive disorder. *Journal of Abnormal Psychology, 129*, 810–823.

Nawijn, L., van Zuiden, M., Frijling, J. L., Koch, S. B., Veltman, D. J., & Olff, M. (2015). Reward functioning in PTSD: A systematic review exploring the mechanisms underlying anhedonia. *Neuroscience & Biobehavioral Reviews, 51*, 189–204.

O'Connor, S. L., Aston-Jones, G., & James, M. H. (2021). The sensation-seeking trait confers a dormant susceptibility to addiction that is revealed by intermittent cocaine self-administration in rats. *Neuropharmacology, 195*, 108566.

Odum, A. L. (2011). Delay discounting: I'm a k, you're a k. *Journal of the Experimental Analysis of Behavior, 96*, 427–439.

Owen, A. M., Downes, J. J., Sahakian, B. J., Polkey, C. E., & Robbins, T. W. (1990). Planning and spatial working memory following frontal lobe lesions in man. *Neuropsychologia, 28*, 1021–1034.

Pattij, T., Schetters, D., Janssen, M. C., Wiskerke, J., & Schoffelmeer, A. N. (2009). Acute effects of morphine on distinct forms of impulsive behavior in rats. *Psychopharmacology, 205*, 489–502.

Perry, J. L., & Carroll, M. E. (2008). The role of impulsive behavior in drug abuse. *Psychopharmacology, 200*, 1–26.

Perry, J. L., Nelson, S. E., & Carroll, M. E. (2008). Impulsive choice as a predictor of acquisition of IV cocaine self- administration and reinstatement of cocaine-seeking behavior in male and female rats. *Experimental and Clinical Psychopharmacology, 16*, 165–177.

Pizzagalli, D. A., Evins, A. E., Schetter, E. C., Frank, M. J., Pajtas, P. E., Santesso, D. L., et al. (2008). Single dose of a dopamine agonist impairs reinforcement learning in humans: Behavioral evidence from a laboratory-based measure of reward responsiveness. *Psychopharmacology, 196*, 221–232.

Pizzagalli, D. A., Jahn, A. L., & O'Shea, J. P. (2005). Toward an objective characterization of an anhedonic phenotype: A signal-detection approach. *Biological Psychiatry, 57*, 319–327.

Poulos, C. X., Le, A. D., & Parker, J. L. (1995). Impulsivity predicts individual susceptibility to high levels of alcohol self-administration. *Behavioural Pharmacology, 6*, 810–814.

Powell, G. L., Beckmann, J. S., Marusich, J. A., & Gipson, C. D. (2020). Nicotine reduction does not alter essential value of nicotine or reduce cue-induced reinstatement of nicotine seeking. *Drug and Alcohol Dependence, 212*, 108020.

Rasmussen, N. (2011). Medical science and the military: The Allies' use of amphetamine during world war II. *Journal of Interdisciplinary History, 42*, 205–233.

Richards, J. B., Mitchell, S. H., de Wit, H., & Seiden, L. S. (1997). Determination of discount functions in rats with an adjusting-amount procedure. *Journal of the Experimental Analysis of Behavior, 67*, 353–366.

Robbins, T. W. (2002). The 5-choice serial reaction time task: Behavioural pharmacology and functional neurochemistry. *Psychopharmacology, 163*, 362–380.

Robbins, T. W. (2017). Cross-species studies of cognition relevant to drug discovery: A translational approach. *British Journal of Pharmacology, 174*, 3191–3199.

Roberts, B. Z., Young, J. W., He, Y. V., Cope, Z. A., Shilling, P. D., & Feifel, D. (2019). Oxytocin improves probabilistic reversal learning but not effortful motivation in Brown Norway rats. *Neuropharmacology, 150*, 15–26.

Romach, M. K., Schoedel, K. A., & Sellers, E. M. (2014). Human abuse liability evaluation of CNS stimulant drugs. *Neuropharmacology, 87*, 81–90.

Rotolo, R. A., Dragacevic, V., Kalaba, P., Urban, E., Zehl, M., Roller, A., et al. (2019). The novel atypical dopamine uptake inhibitor (S)-CE-123 partially reverses the effort-related effects of the dopamine depleting agent tetrabenazine and increases progressive ratio responding. *Frontiers in Pharmacology, 10*, 682.

Rychlik, M., Bollen, E., & Rygula, R. (2017). Ketamine decreases sensitivity of male rats to misleading negative feedback in a probabilistic reversal-learning task. *Psychopharmacology, 234*, 613–620.

Setlow, B., Mendez, I. A., Mitchell, M. R., & Simon, N. W. (2009). Effects of chronic administration of drugs of abuse on impulsive choice (delay discounting) in animal models. *Behavioural Pharmacology, 20*, 380–389.

Shannon, H. E., & Eberle, E. L. (2006). Effects of biasing the location of stimulus presentation, and the muscarinic cholinergic receptor antagonist scopolamine, on performance of a 5-choice serial reaction time attention task in rats. *Behavioural Pharmacology, 17*, 71–85.

Silber, B. Y., Croft, R. J., Papafotiou, K., & Stough, C. (2006). The acute effects of d-amphetamine and methamphetamine on attention and psychomotor performance. *Psychopharmacology, 187*, 154–169.

Slezak, J. M., Desai, R. I., & Katz, J. L. (2017). Further delineation between typical and atypical dopamine uptake inhibitors: Effects on food-maintained behavior and food consumption. *Behavioural Pharmacology, 28*, 74–82.

Smith, J. L., Mattick, R. P., Jamadar, S. D., & Iredale, J. M. (2014). Deficits in behavioural inhibition in substance abuse and addiction: A meta-analysis. *Drug and Alcohol Dependence, 145*, 1–33.

Soto, P. L., Dallery, J., Ator, N. A., & Katz, B. R. (2013). A critical examination of best dose analysis for determining cognitive-enhancing potential of drugs: Studies with rhesus monkeys and computer simulations. *Psychopharmacology, 228*, 611–622.

Stafford, D., & Branch, M. N. (1998). Effects of step size and break-point criterion on progressive-ratio performance. *Journal of the Experimental Analysis of Behavior, 70*, 123–138.

Stolerman, I. P., Mirza, N. R., Hahn, B., & Shoaib, M. (2000). Nicotine in an animal model of attention. *European Journal of Pharmacology, 393*, 147–154.

Strickland, J. C., & Lacy, R. T. (2020). Behavioral economic demand as a unifying language for addiction science: Promoting collaboration and integration of animal and human models. *Experimental and Clinical Psychopharmacology, 28*, 404–416.

Taffe, M. A., Davis, S. A., Gutierrez, T., & Gold, L. H. (2002). Ketamine impairs multiple cognitive domains in rhesus monkeys. *Drug and Alcohol Dependence, 68*, 175–187.

Taffe, M. A., Davis, S. A., Yuan, J., Schroeder, R., Hatzidimitriou, G., Parsons, L. H., et al. (2002). Cognitive performance of MDMA-treated rhesus monkeys: Sensitivity to serotonergic challenge. *Neuropsychopharmacology, 27*, 993–1005.

Taffe, M. A., Weed, M. R., & Gold, L. H. (1999). Scopolamine alters rhesus monkey performance on a novel neuropsychological test battery. *Cognitive Brain Research, 8*, 203–212.

Thompson, D. M. (1973). Repeated acquisition as a behavioral base line for studying drug effects. *Journal of Pharmacology and Experimental Therapeutics, 184*, 506–514.

Thompson, D. M., & Winsauer, P. J. (1985). Delta-9-tetrahydrocannabinol potentiates the disruptive effects of phencyclidine on repeated acquisition in monkeys. *Pharmacology, Biochemistry, and Behavior, 23*, 1051–1057.

Towers, E. B., Bakhti-Suroosh, A., & Lynch, W. J. (2021). Females develop features of an addiction-like phenotype sooner during withdrawal than males. *Psychopharmacology, 238*, 2213–2224.

Von Huben, S. N., Davis, S. A., Lay, C. C., Katner, S. N., Crean, R. D., & Taffe, M. A. (2006). Differential contributions of dopaminergic D1- and D2-like receptors to cognitive function in rhesus monkeys. *Psychopharmacology, 188*, 586–596.

Vrieze, E., Pizzagalli, D. A., Demyttenaere, K., Hompes, T., Sienaert, P., de Boer, P., et al. (2013). Reduced reward learning predicts outcome in major depressive disorder. *Biological Psychiatry, 73*, 639–645.

Warren, J. M. (1965). Primate learning in comparative perspective. In A. M. Schrier, H. F. Harlow, & F. Stollnitz (Eds.), *Vol. 1. Behavior of nonhuman primates* (pp. 249–281). New York: Academic.

Weed, M. R., Gold, L. H., Polis, I., Koob, G. F., Fox, H. S., & Taffe, M. A. (2004). Impaired performance on a rhesus monkey neuropsychological testing battery following simian immunodeficiency virus infection. *AIDS Research and Human Retroviruses*, *20*, 77–89.

Weed, M. R., Taffe, M. A., Polis, I., Roberts, A. C., Robbins, T. W., Koob, G. F., et al. (1999). Performance norms for a rhesus monkey neuropsychological testing battery: Acquisition and long-term performance. *Cognitive Brain Research*, *8*, 185–201.

Weiss, B., & Laties, V. G. (1975). *Behavioral toxicology*. New York: Plenum Press.

White, K. G. (1985). Characteristics of forgetting functions in delayed matching to sample. *Journal of the Experimental Analysis of Behavior*, *44*, 15–34.

Whitton, A. E., Treadway, M. T., & Pizzagalli, D. A. (2015). Reward processing dysfunction in major depression, bipolar disorder and schizophrenia. *Current Opinion in Psychiatry*, *28*, 7–12.

Wightman, R., Perrone, J., Portelli, I., & Nelson, L. (2012). Likeability and abuse liability of commonly prescribed opioids. *Journal of Medical Toxicology*, *8*, 335–340.

Wilkinson, M. P., Grogan, J. P., Mellor, J. R., & Robinson, E. (2020). Comparison of conventional and rapid-acting antidepressants in a rodent probabilistic reversal learning task. *Brain and Neuroscience Advances*, *4*, 2398212820907177.

Winsauer, P. J., Lambert, P., & Moerschbaecher, J. M. (1999). Cannabinoid ligands and their effects on learning and performance in rhesus monkeys. *Behavioural Pharmacology*, *10*, 497–511.

Winsauer, P. J., Silvester, K. R., Moerschbaecher, J. M., & France, C. P. (2000). Cocaine self-administration in monkeys: Effects on the acquisition and performance of response sequences. *Drug and Alcohol Dependence*, *59*, 51–61.

Withey, S. L., Doyle, R. J., Porter, E. N., Bergman, J., & Kangas, B. D. (2020). Discrimination learning in oxycodone-treated nonhuman primates. *Drug and Alcohol Dependence*, *207*, 107778.

Withey, S. L., Kangas, B. D., Charles, S., Gumbert, A. B., Eisold, J. E., George, S. R., et al. (2021). Effects of daily Δ9-tetrahydrocannabinol (THC) alone or combined with cannabidiol (CBD) on cognition-based behavior and activity in adolescent nonhuman primates. *Drug and Alcohol Dependence*, *221*, 108629.

Woodworth, R. S. (1921). *Psychology*. New York, NY: Holt.

Wooldridge, L. M., Bergman, J., Pizzagalli, D. A., & Kangas, B. D. (2021). Translational assessments of reward responsiveness in the marmoset. *International Journal of Neuropsychopharmacology*, *24*, 409–418.

Wooldridge, L. M., Ji, L., Liu, Y., Nikas, S. P., Makriyannis, A., Bergman, J., et al. (2020). Antiemetic effects of cannabinoid agonists in nonhuman primates. *Journal of Pharmacology and Experimental Therapeutics*, *374*, 462–468.

Wright, M. J., Jr., Vandewater, S. A., & Taffe, M. A. (2013). Cannabidiol attenuates deficits of visuospatial associative memory induced by Δ(9) tetrahydrocannabinol. *British Journal of Pharmacology*, *170*, 1365–1373.

CHAPTER NINE

Receptor mechanisms underlying the CNS effects of cannabinoids: CB_1 receptor and beyond

Briana Hempel and Zheng-Xiong Xi*
Addiction Biology Unit, Molecular Targets and Medications Discovery Branch, Intramural Research Program, National Institute on Drug Abuse, Baltimore, MD, United States
*Corresponding author: e-mail address: zxi@mail.nih.gov

Contents

1. Introduction 276
2. Cannabinoid receptors 277
   2.1 CB_1 receptor 279
   2.2 CB_2 receptor 283
   2.3 GPR55 286
   2.4 Peroxisome proliferator-activated receptors (PPARs) 286
   2.5 Transient receptor potential vanilloid 1 (TRPV1) channel 287
   2.6 Other targets 287
3. Cannabinoid tetrad effects 288
   3.1 Analgesia 289
   3.2 Hypothermia 294
   3.3 Catalepsy 295
   3.4 Hypolocomotion 297
4. Cannabinoid subjective effects 299
   4.1 Cannabinoid reward 300
   4.2 Cannabinoid aversion 303
5. Cannabinoid effects on anxiety 304
   5.1 Anxiolytic 305
   5.2 Anxiogenic 306
6. Cannabinoid cognitive effects 309
   6.1 Spatial memory 312
   6.2 Short-term memory 313
7. Conclusion 314
Acknowledgments 314
Conflict of interest 315
References 315

Advances in Pharmacology, Volume 93
ISSN 1054-3589
https://doi.org/10.1016/bs.apha.2021.10.006

Abstract

Cannabis legalization continues to progress in many US states and other countries. Δ^9-tetrahydrocannabinol (Δ^9-THC) is the major psychoactive constituent in cannabis underlying both its abuse potential and the majority of therapeutic applications. However, the neural mechanisms underlying cannabis action are not fully understood. In this chapter, we first review recent progress in cannabinoid receptor research, and then examine the acute CNS effects of Δ^9-THC or other cannabinoids (WIN55212-2) with a focus on their receptor mechanisms. In experimental animals, Δ^9-THC or WIN55212-2 produces classical pharmacological effects (analgesia, catalepsy, hypothermia, hypolocomotion), biphasic changes in affect (reward vs. aversion, anxiety vs. anxiety relief), and cognitive deficits (spatial learning and memory, short-term memory). Accumulating evidence indicates that activation of CB_1Rs underlies the majority of Δ^9-THC or WIN55121-2's pharmacological and behavioral effects. Unexpectedly, glutamatergic CB_1Rs preferentially underlie cannabis action relative to GABAergic CB_1Rs. Functional roles for CB_1Rs expressed on astrocytes and mitochondria have also been uncovered. In addition, Δ^9-THC or WIN55212-2 is an agonist at CB_2R, GPR55 and PPARγ receptors and recent studies implicate these receptors in a number of their CNS effects. Other receptors (such as serotonin, opioid, and adenosine receptors) also modulate Δ^9-THC's actions and their contributions are detailed. This chapter describes the neural mechanisms underlying cannabis action, which may lead to new discoveries in cannabis-based medication development for the treatment of cannabis use disorder and other human diseases.

Abbreviations

Δ^9-THC Δ^9-tetrahydrocannabinol
AEA anandamide
2-AG 2-arachidonoyl glycerol
ChR2 channelrhodopsin 2
GABA gamma-aminobutyric acid
GPR55 G protein-coupled receptor 55
GPCR G protein-coupled receptor
ISH in situ hybridization
NAc nucleus accumbens
oICSS optical intracranial self-stimulation
PPARα peroxisome proliferator-activated nuclear receptor alpha
PPARγ peroxisome proliferator-activated nuclear receptor gamma
TRPV1 transient receptor potential vanilloid 1 channel
VTA ventral tegmental area

1. Introduction

Cannabis is the most commonly abused drug worldwide and accounts for half of all drug seizures by law enforcement (WHO, 2021). Since the

2000s, the general public has reported less perceived risk from cannabis, while diagnoses of cannabis use disorder (CUD) climb (Carliner, Brown, Sarvet, & Hasin, 2017). An estimated 147 million people in the world are cannabis users WHO, 2021. Recreational use remains the most prevalent (53.4%), but a growing community of individuals report purely medical use (10.5%) or a combination of medical and recreational use (36.1%; Schauer, King, Bunnell, Promoff, & McAfee, 2016). Therapeutic use of cannabis has a long history and an accumulating body of work has supported cannabinoids in the treatment of chronic spasticity and pain (Whiting et al., 2015). In this chapter, we explore the acute effects of cannabis from a neurobiological viewpoint. The majority of work in this vein has focused on Δ^9-tetrahydrocannabinol (Δ^9-THC), the primary psychoactive phytocannabinoid in cannabis that underlies its rewarding effects, but also the majority of therapeutic uses. Δ^9-THC was first isolated from hashish by Rafael Mechoulam in 1964 (Gaoni & Mechoulam, 1964). This compound produces a number of physiological and behavioral changes in preclinical animal models including the classic tetrad effects (analgesia, catalepsy, hypothermia, hypolocomotion), a change in affective state either positive (reward, anxiety relief) or negative (aversion, anxiogenesis), and deleterious effects on cognition. Systemic reviews on the endocannabinoid system, pharmacology of cannabinoids, and their involvement and implications in various human diseases have previously been conducted and are beyond the scope of this chapter (Alexander, 2016; Leung, 2011; Mechoulam & Parker, 2013; Pertwee, 2005, 2006). Here we focus on research progress investigating the neural mechanisms underlying the behavioral effects of Δ^9-THC and other cannabinoids in experimental animals. We first describe the receptor systems where cannabinoids bind followed by detailed region- and cell type-specific receptor mechanisms underlying Δ^9-THC's CNS effects.

2. Cannabinoid receptors

There are at least two types of cannabinoid receptors (CB_1R and CB_2R) identified. Δ^9-THC, synthetic cannabinoids (WIN55,212-2, CP55940, HU-210), and the endocannabinoids (anandamide, AEA; 2-arachidonoyl glycerol, 2-AG) have high binding affinities at both the GPCR-coupled receptors. Cannabinoids also bind and activate other putative cannabinoid receptors, including G protein-coupled receptor 55 (GPR55), transient receptor potential vanilloid 1 (TRPV1) channel, and peroxisome proliferator-activated nuclear receptors (PPARs) (Fig. 1). In addition,

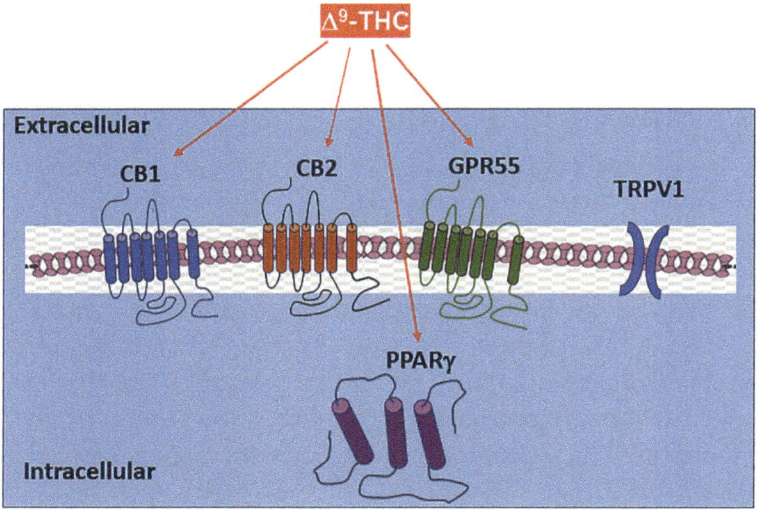

Fig. 1 Major targets of Δ^9-THC based on their receptor binding and functional assays as shown in Table 1.

Table 1 Receptor binding profiles of several major cannabinoids on CB1, CB2 and other putative cannabinoid receptors.

Drug	CB_1 (Ki, nM)	CB_2 (Ki, nM)	GPR55 (EC_{50}, nM)	TRPV1 (EC_{50}, μM)	PPARγ (EC_{50}, μM)
Anandamide (AEA)	61–543	279–1940	18	0.16–1.15	8–10
2-Arachidonoylglycerol (2-AG)	58–472	145, 1400	3	8.4–26	10–30
Δ^9-Tetrahydrocannabinol (THC)	5.05–80.3	3.13–75.3	8	>100	0.3
WIN55,212-2 (WIN)	1.89–123	0.28–16.2	N.D.	>100	10
CP55940	0.5–5.0	0.69–2.8	5	>100	10
HU-210	0.06–0.73	0.17–0.52	26	1.2	N.D.

Based on Pertwee (2008a) and Pertwee et al. (2010).

cannabinoids may also indirectly act on other receptor systems such as opioid, adenosine, and serotonin receptors by diverse ways.

Table 1 shows the receptor binding profiles of those commonly used cannabinoids to both CB_1 and CB_2 receptors and other putative receptors as shown in Fig. 1. In brief, these compounds are classified into four categories based on their chemical structures: classical, nonclassical, eicosanoid, and aminoalkylindole (Pertwee, 2008a, 2008b; Pertwee et al., 2010).

The classical category includes dibenzopyran derivatives such as Δ^9-THC and HU-210. Δ^9-THC is a weak partial agonist at both the CB_1R and CB_2R with greater CB_1R affinity and activity at GPR55 and PPARγ (Pertwee, 2008a, 2008b). HU-210 is a synthetic analog of Δ^8-THC with 100–800-fold greater potency than Δ^9-THC at the CB_1R and CB_2R, a prolonged duration of action, and activity at GPR55 and TRPV1 (Devane et al., 1992; Pertwee et al., 2010). CP55940 fits within the nonclassical nomenclature, containing compounds that are Δ^9-THC derivatives and lack a pyran ring (Howlett et al., 2002). CP55940 has marginally lower affinity than HU-210 at the CB_1R and CB_2Rs and binds to GPR55, TRPV1 and PPARγ (Pertwee et al., 2010). Within the eicosanoid classification are the two main endocannabinoids: 2-AG and AEA. AEA is a partial agonist at both the cannabinoid receptors with even lower CB_2R affinity than Δ^9-THC (Pertwee, 2005). 2-AG has high affinity at the CB_1R and somewhat less at the CB_2R with greater efficacy observed at CB_1Rs than CP55940. Both AEA and 2-AG bind to GPR55, TRVP1, and PPARγ (Pertwee et al., 2010). The fourth and final category, the aminoalkylindoles, have the most distinct chemical structures relative to the other subtypes (Ferraro et al., 2001). The aminoalkylindole WIN 55,212-2 is a full agonist at both the CB_1R and CB_2R with greater affinity than Δ^9-THC at the CB_1R and activity at TRVP1, PPARα and PPARγ (Howlett et al., 2002).

2.1 CB_1 receptor

As stated above, Δ^9-THC acts as a partial agonist at G-protein coupled CB_1R (Iwamura, Suzuki, Ueda, Kaya, & Inaba, 2001). This receptor recruits $G_{i/o}$ proteins and inhibits adenylate cyclase while increasing mitogen-activated protein kinase (Howlett, 2005; Pertwee, 2008a, 2008b). CB_1R can also inhibit N-type and P/Q-type calcium currents, stimulate A-type outward potassium channels, and use G_s proteins to signal (Howlett et al., 2002; Jarrahian, Watts, & Barker, 2004).

Regional distribution of CB_1R: The first CB_1R distribution studies used autoradiography with [^{3}H]-CP55,940, a tritiated CB_1R agonist (Herkenham et al., 1991, 1990) and found extraordinarily high levels of CB1Rs in the substantia nigra, globus pallidus, hippocampus, cerebellum, and cortex (Fig. 2). Autoradiographic studies using [^{3}H]-WIN55,212-2 further confirmed this pattern in rat (Jansen, Haycock, Ward, & Seybold, 1992) and human brains (Glass, Faull, & Dragunow, 1997; Mato, Del Olmo, & Pazos, 2003). *In situ* hybridization (ISH) and immunohistochemistry (IHC) assays corroborated

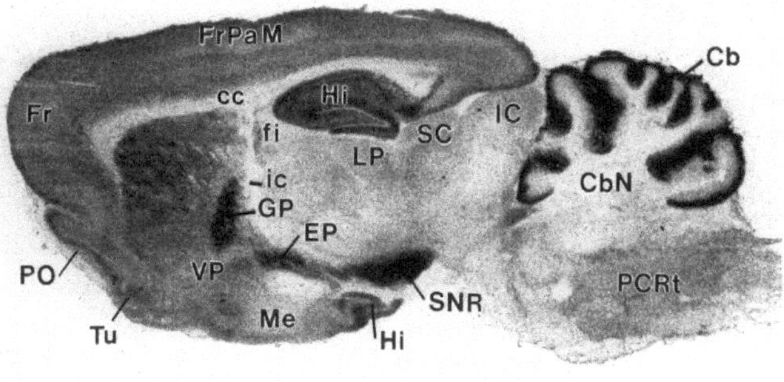

Fig. 2 [^{3}H]CP55,940 autoradiography demonstrating CB_1R distribution in the rat brain. A high density of CB_1Rs is expressed in the SNR, GP, Hi, and cerebellum. Fr, Frontal cortex; FrPaM, frontal primary motor cortex; PO, pre-olfactory bulb; *Tu*, olfactory tubercle; Hi, hippocampus; *VP*, ventral pallidum; Me, Median eminence; fi, fimbria of the hippocampus; ic, internal capsule; LP, lateral post thalamus nuclei; SC, superior colliculus; IC, inferior colliculus; *Cb*, cerebellum; *CbN*, cerebellar nuclei; *CC*, corpus cal losum; *GP*, globus pallidus; *EP*, entopeduncular nucleus (homolog of GPi); *SNR*, substantia nigra pars reticulata; PCRt, parvicellular reticular nuclei. (This image was provided by Dr. Miles Herkenham at NIMH, USA)

the autoradiographic reports and revealed that CB_1Rs are highly expressed in a restricted set of forebrain neurons, particularly in the cortex, amygdala, and hippocampus (see reviews by Galaj & Xi, 2019; Hu & Mackie, 2015). These neurons project widely throughout the CNS, resulting in a dense network of CB_1-positive axons (Bodor et al., 2005; Mackie, 2008). Double-label immunostaining and ISH experiments revealed that the cells expressing CB1Rs in the forebrain are primarily GABAergic and CCK-positive interneurons (Katona et al., 1999; Tsou, Mackie, Sañudo-Peña, & Walker, 1999).

Neuronal CB_1R: RNAscope ISH is a highly sensitive and selective assay that we and others have used to characterize the cellular distributions of CB_1Rs in the brain. High densities of CB_1 mRNA have been detected in the cell bodies of both GABA and glutamate neurons in multiple brain regions including the cortex, thalamus, midbrain and cerebellum (Fig. 3; Han et al., 2017; Humburg et al., 2021; Vickstrom et al., 2021). This CB_1 mRNA signal is highly specific as selective deletion of CB_1Rs from either GABAergic neurons or glutamatergic neurons abolished CB_1 mRNA staining in the corresponding cell types. Functional studies provide further information regarding cellular localization of CB_1R. For example, electrophysiological assays demonstrate that CB_1R activation inhibits GABA release in the midbrain, which may lead to postsynaptic (dopamine) neuron disinhibition (or activation; Lupica & Riegel, 2005; Szabo,

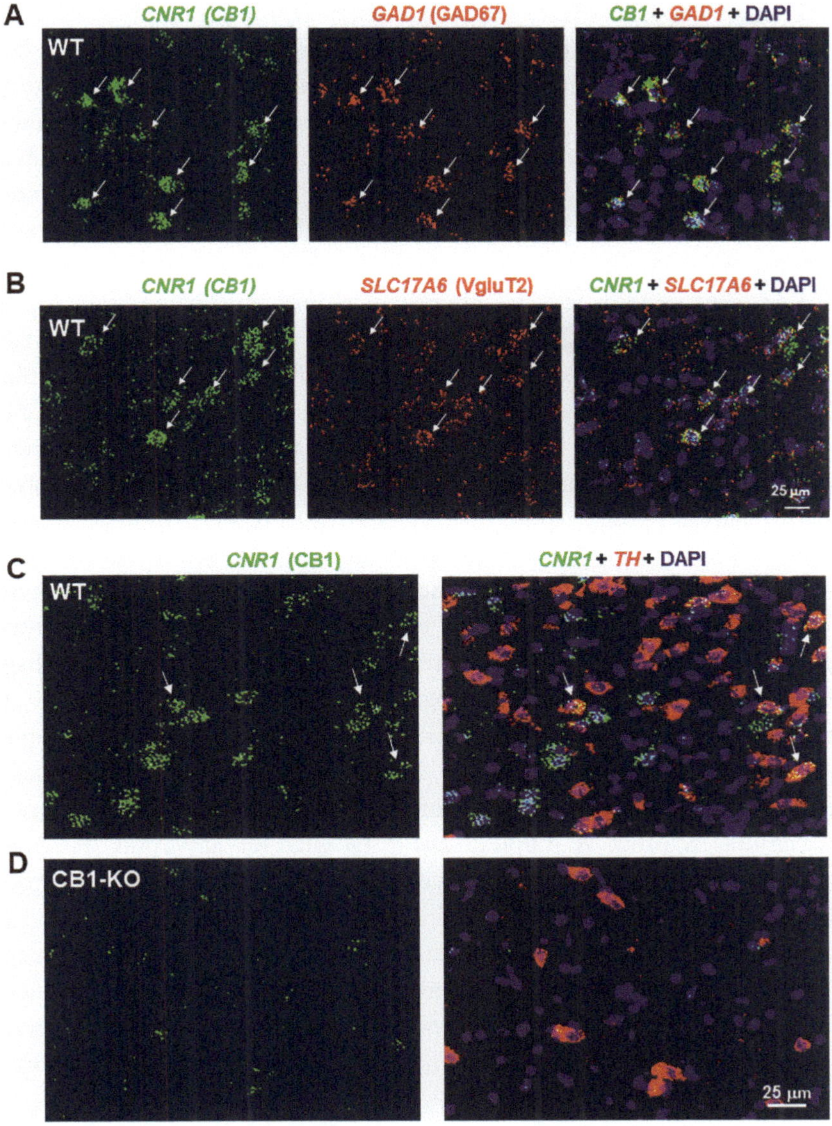

Fig. 3 RNAscope ISH results, illustrating the cellular distributions of CB_1Rs in the midbrain ventral tegmental area. CB_1 mRNA was detected in GAD1-labeled GABAergic neurons (A), VgluT2-labeled glutamate neurons (B) and a small population of TH-labeled DA neurons (C) in the midbrain of WT, but not CB_1-KO mice (D).

Siemes, & Wallmichrath, 2002). This suggests that activation of GABAergic CB1Rs has functional consequences. Electrophysiological assays also demonstrate functional CB1R expression in glutamatergic neurons or their terminals in the midbrain and many other brain regions (Melis, Gessa, & Diana, 2000;

Melis et al., 2004). We have examined CB_1R expression in midbrain dopamine (DA) neurons. Under high magnification, CB_1-immunostaining was found mainly in cell membranes and nerve fibers, but not in neuronal cell bodies (Han et al., 2017). Since nerve fibers from different neuronal types are always intertwined, IHC assays alone are not sufficient to identify whether midbrain DA neurons express CB_1Rs. However, RNAscope ISH assays indicate that a subpopulation of midbrain DA neurons expresses CB_1 mRNA (Fig. 3).

Endocannabinoids regulate physiological functions in the brain mainly through activation of CB_1Rs that inhibit presynaptic GABA or glutamate release via a retrograde endocannabinoid-CB_1R mechanism (Castillo, Younts, Chávez, & Hashimotodani, 2012; Piomelli, 2003). Specifically, presynaptic neuronal excitation increases glutamate release at excitatory synapses by activation of voltage-dependent Ca^{++} channels, which subsequently activates postsynaptic AMPA and NMDA receptors and depolarizes post-synaptic neurons. Meanwhile, glutamate may also activate postsynaptic mGluR1 or mGluR5, causing an increase in 2-AG synthesis in postsynaptic neurons. Postsynaptic neuronal depolarization may also elevate intracellular Ca^{++} and elicit 2-AG production. After being released from postsynaptic neurons, 2-AG retrogradely travels across the synapse to activate presynaptic CB_1Rs. Presynaptic CB1Rs are $G_{i/o}$ protein-coupled receptors (Howlett, 2005; Pertwee, 2008a, 2008b). Their activation leads to inhibition of presynaptic glutamate or GABA release (Hoffman, Laaris, Kawamura, Masino, & Lupica, 2010; Howlett et al., 2002; Howlett, Blume, & Dalton, 2010; Jarrahian et al., 2004; Laaris, Good, & Lupica, 2010). This neuronal CB_1R-mediated inhibition leads to several types of short-term or long-term synaptic plasticity, such as depolarization-induced suppression of excitation at excitatory synapses, depolarization-induced suppression of inhibition at inhibitory synapses, or long-term depression, which are associated with endocannabinoid involvement in various brain functions (Galaj & Xi, 2019).

Glial CB_1R: CB_1R has also been detected on non-neuronal cells such as astrocytes (Djeungoue-Petga & Hebert-Chatelain, 2017; Han et al., 2012; Oliveira da Cruz, Robin, Drago, Marsicano, & Metna-Laurent, 2016; Stella, 2010). Astrocytes were traditionally thought to provide nutrients to neurons and to maintain a functional homeostasis for neuronal functions. However, recent studies have indicated that astrocytes can regulate synaptic transmission and brain functions. For example, electrical stimulation of adjacent neurons can increase intracellular Ca^{++} levels in hippocampal astrocytes that express CB_1R (Navarrete & Araque, 2008). This effect is mediated by a $G\alpha q$ protein-phospholipase C signal pathway, rather than the $G\alpha_{i/o}$ protein-cAMP signal pathway observed in neurons. The increase in astrocyte Ca^{++} induces gliotransmitter release (Metna-Laurent & Marsicano, 2015; Mothet et al., 2000) and results in hetero-synaptic potentiation at excitatory or inhibitory synapses. Thus, glial CB_1R-mediated neuronal excitation differs significantly from neuronal CB_1R-mediated homosynaptic inhibition.

Less is known regarding CB_1R present on microglia and mitochondria. Microglia are the immune cells of the CNS. They act as macrophages and can change phenotype based on their microenvironment. Microglia in an activated state dispense a substantial amount of nitric oxide (NO). Interestingly, administration of a CB_1R agonist blocks this effect (Waksman, Olson, Carlisle, & Cabral, 1999) and microglia contain an anandamide binding site coupled to NO release (Stefano, Liu, & Goligorsky, 1996). As such, changes in NO production may mediate the effects of cannabinoids via microglial CB_1Rs. On the other hand, mitochondria are organelles responsible for a cell's energy production. They support basic brain functioning primarily via the process of mitochondrial respiration i.e., the conversion of oxygen and nutrients into ATP. CB_1R on mitochondria ($mtCB_1Rs$) modulates mitochondrial respiration (Bénard et al., 2012) and are neuroprotective (Ma et al., 2015). Further, $mtCB_1R$ mediates depolarization-induced suppression of inhibition, a form of short term synaptic plasticity in which glutamatergic neurons in the hippocampus are depolarized leading to the release of endocannabinoids and subsequent CB_1R activation and decreased GABAergic activity (Bénard et al., 2012).

2.2 CB_2 receptor

The cannabinoid CB_2R was cloned in 1993 from human leukemia cells (Munro, Thomas, & Abu-Shaar, 1993). CB2R has 44% sequence homology with CB_1Rs (Pertwee, 1997). They are G-protein coupled ($G_{i/o}$) and inhibit adenylate cyclase, leading to a decrease in cAMP signaling and neuronal inhibition (Patel, Davison, Pittman, & Sharkey, 2010). CB_2R activation can also stimulate p42/p44 MAP kinase and elevate intracellular calcium (Cabral & Griffin-Thomas, 2008). Δ^9-THC is a partial agonist at CB_2R with relatively high affinity (Table 1; Iwamura et al., 2001).

Regional distribution of CB_2R: CB_2R was initially referred to as "peripheral cannabinoid receptors" due to their predominant expression in peripheral tissues including immune cells, spleen, tonsils, lymph nodes, liver, and the gastrointestinal tract (Galiègue et al., 1995; Onaivi et al., 1999) and the failure to detect CB_2R in the CNS. However, more advanced techniques such as RNAscope ISH and fluorescence-activated cell sorting (FACS) followed by RT-PCR assays have unearthed CB_2R expression in the CNS including the spinal cord (Nent, Nozaki, Schmöle, Otte, & Zimmer, 2019), brain stem (Van Sickle et al., 2005), hippocampus (Li & Kim, 2015), ventral tegmental area (Zhang et al., 2017), and cerebellum (Gong et al., 2006).

Cellular distribution of CB_2R: The specific cell types within the CNS that express CB_2R are somewhat controversial. The majority of work assumes that CB_2Rs are expressed on microglia although more direct anatomical evidence is still needed. Recent studies have revealed neuronal CB_2R expression on DA neurons in the midbrain (Zhang et al., 2015; Zhang et al., 2017), glutamate neurons in the red nucleus and hippocampus (Li & Kim, 2015; Stempel et al., 2016; Zhang et al., 2021) and GABA neurons in the striatum and cerebellum (Fig. 4; Li & Kim, 2015; Zhang, De Biase, et al., 2021) (Fig. 4). CB_2Rs in the brain are located on the post-synaptic cells (Brusco, Tagliaferro, Saez, & Onaivi, 2008a, 2008b) and are inducible, showing upregulation under neuroinflammatory conditions (Atwood & Mackie, 2010; Maresz, Carrier, Ponomarev, Hillard, & Dittel, 2005).

CB_2R transcripts: An important finding in recent research is the unique distribution patterns of CB_2 transcript (mRNA) isoforms (CB_{2A}, CB_{2B}, CB_{2C}, CB_{2D}) across species and tissue types (Liu et al., 2009; Zhang et al., 2015), which may, in part, explain why early assessments failed to detect CB_2 mRNA in the brain (Galiègue et al., 1995; Munro et al., 1993; Schatz, Lee, Condie, Pulaski, & Kaminski, 1997). In humans and mice the CB_{2A} isoform was found primarily in the testis and brain, whereas CB_{2B} was expressed in the spleen and leukocytes (Liu et al., 2009). CB_{2C} and CB_{2D} isoforms were only detected in rats (Zhang et al., 2015). On the whole, CB_{2A} is the predominant subtype (20–30-fold higher than CB_{2B}; Zhang et al., 2014). However, in the mouse spleen CB_{2A} is only about 3-fold higher than CB_{2B} (Zhang et al., 2014). A direct comparison of brain and spleen CB_{2A} mRNA levels revealed considerably greater expression in the spleen (50–100-fold). These findings suggest that brain CB_2 mRNA is more likely to be detected with a probe that targets CB_{2A} rather than CB_{2B} transcript. However, brain CB2 expression is still detectable using riboprobes that recognize the encoding sequences on both CB_{2A} and CB_{2B} isoforms, by which CB_2 mRNA was discovered in the cortex,

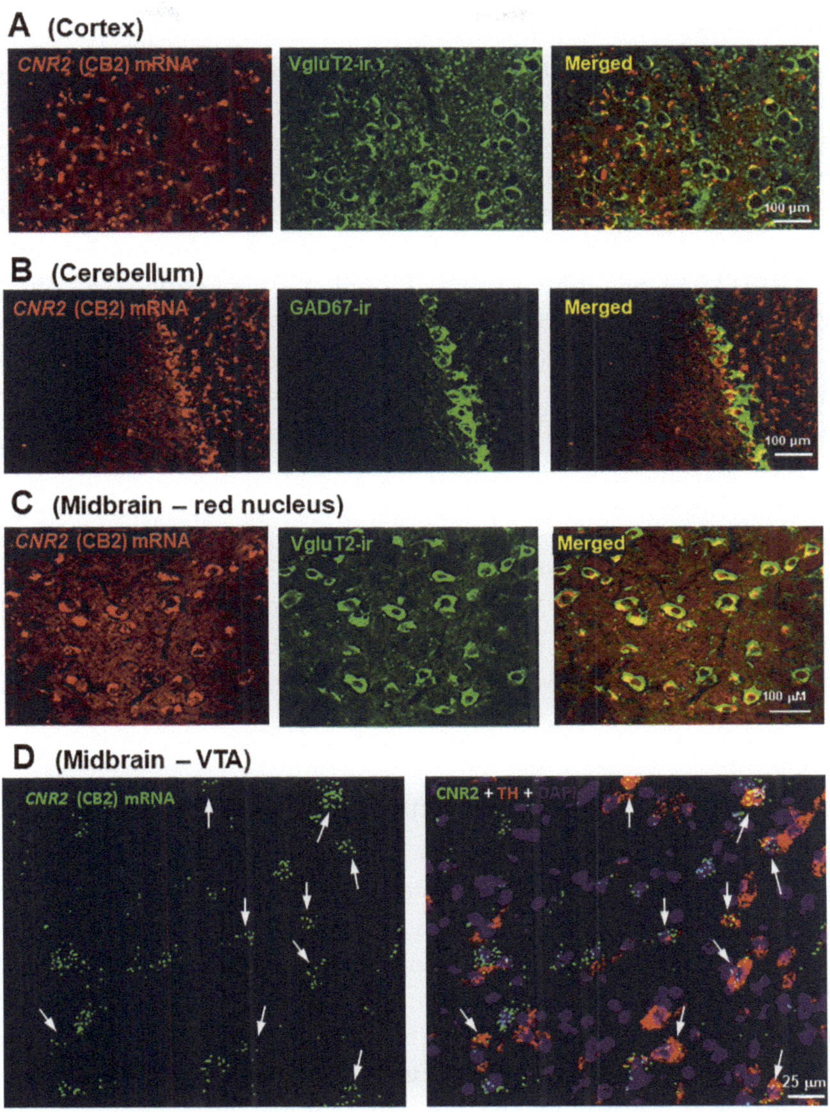

Fig. 4 Conventional (A, B, C) and RNAscope (D) ISH results, illustrating the cellular distributions of CB_2Rs in mouse brain. CB_2 mRNA was detected in cortical VgluT2-labeled glutamatergic neurons (A), cerebellar GAD1-labeled GABAergic neurons (B), red nucleus VgluT2-labeled glutamatergic neurons (C), and VTA TH-labeled dopaminergic neurons (D).

hippocampus, and globus pallidus of non-human primates (Lanciego et al., 2011; Sierra et al., 2015). These findings indicate that expression of the CB_2 gene is dependent on the isoform subtype and varies by species and region.

2.3 GPR55

Δ^9-THC is an agonist at the orphan receptor GPR55 (Table 1). This receptor has been put forward as a putative "CB3 cannabinoid receptor," given that both endocannabinoids (AEA, 2-AG) and synthetic cannabinoids (HU-210, CP55,940) are also able to bind (Table 1). However, GPR55 does not contain a quintessential cannabinoid binding pocket (Baker, Pryce, Davies, & Hiley, 2006) and has minimal receptor homology with CB1R (13.5%) or CB2R (14.4%; Elbegdorj, Westkaemper, & Zhang, 2013). GPR55 couples to G_{12} and G_{13} proteins and activates RhoA and Ca^{++} (Henstidge et al., 2009; Ryberg et al., 2007). GPR55 is distributed throughout the nervous system. In the periphery, it was been uncovered in the GI tract (Li et al., 2013), liver (Romero-Zerbo et al., 2011), pancreas (McKillop, Moran, Abdel-Wahab, & Flatt, 2013), and adipose tissue (Imbernon et al., 2014). QT-PCR assays indicate GPR55 mRNA expression in the striatum, substantia nigra, frontal cortex, hippocampus and cerebellum (Celorrio et al., 2017; Ryberg et al., 2007; Wu et al., 2013). In cell cultures, GPR55 and microglia colocalize (Pietr et al., 2009). In striatal or substantia nigra (SN) brain tissues, GPR55 mRNA was detected in neurons (colocalized with a neuronal marker), but not in microglia or astrocytes (Celorrio et al., 2017).

2.4 Peroxisome proliferator-activated receptors (PPARs)

PPARs are nuclear receptors with 3 isoforms (α, β, γ) that regulate gene expression (O'Sullivan, 2016). Activated PPARs dimerize retinoid X receptors and bind to DNA sequences termed PPAR response elements (Bishop-Bailey, 2000). Δ^9-THC is an agonist at PPARγ (EC50 ~0.3 μM; O'Sullivan, Tarling, Bennett, Kendall, & Randall, 2005) (Table 1), but does not bind to PPARα (Sun et al., 2007). However, one report demonstrated that Δ^9-THC administration increased PPARα transcriptional activity (Takeda et al., 2014). PPARs are also activated by endocannabinoids (AEA, 2-AG) and fatty acids (oleic acid, arachidonic acid) and may function as lipid sensors, monitoring metabolic activity *in vivo* (Pertwee et al., 2010). PPARγ expression predominates in adipose tissue, but is also observed in the liver, large intestine, and spleen (Lehrke & Lazar, 2005; Vidal-Puig et al., 1996; Villapol, 2018). Within the CNS, PPARγ expression has been detected in the piriform cortex, ventral pallidum, caudate putamen (Moreno, Farioli-Vecchioli, & Cerù, 2004), and to a lesser extent the prefrontal cortex (PFC), nucleus accumbens (NAc), and amygdala

(Warden et al., 2016). Immunohistochemical images showed colocalization of PPARγ in neurons, some staining in astrocytes, but not in microglia (Warden et al., 2016).

2.5 Transient receptor potential vanilloid 1 (TRPV1) channel

Six families of transient receptor potential channels (TRP) have been identified: canonical, vanilloid (TRPV), melastatin (TRPM), polycystin, mucolipin and ankyrin (TRPA). TRPs are ion channels with a nonselective cation pore and six transmembrane domains that are involved in sensory transduction. Δ^9-THC has no effect on TRPV1 functional activity at 100 μM, while AEA is a potent TRPV1 agonist with a EC_{50} value of 0.16–1.15 μM (Table 1). Δ^9-THC is a mild agonist at TRPV2 (EC_{50}: ~0.65 μM) and has intermediate effects at TRPA1 (EC_{50}: ~0.23 μM) and TRPM8 (IC50: ~0.16 μM; De Petrocellis et al., 2011). TRPV2 is activated by elevations in temperature and inflammation (De Petrocellis, Nabissi, Santoni, & Ligresti, 2017) and distributed in the paraventricular nucleus, arcuate nucleus, nucleus of the solitary tract, locus coeruleus as well as a number of other regions in the rat forebrain and hindbrain (Nedungadi, Dutta, Bathina, Caterina, & Cunningham, 2012). TRPV2 is colocalized with neurons and to a lesser extent, astrocytes (Nedungadi et al., 2012; Shibasaki, Ishizaki, & Mandadi, 2013).

2.6 Other targets

Beyond the five main receptor systems described above, cannabinoids may also interact with other targets possibly by forming heterodimers or functioning as opioid receptor allosteric modulators. For the purposes of this book chapter, we will only discuss the few receptors implicated in cannabinoid action in later Sections 3–6.

Opioid receptors: A significant amount of work indicates cross-talk between the endocannabinoid and endogenous opioid system. Opioid receptors are inhibitory GPCRs. There are four receptor subtypes: μ, δ, κ, and nociception, with endorphins, enkephalins, dynorphins, and nociceptin as the endogenous ligands, respectively. CB_1R was reported to form heterodimers with μ, δ, and κ opioid receptors and signaling at μ opioid receptors (MORs) is reduced by CB_1R agonism (Rios, Gomes, & Devi, 2006). Colocalization of CB_1Rs and MORs has also been detected in striatal medium-spiny neurons and the dorsal horn of the spinal cord (Rodriguez, Mackie, & Pickel, 2001; Salio et al., 2001). In addition, Δ^9-THC was reported to increase the rate of dissociation of MOR and δ opioid receptor (DOR) ligands from their orthosteric binding sites designating THC as an allosteric modulator at these receptors (Kathmann, Flau, Redmer, Tränkle, & Schlicker, 2006).

Adenosine receptors: Cannabinoids also have activity at the adenosine receptors, which are divided into four subtypes: A_1, A_{2A}, A_{2B} and A_3. Prior work has demonstrated that CB_1R antagonism prevents A_1R activation (Savinainen, Saario, Niemi, Järvinen, & Laitinen, 2003). Heteromeric complexes between CB_1Rs and $A_{2A}Rs$ have been detected in the striatum (Ferre et al., 2011; Ferreira et al., 2015) and hippocampus (Aso et al., 2019). The endocannabinoids (2-AG, AEA), but not synthetic cannabinoids (WIN55,212-2, CP55940), were reported to function as negative allosteric modulators at the A_3 receptor (Lane, Beukers, Mulder-Krieger, & Ijzerman, 2010).

Serotonin receptors: Additionally, a subset of serotonergic receptors is targeted by cannabinoids. There are seven families of 5-HT receptors (5-$HT_{1\text{-}7}$) and further subcategories within these classes. The majority of 5-HT receptors are GPCRs, not including the 5HT_3R. CB_1-5HT_{2A} heterodimers have been identified in the hippocampus, caudate putamen, and somatosensory cortex (Viñals et al., 2015). The Δ^9-THC metabolites, 11-hydroxy-Δ^8-THC and 11-oxo-Δ^8-THC, attenuated serotonin binding to 5-HT_{1A}, 5-HT_{1B}, 5-HT_{1D}, 5-HT_{1E}, and 5-HT_{2C} receptors (Kimura, Ohta, Watanabe, Yoshimura, & Yamamoto, 1998; Kimura, Yamamoto, Ohta, Yoshida, & Watanabe, 1996). Similarly, AEA weakened radioligand binding of 5-HT to 5-HT_{2A}, 5-HT_{2B}, and 5-HT_{2C} (Kimura et al., 1998). On the other hand, HU210 increased 5-HT binding to 5-HT_2Rs on rat cortical membranes (Cheer, Cadogan, Marsden, Fone, & Kendall, 1999). In addition, CB_1R may also form heterodimers with dopamine D_2Rs in the striatum (Marcellino et al., 2008)

3. Cannabinoid tetrad effects

High doses of cannabinoids such as Δ^9-THC or WIN55,212-2 (a potent CB_1R and CB_2R agonist) produce classical tetrad effects—analgesia, hypothermia, catalepsy, and hypolocomotion, which are often used to determine whether a novel compound is cannabimimetic in nature. The receptor mechanisms mediating cannabinoid effects in the tetrad are not fully understood. However, transgenic mice with conditional knockouts of different cannabinoid receptors have been widely used to identify the neuronal populations that mediate Δ^9-THC or other cannabinoid effects. Significant progress has been made. Here, we discuss each assay within the tetrad and the current knowledge regarding the neural underpinnings of Δ^9-THC- or WIN55,212-2-induced changes.

3.1 Analgesia

In pre-clinical work, Δ^9-THC induces a strong antinociceptive effect across multiple behavioral tests (hot plate, tail flick test, formalin test) and models of chronic pain (inflammatory pain, neuropathic pain; Casey, Atwal, & Vaughan, 2017; Craft, Haas, Wiley, Yu, & Clowers, 2017; Finn et al., 2004; Wang et al., 2020).

CB_1R mechanisms: Early work demonstrated that pharmacological blockade or genetic deletion of CB_1Rs in CB_1-KO mice blocked Δ^9-THC- or WIN55,212-2-induced analgesia (Compton, Aceto, Lowe, & Martin, 1996; Ledent et al., 1999; Rinaldi-Carmona et al., 1994; Varvel et al., 2005; Wiley & Martin, 2003; Zimmer, Zimmer, Hohmann, Herkenham, & Bonner, 1999). To address the anatomical locus and the cell type-specific receptor mechanisms underlying cannabinoid modulation of pain, multiple cell-type specific CB_1-KO mice have been developed with CB_1R deleted from a restricted neuronal population. As stated above, CB_1Rs are highly expressed on GABA and glutamatergic neurons. However, selective deletion of CB_1Rs on cortical glutamatergic neurons (Glu-CB_1-KO, generated by crossing CB_1-floxed mice with NEX-Cre mice), forebrain GABAergic interneurons (GABA-CB_1-KO, generated by crossing CB_1-floxed mice with Dlx5/6-Cre mice), or dopamine D_1 receptor-expressing neurons (Drd_1-CB_1-KO, generated by crossing CB_1-floxed mice with D_1-Cre mice) failed to alter Δ^9-THC antinociception (Table 2; Monory et al., 2007). These findings indicate that CB_1Rs on cortical GABAergic or glutamatergic neurons as well as D_1-expressing neurons do not mediate cannabinoid antinociception.

In a more recent report, De Giacomo and colleagues (2020) used a conditional rescue model in which CB_1Rs are restored only in distinct neuronal subpopulations in full CB_1-KO mice and compared to full CB_1R-KO mice to determine whether CB_1Rs in a given region can reproduce Δ^9-THC antinociception. In line with the findings from conditional CB_1-KO mice, the rescue of CB_1R expression in dorsal telencephalic glutamate neurons (Glu-CB_1-RS) or forebrain GABA neurons (GABA-CB_1-RS) did not re-establish Δ^9-THC-induced analgesia (De Giacomo et al., 2020),

Table 2 Summary of cannabinoid (THC, WIN55,212-2, JWH133)-induced tetrad effects in transgenic animals.

Transgenic mouse line	Analgesia	Hypothermia	Catalepsy	Hypoactivity	References
Wildtype	Normal THC or WIN effect	Normal effect	Normal effect	Normal effect	Monory et al. (2007) andWang et al. (2020)
Global CB_1-KO	No effect (to THC or WIN)	No effect	No effect	No effect	Ledent et al. (1999), Monory et al. (2007), Wang et al. (2020), and Zimmer, Zimmer, Hohmann, Herkenham, and Bonner (1999)
CaMK-CB_1-KO (CB_1^{flox} x CaMK-Cre)	↓ THC effect	No effect	No effect	No effect	Monory et al. (2007)
Glu-CB_1-KO (CB_1^{flox} x NEX-Cre)	Normal THC effect	↓ THC effect	Normal effect	↓ THC effect	Monory et al. (2007)
GABA-CB_1-KO (CB_1^{flox} x Dlx5/6-Cre)	Normal THC effect	Normal effect	Normal effect	Normal effect	Monory et al. (2007)
D1-CB_1-KO (CB_1^{flox} x Drd1-Cre)	Normal THC effect	↓ THC effect	↓ THC effect	Normal effect	Monory et al. (2007)
SNS-CB_1-KO (CB_1^{flox} x Nav1.8-Cre)	↓ WIN effect	N/D	Normal effect	N/D	Agarwal et al. (2007)
Global CB_2-KO	↓ THC or WIN effect	Normal effect	↓ THC or WIN effect	Normal effect (rotarod) ↓ THC effect (open-field)	Wang et al. (2020) and Li et al. (2021)
DA-CB_2-KO (CB_2^{flox} x DAT-Cre)	Normal effect (to WIN)	Normal effect	↓ WIN effect	Normal effect	Liu et al. (2017))
CX3CR1-CB_2-KO (CB_2^{flox} x CX3CR1-Cre)	Normal effect (to WIN, ACEA)	Normal effect	Normal effect	Normal effect	Liu, Canseco-Alba, Liang, Ishiguro, and Onaivi (2020)

Immune-CB_2-KO ($CB2^{flox}$ x LysM-Cre)	Normal JWH133 effect	N/D	N/D	N/D	Cabañero et al. (2020)
Syn-CB_2-KO (CB_2^{flox} x Syn-Cre)	↓ JWH133 effect	N/D	N/D	N/D	Cabañero et al. (2020)
SNS-CB_2-KO (CB_2^{flox} x Nav1.8-Cre)	↓ JWH133 effect in thermal pain	N/D	N/D	N/D	Cabañero et al. (2020)
GPR55-KO	Normal THC effect ↑ WIN effect	↑ THC effect	↑ THC effect	↑ THC effect	Wang et al. (2020)

Abbreviations: CaMK—Ca^{++}/calmodulin-dependent protein kinase II; $CB1^{flox}$—CB1-floxed mice; NEX—a gene encodes neuronal helix-loop-helix protein (a transcription factor), expressed in pyramidal neurons of the dorsal telencephalon during embryonic development; Dlx5/6—distal-less homeobox genes 5/6, expressed in forebrain GABAergic neurons during embryotic development; SNS—sensory neurons expressing $Na_v1.8$ channel; DA—dopamine; LysM—lymphocytes/monocytes; Syn—Synapsin (a neuronal marker).

suggesting that activation of CB_1Rs in forebrain GABA or glutamate neurons is insufficient to produce analgesic effects. In contrast, mice lacking CB_1Rs on CaMKIIα-positive neurons (CaMK-CB_1-KO, generated by CB_1-floxed mice with CaMKIIα-Cre mice) demonstrated attenuated (but not abolished) Δ^9-THC-induced analgesia (Monory et al., 2007), suggesting that CB_1Rs in CaMKIIα-expressing neurons partially mediate Δ^9-THC-induced analgesia. In addition, CB_1Rs may still be expressed by GABAergic neurons in other brain regions in the forebrain of GABA-CB_1-KO mice since the *Dlx5/6* (distal-less homeobox 5 and 6) genes are expressed in progenitors of GABAergic interneurons only in developing forebrain and their expression strongly diminishes after birth (Dimidschstein et al., 2016). Moreover, in the striatum these genes are not GABA specific. Similarly, CB_1Rs may still be expressed in glutamatergic neurons in other brain regions in the forebrain Glu-CB_1-KO mice since the NEX gene is mainly expressed in pyramidal neurons of the dorsal telencephalon during embryonic development (Schwab et al., 2000). Thus, more studies are required to determine the role of CB_1Rs in GABA or glutamate neurons of other non-forebrain regions in cannabinoid antinociception.

The major site of pain perception is the sensory nervous system, to be more precise, the sensory neurons in the dorsal root ganglia (DRG) as well as the dorsal horn neurons in the spinal cord, which also contain high densities of CB1Rs (Ahluwalia, Urban, Capogna, Bevan, & Nagy, 2000; Farquhar-Smith et al., 2000). To determine the role of CB_1Rs in primary sensory neurons, a peripheral CB_1-KO mouse line was developed, in which CB1Rs in DRG nociceptive ($Na_v1.8$-expressing) sensory neurons were deleted (SNS-CB1-KO, generated by crossing CB_1-floxed mice with SNS-Cre mice; Agarwal et al., 2007). The nociceptor-specific loss of CB_1Rs substantially reduced analgesia produced by local and systemic, but not intrathecal, delivery of WIN55,212-2 (Table 2; Agarwal et al., 2007). This suggests that CB_1Rs expressed on the peripheral terminals of nociceptors (DRG sensory neurons) are critical in cannabinoid-induced analgesia (Fig. 5). These findings are consistent with work demonstrating that systemic administration of a novel peripherally acting CB_1R agonist, AZ11713908, produced robust analgesia (Yu et al., 2010). Interestingly, CaMKIIα is also highly expressed in DRG neurons (Carlton & Hargett, 2002), suggesting that a peripheral CB_1R mechanism could also contribute to the reduction of Δ^9-THC-induced analgesia observed in CaMK-CB_1-KO mice. Thus, CB1R mechanisms in peripheral sensory neurons appear to be the primary mechanism underlying cannabinoid analgesic effects (Fig. 5).

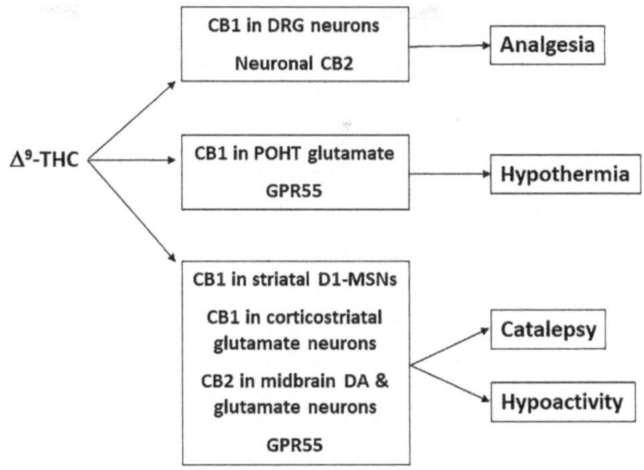

Fig. 5 A summary of the major neural mechanisms underlying THC-induced tetrad effects.

CB_2R mechanisms: Although CB_1R activation appears to be the primary mechanism underlying Δ^9-THC's analgesic effects, other targets have been discovered. For instance, CB_2R agonists have been demonstrated to produce potent analgesic effects in animal models of chronic inflammatory and neuropathic pain (Maldonado, Baños, & Cabañero, 2016; Shang & Tang, 2017). Further, we have recently reported that deletion of CB_2Rs in CB_2-KO mice significantly reduces Δ^9-THC- or WIN55,212-2-induced analgesia, implicating CB_2Rs in cannabinoid antinociception (Wang et al., 2020). However, the anatomical substrates underlying CB_2R-mediated analgesia are still unclear. Recently, it was reported that mice can learn to self-administer the CB_2R agonist JWH133 to inhibit neuropathic pain (Cabañero et al., 2020). This behavior was blocked by global CB_2-KO mice, suggesting a CB_2R-mediated effect. Interestingly, selective deletion of CB_2R from neurons in neuronal CB_2-KO mice (CB_2-floxed X Syn-Cre) caused an increase in JWH133 self-administration, while selective deletion of CB_2R from immune cells in monocyte-specific CB_2-KO mice (CB_2-floxed X LysM-Cre) did not alter JWH133 self-administration, suggesting that increased spontaneous pain occurs in neuronal CB_2-KO mice and high doses of JWH133 are required to relieve neuropathic pain (Cabañero et al., 2020) (Table 2). These findings provide clear evidence supporting a neuronal CB_2R mechanism underlying CB2R-induced analgesia. However, selective deletion of CB_2R from DGR neurons in peripheral neuronal CB_2-KO mice (CB_2-loxed X Nav1.8-Cre) did not significantly alter JWH133-produced analgesic effects, suggesting that a

neuronal CB_2R mechanism in the brain play a dominant role in JWH133- or other cannabinoid-induced analgesia (Fig. 5).

Other mechanisms: Additionally, the TRPA1 channel is a receptor critically involved in thermal pain perception. Evidence has shown that TRPA1 is implicated in cannabinoid antinociception. Specifically, Akopian et al. (2008) found that WIN55,212-2 induces analgesia in a peripheral capsaicin pain model, which is absent in TRPA1-KO mice. JWH133 produced a significant reduction in either mechanical or thermal hypernociception in a neuropathic pain model (Cabañero et al., 2020). Genetic deletion of TRPA1 blocked JWH133-induced reduction in thermal, but not, mechanical, pain, suggesting possible involvement of TRPA1 in cannabinoid analgesia. In addition, the opioid system was reported to be involved in cannabinoid analgesia. Specifically, κ-opioid receptors (KORs) are involved in Δ^9-THC-induced analgesia as the κ agonist dynorphin was increased by Δ^9-THC administration and mice with a genetic deletion of dynorphin showed attenuated Δ^9-THC-induced analgesia (Houser, Eads, Embrey, & Welch, 2000; Zimmer et al., 2001). However, KOR-KO mice displayed no change in Δ^9-THC antinociception (Ghozland et al., 2002). Given that Δ^9-THC does not bind to KORs, dynorphin may indirectly alter Δ^9-THC's action against pain. Unexpectedly, genetic deletion of GPR55 produced an opposite enhancement in WIN55,212-2-induced analgesia (Wang et al., 2020), suggesting involvement of GPR55 mechanism in cannabinoid analgesia.

3.2 Hypothermia

Intermediate to high doses of Δ^9-THC produce a drop in body temperature across different routes of administration and species (Hayakawa et al., 2007; McMahon, Amin, & France, 2005; Taffe, Kevin, Creehan, & Vandewater, 2015; Taffe, Creehan, Vandewater, Kerr, & Cole, 2021; Varvel et al., 2006).

CB_1R mechanism: CB_1Rs mediate the hypothermic effects of Δ^9-THC as pharmacological antagonism or genetic deletion of CB_1Rs blocks Δ^9-THC-induced decreases in temperature (Hayakawa et al., 2007; Ledent et al., 1999; McMahon et al., 2005; Varvel et al., 2005; Zimmer et al., 1999). In contrast to the analgesic effects, hypothermic responses to Δ^9-THC were significantly attenuated in CaMK-CB_1-KO and forebrain Glu-CB_1-KO mice, but not forebrain GABA-CB_1-KO mice, implicating cortical glutamatergic neurons in Δ^9-THC-induced hypothermia (Monory et al., 2007). The hypothermic effects of Δ^9-THC are likely mediated mainly by CB_1Rs expressed in the preoptic anterior hypothalamus (POAH),

a major thermoregulatory brain area (Fitton & Pertwee, 1982; Rawls, Cabassa, Geller, & Adler, 2002). In forebrain Glu-CB_1-RS and GABA-CB_1-RS mice, CB_1R expression is rescued in the hypothalamus relative to full CB_1-KO mice (Gutiérrez-Rodríguez et al., 2017; Remmers et al., 2017; Ruehle et al., 2013). Consistent with the data from conditional knockout mice, Glu-CB_1-RS, but not GABA-CB_1-RS, mice showed a partial rescue of Δ^9-THC hypothermia. As such, glutamatergic CB_1Rs may play a dominant role in Δ^9-THC-mediated hypothermia. Glutamate tonically increases body temperature by binding to NMDA receptors in the preoptic hypothalamus (Sengupta, Jaryal, & Mallick, 2016). One report found that the hypothermic response to WIN55,212-2 is synergistically enhanced by NMDA receptor antagonism (Rawls, Cowan, Tallarida, Geller, & Adler, 2002). Microinjections of WIN55,212-2 into the POAH induced hypothermia (Rawls, Cabassa, et al., 2002). These findings suggest that cannabinoids may act on a glutamatergic pathway in the POAH to produce hypothermia (Fig. 5).

Non-CB_1R mechanisms: Additional non-CB_1R receptor mechanisms have been implicated in Δ^9-THC-induced temperature shifts. We found that blockade or deletion of CB_2Rs in global CB_2-KO mice or selective deletion of CB2Rs in midbrain DA neurons failed to alter Δ^9-THC- or WIN55,121-2-induced hypothermia (Liu et al., 2017; Wang et al., 2020). In contrast, selective antagonism or genetic deletion of GPR55 receptors augmented hypothermia in response to Δ^9-THC or WIN55,212-2 (Wang et al., 2020), suggesting that activation of GPR55 has a suppressive effect on Δ^9-THC-induced hypothermia. No prior work has established a role for GPR55 in temperature control. However, knowledge of this receptor is limited, and future work should investigate this possibility. In addition, serotonergic 5-HT_{1A} receptors and dopamine D_2 receptors also regulate Δ^9-THC-induced hypothermia in an opposing manner such that D_2 receptor antagonists attenuate and 5-HT_{1A} receptor antagonists potentiate Δ^9-THC's hypothermic effects and vice versa with their respective agonists (Malone & Taylor, 2001; Nava, Carta, & Gessa, 2000). Although Δ^9-THC has no direct binding affinity at 5-HT_{1A} and D2 receptors, these effects could be mediated indirectly via Δ^9-THC metabolite activity at the 5-HT_{1A}R and CB_1-D_2 heterodimer interactions.

3.3 Catalepsy

In rodents, Δ^9-THC induces catalepsy at high doses (10 mg/kg and above; Long et al., 2010; Metna-Laurent, Mondésir, Grel, Vallée, & Piazza, 2017). The most common behavioral assay of catalepsy is the bar test in which an animals forepaws are placed on a horizontal bar and the amount of time it takes them to move out of this unusual conformation and put both paws on the ground is recorded (Sanberg, Bunsey, Giordano, & Norman, 1988).

CB_1R mechanism: As with Δ^9-THC induced hypothermia, blockage or deletion of CB_1Rs effectively abolishes Δ^9-THC's cataleptic effects (Ledent et al., 1999; Lichtman & Martin, 1997; Tseng & Craft, 2004; Varvel et al., 2005; Zimmer, Zimmer, Hohmann, Herkenham, & Bonner, 1999). An early study found that deletion of CB_1Rs on forebrain GABA or glutamate neurons failed to alter the cataleptic effects of Δ^9-THC (Monory et al., 2007), demonstrating that CB_1Rs on both neuronal cell types in the cortex do not mediate Δ^9-THC-induced catalepsy. This is consistent with findings from conditional rescue mice in which neither dorsal telencephalic glutamatergic CB_1Rs nor forebrain GABAergic CB_1Rs were sufficient to rescue the cataleptic effect of Δ^9-THC (De Giacomo et al., 2020).

Interestingly, deletion of CB_1Rs from CaMKIIα (CaMK-CB_1-KO) or D_1-expressing neurons (Drd1-CB_1-KO) abolished Δ^9-THC-induced catalepsy (Monory et al., 2007), suggesting that CB1Rs on both types of neurons play a critically important role in catalepsy produced by cannabinoids. CaMKIIα is expressed in numerous neuronal cell types that project to a myriad of brain regions. Therefore, it is unknown exactly how CB_1Rs in CaMKIIα-expressing neurons underlie cannabinoid-induced catalepsy. In contrast, D1Rs are mainly distributed in one population of GABAergic medium-spiny neurons (D_1-MSNs) in the striatum and glutamatergic neurons in the cortex. It is well known that D_1-MSNs regulate voluntary motor movements (van der Stelt & Di Marzo, 2003). Activation of CB_1Rs on D_1-MSNs likely inhibits GABAergic MSNs in the striatum, producing motor impairment. This is supported by the finding that microinjections of Δ^9-THC into the nucleus accumbens (NAc) produced catalepsy (Sano et al., 2008) that was inhibited by both serotoninergic agonists and NMDA receptor antagonists (Nobuaki Egashira et al., 2006; Kinoshita et al., 1994). These findings suggest that CB_1R expression in the striatum may be a primary brain region underlying Δ^9-THC-induced catalepsy (Fig. 5).

CB_2R mechanism: In addition to CB_1R, CB_2R also plays a role in the cataleptic effects of Δ^9-THC or WIN55212-2. Indeed, deletion and pharmacological antagonism of CB_2Rs attenuated cataleptic behavior following Δ^9-THC or WIN55,212-2 administration (Wang et al., 2020). Furthermore, selective deletion of CB_2Rs from midbrain DA neurons attenuated WIN55,212-2-induced catalepsy (Liu et al., 2017), while deletion of

CB_2R from microglia (CB_2-floxed X CX3CR1-Cre) had no effect on WIN55,212-2-induced catalepsy (Liu, Canseco-Alba, Liang, Ishiguro, & Onaivi, 2020), suggesting that a neuronal, not microglial, CB_2R mechanism underlies cannabinoid-induced catalepsy. In addition, it was recently reported that CB_2Rs are highly expressed in glutamate neurons in the red nucleus of the midbrain and modulate locomotor activity (Zhang, Shen, et al., 2021). These findings together suggest that activation of CB_2Rs in the mesolimbic DA neurons and the motor circuit glutamate neurons at least in part underlies cannabinoid-induced catalepsy (Fig. 5).

GPR55 mechanism: On the other hand, it was recently reported that GPR55 receptors are densely distributed in the striatum and administration of a GPR55 agonist (abnormal-cannabidiol) has been shown to block catalepsy produced by haloperidol (Marichal-Cancino, Fajardo-Valdez, E. Ruiz-Contreras, Mendez-Díaz, & Prospero-García, 2017; Celorrio et al., 2017), while pharmacological blockade of GPR55 potentiate Δ^9-THC-induced catalepsy (Wang et al., 2020). Similarly, mice lacking GPR55 demonstrated enhanced Δ^9-THC- or WIN55,212-2-induced catalepsy (Wang et al., 2020). These findings suggest that GPR55 activation may produce an anti-cataleptic effect. As such, the final behavioral expression of cannabinoid-induced catalepsy may depend on the respective contributions of CB_1R, CB_2R, and GPR55.

3.4 Hypolocomotion

Δ^9-THC suppresses locomotor activity at doses of 3 mg/kg and above. The open field locomotion test is most often utilized to measure changes in movement. Mice are placed in a large, empty container and the distance they travel is monitored. The rotarod test is another measure of locomotor performance, particularly motor coordination, in which mice are placed on an elevated revolving rod and the time it takes them to fall is recorded.

CB_1R mechanism: Like the other assays within the tetrad, Δ^9-THC or WIN55,212-2 alters locomotor activity via activation of CB_1Rs as deletion of CB_1Rs abolished Δ^9-THC and other cannabinoids-induced locomotor impairment (Ledent et al., 1999; Nguyen et al., 2016; Taffe, Creehan, & Vandewater, 2015; Zimmer et al., 1999). Findings from three different conditional CB_1-KO mice strains (Glu-CB_1-KO, CaMK-CB_1-KO and VgluT2-CB_1-KO) implicate glutamatergic neurons in Δ^9-THC's effects on locomotion (Monory et al., 2007; Han et al., 2017). These findings parallel work with conditional rescue mice in which restoration of CB1R

expression in dorsal telencephalic glutamatergic neurons (Glu-CB_1-RS mice) reestablished Δ^9-THC-induced locomotor suppression (De Giacomo et al., 2020). In contrast, deletion of CB_1Rs in forebrain GABA neurons failed to alter Δ^9-THC-induced locomotor impairment (Monory et al., 2007). Similarly, GABA-CB_1-RS mice with CB_1R expression rescued in forebrain GABAergic neurons showed no evidence of Δ^9-THC locomotor inhibition (De Giacomo et al., 2020). Previous work has demonstrated that cannabinoids attenuate excitatory glutamatergic input in the striatum (Brown, Brotchie, & Fitzjohn, 2003). Thus, CB_1Rs on corticostriatal glutamatergic projection neurons likely mediate hypolocomotion produced by Δ^9-THC (Monory et al., 2007) (Fig. 5).

The basal ganglia contains two major GABAergic neuronal populations—D_1-MSNs and D_2-MSNs. Both populations of neurons express CB_1Rs (Hermann, Marsicano, & Lutz, 2002) and control basal ganglia motoric output (Graybiel, 2000). Activation of D_1-MSNs enhances, while activation of D_2-MSNs inhibits locomotion (Calabresi, Picconi, Tozzi, Ghiglieri, & Di Filippo, 2014; Kravitz et al., 2010). The D_1-expressing MSNs have become a locus of interest since Δ^9-THC treatment may directly inhibit this locomotor-enhancing population of neurons. However, CB_1R deletion from D_1-MSNs had no effect on Δ^9-THC-induced hypolocomotion (Monory et al., 2007). Interestingly, the effects of Δ^9-THC on overall locomotor activity (open field test) vs. motor coordination (rotarod) may have distinct neural underpinnings. Indeed, Blazquez and colleagues (2020) found that Glu-CB_1-KO and WT mice had comparable deficits in motor coordination following Δ^9-THC in direct contrast to the findings described above using the open-field. Further, the motor dyscoordinating effects of Δ^9-THC were absent in Drd1-CB_1-KO mice, indicating that D_1-MSNs are critical for Δ^9-THC-induced deficits in motor coordination (Blázquez et al., 2020) (Fig. 5).

CB_2R mechanism: In addition to CB_1R mechanisms, dopaminergic CB_2Rs may also underlie Δ^9-THC-induced locomotor depression. We have previously reported that CB_1 and CB_2 receptors modulate locomotor activity in opposite directions (Li et al., 2021; Li et al., 2009; Wang et al., 2020; Xi et al., 2011). Specifically, genetic deletion of CB_1Rs decreased basal locomotor activity, while genetic deletion of CB_2Rs produced a moderate increase, indicating that activation of CB_2Rs inhibits locomotor behavior (Li et al., 2021; Wang et al., 2020). Systemic or intra-NAc administration of JWH133, a selective CB_2R agonist, inhibits basal level

locomotion and decreases cocaine's locomotor activating effects in a dose-dependent manner (Xi et al., 2011). Further, genetic deletion of CB_2Rs blocked the Δ^9-THC-induced reduction in open-field locomotion (Li et al., 2021; Wang et al., 2020), implicating CB2Rs in Δ^9-THC's locomotor suppressant effects. When CB_2Rs are selectively deleted from midbrain DA neurons, mice show an increase in basal locomotor activity (Canseco-Alba et al., 2019). These findings suggest that dopaminergic CB_2Rs contribute to Δ^9-THC-induced hypolocomotion (Galaj & Xi, 2019; Jordan & Xi, 2019) (Fig. 5).

GPR55 mechanism: Finally, GPR55-KO mice showed heightened Δ^9-THC or WIN55,212-2-induced deficits in motor coordination on the rotarod (Wang et al., 2020). These findings complement prior work in which administration of a GPR55 agonist improved performance on the rotarod following selective lesions of striatal DA neurons (Fatemi, Abdollahi, Shamsizadeh, Allahtavakoli, & Roohbakhsh, 2021). This work demonstrates that GPR55 agonism is involved in motor coordination and has an obverse effect on Δ^9-THC hypomotility in the tetrad, although the cell types and brain regions responsible are unknown.

In summary, Δ^9-THC and other cannabinoids produce classical tetrad effects through multiple receptor mechanisms, including CB_1R, CB_2R and GPR55 with CB_1R predominant (Table 2). Technical advances in detecting low level gene expression and the development of conditional transgenic animals have begun to uncover the region and cell type-specific subpopulations that underlie Δ^9-THC's effects in the tetrad. In brief, CB_1R in peripheral primary sensory neurons of the DRG and CB_2R in super-spinal neurons appear to be the major targets underlying THC-induced analgesia, while glutamatergic CB_1Rs in the preoptic anterior hypothalamus are not only necessary, but also sufficient for Δ^9-THC-induced hypothermia. The cataleptic and locomotor suppressant effects of Δ^9-THC are likely mediated mainly by activation of CB_1Rs on corticostriatal glutamatergic projection neurons and CB_2Rs on midbrain DA neurons and red nucleus glutamate neurons (Fig. 5).

4. Cannabinoid subjective effects

The subjective experience of cannabis varies on the affective spectrum from person to person. The majority of human users report enjoyment, relaxation and laughter, while others describe paranoia, anxiety and depression (Green, Kavanagh, & Young, 2003). In preclinical work, negative or aversive effects of Δ^9-THC are most commonly observed, particularly at high doses, whereas reward is rarer, difficult to replicate and only observed with low doses. A number of preclinical models of drug reward are utilized in addiction research. The gold standard is intravenous self-administration where animals are implanted with a jugular catheter and trained to make operant responses for drug infusions. Another commonly used model is place conditioning in which the amount of time spent in a context formerly associated with drug exposure is used as a measure of reward. Aversion can also be assessed in this model if time in the drug paired context drops considerably after conditioning. Lastly, intracranial self-stimulation (ICSS) is a behavioral test that assesses how drugs of abuse alter operant responding for electrical stimulation of the median forebrain bundle or optical stimulation of a specific phenotype of neurons such as DA neurons or glutamate neurons. A decrease or increase in brain-stimulation reward (BSR) thresholds denotes a rewarding or aversive drug effect, respectively. The following section will walk through studies investigating the neural mechanisms underlying Δ^9-THC reward *versus* aversion using these behavioral models.

4.1 Cannabinoid reward

Self-administration of Δ^9-THC has been demonstrated in squirrel monkeys at low doses (4 μg/kg/infusion), but not in rhesus monkeys, an effect that can be blocked by rimonabant, a selective CB1R blocker (John et al., 2018; Justinova, Tanda, Redhi, & Goldberg, 2003; Mansbach, Nicholson, Martin, & Balster, 1994; Tanda, Munzar, & Goldberg, 2000). However, in rodents (rats and mice), Δ^9-THC or WIN55,212-2 alone cannot maintain reliable self-administration possibly due to the limited reinforcing efficacy and anxiogenic effects of cannabinoids (Lefever, Marusich, Antonazzo, & Wiley, 2014; Takahashi & Singer, 1979). Interestingly, it was recently reported that passive Δ^9-THC pre-exposure or co-administration of Δ^9-THC with cannabidiol (CBD), a phytocannabinoid devoid of psychotomimetic effects, improved cannabinoid self-administration in rats (Spencer et al., 2018). A small number of studies have demonstrated Δ^9-THC-induced place preferences and decreases in BSR thresholds at the low end of the dose range (0.075–1 mg/kg), which are absent in the presence of a CB_1R antagonist or in CB_1-KO mice (Braida, Iosue, Pegorini, & Sala, 2004; Foll, Wiggins, & Goldberg, 2006; Gardner et al., 1988; Ghozland et al., 2002; Katsidoni, Kastellakis, & Panagis, 2013; Lepore, Liu, Savage, Matalon, & Gardner, 1996; Lepore, Vorel, Lowinson, & Gardner, 1995;

Li et al., 2021; Soria et al., 2004; Valjent & Maldonado, 2000). Microinjections of Δ^9-THC directly into the NAc shell and posterior ventral tegmental area (VTA) also support place preferences in rats, implicating these brain regions in Δ^9-THC-induced reward (Zangen, Solinas, Ikemoto, Goldberg, & Wise, 2006).

GABAergic CB_1R mechanism: Δ^9-THC administration produces a rise in DA concentration in the NAc (Tanda, Pontieri, & Chiara, 1997) and increases the firing rate of dopaminergic neurons in the VTA (French, Dillon, & Wu, 1997). Thus, it was hypothesized that CB_1Rs on GABA neurons mediate the rewarding effects of Δ^9-THC via disinhibition of VTA DA neurons (Fig. 6). This hypothesis is supported by electrophysiological data demonstrating decreased GABA activity in midbrain slices in the presence of Δ^9-THC and WIN55,212-2 (Friend et al., 2017; Szabo et al., 2002). Additionally, transgenic $FAAH^{C/A}$ knock-in mice,

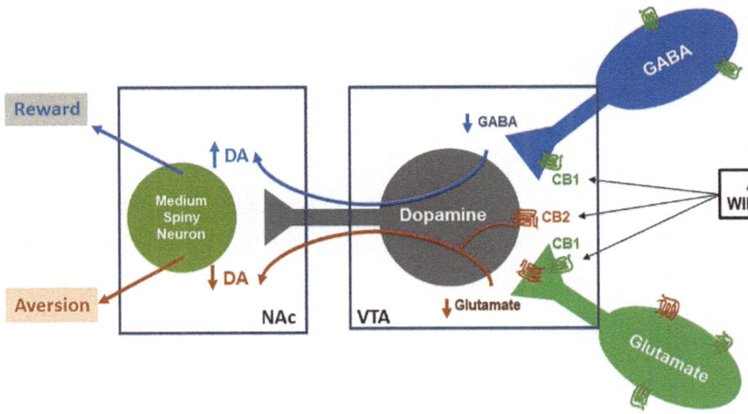

Fig. 6 Neural mechanisms underlying cannabinoid reward vs. aversion. CB_1Rs are expressed in VTA GABAergic neurons and glutamatergic neurons as well as their afferents projected from other brain regions to VTA DA neurons (data shown). CB_2Rs are found in VTA DA neurons. Cannabinoids modulate the mesolimbic DA system via activation of brain CB_1Rs and CB_2Rs. Cannabinoids such as Δ^9-THC or WIN55,212-2 produce rewarding effects by binding to CB_1Rs on VTA GABAergic interneurons and/or their afferents, thereby reducing GABA-mediated disinhibition of VTA DA neurons and cannabinoid reward. Conversely, Δ^9-THC or WIN55,212-2 may also produce aversive effects by activating CB_1Rs on glutamatergic neurons in the VTA or glutamatergic afferents, and CB_2Rs on midbrain DA neurons, thereby inhibiting VTA DA release to the NAc. The subjective effects of cannabinoids may thus depend on the balance of opposing CB1R and CB_2R effects and individual differences in expression of cannabinoid receptors. *DA,* dopamine; GABA, γ-aminobutyric acid; *NAc,* nucleus accumbens; *VTA,* ventral tegmental area.

which recapitulate the FAAH (fatty acid amide hydrolase) polymorphism and display decreased FAAH expression and elevated circulating AEA, produced an enhanced place preference in adolescent female $FAAH^{C/A}$ mice relative to controls (Burgdorf et al., 2020). Importantly, this increase in cannabinoid reward was accompanied by greater expression of GABAergic CB_1Rs and lower expression of glutamatergic CB_1Rs in the VTA (Burgdorf et al., 2020).

Non-CB_1R mechanisms: Other work has evaluated whether non-cannabinoid receptor systems are involved in the rewarding effects of Δ^9-THC. In one report, the MOR antagonist, naltrexone, decreased Δ^9-THC self-administration (Justinova, Tanda, Munzar, & Goldberg, 2004) and Δ^9-THC place preferences were absent in MOR-KO mice (Ghozland et al., 2002). Δ^9-THC increases β-endorphin release in the VTA, which could explain the lack of rewarding effects when MORs are antagonized or deleted (Solinas, Zangen, Thiriet, & Goldberg, 2004). Another series of studies implicated A_{2A} adenosine receptors ($A_{2A}Rs$) in the rewarding effects of Δ^9-THC. CB_1Rs form heterodimers with $A_{2A}Rs$ on presynaptic cells and activation of $A_{2A}Rs$ counteracts the inhibitory effects of CB_1Rs on glutamate release in corticostriatal terminals (Ferreira et al., 2015; Köfalvi et al., 2020). Antagonism of presynaptic $A_{2A}Rs$ was shown to reduce Δ^9-THC self-administration in squirrel monkeys, indicating that a decrease in cortical striatal glutamate attenuates Δ^9-THC reward (Justinová et al., 2011). Similarly, inhibition of postsynaptic $A_{2A}Rs$ potentiated Δ^9-THC self-administration (Justinová, Redhi, Goldberg, & Ferré, 2014). These findings suggest that excess glutamate in corticostriatal brain regions, perhaps the NAc, may also contribute to the rewarding effects of Δ^9-THC likely by stimulating dopamine release in the striatum. Finally, α7 nicotinic acetylcholine receptors (α7nAChRs) also play a role in Δ^9-THC reward. Kynurenic acid (KYNA) acts as a negative allosteric modulator of α7nAChRs and increased levels of KYNA inhibit Δ^9-THC-induced increases in NAc dopamine and Δ^9-THC self-administration in squirrel monkeys (Justinova et al., 2013). α7nAChRs are located on glutamatergic neurons that project to the NAc shell (Dani & Bertrand, 2007; Secci et al., 2019). As such, suppression of glutamatergic activity by KYNA and subsequent decreases in NAc DA likely underlie the decrease in Δ^9-THC reward. This work by Justinova and colleagues provides further evidence in support of a glutamatergic accumbal mechanism meditating Δ^9-THC's rewarding properties perhaps in conjunction with disinhibition of GABAergic tone in the VTA.

4.2 Cannabinoid aversion

The aversive effects of Δ^9-THC are well documented in preclinical work. Subjects develop robust place aversions and increases in BSR thresholds in ICSS particularly at intermediate to high doses (3–20 mg/kg; Braida et al., 2004; Hempel, Clasen, Nelson, Woloshchuk, & Riley, 2018; Katsidoni et al., 2013; Li et al., 2021; Mallet & Beninger, 1998a, b; Schramm-Sapyta et al., 2007; Spiller et al., 2019; Valjent & Maldonado, 2000; Vann et al., 2008; Wiebelhaus et al., 2015). We have recently tested cannabinoids in a new assay, optogenetic ICSS (oICSS), to further evaluate the rewarding (or reward-enhancing) *versus* aversive (or reward-attenuating) effects of a given drug (Han et al., 2017; Jordan et al., 2019; Newman et al., 2019). In this procedure, an adeno-associated virus (AAV) carrying a Cre-dependent channelrhodopsin 2 (ChR2) gene is microinjected into the VTA to express light-sensitive ChR2 in DA neurons of transgenic DA transporter (DAT)-Cre mice or glutamatergic neurons in VgluT2-Cre mice. Using this assay, we found that systemic administration of Δ^9-THC or WIN55,212-2 dose-dependently inhibited oICSS maintained by optical stimulation of VTA DA neurons and shifted the stimulation-response curve rightward or downward (Humburg et al., 2021), suggesting that cannabinoids are aversive in mice.

Glutamatergic CB_1R mechanism: The receptor mechanisms underlying Δ^9-THC's aversive effects are not fully understood. In prior work, cannabinoid-induced reductions in BSR thresholds were prevented by CB_1R antagonism (SR141716A or AM251; Katsidoni, Kastellakis, & Panagis, 2013; Spiller et al., 2019), pointing to a CB_1R mechanism in cannabinoid-induced aversion. To determine the specific cell types involved, we have recently used optogenetics to stimulate VTA glutamate neurons in VgluT2-Cre mice (Han et al., 2017). Unexpectedly, Δ^9-THC significantly inhibited oICSS maintained by optical stimulation of VTA glutamatergic neurons, but this effect was absent in VgluT2-CB_1-KO mice. Similarly, deletion of CB_1Rs on glutamate neurons prevented the expression of Δ^9-THC place aversions (Han et al., 2017). These findings suggest that CB_1Rs on VTA glutamate neurons are involved in Δ^9-THC-induced aversion (Fig. 6). This fits with the model of Δ^9-THC's affective properties described above wherein increased expression of CB_1Rs on GABA neurons and lower expression of CB_1Rs on glutamate neurons shifts the affective properties of Δ^9-THC towards reward (Burgdorf et al., 2020).

Dopaminergic CB_2R mechanism: Beyond CB_1Rs, Δ^9-THC's aversive effects were also blocked by CB_2R antagonism, as assessed by an increase in BSR thresholds in rats (Spiller et al., 2019). Additionally, genetic deletion of CB_2Rs shifted Δ^9-THC place conditioning from a place aversion in wildtype mice to a place preference in CB_2-KO mice (Li et al., 2021), indicating that CB_2Rs play a role in the initial aversive effects of Δ^9-THC. CB_2Rs are expressed on VTA dopaminergic neurons (Zhang et al., 2014; Zhang et al., 2017; Zhang et al., 2019) and can decrease the firing rate of these cells as well as diminish DA release in the NAc (Ma et al., 2019; Zhang et al., 2014; Zhang et al., 2017). These findings implicate CB_2Rs on mesolimbic DA neurons in THC-induced aversion (Fig. 6).

PPAR mechanisms: Little is known regarding the role of PPARs in cannabinoid action. However, we have recently explored the function of PPARs in Δ^9-THC induced aversion using oICSS (Hempel, Bi, Klein, & Xi, 2021). Administration of Δ^9-THC decreased responding for optical stimulation of VTA DA neurons in DAT-cre mice and this effect was attenuated by administration of a PPARα or PPARγ antagonist. As previously stated, Δ^9-THC is a potent PPARγ agonist (Table 1), which delineates how PPARγ antagonism reduced Δ^9-THC action on oICSS. PPARα receptors have been detected in the VTA and NAc at low levels (Warden et al., 2016). However, the mechanism through which PPARα modulates Δ^9-THC's aversive effects is still unclear. While Δ^9-THC administration does produce changes in PPARα gene transcription, it does not bind to the α isoform.

Kappa opioid receptor mechanism: Finally, κ-opioid receptors (KORs) have been investigated as a potential receptor target mediating Δ^9-THC aversion. Mice with elevated expression of the opioid encoding gene prodynorphin, a precursor of the KOR agonist dynorphin, demonstrated enhanced Δ^9-THC place aversions relative to controls (Cheng, Laviolette, van der Kooy, & Penninger, 2004). In the same vein, dynorphin-deficient and KOR-KO mice developed attenuated Δ^9-THC place aversions as did mice administered a KOR antagonist prior to assessments of Δ^9-THC aversion (Clasen et al., 2017; Ghozland et al., 2002; Zimmer et al., 2001). Microinjections of Δ^9-THC into the posterior NAc shell produced a significant place aversion that was attenuated by KOR antagonism, implicating NAc KORs in the expression of Δ^9-THC aversion (Norris, Szkudlarek, Pereira, Rushlow, & Laviolette, 2019).

5. Cannabinoid effects on anxiety

One of the most commonly cited reasons for cannabis use in humans is the relaxing effects of the drug (Ewusi Boisvert et al., 2020; Green,

Kavanagh, & Young, 2003); however, some individuals experience anxiety under the influence (Spindle et al., 2018). In preclinical models, Δ^9-THC has a biphasic effect on anxiety: anxiolytic at low doses and anxiogenic at high doses. The elevated plus maze (EPM) is a frequently used animal model in which rodents are placed on a raised apparatus containing two crossed arms – one of which is enclosed by walls and the other is open. Greater time spent in the open arms is a measure of decreased anxiety. The light dark test is another assay of anxiety that takes advantage of rodents' preference for dark, enclosed spaces. Subjects have access to two compartments separated by a door – one compartment is open and well-lit and the other is dark and enclosed. Anxiolytic drugs increase the proportion of time spent in the light compartment. The following subsections will update the current understanding of the receptor mechanisms underlying the anxiolytic and anxiogenic effects of Δ^9-THC.

5.1 Anxiolytic

As with the majority of cannabinoid effects on the central nervous system, administration of a CB_1 antagonist blocks Δ^9-THC-induced anxiolytic properties (Berrendero & Maldonado, 2002; Rubino et al., 2007). CB_1Rs in the amygdala and prefrontal cortex (PFC) underlie this effect (Tiziana Rubino et al., 2007). CP55,940 also produces an anxiolytic-like response at a low dose (1 μg/kg), which is absent in Glu-CB_1-KO, but not GABA-CB_1-KO mice (Rey, Purrio, Viveros, & Lutz, 2012), suggesting that glutamatergic CB_1Rs in the PFC and amygdala mediate the initial anxiolytic effects of Δ^9-THC. However, further work is needed to confirm this.

CB_1R and CB_2R mechanisms: One study found that brief exposure to a predator odor produced an anxiety-like state in rats that was blocked by the selective monoacylglycerol lipase (MGL) inhibitors, KML29 and JZL184 (Ivy et al., 2020). MGL inhibitors prevent 2-AG degradation and elevate brain 2-AG concentrations, indicating that increased levels of 2-AG were anxiolytic in this model. Unexpectedly, the behavioral response to JZL184 was abolished by a CB_2R, but not CB_1R, antagonist. Specifically, the selective CB_2R agonist, JWH133, produced anxiolytic-like effects in rats exposed to a predator odor stressor and this response was blocked by the CB_2R antagonist AM630 (Ivy et al., 2020). However, early studies demonstrated that JZL184 produced marked anti-anxiety effects that were prevented by administration of the CB_1R antagonist SR141716A

(Kinsey, O'Neal, Long, Cravatt, & Lichtman, 2011; Sciolino, Zhou, & Hohmann, 2011). Thus, 2-AG relieves anxiety potentially through activation of both CB_1Rs and CB_2Rs.

Other receptor mechanisms: Outside of the cannabinoid receptor family, other systems also modulate Δ^9-THC's anti-anxiety effect (Table 3). For instance, antagonism of the MOR and DOR suppressed the anxiolytic response to Δ^9-THC, although no additional work has investigated this neurobiological mechanism (Berrendero & Maldonado, 2002). Additionally, serotonergic receptors are known to regulate anxiety and have been investigated in this context. Administration of a 5-HT_{1A} receptor antagonist abolished the anxiolytic effect of Δ^9-THC (Braida, Limonta, Malabarba, Zani, & Sala, 2007). Similarly, genetic deletion of 5-HT_{2A} receptors (5-HT_{2A}Rs) blocked the anxiolytic response to Δ^9-THC (Viñals et al., 2015). Viñals et al. (2015) further demonstrated that CB1Rs form heterodimeric complexes with 5-HT_{2A}Rs and perturbation of this relationship via transmembrane helix interference peptides suppressed the anti-anxiety effect of Δ^9-THC. These heterodimers were found in the cortex, hippocampus and striatum, although it's unknown exactly which regions mediate the anxiolytic effects of Δ^9-THC.

5.2 Anxiogenic

CB_1Rs in the basolateral amygdala mediate the anxiogenic effects of Δ^9-THC, as prior work has demonstrated that microinjections of Δ^9-THC into this brain region produced anxiety that was attenuated by pretreatment with the CB_1R antagonist AM251 (Rubino et al., 2008). Interestingly, mice lacking CB_1Rs on GABAergic, but not glutamatergic neurons, failed to demonstrate anxiety in response to CP55,940 (50 μg/kg; Rey, Purrio, Viveros, & Lutz, 2012). A $GABA_B$ receptor-related mechanism may also contribute to the anxiogenic effect as positive allosteric modulation of $GABA_B$ receptors blocked CP55,940-induced anxiety. Whether these findings extend to Δ^9-THC's anxiogenic response is unknown. In addition, we have recently discovered that inhibition of PPARα can attenuate the anxiety produced by 5 mg/kg Δ^9-THC (Hempel et al., 2021). PPARα is expressed brain regions that regulate anxiety including the amygdala and hippocampus (Kainu, Wikström, Gustafsson, & Pelto-Huikko, 1994; Warden et al., 2016). However, the function of PPARα in the CNS is still being explored and very little is currently known.

Table 3 Receptor mechanisms underlying Δ^9-THC's affective properties.

Assay	Target	Antagonist	Knockout mouse	Results	References
Reward					
IVSA	CB_1Rs	AM251 SR141716A	N/A	Blocked	Freels et al. (2020, Justinova, Tanda, Redhi, and Goldberg (2003), and Spencer et al. (2018)
CPP	CB_1Rs	SR141716A	CB1-KO	Blocked	Braida, Iosue, Pegorini, and Sala (2004), Li et al. (2021)
ICSS	CB_1Rs	SR141716A	N/A	Blocked	Katsidoni, Kastellakis, and Panagis (2013)
IVSA	MORs	Naltrexone	N/A	Attenuated	Justinova, Tanda, Munzar, & Goldberg, 2004
CPP	MORs	N/A	MOR-KO	Blocked	Ghozland et al. (2002)
IVSA	$A_{2A}Rs$	MSX-3	N/A	Attenuated	Justinová et al. (2011)
IVSA	Presynaptic $A_{2A}Rs$ Postsynaptic $A_{2A}Rs$	SCH-442416 KW-6002	N/A	Attenuated Enhanced	Justinová et al. (2011) and Justinová, Redhi, Goldberg, and Ferré (2014)
IVSA	α7nAChRs	Ro 61-8048	N/A	Attenuated	Justinova et al. (2013)
Aversion					
ICSS	CB_1Rs	SR141716A	N/A	Blocked	Katsidoni, Kastellakis, and Panagis (2013)
ICSS	CB_2Rs	AM630	N/A	Blocked	Spiller et al. (2019)
oICSS	PPARα/PPARγ	GW6471 GW9662	N/A	Attenuated	Hempel et al. (2021)
oICSS CPA	Subcortical glutamate-CB1Rs	N/A	VgluT2-CB1-KO	Attenuated Blocked	Han et al. (2017)
CPA	CB_2Rs	N/A	CB2-KO	Blocked	Li et al. (2021)

Continued

Table 3 Receptor mechanisms underlying Δ^9-THC's affective properties.—cont'd

Assay	Target	Antagonist	Knockout mouse	Results	References
CPA	Prodynorphin gene	N/A	Dream-KO	Enhanced	Cheng, Laviolette, van der Kooy, and Penninger (2004)
CPA	Prodynorphin gene	N/A	Pdyn-KO	Attenuated	Zimmer et al. (2001))
CPA	KORs	Nor-BNI	KOR-KO	Blocked	Clasen et al. (2017), Ghozland et al. (2002) and Norris, Szkudlarek, Pereira, Rushlow, and Laviolette (2019)
Anxiolytic effect					
LDB EPM	CB1Rs	SR141716A	N/A	Blocked	Berrendero and Maldonado (2002) and Rubino et al. (2007)
LDB	MORs DORs	β-funaltrexamine Naltrindole	N/A	Blocked	Berrendero and Maldonado (2002)
EPM	$5\text{-}HT_{1A}Rs$	WAY100635	N/A	Blocked	Braida, Limonta, Malabarba, Zani, and Sala (2007)
EPM	$5\text{-}HT_{2A}Rs$	N/A	$5\text{-}HT_{2A}R$-KO	Blocked	Viñals et al. (2015)
EPM	CB_2Rs	AM630	N/A	Blocked	Ivy et al. (2020)
Anxiogenic effect					
EPM	CB_1Rs	AM251	N/A	Blocked	Rubino et al. (2008)
EPM	PPARα	GW6471	N/A	Attenuated	Hempel et al. (2021)
EPM Open field	Unknown	CBD	N/A	Attenuated	Liu et al. (2017), Murphy et al. (2017), and Todd and Arnold (2016)

Abbreviations: IVSA—intravenous self-administration, CPP—conditioned place preference, CPA—conditioned place aversion, ICSS—intracranial self-stimulation, oICS-S—optical ICSS, LDB—Light dark box, EPM—elevated plus maze, DREAM—downstream regulatory element antagonistic modulator, Pdyn, prodynorphin.

A number of studies have demonstrated that co-administration of CBD can inhibit the anxiogenic effects of Δ^9-THC (Liu, Scott, & Burnham, 2021; Murphy et al., 2017; Szkudlarek et al., 2019; Todd & Arnold, 2016; Zuardi, Shirakawa, Finkelfarb, & Karniol, 1982). CBD targets a number of receptors, but could suppress the effects of Δ^9-THC on anxiety via negative allosteric modulation of the CB1R or 5-HT_{1A}R activation (Campos & Guimarães, 2008; Galaj & Xi, 2021; Laprairie, Bagher, Kelly, & Denovan-Wright, 2015; Russo, Burnett, Hall, & Parker, 2005). Prior work has demonstrated that CBD can block anxiety caused by restraint stress via activity at the 5-HT_{1A}R (Resstel et al., 2009). Along these lines, Szkudlarek et al. (2019) found that intra-PFC injections of CBD suppressed Δ^9-THC-induced anxiety in the EPM and 5-HT_{1A}Rs are highly expressed in PFC neurons. Further work is needed to ascertain if direct 5-HT_{1A}R activation mediates CBD's inhibitory effect on Δ^9-THC in preclinical models of anxiety (for a summary see Table 3).

6. Cannabinoid cognitive effects

Acute exposure to cannabis impairs executive functions in human users across a number of domains such as attention, inhibitory control, psychomotor control, short term episodic memory, working memory and spatial memory (Crane, Schuster, Fusar-Poli, & Gonzalez, 2013; Crean, Crane, & Mason, 2011; Ranganathan & D'Souza, 2006). In animals, deficits in learning and memory are observed in spatial learning and memory, short term memory, repeated acquisition, habit formation, and fear conditioning (Goodman & Packard, 2015; Kangas et al., 2016; Prini et al., 2020; Resstel, Moreira, & Guimarães, 2009). A comprehensive review of the literature regarding the neurobiology of cannabinoids and cognition is beyond the scope of the present work. Here, we will focus on the neural mechanisms underlying acute effects of the most consistent Δ^9-THC-induced neurocognitive impairments, namely spatial learning and memory and short-term memory. A number of different animal models have been used in this context. Two commonly employed tests are the Morris water maze (MWM) and the novel object recognition task (NOR). The MWM assesses spatial learning and memory and in this task, animals are placed in a tank filled with cloudy liquid and must find a hidden platform to escape. In the NOR, subjects are initially exposed to two objects and in a subsequent session they are presented with one familiar and one novel object. Time spent exploring the new object is a measure of short-term memory impairment (for a summary see Table 4).

Table 4 Receptor mechanisms underlying Δ^9-THC-induced learning and memory impairments.

Assay	Target	Antagonist	Knockout mouse	Results	References
Spatial learning and memory					
RAM	CB_1R	SR141716A	N/A	Blocked	Lichtman and Martin (1996)
MWM	CB_1R	SR141716A	CB1-KO	Blocked	Varvel and Lichtman (2002)
MWM	Cell-type specific CB_1Rs	N/A	GABA-CB1-KO Glu-CB1-KO GFAP-CB1-KO	No effect No effect Blocked	Han et al. (2012)
MWM	NDMARs	AP-5	N/A	Blocked	Han et al. (2012)
MWM	COX-2	NS-398	$COX\text{-}2\text{-}KO^-$	Blocked	Chen et al. (2013)
MWM	A_1R	Caffeine	N/A	Enhanced	Sousa et al. (2011)
RAM	5-HT	Clomipramine 5-MeODMT	N/A	Attenuated Attenuated	Egashira et al. (2002)
RAM	$5\text{-}HT_2$	DOI	N/A	Attenuated	Egashira et al. (2002)
RAM	$5\text{-}HT_{1A}$	8-OHDPAT	N/A	Reversed	Inui et al. (2004)
RAM	AchE	Physostigmine Tetrahydroaminoacridine	N/A	Attenuated Attenuated	Mishima, Egashira, Matsumoto, Iwasaki, and Fujiwara (2002)
Short-term memory					
DNMS	CB_1R	SR141617A	N/A	Blocked	Hampson and Deadwyler (2000)
DNMP	CB_1R	SR141617A	N/A	Attenuated	Hampson and Deadwyler (2000) and Mallet and Beninger (1998a, b)

NOR	Mitochondria-specific CB_1R	N/A	DN22-CB1	Blocked	Hebert-Chatelain et al. (2016)
NOR	PKC	NPC CHE	N/A	Blocked Blocked	Busquets-Garcia et al. (2018)
DNMP	A_1R	Caffeine CPT	N/A	Enhanced Enhanced	Panlilio et al. (2012)
NOR	$A_{2A}R$	SCH442416 KW-6002	N/A	Attenuated No effect	Aso et al. (2019)
NOR	5-$HT_{2A}R$	MDL 100907	N/A	Reversed	Viñals et al. (2015)
NOR	5-$HT_{2A}R$	N/A	5-$HT_{2A}R$-KO	Attenuated	Viñals et al. (2015)
DNMS	ACHe	Rivastigmine	N/A	Blocked	Goonawardena, Robinson, Hampson, and Riedel (2010)

Abbreviations: RAM—radial arm maze, MWM—Morris water maze, DNMS—delayed nonmatch to sample, DNMP—delayed nonmatch to position, NOR—novel object recognition.

6.1 Spatial memory

CB_1Rs mediate the impairment in spatial memory after acute administration of Δ^9-THC as demonstrated by work in which CB_1Rs are antagonized or genetically deleted (Lichtman & Martin, 1996; Varvel & Lichtman, 2002). Intracerebral microinjection studies have established that CB1Rs in the hippocampus and medial PFC (mPFC) underlie this effect (Egashira, Mishima, Iwasaki, & Fujiwara, 2002). Moreover, the synthetic cannabinoid, HU210, produced deficits in spatial memory that were present in the forebrain GABA-CB_1-KO and Glu-CB_1-KO mice, but absent in mice with a conditional deletion of CB_1Rs in astrocytes (Han et al., 2012). In this report, antagonism of glutamatergic NMDA receptors (NMDARs) blocked the effects of HU210 on spatial memory and long-term synaptic depression in the hippocampus (Han et al., 2012). These findings indicate that cannabinoid-induced changes in spatial memory rely on stimulation of CB_1Rs on astrocytes and subsequent release of glutamate and changes in NMDAR signaling that induce LTD. It's unknown whether a similar pathway underlies the effects of Δ^9-THC in the MWM. However, antagonism and genetic ablation of cyclooxygenase-2 (COX-2), an enzyme responsible for the conversion of arachidonic acid to prostanoids, blocked Δ^9-THC impairments in spatial memory (Chen et al., 2013). These findings tie in with the astrocytic CB_1R mechanism as COX-2 enhances prostaglandin E_2 (PGE_2) release from astrocytes (Chen et al., 2013) and PGE_2 signaling can facilitate glutamatergic gliotransmission (Cali, Lopatar, Petrelli, Pucci, & Bezzi, 2014). Overall, astrocytic glutamate release appears to play a pivotal role in the expression of cannabinoid memory impairment.

A number of other pathways are involved in the effects of Δ^9-THC on spatial memory. For instance, pretreatment with an adenosine A_1 receptor (A_1R) agonist (caffeine) significantly elevated the Δ^9-THC-induced deficit in spatial memory (Sousa et al., 2011). A_1Rs were detected on glutamatergic terminals in the hippocampus and stimulation of A_1Rs disinhibited CB_1R suppression of hippocampal glutamatergic signaling (Sousa et al., 2011). Activation of the serotonergic system had the opposite effect on Δ^9-THC spatial memory impairments, i.e. the deficit was reversed by 5-HT_{1A} and $5HT_2$ receptor agonism (Egashira et al., 2002; Inui et al., 2004). Δ^9-THC also attenuated acetylcholine release in the dorsal hippocampus, which was blocked by administration of a 5-$HT_{1A}R$ agonist in agreement with prior work in which facilitation of acetylcholine release rescued Δ^9-THC-induced memory deficits (Inui et al., 2004; Mishima, Egashira,

Matsumoto, Iwasaki, & Fujiwara, 2002). These systems may work in concert with astrocyte mediated glutamate release to mediate Δ^9-THC's effects on spatial memory.

6.2 Short-term memory

Unsurprisingly, activation of CB_1Rs mediates the Δ^9-THC-induced deficits in short-term memory as confirmed by CB_1R antagonism studies (Hampson & Deadwyler, 2000; Mallet & Beninger, 1998a, b). The hippocampus appears to be a locus of interest in this respect as *in vivo* recording from groups of hippocampal neurons during performance of a short-term memory task revealed attenuated firing strength following Δ^9-THC administration (Hampson & Deadwyler, 2000). One group has demonstrated that mice lacking CB_1Rs in hippocampal mitochondria fail to demonstrate a disruption in short-term memory following WIN55,212-2 administration (Hebert-Chatelain et al., 2016). CB_1Rs on mitochondria inhibit soluble-adenylyl cyclase, which decreases protein kinase A phosphorylation and has downstream impacts on mitochondrial energetic activity (Hebert-Chatelain et al., 2016). However, recent work has shown that intra-hippocampal injections of a protein kinase C inhibitor blocked Δ^9-THC's effects on short-term memory (Busquets-Garcia et al., 2018). It's not clear whether the differential activity at these two protein kinase families works in conjunction to produce cannabinoid memory deficits or if the cannabinoid agent selected drives activity at one or the other group of enzymes.

The adenosine system has also been implicated in Δ^9-THC's inhibitory effect on short-term memory. Administration of caffeine or a selective A_1R antagonist potentiated Δ^9-THC-induced short-term memory impairments (Panlilio et al., 2012). On the other hand, $A_{2A}R$ antagonism mediated the therapeutic effect of CBD on Δ^9-THC short-term memory deficits (Aso et al., 2019). A_1 and $A_{2A}R$ antagonists have recently been shown to differentially regulate synaptic plasticity in the hippocampus, which could underlie their opposing actions on cannabinoid memory changes (Reis et al., 2019). As described earlier, CB_1Rs form heterodimers with $5HT_{2A}Rs$ and evidence of these structures has been detected in the hippocampus (Viñals et al., 2015). Both genetic deletion and pharmacological antagonism of $5HT_{2A}Rs$ reversed Δ^9-THC-induced changes in short-term memory (Viñals et al., 2015). Finally, cholinergic hypofunction has been hypothesized to play a role in the cognitive deficits produced by cannabinoids. Goonawardena, Robinson, Hampson, and Riedel (2010) found that an acetylcholinesterase inhibitor blocked WIN55,212-2-induced memory impairing properties and restored the normal firing patterns of hippocampal neurons. Whether these findings can be applied to Δ^9-THC is unknown.

7. Conclusion

The majority of Δ^9-THC's pharmacological and behavioral effects are mediated by activation of CB_1Rs (Tables 2–4). However, the cell types and brain regions expressing these receptors varies depending on the behavior assessed. Despite the widespread expression of CB_1Rs on GABAergic neurons, glutamatergic CB_1Rs preferentially underlie many of Δ^9-THC's effects including hypothermia, hypolocomotion, aversion, and anxiety relief. New research has discovered functional roles for CB_1Rs expressed on astrocytes and mitochondria in cannabinoid-induced cognitive impairments. This represents an exciting and promising area for future work, as non-neuronal CB_1R expression has been mostly ignored. Similarly, Δ^9-THC binds to a number of other targets such as CB_2R, GPR55, PPARs. The data from our lab has demonstrated that activation of these non-CB_1 receptors also modulate Δ^9-THC-induced behavior (Hempel et al., 2021; Li et al., 2021; Spiller et al., 2019; Wang et al., 2020). A host of additional non-cannabinoid receptor systems have been implicated in Δ^9-THC's behavioral effects primarily serotonergic (5-$HT_{1A}Rs$ & 5-$HT_{2A}Rs$), opioidergic (MORs & KORs), and adenosinergic (A_1Rs & $A_{2A}Rs$) signaling. Activity at these receptors may stem from downstream activity following CB_1R or CB_2R stimulation. Given the increasing use of cannabis for both recreational and medicinal purposes, understanding the neurobiology of Δ^9-THC's CNS effects is of vital concern. Moreover, this research provides a basis for the design of pharmacotherapeutics for substance use disorders including cannabis use disorder as well as non-psychoactive alternatives for medical marijuana users.

Acknowledgments

This work was supported by the Intramural Research Program (IRP) at the National Institute on Drug Abuse (NIDA; DA000620-02), National Institutes of Health, U.S. Public Health Service, USA. We thank Dr. Mikes Herkenham at Section on Functional Neuroanatomy, Laboratory of Cellular and Molecular Regulation, National Institute on Mental Health (NIMH), Bethesda, MD, USA, for providing the original high quality image in Fig. 2.

Conflict of interest

The authors have no conflicts of interest to declare.

References

Agarwal, N., Pacher, P., Tegeder, I., Amaya, F., Constantin, C. E., Brenner, G. J., et al. (2007). Cannabinoids mediate analgesia largely via peripheral type 1 cannabinoid receptors in nociceptors. *Nature Neuroscience*, *10*(7), 870–879. https://doi.org/10.1038/nn1916.

Ahluwalia, J., Urban, L., Capogna, M., Bevan, S., & Nagy, I. (2000). Cannabinoid 1 receptors are expressed in nociceptive primary sensory neurons. *Neuroscience*, *100*(4), 685–688. https://doi.org/10.1016/S0306-4522(00)00389-4.

Akopian, A. N., Ruparel, N. B., Patwardhan, A., & Hargreaves, K. M. (2008). Cannabinoids desensitize capsaicin and mustard oil responses in sensory neurons via TRPA1 activation. *The Journal of Neuroscience*, *28*(5), 1064–1075. https://doi.org/10.1523/jneurosci.1565-06.2008.

Alexander, S. P. H. (2016). Therapeutic potential of cannabis-related drugs. *Progress in Neuro-Psychopharmacology and Biological Psychiatry*, *64*, 157–166. https://doi.org/10.1016/j.pnpbp.2015.07.001.

Aso, E., Fernández-Dueñas, V., López-Cano, M., Taura, J., Watanabe, M., Ferrer, I., et al. (2019). Adenosine A2A-cannabinoid CB1 receptor heteromers in the hippocampus: Cannabidiol blunts Δ9-tetrahydrocannabinol-induced cognitive impairment. *Molecular Neurobiology*, *56*(8), 5382–5391. https://doi.org/10.1007/s12035-018-1456-3.

Atwood, B. K., & Mackie, K. (2010). CB2: A cannabinoid receptor with an identity crisis. *British Journal of Pharmacology*, *160*(3), 467–479. https://doi.org/10.1111/j.1476-5381.2010.00729.x.

Baker, D., Pryce, G., Davies, W. L., & Hiley, C. R. (2006). In silico patent searching reveals a new cannabinoid receptor. *Trends in Pharmacological Sciences*, *27*(1), 1–4. https://doi.org/10.1016/j.tips.2005.11.003.

Bénard, G., Massa, F., Puente, N., Lourenço, J., Bellocchio, L., Soria-Gómez, E., et al. (2012). Mitochondrial CB1 receptors regulate neuronal energy metabolism. *Nature Neuroscience*, *15*(4), 558–564. https://doi.org/10.1038/nn.3053.

Berrendero, F., & Maldonado, R. (2002). Involvement of the opioid system in the anxiolytic-like effects induced by Δ9-tetrahydrocannabinol. *Psychopharmacology*, *163*(1), 111–117. https://doi.org/10.1007/s00213-002-1144-9.

Bishop-Bailey, D. (2000). Peroxisome proliferator-activated receptors in the cardiovascular system. *British Journal of Pharmacology*, *129*(5), 823–834. https://doi.org/10.1038/sj.bjp.0703149.

Blázquez, C., Ruiz-Calvo, A., Bajo-Grañeras, R., Baufreton, J. M., Resel, E., Varilh, M., et al. (2020). Inhibition of striatonigral autophagy as a link between cannabinoid intoxication and impairment of motor coordination. *eLife*, *9*, e56811. https://doi.org/10.7554/eLife.56811.

Bodor, A. L., Katona, I., Nyíri, G., Mackie, K., Ledent, C., Hájos, N., et al. (2005). Endocannabinoid signaling in rat somatosensory cortex: Laminar differences and involvement of specific interneuron types. *The Journal of Neuroscience*, *25*(29), 6845–6856. https://doi.org/10.1523/jneurosci.0442-05.2005.

Braida, D., Iosue, S., Pegorini, S., & Sala, M. (2004). Delta9-tetrahydrocannabinol-induced conditioned place preference and intracerebroventricular self-administration in rats. *European Journal of Pharmacology*, *506*(1), 63–69. https://doi.org/10.1016/j.ejphar.2004.10.043.

Braida, D., Limonta, V., Malabarba, L., Zani, A., & Sala, M. (2007). 5-HT1A receptors are involved in the anxiolytic effect of Δ9-tetrahydrocannabinol and AM 404, the anandamide transport inhibitor, in Sprague–Dawley rats. *European Journal of Pharmacology, 555*(2), 156–163. https://doi.org/10.1016/j.ejphar.2006.10.038.
Brown, T. M., Brotchie, J. M., & Fitzjohn, S. M. (2003). Cannabinoids decrease corticostriatal synaptic transmission via an effect on glutamate uptake. *The Journal of Neuroscience, 23*(35), 11073–11077. https://doi.org/10.1523/jneurosci.23-35-11073.2003.
Brusco, A., Tagliaferro, P., Saez, T., & Onaivi, E. S. (2008a). Postsynaptic localization of CB2 cannabinoid receptors in the rat hippocampus. *Synapse, 62*(12), 944–949. https://doi.org/10.1002/syn.20569.
Brusco, A., Tagliaferro, P., Saez, T., & Onaivi, E. S. (2008b). Ultrastructural localization of neuronal brain CB2 cannabinoid receptors. *Annals of the New York Academy of Sciences, 1139*(1), 450–457.
Burgdorf, C. E., Jing, D., Yang, R., Huang, C., Hill, M. N., Mackie, K., et al. (2020). Endocannabinoid genetic variation enhances vulnerability to THC reward in adolescent female mice. *Science Advances, 6*(7), eaay1502. https://doi.org/10.1126/sciadv.aay1502.
Busquets-Garcia, A., Gomis-González, M., Salgado-Mendialdúa, V., Galera-López, L., Puighermanal, E., Martín-García, E., et al. (2018). Hippocampal protein kinase C signaling mediates the short-term memory impairment induced by Delta9-tetrahydrocannabinol. *Neuropsychopharmacology, 43*(5), 1021–1031. https://doi.org/10.1038/npp.2017.175.
Cabañero, D., Ramírez-López, A., Drews, E., Schmöle, A., Otte, D. M., Wawrzczak-Bargiela, A., et al. (2020). Protective role of neuronal and lymphoid cannabinoid CB2 receptors in neuropathic pain. *eLife, 9*, e55582.
Cabral, G. A., & Griffin-Thomas, L. (2008). Cannabinoids as therapeutic agents for ablating neuroinflammatory disease. *Endocrine, Metabolic & Immune Disorders Drug Targets, 8*(3), 159–172. https://doi.org/10.2174/187153008785700118.
Calabresi, P., Picconi, B., Tozzi, A., Ghiglieri, V., & Di Filippo, M. (2014). Direct and indirect pathways of basal ganglia: a critical reappraisal. *Nature Neuroscience, 17*(8), 1022–1030. https://doi.org/10.1038/nn.3743.
Cali, C., Lopatar, J., Petrelli, F., Pucci, L., & Bezzi, P. (2014). G-protein coupled receptor-evoked glutamate exocytosis from astrocytes: Role of prostaglandins. *Neural Plasticity, 2014*, 254574. https://doi.org/10.1155/2014/254574.
Campos, A. C., & Guimarães, F. S. (2008). Involvement of 5HT1A receptors in the anxiolytic-like effects of cannabidiol injected into the dorsolateral periaqueductal gray of rats. *Psychopharmacology, 199*(2), 223. https://doi.org/10.1007/s00213-008-1168-x.
Canseco-Alba, A., Schanz, N., Sanabria, B., Zhao, J., Lin, Z., Liu, Q.-R., et al. (2019). Behavioral effects of psychostimulants in mutant mice with cell-type specific deletion of CB2 cannabinoid receptors in dopamine neurons. *Behavioural Brain Research, 360*, 286–297. https://doi.org/10.1016/j.bbr.2018.11.043.
Carliner, H., Brown, Q. L., Sarvet, A. L., & Hasin, D. S. (2017). Cannabis use, attitudes, and legal status in the U.S.: A review. *Preventive Medicine, 104*, 13–23. https://doi.org/10.1016/j.ypmed.2017.07.008.
Carlton, S. M., & Hargett, G. L. (2002). Stereological analysis of Ca2+/calmodulin-dependent protein kinase IIα-containing dorsal root ganglion neurons in the rat: Colocalization with isolectin Griffonia simplicifolia, calcitonin gene-related peptide, or vanilloid receptor 1. *Journal of Comparative Neurology, 448*(1), 102–110. https://doi.org/10.1002/cne.10250.
Casey, S. L., Atwal, N., & Vaughan, C. W. (2017). Cannabis constituent synergy in a mouse neuropathic pain model. *Pain, 158*(12), 2452–2460. https://doi.org/10.1097/j.pain.0000000000001051.

Castillo, P. E., Younts, T. J., Chávez, A. E., & Hashimotodani, Y. (2012). Endocannabinoid signaling and synaptic function. *Neuron, 76*(1), 70–81. https://doi.org/10.1016/j.neuron.2012.09.020.

Celorrio, M., Rojo-Bustamante, E., Fernández-Suárez, D., Sáez, E., Estella-Hermoso de Mendoza, A., Müller, C. E., et al. (2017). GPR55: A therapeutic target for Parkinson's disease? *Neuropharmacology, 125*, 319–332. https://doi.org/10.1016/j.neuropharm.2017.08.017.

Cheer, J. F., Cadogan, A. K., Marsden, C. A., Fone, K. C. F., & Kendall, D. A. (1999). Modification of 5-HT2 receptor mediated behaviour in the rat by oleamide and the role of cannabinoid receptors. *Neuropharmacology, 38*(4), 533–541. https://doi.org/10.1016/S0028-3908(98)00208-1.

Chen, R., Zhang, J., Fan, N., Teng, Z.-Q., Wu, Y., Yang, H., et al. (2013). Δ9-THC-caused synaptic and memory impairments are mediated through COX-2 signaling. *Cell, 155*(5), 1154–1165. https://doi.org/10.1016/j.cell.2013.10.042.

Cheng, H.-Y. M., Laviolette, S. R., van der Kooy, D., & Penninger, J. M. (2004). DREAM ablation selectively alters THC place aversion and analgesia but leaves intact the motivational and analgesic effects of morphine. *The European Journal of Neuroscience, 19*(11), 3033–3041. https://doi.org/10.1111/j.0953-816X.2004.03435.x.

Clasen, M. M., Flax, S. M., Hempel, B. J., Cheng, K., Rice, K. C., & Riley, A. L. (2017). Antagonism of the kappa opioid receptor attenuates THC-induced place aversions in adult male Sprague-Dawley rats. *Pharmacology Biochemistry and Behavior, 163*, 30–35. https://doi.org/10.1016/j.pbb.2017.10.010.

Compton, D. R., Aceto, M. D., Lowe, J., & Martin, B. R. (1996). In vivo characterization of a specific cannabinoid receptor antagonist (SR141716A): Inhibition of delta 9-tetrahydrocannabinol-induced responses and apparent agonist activity. *The Journal of Pharmacology and Experimental Therapeutics, 277*(2), 586–594.

Craft, R. M., Haas, A. E., Wiley, J. L., Yu, Z., & Clowers, B. H. (2017). Gonadal hormone modulation of Δ9-tetrahydrocannabinol-induced antinociception and metabolism in female versus male rats. *Pharmacology Biochemistry and Behavior, 152*, 36–43. https://doi.org/10.1016/j.pbb.2016.09.006.

Crane, N. A., Schuster, R. M., Fusar-Poli, P., & Gonzalez, R. (2013). Effects of cannabis on neurocognitive functioning: recent advances, neurodevelopmental influences, and sex differences. *Neuropsychology Review, 23*(2), 117–137. https://doi.org/10.1007/s11065-012-9222-1.

Crean, R. D., Crane, N. A., & Mason, B. J. (2011). An evidence based review of acute and long-term effects of cannabis use on executive cognitive functions. *Journal of Addiction Medicine, 5*(1), 1–8. https://doi.org/10.1097/ADM.0b013e31820c23fa.

Dani, J. A., & Bertrand, D. (2007). Nicotinic acetylcholine receptors and nicotinic cholinergic mechanisms of the central nervous system. *Annual Review of Pharmacology and Toxicology, 47*(1), 699–729. https://doi.org/10.1146/annurev.pharmtox.47.120505.105214.

De Giacomo, V., Ruehle, S., Lutz, B., Häring, M., & Remmers, F. (2020). Differential glutamatergic and GABAergic contributions to the tetrad effects of Δ(9)-tetrahydrocannabinol revealed by cell-type-specific reconstitution of the CB1 receptor. *Neuropharmacology, 179*, 108287. https://doi.org/10.1016/j.neuropharm.2020.108287.

De Petrocellis, L., Ligresti, A., Moriello, A. S., Allarà, M., Bisogno, T., Petrosino, S., et al. (2011). Effects of cannabinoids and cannabinoid-enriched Cannabis extracts on TRP channels and endocannabinoid metabolic enzymes. *British Journal of Pharmacology, 163*(7), 1479–1494. https://doi.org/10.1111/j.1476-5381.2010.01166.x.

De Petrocellis, L., Nabissi, M., Santoni, G., & Ligresti, A. (2017). Chapter Eight—Actions and regulation of ionotropic cannabinoid receptors. In D. Kendall, & S. P. H. Alexander (Eds.), *Vol. 80. Advances in pharmacology* (pp. 249–289). Academic Press.

Devane, W. A., Breuer, A., Sheskin, T., Jaerbe, T. U., Eisen, M. S., & Mechoulam, R. (1992). A novel probe for the cannabinoid receptor. *Journal of Medicinal Chemistry*, *35*(11), 2065–2069.

Dimidschstein, J, Chen, Q, Tremblay, R, Rogers, SL, Saldi, GA, Guo, L, et al. (2016). A viral strategy for targeting and manipulating interneurons across vertebrate species. *Nature Neuroscience*, *19*(12), 1743–1749.

Djeungoue-Petga, M.-A., & Hebert-Chatelain, E. (2017). Linking mitochondria and synaptic transmission: The CB1 receptor. *BioEssays*, *39*(12), 1700126. https://doi.org/10.1002/bies.201700126.

Egashira, N., Matsuda, T., Koushi, E., Mishima, K., Iwasaki, K., Shoyama, Y., et al. (2006). Involvement of 5-hydroxytryptamine1A receptors in Δ9-tetrahydrocannabinol-induced catalepsy-like immobilization in mice. *European Journal of Pharmacology*, *550*(1), 117–122. https://doi.org/10.1016/j.ejphar.2006.08.051.

Egashira, N., Mishima, K., Iwasaki, K., & Fujiwara, M. (2002). Intracerebral microinjections of delta 9-tetrahydrocannabinol: search for the impairment of spatial memory in the eight-arm radial maze in rats. *Brain Research*, *952*(2), 239–245. https://doi.org/10.1016/s0006-8993(02)03247-x.

Egashira, N., Mishima, K., Katsurabayashi, S., Yoshitake, T., Matsumoto, Y., Ishida, J., et al. (2002). Involvement of 5-hydroxytryptamine neuronal system in Δ9-tetrahydrocannabinol-induced impairment of spatial memory. *European Journal of Pharmacology*, *445*(3), 221–229. https://doi.org/10.1016/S0014-2999(02)01755-7.

Elbegdorj, O., Westkaemper, R. B., & Zhang, Y. (2013). A homology modeling study toward the understanding of three-dimensional structure and putative pharmacological profile of the G-protein coupled receptor GPR55. *Journal of Molecular Graphics and Modelling*, *39*, 50–60. https://doi.org/10.1016/j.jmgm.2012.10.005.

Ewusi Boisvert, E., Bae, D., Pang, R. D., Davis, J. P., Kelley-Quon, L. I., Barrington-Trimis, J. L., et al. (2020). Subjective effects of combustible, vaporized, and edible cannabis: Results from a survey of adolescent cannabis users. *Drug and Alcohol Dependence*, *206*, 107716. https://doi.org/10.1016/j.drugalcdep.2019.107716.

Farquhar-Smith, W. P., Egertová, M., Bradbury, E. J., McMahon, S. B., Rice, A. S. C., & Elphick, M. R. (2000). Cannabinoid CB1 receptor expression in rat spinal cord. *Molecular and Cellular Neuroscience*, *15*(6), 510–521. https://doi.org/10.1006/mcne.2000.0844.

Fatemi, I., Abdollahi, A., Shamsizadeh, A., Allahtavakoli, M., & Roohbakhsh, A. (2021). The effect of intra-striatal administration of GPR55 agonist (LPI) and antagonist (ML193) on sensorimotor and motor functions in a Parkinson's disease rat model. *Acta Neuropsychiatrica*, *33*(1), 15–21. https://doi.org/10.1017/neu.2020.30.

Ferraro, L., Tomasini, M. C., Gessa, G. L., Bebe, B. W., Tanganelli, S., & Antonelli, T. (2001). The cannabinoid receptor agonist WIN 55,212-2 regulates glutamate transmission in rat cerebral cortex: An in vivo and in vitro study. *Cerebral Cortex*, *11*(8), 728–733. https://doi.org/10.1093/cercor/11.8.728.

Ferre, S., Quiroz, C., Orru, M., Guitart, X., Navarro, G., Cortes, A., et al. (2011). Adenosine A2A receptors and A2A receptor heteromers as key players in striatal function. *Frontiers in Neuroanatomy*, *5*(36). https://doi.org/10.3389/fnana.2011.00036.

Ferreira, S. G., Gonçalves, F. Q., Marques, J. M., Tomé, Â. R., Rodrigues, R. J., Nunes-Correia, I., et al. (2015). Presynaptic adenosine A2A receptors dampen cannabinoid CB1 receptor-mediated inhibition of corticostriatal glutamatergic transmission. *British Journal of Pharmacology*, *172*(4), 1074–1086. https://doi.org/10.1111/bph.12970.

Finn, D. P., Beckett, S. R., Roe, C. H., Madjd, A., Fone, K. C., Kendall, D. A., et al. (2004). Effects of coadministration of cannabinoids and morphine on nociceptive behaviour, brain monoamines and HPA axis activity in a rat model of persistent pain. *The European Journal of Neuroscience*, *19*(3), 678–686. https://doi.org/10.1111/j.0953-816x.2004.03177.x.

Fitton, A. G., & Pertwee, R. G. (1982). Changes in body temperature and oxygen consumption rate of conscious mice produced by intrahypothalamic and intracerebroventricular injections of Δ9-tetrahydrocannabinol. *British Journal of Pharmacology, 75*(2), 409–414. https://doi.org/10.1111/j.1476-5381.1982.tb08802.x.

Foll, B. L., Wiggins, M., & Goldberg, S. R. (2006). Nicotine pre-exposure does not potentiate the locomotor or rewarding effects of Δ-9-tetrahydrocannabinol in rats. *Behavioural Pharmacology, 17*(2). Retrieved from http://journals.lww.com/behaviouralpharm/Fulltext/2006/03000/Nicotine_pre_exposure_does_not_potentiate_the.10.aspx.

Freels, T. G., Baxter-Potter, L. N., Lugo, J. M., Glodosky, N. C., Wright, H. R., Baglot, S. L., et al. (2020). Vaporized cannabis extracts have reinforcing properties and support conditioned drug-seeking behavior in rats. *The Journal of Neuroscience, 40*(9), 1897–1908. https://doi.org/10.1523/jneurosci.2416-19.2020.

French, E. D., Dillon, K., & Wu, X. (1997). Cannabinoids excite dopamine neurons in the ventral tegmentum and substantia nigra. *Neuroreport, 8*(3). Retrieved from http://journals.lww.com/neuroreport/Fulltext/1997/02100/Cannabinoids_excite_dopamine_neurons_in_the.14.aspx.

Friend, L., Weed, J., Sandoval, P., Nufer, T., Ostlund, I., & Edwards, J. G. (2017). CB1-dependent long-term depression in ventral tegmental area GABA neurons: A novel target for marijuana. *The Journal of Neuroscience, 37*(45), 10943–10954. https://doi.org/10.1523/jneurosci.0190-17.2017.

Galaj, E., & Xi, Z.-X. (2019). Potential of cannabinoid receptor ligands as treatment for substance use disorders. *CNS Drugs, 33*(10), 1001–1030. https://doi.org/10.1007/s40263-019-00664-w.

Galaj, E., & Xi, Z.-X. (2021). Possible receptor mechanisms underlying cannabidiol effects on addictive-like behaviors in experimental animals. *International Journal of Molecular Sciences, 22*(1), 134. Retrieved from https://www.mdpi.com/1422-0067/22/1/134.

Galiègue, S., Mary, S., Marchand, J., Dussossoy, D., Carrière, D., Carayon, P., et al. (1995). Expression of central and peripheral cannabinoid receptors in human immune tissues and leukocyte subpopulations. *European Journal of Biochemistry, 232*(1), 54–61. https://doi.org/10.1111/j.1432-1033.1995.tb20780.x.

Gaoni, Y., & Mechoulam, R. (1964). Isolation, structure, and partial synthesis of an active constituent of hashish. *Journal of the American Chemical Society, 86*(8), 1646–1647.

Gardner, E. L., Paredes, W., Smith, D., Donner, A., Milling, C., Cohen, D., et al. (1988). Facilitation of brain stimulation reward by delta 9-tetrahydrocannabinol. *Psychopharmacology, 96*(1), 142–144.

Ghozland, S., Matthes, H. W. D., Simonin, F., Filliol, D., Kieffer, B. L., & Maldonado, R. (2002). Motivational effects of cannabinoids are mediated by mu-opioid and kappa-opioid receptors. *The Journal of Neuroscience: The Official Journal of the Society for Neuroscience, 22*(3), 1146–1154.

Glass, M., Faull, R. L. M., & Dragunow, M. (1997). Cannabinoid receptors in the human brain: A detailed anatomical and quantitative autoradiographic study in the fetal, neonatal and adult human brain. *Neuroscience*, 77(2), 299–318. https://doi.org/10.1016/S0306-4522(96)00428-9.

Gong, J.-P., Onaivi, E. S., Ishiguro, H., Liu, Q.-R., Tagliaferro, P. A., Brusco, A., et al. (2006). Cannabinoid CB2 receptors: Immunohistochemical localization in rat brain. *Brain Research, 1071*(1), 10–23. https://doi.org/10.1016/j.brainres.2005.11.035.

Goodman, J., & Packard, M. G. (2015). The influence of cannabinoids on learning and memory processes of the dorsal striatum. *Neurobiology of Learning and Memory, 125*, 1–14. https://doi.org/10.1016/j.nlm.2015.06.008.

Goonawardena, A. V., Robinson, L., Hampson, R. E., & Riedel, G. (2010). Cannabinoid and cholinergic systems interact during performance of a short-term memory task in the rat. *Learning & Memory, 17*(10), 502–511.

Graybiel, A. M. (2000). The basal ganglia. *Current Biology, 10*(14), R509–R511.

Green, B., Kavanagh, D., & Young, R. (2003). Being stoned: A review of self-reported cannabis effects. *Drug and Alcohol Review, 22*(4), 453–460. https://doi.org/10.1080/09595230310001613976.

Gutiérrez-Rodríguez, A., Puente, N., Elezgarai, I., Ruehle, S., Lutz, B., Reguero, L., et al. (2017). Anatomical characterization of the cannabinoid CB1 receptor in cell-type–specific mutant mouse rescue models. *Journal of Comparative Neurology, 525*(2), 302–318. https://doi.org/10.1002/cne.24066.

Hampson, R. E., & Deadwyler, S. A. (2000). Cannabinoids reveal the necessity of hippocampal neural encoding for short-term memory in rats. *The Journal of Neuroscience, 20*(23), 8932–8942. https://doi.org/10.1523/jneurosci.20-23-08932.2000.

Han, X., He, Y., Bi, G.-H., Zhang, H.-Y., Song, R., Liu, Q.-R., et al. (2017). CB1 receptor activation on VgluT2-expressing glutamatergic neurons underlies Δ 9-tetrahydrocannabinol (Δ 9-THC)-induced aversive effects in mice. *Scientific Reports, 7*(1), 1–15.

Han, J., Kesner, P., Metna-Laurent, M., Duan, T., Xu, L., Georges, F., et al. (2012). Acute cannabinoids impair working memory through astroglial CB1 receptor modulation of hippocampal LTD. *Cell, 148*(5), 1039–1050. https://doi.org/10.1016/j.cell.2012.01.037.

Hayakawa, K., Mishima, K., Nozako, M., Hazekawa, M., Ogata, A., Fujioka, M., et al. (2007). Δ9-tetrahydrocannabinol (Δ9-THC) prevents cerebral infarction via hypothalamic-independent hypothermia. *Life Sciences, 80*(16), 1466–1471. https://doi.org/10.1016/j.lfs.2007.01.014.

Hebert-Chatelain, E., Desprez, T., Serrat, R., Bellocchio, L., Soria-Gomez, E., Busquets-Garcia, A., et al. (2016). A cannabinoid link between mitochondria and memory. *Nature, 539*(7630), 555–559. https://doi.org/10.1038/nature20127.

Hempel, B., Bi, G. H., Klein, B., & Xi, Z. X. (2021). Peroxisome proliferator-activated receptors modulate optical brain-stimulation reward in DAT-Cre mice. *Under review.*

Hempel, B. J., Clasen, M. M., Nelson, K. H., Woloshchuk, C. J., & Riley, A. L. (2018). An assessment of concurrent cannabidiol and Δ^9-tetrahydrocannabinol administration in place aversion and taste avoidance conditioning. *Experimental and Clinical Psychopharmacology, 26*(2), 205–213. https://doi.org/10.1037/pha0000188.

Henstidge, C. M., Balenga, N. A. B., Ford, L. A., Ross, R. A., Waldhoer, M., & Irving, A. J. (2009). The GPR55 ligand L-α-lysophosphatidylinositol promotes RhoA-dependent Ca2+ signaling and NFAT activation. *The FASEB Journal, 23*(1), 183–193. https://doi.org/10.1096/fj.08-108670.

Herkenham, M., Lynn, A., Johnson, M., Melvin, L., de Costa, B., & Rice, K. (1991). Characterization and localization of cannabinoid receptors in rat brain: a quantitative in vitro autoradiographic study. *The Journal of Neuroscience, 11*(2), 563–583. https://doi.org/10.1523/jneurosci.11-02-00563.1991.

Herkenham, M., Lynn, A. B., Little, M. D., Johnson, M. R., Melvin, L. S., de Costa, B. R., et al. (1990). Cannabinoid receptor localization in brain. *Proceedings of the National Academy of Sciences, 87*(5), 1932–1936. Retrieved from https://www.pnas.org/content/pnas/87/5/1932.full.pdf.

Hermann, H., Marsicano, G., & Lutz, B. (2002). Coexpression of the cannabinoid receptor type 1 with dopamine and serotonin receptors in distinct neuronal subpopulations of the adult mouse forebrain. *Neuroscience, 109*(3), 451–460. https://doi.org/10.1016/S0306-4522(01)00509-7.

Hoffman, A. F., Laaris, N., Kawamura, M., Masino, S. A., & Lupica, C. R. (2010). Control of cannabinoid CB_1 receptor function on glutamate axon terminals by endogenous adenosine acting at A_1 receptors. *The Journal of Neuroscience, 30*(2), 545–555. https://doi.org/10.1523/jneurosci.4920-09.2010.

Houser, S. J., Eads, M., Embrey, J. P., & Welch, S. P. (2000). Dynorphin B and spinal analgesia: induction of antinociception by the cannabinoids CP55,940, Delta(9)-THC and anandamide. *Brain Research*, *857*(1-2), 337–342. https://doi.org/10.1016/s0006-8993(00)01981-8.

Howlett, A. C. (2005). Cannabinoid receptor signaling. In R. G. Pertwee (Ed.), *Cannabinoids* (pp. 53–79). Berlin, Heidelberg: Springer Berlin Heidelberg.

Howlett, A. C., Barth, F., Bonner, T. I., Cabral, G., Casellas, P., Devane, W. A., et al. (2002). International union of pharmacology. XXVII. Classification of cannabinoid receptors. *Pharmacological Reviews*, *54*(2), 161–202. https://doi.org/10.1124/pr.54.2.161.

Howlett, A. C., Blume, L. C., & Dalton, G. D. (2010). CB1 cannabinoid receptors and their associated proteins. *Current Medicinal Chemistry*, *17*(14), 1382–1393.

Hu, S. S.-J., & Mackie, K. (2015). Distribution of the endocannabinoid system in the central nervous system. In R. G. Pertwee (Ed.), *Endocannabinoids* (pp. 59–93). Cham: Springer International Publishing.

Humburg, B. A., Jordan, C. J., Zhang, H.-Y., Shen, H., Han, X., Bi, G.-H., et al. (2021). Optogenetic brain-stimulation reward: A new procedure to re-evaluate the rewarding versus aversive effects of cannabinoids in dopamine transporter-Cre mice. *Addiction Biology*, *26*(4), e13005. https://doi.org/10.1111/adb.13005.

Imbernon, M., Whyte, L., Diaz-Arteaga, A., Russell, W. R., Moreno, N. R., Vazquez, M. J., et al. (2014). Regulation of GPR55 in rat white adipose tissue and serum LPI by nutritional status, gestation, gender and pituitary factors. *Molecular and Cellular Endocrinology*, *383*(1), 159–169. https://doi.org/10.1016/j.mce.2013.12.011.

Inui, K., Egashira, N., Mishima, K., Yano, A., Matsumoto, Y., Hasebe, N., et al. (2004). The serotonin1A receptor agonist 8-OHDPAT reverses delta 9-tetrahydrocannabinol-induced impairment of spatial memory and reduction of acetylcholine release in the dorsal hippocampus in rats. *Neurotoxicity Research*, *6*(2), 153–158. https://doi.org/10.1007/bf03033218.

Ivy, D., Palese, F., Vozella, V., Fotio, Y., Yalcin, A., Ramirez, G., et al. (2020). Cannabinoid CB2 receptors mediate the anxiolytic-like effects of monoacylglycerol lipase inhibition in a rat model of predator-induced fear. *Neuropsychopharmacology*, *45*(8), 1330–1338. https://doi.org/10.1038/s41386-020-0696-x.

Iwamura, H., Suzuki, H., Ueda, Y., Kaya, T., & Inaba, T. (2001). In vitro and in vivo pharmacological characterization of JTE-907, a novel selective ligand for cannabinoid CB_2 receptor. *Journal of Pharmacology and Experimental Therapeutics*, *296*(2), 420–425. Retrieved from https://jpet.aspetjournals.org/content/jpet/296/2/420.full.pdf.

Jansen, E. M., Haycock, D. A., Ward, S. J., & Seybold, V. S. (1992). Distribution of cannabinoid receptors in rat brain determined with aminoalkylindoles. *Brain Research*, *575*(1), 93–102. https://doi.org/10.1016/0006-8993(92)90428-C.

Jarrahian, A., Watts, V. J., & Barker, E. L. (2004). D2 dopamine receptors modulate Galpha-subunit coupling of the CB1 cannabinoid receptor. *The Journal of Pharmacology and Experimental Therapeutics*, *308*(3), 880–886. https://doi.org/10.1124/jpet.103.057620.

John, W. S., Martin, T. J., Solingapuram Sai, K. K., Nader, S. H., Gage, H. D., Mintz, A., et al. (2018). Chronic Δ^9-THC in rhesus monkeys: Effects on cognitive performance and dopamine D2/D3 receptor availability. *Journal of Pharmacology and Experimental Therapeutics*, *364*(2), 300–310. https://doi.org/10.1124/jpet.117.244194.

Jordan, C. J., Humburg, B., Rice, M., Bi, G.-H., You, Z.-B., Shaik, A. B., et al. (2019). The highly selective dopamine D3R antagonist, R-VK4-40 attenuates oxycodone reward and augments analgesia in rodents. *Neuropharmacology*, *158*, 107597. https://doi.org/10.1016/j.neuropharm.2019.04.003.

Jordan, C. J., & Xi, Z. X. (2019). Progress in brain cannabinoid CB(2) receptor research: From genes to behavior. *Neuroscience and Biobehavioral Reviews*, *98*, 208–220. https://doi.org/10.1016/j.neubiorev.2018.12.026.

Justinová, Z., Ferré, S., Redhi, G. H., Mascia, P., Stroik, J., Quarta, D., et al. (2011). Reinforcing and neurochemical effects of cannabinoid CB1 receptor agonists, but not cocaine, are altered by an adenosine A2A receptor antagonist. *Addiction Biology*, *16*(3), 405–415. https://doi.org/10.1111/j.1369-1600.2010.00258.x.

Justinova, Z., Mascia, P., Wu, H.-Q., Secci, M. E., Redhi, G. H., Panlilio, L. V., et al. (2013). Reducing cannabinoid abuse and preventing relapse by enhancing endogenous brain levels of kynurenic acid. *Nature Neuroscience*, *16*(11), 1652.

Justinová, Z., Redhi, G. H., Goldberg, S. R., & Ferré, S. (2014). Differential effects of presynaptic versus postsynaptic adenosine A_{2A} receptor blockade on Δ_9-tetrahydrocannabinol (THC) self-administration in squirrel monkeys. *The Journal of Neuroscience*, *34*(19), 6480–6484. https://doi.org/10.1523/jneurosci.5073-13.2014.

Justinova, Z., Tanda, G., Munzar, P., & Goldberg, S. R. (2004). The opioid antagonist naltrexone reduces the reinforcing effects of Delta 9 tetrahydrocannabinol (THC) in squirrel monkeys. *Psychopharmacology*, *173*(1-2), 186–194. https://doi.org/10.1007/s00213-003-1693-6.

Justinova, Z., Tanda, G., Redhi, G. H., & Goldberg, S. R. (2003). Self-administration of delta9-tetrahydrocannabinol (THC) by drug naive squirrel monkeys. *Psychopharmacology*, *169*(2), 135–140. https://doi.org/10.1007/s00213-003-1484-0.

Kainu, T., Wikström, A. C., Gustafsson, J. A., & Pelto-Huikko, M. (1994). Localization of the peroxisome proliferator-activated receptor in the brain. *Neuroreport*, *5*(18), 2481–2485. https://doi.org/10.1097/00001756-199412000-00019.

Kangas, B. D., Leonard, M. Z., Shukla, V. G., Alapafuja, S. O., Nikas, S. P., Makriyannis, A., et al. (2016). Comparisons of Δ_9-tetrahydrocannabinol and anandamide on a battery of cognition-related behavior in nonhuman primates. *Journal of Pharmacology and Experimental Therapeutics*, *357*(1), 125–133. https://doi.org/10.1124/jpet.115.228189.

Kathmann, M., Flau, K., Redmer, A., Tränkle, C., & Schlicker, E. (2006). Cannabidiol is an allosteric modulator at mu-and delta-opioid receptors. *Naunyn-Schmiedeberg's Archives of Pharmacology*, *372*(5), 354–361.

Katona, I., Sperlágh, B., Sı́k, A., Käfalvi, A., Vizi, E. S., Mackie, K., et al. (1999). Presynaptically located CB1 cannabinoid receptors regulate GABA release from axon terminals of specific hippocampal interneurons. *The Journal of Neuroscience*, *19*(11), 4544–4558. https://doi.org/10.1523/jneurosci.19-11-04544.1999.

Katsidoni, V., Kastellakis, A., & Panagis, G. (2013). Biphasic effects of Delta9-tetrahydrocannabinol on brain stimulation reward and motor activity. *The international journal of neuropsychopharmacology/official scientific journal of the Collegium Internationale Neuropsychopharmacologicum (CINP)*, *16*(10), 2273–2284. https://doi.org/10.1017/S1461145713000709.

Kimura, T., Ohta, T., Watanabe, K., Yoshimura, H., & Yamamoto, I. (1998). Anandamide, an endogenous cannabinoid receptor ligand, also interacts with 5-hydroxytryptamine (5-HT) receptor. *Biological and Pharmaceutical Bulletin*, *21*(3), 224–226.

Kimura, T., Yamamoto, I., Ohta, T., Yoshida, H., & Watanabe, K. (1996). Changes in 5-HT receptor binding induced by tetrahydrocannabinol metabolites in bovine cerebral cortex. *Research Communications in Alcohol and Substances of Abuse*, *17*(1-2), 57–69.

Kinoshita, H., Hasegawa, T., Katsumata, Y., Kameyama, T., Yamamoto, I., & Nabeshima, T. (1994). Effect of dizocilpine (MK-801) on the catalepsy induced by Δ9-tetrahydrocannabinol in mice. *Journal of Neural Transmission/General Section JNT*, *95*(2), 137–143. https://doi.org/10.1007/BF01276432.

Kinsey, S. G., O'Neal, S. T., Long, J. Z., Cravatt, B. F., & Lichtman, A. H. (2011). Inhibition of endocannabinoid catabolic enzymes elicits anxiolytic-like effects in the marble burying assay. *Pharmacology Biochemistry and Behavior*, *98*(1), 21–27. https://doi.org/10.1016/j.pbb.2010.12.002.

Köfalvi, A., Moreno, E., Cordomí, A., Cai, N.-S., Fernández-Dueñas, V., Ferreira, S. G., et al. (2020). Control of glutamate release by complexes of adenosine and cannabinoid receptors. *BMC Biology*, *18*(1), 9. https://doi.org/10.1186/s12915-020-0739-0.

Kravitz, A. V., Freeze, B. S., Parker, P. R. L., Kay, K., Thwin, M. T., Deisseroth, K., et al. (2010). Regulation of parkinsonian motor behaviours by optogenetic control of basal ganglia circuitry. *Nature*, *466*(7306), 622–626. https://doi.org/10.1038/nature09159.

Laaris, N., Good, C. H., & Lupica, C. R. (2010). Δ9-tetrahydrocannabinol is a full agonist at CB1 receptors on GABA neuron axon terminals in the hippocampus. *Neuropharmacology*, *59*(1), 121–127. https://doi.org/10.1016/j.neuropharm.2010.04.013.

Lanciego, J. L., Barroso-Chinea, P., Rico, A. J., Conte-Perales, L., Callén, L., Roda, E., et al. (2011). Expression of the mRNA coding the cannabinoid receptor 2 in the pallidal complex of Macaca fascicularis. *Journal of Psychopharmacology*, *25*(1), 97–104. https://doi.org/10.1177/0269881110367732.

Lane, J. R., Beukers, M. W., Mulder-Krieger, T., & Ijzerman, A. P. (2010). The endocannabinoid 2-arachidonylglycerol is a negative allosteric modulator of the human A3 adenosine receptor. *Biochemical Pharmacology*, *79*(1), 48–56. https://doi.org/10.1016/j.bcp.2009.07.024.

Laprairie, R. B., Bagher, A. M., Kelly, M. E. M., & Denovan-Wright, E. M. (2015). Cannabidiol is a negative allosteric modulator of the cannabinoid CB1 receptor. *British Journal of Pharmacology*, *172*(20), 4790–4805. https://doi.org/10.1111/bph.13250.

Ledent, C., Valverde, O., Cossu, G., Petitet, F., Aubert, J. F., Beslot, F., et al. (1999). Unresponsiveness to cannabinoids and reduced addictive effects of opiates in CB1 receptor knockout mice. *Science*, *283*(5400), 401–404. https://doi.org/10.1126/science.283.5400.401.

Lefever, T. W., Marusich, J. A., Antonazzo, K. R., & Wiley, J. L. (2014). Evaluation of WIN 55,212-2 self-administration in rats as a potential cannabinoid abuse liability model. *Pharmacology, Biochemistry, and Behavior*, *118*, 30–35. https://doi.org/10.1016/j.pbb.2014.01.002.

Lehrke, M., & Lazar, M. A. (2005). The many faces of PPARγ. *Cell*, *123*(6), 993–999. https://doi.org/10.1016/j.cell.2005.11.026.

Lepore, M., Liu, X., Savage, V., Matalon, D., & Gardner, E. L. (1996). Genetic differences in Δ9-tetrahydrocannabinol-induced facilitation of brain stimulation reward as measured by a rate-frequency curve-shift electrical brain stimulation paradigm in three different rat strains. *Life Sciences*, *58*(25), PL365–PL372. https://doi.org/10.1016/0024-3205(96)00237-8.

Lepore, M., Vorel, S. R., Lowinson, J., & Gardner, E. L. (1995). Conditioned place preference induced by !D–9-tetrahydrocannabinol: Comparison with cocaine, morphine, and food reward. *Life Sciences*, *56*(23-24), 2073–2080. https://doi.org/10.1016/0024-3205(95)00191-8.

Leung, L. (2011). Cannabis and its derivatives: Review of medical use. *The Journal of the American Board of Family Medicine*, *24*(4), 452–462. https://doi.org/10.3122/jabfm.2011.04.100280.

Li, K., Fichna, J., Schicho, R., Saur, D., Bashashati, M., Mackie, K., et al. (2013). A role for O-1602 and G protein-coupled receptor GPR55 in the control of colonic motility in mice. *Neuropharmacology*, *71*, 255–263. https://doi.org/10.1016/j.neuropharm.2013.03.029.

Li, X., Hempel, B. J., Yang, H.-J., Han, X., Bi, G.-H., Gardner, E. L., et al. (2021). Dissecting the role of CB1 and CB2 receptors in cannabinoid reward versus aversion using transgenic CB1- and CB2-knockout mice. *European Neuropsychopharmacology, 43*, 38–51. https://doi.org/10.1016/j.euroneuro.2020.11.019.

Li, X., Hoffman, A. F., Peng, X. Q., Lupica, C. R., Gardner, E. L., & Xi, Z. X. (2009). Attenuation of basal and cocaine-enhanced locomotion and nucleus accumbens dopamine in cannabinoid CB1-receptor-knockout mice. *Psychopharmacology, 204*(1), 1–11. https://doi.org/10.1007/s00213-008-1432-0.

Li, Y., & Kim, J. (2015). Neuronal expression of CB2 cannabinoid receptor mRNAs in the mouse hippocampus. *Neuroscience, 311*, 253–267. https://doi.org/10.1016/j.neuroscience.2015.10.041.

Lichtman, A. H., & Martin, B. R. (1996). Delta 9-tetrahydrocannabinol impairs spatial memory through a cannabinoid receptor mechanism. *Psychopharmacology, 126*(2), 125–131. https://doi.org/10.1007/bf02246347.

Lichtman, A. H., & Martin, B. R. (1997). The selective cannabinoid antagonist SR 141716A blocks cannabinoid-induced antinociception in rats. *Pharmacology Biochemistry and Behavior, 57*(1), 7–12. https://doi.org/10.1016/S0091-3057(96)00121-9.

Liu, QR, Canseco-Alba, A, Liang, Y, Ishiguro, H, & Onaivi, ES. (2020). Low basal CB2R in dopamine neurons and microglia influences cannabinoid tetrad effects. *International Journal of Molecular Sciences, 21*(24), 9763. https://doi.org/10.3390/ijms21249763.

Liu, Q. R., Canseco-Alba, A., Liang, Y., Ishiguro, H., & Onaivi, E. S. (2020). Low Basal CB2R in Dopamine Neurons and Microglia Influences Cannabinoid Tetrad Effects. *International Journal of Molecular Sciences, 21*(24). https://doi.org/10.3390/ijms21249763.

Liu, Q.-R., Canseco-Alba, A., Zhang, H.-Y., Tagliaferro, P., Chung, M., Dennis, E., et al. (2017). Cannabinoid type 2 receptors in dopamine neurons inhibits psychomotor behaviors, alters anxiety, depression and alcohol preference. *Scientific Reports*, 7(1), 17410. https://doi.org/10.1038/s41598-017-17796-y.

Liu, Q.-R., Pan, C.-H., Hishimoto, A., Li, C.-Y., Xi, Z.-X., Llorente-Berzal, A., et al. (2009). Species differences in cannabinoid receptor 2 (CNR2 gene): Identification of novel human and rodent CB2 isoforms, differential tissue expression and regulation by cannabinoid receptor ligands. *Genes, Brain and Behavior, 8*(5), 519–530. https://doi.org/10.1111/j.1601-183X.2009.00498.x.

Liu, J., Scott, B. W., & Burnham, W. M. (2021). Effects of cannabidiol and Δ9-tetrahydrocannabinol in the elevated plus maze in mice. *Behavioural Pharmacology*. https://doi.org/10.1097/fbp.0000000000000636. Publish Ahead of Print.

Long, L. E., Chesworth, R., Huang, X.-F., McGregor, I. S., Arnold, J. C., & Karl, T. (2010). A behavioural comparison of acute and chronic Delta9-tetrahydrocannabinol and cannabidiol in C57BL/6JArc mice. *The international journal of neuropsychopharmacology/official scientific journal of the Collegium Internationale Neuropsychopharmacologicum (CINP), 13*(7), 861–876. https://doi.org/10.1017/S1461145709990605.

Lupica, C. R., & Riegel, A. C. (2005). Endocannabinoid release from midbrain dopamine neurons: a potential substrate for cannabinoid receptor antagonist treatment of addiction. *Neuropharmacology, 48*(8), 1105–1116. https://doi.org/10.1016/j.neuropharm.2005.03.016.

Ma, Z., Gao, F., Larsen, B., Gao, M., Luo, Z., Chen, D., et al. (2019). Mechanisms of cannabinoid CB(2) receptor-mediated reduction of dopamine neuronal excitability in mouse ventral tegmental area. *eBioMedicine, 42*, 225–237. https://doi.org/10.1016/j.ebiom.2019.03.040.

Ma, L., Jia, J., Niu, W., Jiang, T., Zhai, Q., Yang, L., et al. (2015). Mitochondrial CB1 receptor is involved in ACEA-induced protective effects on neurons and mitochondrial functions. *Scientific Reports, 5*(1), 12440. https://doi.org/10.1038/srep12440.

Mackie, K. (2008). Cannabinoid receptors: where they are and what they do. *Journal of Neuroendocrinology, 20*(Suppl 1), 10–14. https://doi.org/10.1111/j.1365-2826.2008.01671.x.
Maldonado, R., Baños, J. E., & Cabañero, D. (2016). The endocannabinoid system and neuropathic pain. *Pain, 157*, S23–S32. https://doi.org/10.1097/j.pain.0000000000000428.
Mallet, P. E., & Beninger, R. J. (1998a). The cannabinoid CB1 receptor antagonist SR141716A attenuates the memory impairment produced by Δ9-tetrahydrocannabinol or anandamide. *Psychopharmacology, 140*(1), 11–19. https://doi.org/10.1007/s002130050733.
Mallet, P. E., & Beninger, R. J. (1998b). Δ9-Tetrahydrocannabinol, but not the endogenous cannabinoid receptor ligand anandamide, produces conditioned place avoidance. *Life Sciences, 62*(26), 2431–2439. https://doi.org/10.1016/S0024-3205(98)00226-4.
Malone, D. T., & Taylor, D. A. (2001). Involvement of somatodendritic 5-HT1A receptors in Δ9-tetrahydrocannabinol-induced hypothermia in the rat. *Pharmacology Biochemistry and Behavior, 69*(3), 595–601. https://doi.org/10.1016/S0091-3057(01)00567-6.
Mansbach, R. S., Nicholson, K. L., Martin, B. R., & Balster, R. L. (1994). Failure of Delta(9)-tetrahydrocannabinol and CP 55,940 to maintain intravenous self-administration under a fixed-interval schedule in rhesus monkeys. *Behavioural Pharmacology, 5*(2), 219–225.
Marcellino, D., Carriba, P., Filip, M., Borgkvist, A., Frankowska, M., Bellido, I., et al. (2008). Antagonistic cannabinoid CB1/dopamine D2 receptor interactions in striatal CB1/D2 heteromers. A combined neurochemical and behavioral analysis. *Neuropharmacology, 54*(5), 815–823. https://doi.org/10.1016/j.neuropharm.2007.12.011.
Maresz, K., Carrier, E. J., Ponomarev, E. D., Hillard, C. J., & Dittel, B. N. (2005). Modulation of the cannabinoid CB2 receptor in microglial cells in response to inflammatory stimuli. *Journal of Neurochemistry, 95*(2), 437–445. https://doi.org/10.1111/j.1471-4159.2005.03380.x.
Marichal-Cancino, B. A., Fajardo-Valdez, A., Ruiz-Contreras, A. E., Mendez-Díaz, M., & Prospero-García, O. (2017). Advances in the physiology of GPR55 in the central nervous system. *Current Neuropharmacology, 15*(5), 771–778. https://doi.org/10.2174/1570159X14666160729155441.
Mato, S., Del Olmo, E., & Pazos, A. (2003). Ontogenetic development of cannabinoid receptor expression and signal transduction functionality in the human brain. *European Journal of Neuroscience, 17*(9), 1747–1754. https://doi.org/10.1046/j.1460-9568.2003.02599.x.
McKillop, A. M., Moran, B. M., Abdel-Wahab, Y. H. A., & Flatt, P. R. (2013). Evaluation of the insulin releasing and antihyperglycaemic activities of GPR55 lipid agonists using clonal beta-cells, isolated pancreatic islets and mice. *British Journal of Pharmacology, 170*(5), 978–990. https://doi.org/10.1111/bph.12356.
McMahon, L. R., Amin, M. R., & France, C. P. (2005). SR 141716A differentially attenuates the behavioral effects of Δ9-THC in rhesus monkeys. *Behavioural Pharmacology, 16*(5-6), 363–372. Retrieved from https://journals.lww.com/behaviouralpharm/Fulltext/2005/09000/SR_141716A_differentially_attenuates_the.8.aspx.
Mechoulam, R., & Parker, L. A. (2013). The endocannabinoid system and the brain. *Annual Review of Psychology, 64*(1), 21–47. https://doi.org/10.1146/annurev-psych-113011-143739.
Melis, M., Gessa, G. L., & Diana, M. (2000). Different mechanisms for dopaminergic excitation induced by opiates and cannabinoids in the rat midbrain. *Progress in Neuro-Psychopharmacology and Biological Psychiatry, 24*(6), 993–1006. https://doi.org/10.1016/S0278-5846(00)00119-6.
Melis, M., Perra, S., Muntoni, A. L., Pillolla, G., Lutz, B., Marsicano, G., et al. (2004). Prefrontal Cortex Stimulation Induces 2-Arachidonoyl-Glycerol-Mediated Suppression of Excitation in Dopamine Neurons. *The Journal of Neuroscience, 24*(47), 10707–10715. https://doi.org/10.1523/jneurosci.3502-04.2004.

Metna-Laurent, M., & Marsicano, G. (2015). Rising stars: Modulation of brain functions by astroglial type-1 cannabinoid receptors. *Glia*, *63*(3), 353–364. https://doi.org/10.1002/glia.22773.

Metna-Laurent, M., Mondésir, M., Grel, A., Vallée, M., & Piazza, P.-V. (2017). Cannabinoid-Induced Tetrad in Mice. *Current Protocols in Neuroscience*, *80*(1), 9.59.51–59.59.10. https://doi.org/10.1002/cpns.31.

Mishima, K., Egashira, N., Matsumoto, Y., Iwasaki, K., & Fujiwara, M. (2002). Involvement of reduced acetylcholine release in Δ9-tetrahydrocannabinol-induced impairment of spatial memory in the 8-arm radial maze. *Life Sciences*, *72*(4), 397–407. https://doi.org/10.1016/S0024-3205(02)02274-9.

Monory, K., Blaudzun, H., Massa, F., Kaiser, N., Lemberger, T., Schütz, G., et al. (2007). Genetic Dissection of Behavioural and Autonomic Effects of Δ9-Tetrahydrocannabinol in Mice. *PLoS Biology*, *5*(10), e269. https://doi.org/10.1371/journal.pbio.0050269.

Moreno, S., Farioli-Vecchioli, S., & Cerù, M. P. (2004). Immunolocalization of peroxisome proliferator-activated receptors and retinoid x receptors in the adult rat CNS. *Neuroscience*, *123*(1), 131–145. https://doi.org/10.1016/j.neuroscience.2003.08.064.

Mothet, J.-P., Parent, A. T., Wolosker, H., Brady, R. O., Linden, D. J., Ferris, C. D., et al. (2000). d-Serine is an endogenous ligand for the glycine site of the N-methyl-d-aspartate receptor. *Proceedings of the National Academy of Sciences*, *97*(9), 4926–4931. https://doi.org/10.1073/pnas.97.9.4926.

Munro, S., Thomas, K. L., & Abu-Shaar, M. (1993). Molecular characterization of a peripheral receptor for cannabinoids. *Nature*, *365*(6441), 61–65. https://doi.org/10.1038/365061a0.

Murphy, M., Mills, S., Winstone, J., Leishman, E., Wager-Miller, J., Bradshaw, H., et al. (2017). Chronic adolescent Δ9-tetrahydrocannabinol treatment of male mice leads to long-term cognitive and behavioral dysfunction, which are prevented by concurrent cannabidiol treatment. *Cannabis and Cannabinoid Research*, *2*(1), 235–246.

Nava, F., Carta, G., & Gessa, G. L. (2000). Permissive Role of Dopamine D2 Receptors in the Hypothermia Induced by Δ9-Tetrahydrocannabinol in Rats. *Pharmacology Biochemistry and Behavior*, *66*(1), 183–187. https://doi.org/10.1016/S0091-3057(00)00231-8.

Navarrete, M., & Araque, A. (2008). Endocannabinoids mediate neuron-astrocyte communication. *Neuron*, *57*(6), 883–893. https://doi.org/10.1016/j.neuron.2008.01.029.

Nedungadi, T. P., Dutta, M., Bathina, C. S., Caterina, M. J., & Cunningham, J. T. (2012). Expression and distribution of TRPV2 in rat brain. *Experimental Neurology*, *237*(1), 223–237. https://doi.org/10.1016/j.expneurol.2012.06.017.

Nent, E., Nozaki, C., Schmöle, A.-C., Otte, D., & Zimmer, A. (2019). CB2 receptor deletion on myeloid cells enhanced mechanical allodynia in a mouse model of neuropathic pain. *Scientific Reports*, *9*(1), 7468. https://doi.org/10.1038/s41598-019-43858-4. 31097758.

Newman, A. H., Cao, J., Keighron, J. D., Jordan, C. J., Bi, G.-H., Liang, Y., et al. (2019). Translating the atypical dopamine uptake inhibitor hypothesis toward therapeutics for treatment of psychostimulant use disorders. *Neuropsychopharmacology*, *44*(8), 1435–1444. https://doi.org/10.1038/s41386-019-0366-z.

Nguyen, J. D., Aarde, S. M., Vandewater, S. A., Grant, Y., Stouffer, D. G., Parsons, L. H., et al. (2016). Inhaled delivery of Δ9-tetrahydrocannabinol (THC) to rats by e-cigarette vapor technology. *Neuropharmacology*, *109*, 112–120. https://doi.org/10.1016/j.neuropharm.2016.05.021.

Norris, C., Szkudlarek, H. J., Pereira, B., Rushlow, W., & Laviolette, S. R. (2019). The bivalent rewarding and aversive properties of Δ9-tetrahydrocannabinol are mediated through dissociable opioid receptor substrates and neuronal modulation mechanisms in distinct striatal sub-regions. *Scientific Reports*, *9*(1), 9760. https://doi.org/10.1038/s41598-019-46215-7.

O'Sullivan, S. E., Tarling, E. J., Bennett, A. J., Kendall, D. A., & Randall, M. D. (2005). Novel time-dependent vascular actions of Δ9-tetrahydrocannabinol mediated by peroxisome proliferator-activated receptor gamma. *Biochemical and Biophysical Research Communications*, *337*(3), 824–831. https://doi.org/10.1016/j.bbrc.2005.09.121.

Oliveira da Cruz, J. F., Robin, L. M., Drago, F., Marsicano, G., & Metna-Laurent, M. (2016). Astroglial type-1 cannabinoid receptor (CB1): A new player in the tripartite synapse. *Neuroscience*, *323*, 35–42. https://doi.org/10.1016/j.neuroscience.2015.05.002.

Onaivi, E. S., Chaudhuri, G., Abaci, A. S., Parker, M., Manier, D. H., Martin, P. R., et al. (1999). Expression of cannabinoid receptors and their gene transcripts in human blood cells. *Progress in Neuro-Psychopharmacology and Biological Psychiatry*, *23*(6), 1063–1077. https://doi.org/10.1016/S0278-5846(99)00052-4.

O'Sullivan, S. E. (2016). An update on PPAR activation by cannabinoids. *British Journal of Pharmacology*, *173*(12), 1899–1910. https://doi.org/10.1111/bph.13497.

Panlilio, L. V., Ferré, S., Yasar, S., Thorndike, E. B., Schindler, C. W., & Goldberg, S. R. (2012). Combined effects of THC and caffeine on working memory in rats. *British Journal of Pharmacology*, *165*(8), 2529–2538. https://doi.org/10.1111/j.1476-5381.2011.01554.x.

Patel, K. D., Davison, J. S., Pittman, Q. J., & Sharkey, K. A. (2010). Cannabinoid CB2 Receptors in Health and Disease. *Current Medicinal Chemistry*, *17*(14), 1394–1410. https://doi.org/10.2174/092986710790980041.

Pertwee, R. G. (1997). Pharmacology of cannabinoid CB1 and CB2 receptors. *Pharmacology & Therapeutics*, *74*(2), 129–180.

Pertwee, R. (2005). Pharmacological actions of cannabinoids. In R. G. Pertwee (Ed.), *Cannabinoids* (pp. 1–51). Berlin, Heidelberg: Springer Berlin Heidelberg.

Pertwee, R. (2006). Cannabinoid pharmacology: The first 66 years. *British Journal of Pharmacology*, *147*(Suppl. 1), S163–S171. https://doi.org/10.1038/sj.bjp.0706406.

Pertwee, R. G. (2008a). The diverse CB1 and CB2 receptor pharmacology of three plant cannabinoids: delta9-tetrahydrocannabinol, cannabidiol and delta9-tetrahydrocannabivarin. *British Journal of Pharmacology*, *153*(2), 199–215. https://doi.org/10.1038/sj.bjp.0707442.

Pertwee, R. G. (2008b). Ligands that target cannabinoid receptors in the brain: from THC to anandamide and beyond. *Addiction Biology*, *13*(2), 147–159. https://doi.org/10.1111/j.1369-1600.2008.00108.x.

Pertwee, R. G., Howlett, A. C., Abood, M. E., Alexander, S. P. H., Di Marzo, V., Elphick, M. R., et al. (2010). International Union of Basic and Clinical Pharmacology. LXXIX. Cannabinoid Receptors and Their Ligands: Beyond CB_1 and CB_2. *Pharmacological Reviews*, *62*(4), 588–631. https://doi.org/10.1124/pr.110.003004.

Pietr, M., Kozela, E., Levy, R., Rimmerman, N., Lin, Y. H., Stella, N., et al. (2009). Differential changes in GPR55 during microglial cell activation. *FEBS Letters*, *583*(12), 2071–2076. https://doi.org/10.1016/j.febslet.2009.05.028.

Piomelli, D. (2003). The molecular logic of endocannabinoid signalling. *Nature Reviews Neuroscience*, *4*(11), 873–884. https://doi.org/10.1038/nrn1247.

Prini, P., Zamberletti, E., Manenti, C., Gabaglio, M., Parolaro, D., & Rubino, T. (2020). Neurobiological mechanisms underlying cannabis-induced memory impairment. *European Neuropsychopharmacology*, *36*, 181–190. https://doi.org/10.1016/j.euroneuro.2020.02.002.

Ranganathan, M., & D'Souza, D. C. (2006). The acute effects of cannabinoids on memory in humans: a review. *Psychopharmacology*, *188*(4), 425–444. https://doi.org/10.1007/s00213-006-0508-y.

Rawls, S. M., Cabassa, J., Geller, E. B., & Adler, M. W. (2002). CB_1 receptors in the preoptic anterior hypothalamus regulate WIN 55212-2 [(4,5-dihydro-2-methyl-4(4-morpholinylmethyl))-1-(1-naphthalenyl-carbonyl)-6H-pyrrolo[3,2,1ij]quinolin-6-one]-induced hypothermia. *Journal of Pharmacology and Experimental Therapeutics*, *301*(3), 963–968. https://doi.org/10.1124/jpet.301.3.963.

Rawls, S. M., Cowan, A., Tallarida, R. J., Geller, E. B., & Adler, M. W. (2002). N-methyl-d-aspartate antagonists and WIN 55212-2 [4,5-dihydro-2-methyl-4(4-morpholinyl-methyl)-1-(1-naphthalenyl-carbonyl)-6H-pyrrolo[3,2,1-ij]quinolin-6-one], a cannabinoid agonist, interact to produce synergistic hypothermia. *Journal of Pharmacology and Experimental Therapeutics*, *303*(1), 395–402. https://doi.org/10.1124/jpet.102.037473.

Reis, S. L., Silva, H. B., Almeida, M., Cunha, R. A., Simões, A. P., & Canas, P. M. (2019). Adenosine A1 and A2A receptors differently control synaptic plasticity in the mouse dorsal and ventral hippocampus. *Journal of Neurochemistry*, *151*(2), 227–237. https://doi.org/10.1111/jnc.14816.

Remmers, F., Lange, M. D., Hamann, M., Ruehle, S., Pape, H.-C., & Lutz, B. (2017). Addressing sufficiency of the CB1 receptor for endocannabinoid-mediated functions through conditional genetic rescue in forebrain GABAergic neurons. *Brain Structure and Function*, *222*(8), 3431–3452. https://doi.org/10.1007/s00429-017-1411-5.

Resstel, L. B. M., Moreira, F. A., & Guimarães, F. S. (2009). Chapter 16 Endocannabinoid System and Fear Conditioning. In *Vol. 81*. *Vitamins & Hormones* (pp. 421–440). Academic Press.

Resstel, L. B. M., Tavares, R. F., Lisboa, S. F. S., Joca, S. R. L., Corrêa, F. M. A., & Guimarães, F. S. (2009). 5-HT1A receptors are involved in the cannabidiol-induced attenuation of behavioural and cardiovascular responses to acute restraint stress in rats. *British Journal of Pharmacology*, *156*(1), 181–188. https://doi.org/10.1111/j.1476-5381.2008.00046.x.

Rey, A. A., Purrio, M., Viveros, M.-P., & Lutz, B. (2012). Biphasic Effects of Cannabinoids in Anxiety Responses: CB1 and GABAB Receptors in the Balance of GABAergic and Glutamatergic Neurotransmission. *Neuropsychopharmacology*, *37*(12), 2624–2634. https://doi.org/10.1038/npp.2012.123.

Rinaldi-Carmona, M., Barth, F., Héaulme, M., Shire, D., Calandra, B., Congy, C., et al. (1994). SR141716A, a potent and selective antagonist of the brain cannabinoid receptor. *FEBS Letters*, *350*(2-3), 240–244. https://doi.org/10.1016/0014-5793(94)00773-x.

Rios, C., Gomes, I., & Devi, L. A. (2006). μ opioid and CB1 cannabinoid receptor interactions: reciprocal inhibition of receptor signaling and neuritogenesis. *British Journal of Pharmacology*, *148*(4), 387–395. https://doi.org/10.1038/sj.bjp.0706757.

Rodriguez, J. J., Mackie, K., & Pickel, V. M. (2001). Ultrastructural localization of the CB1 cannabinoid receptor in mu-opioid receptor patches of the rat Caudate putamen nucleus. *The Journal of Neuroscience: The Official Journal of the Society for Neuroscience*, *21*(3), 823–833. https://doi.org/10.1523/JNEUROSCI.21-03-00823.2001.

Romero-Zerbo, S., Rafacho, A., Díaz-Arteaga, A., Suárez, J., Quesada, I., Imbernón, M., et al. (2011). A role for the putative cannabinoid receptor GPR55 in the islets of Langerhans. *The Journal of Endocrinology*, *211*(2), 177–185.

Rubino, T., Guidali, C., Vigano, D., Realini, N., Valenti, M., Massi, P., et al. (2008). CB1 receptor stimulation in specific brain areas differently modulate anxiety-related behaviour. *Neuropharmacology*, *54*(1), 151–160. https://doi.org/10.1016/j.neuropharm.2007.06.024.

Rubino, T., Sala, M., Viganò, D., Braida, D., Castiglioni, C., Limonta, V., et al. (2007). Cellular mechanisms underlying the anxiolytic effect of low doses of peripheral [Delta]9-tetrahydrocannabinol in rats. *Neuropsychopharmacology*, *32*(9), 2036–2045. https://doi.org/10.1038/sj.npp.1301330.

Ruehle, S., Remmers, F., Romo-Parra, H., Massa, F., Wickert, M., Wörtge, S., et al. (2013). Cannabinoid CB1 receptor in dorsal telencephalic glutamatergic neurons: Distinctive sufficiency for hippocampus-dependent and amygdala-dependent synaptic and behavioral functions. *The Journal of Neuroscience*, *33*(25), 10264–10277. https://doi.org/10.1523/jneurosci.4171-12.2013.

Russo, E. B., Burnett, A., Hall, B., & Parker, K. K. (2005). Agonistic properties of cannabidiol at 5-HT1a receptors. *Neurochemical Research*, *30*(8), 1037–1043. https://doi.org/10.1007/s11064-005-6978-1.

Ryberg, E., Larsson, N., Sjögren, S., Hjorth, S., Hermansson, N. O., Leonova, J., et al. (2007). The orphan receptor GPR55 is a novel cannabinoid receptor. *British Journal of Pharmacology*, *152*(7), 1092–1101. https://doi.org/10.1038/sj.bjp.0707460.

Salio, C., Fischer, J., Franzoni, M. F., Mackie, K., Kaneko, T., & Conrath, M. (2001). CB1-cannabinoid and μ-opioid receptor co-localization on postsynaptic target in the rat dorsal horn. *Neuroreport*, *12*(17), 3689–3692. Retrieved from https://journals.lww.com/neuroreport/Fulltext/2001/12040/CB1_cannabinoid_and___opioid_receptor.17.aspx.

Sanberg, P. R., Bunsey, M. D., Giordano, M., & Norman, A. B. (1988). The catalepsy test: its ups and downs. *Behavioral Neuroscience*, *102*(5), 748–759. https://doi.org/10.1037//0735-7044.102.5.748.

Sano, K., Mishima, K., Koushi, E., Orito, K., Egashira, N., Irie, K., et al. (2008). Δ9-Tetrahydrocannabinol-induced catalepsy-like immobilization is mediated by decreased 5-HT neurotransmission in the nucleus accumbens due to the action of glutamate-containing neurons. *Neuroscience*, *151*(2), 320–328. https://doi.org/10.1016/j.neuroscience.2007.10.026.

Savinainen, J. R., Saario, S. M., Niemi, R., Järvinen, T., & Laitinen, J. T. (2003). An optimized approach to study endocannabinoid signaling: Evidence against constitutive activity of rat brain adenosine A1 and cannabinoid CB1 receptors. *British Journal of Pharmacology*, *140*(8), 1451–1459. https://doi.org/10.1038/sj.bjp.0705577.

Schatz, A. R., Lee, M., Condie, R. B., Pulaski, J. T., & Kaminski, N. E. (1997). Cannabinoid receptors CB1 and CB2: a characterization of expression and adenylate cyclase modulation within the immune system. *Toxicology and Applied Pharmacology*, *142*(2), 278–287. https://doi.org/10.1006/taap.1996.8034.

Schauer, G. L., King, B. A., Bunnell, R. E., Promoff, G., & McAfee, T. A. (2016). Toking, vaping, and eating for health or fun: marijuana use patterns in adults, U.S., 2014. *American Journal of Preventive Medicine*, *50*(1), 1–8. https://doi.org/10.1016/j.amepre.2015.05.027.

Schramm-Sapyta, N., Cha, Y., Chaudhry, S., Wilson, W., Swartzwelder, H. S., & Kuhn, C. (2007). Differential anxiogenic, aversive, and locomotor effects of THC in adolescent and adult rats. *Psychopharmacology*, *191*(4), 867–877. https://doi.org/10.1007/s00213-006-0676-9.

Schwab, MH, Bartholomae, A, Heimrich, B, Feldmeyer, D, Druffel-Augustin, S, Goebbels, S, et al. (2000). Neuronal basic helix-loop-helix proteins (NEX and BETA2/Neuro D) regulate terminal granule cell differentiation in the hippocampus. *Journal of Neuroscience*, *20*(10), 3714–3724.

Sciolino, N. R., Zhou, W., & Hohmann, A. G. (2011). Enhancement of endocannabinoid signaling with JZL184, an inhibitor of the 2-arachidonoylglycerol hydrolyzing enzyme monoacylglycerol lipase, produces anxiolytic effects under conditions of high environmental aversiveness in rats. *Pharmacological Research*, *64*(3), 226–234. https://doi.org/10.1016/j.phrs.2011.04.010.

Secci, M. E., Mascia, P., Sagheddu, C., Beggiato, S., Melis, M., Borelli, A. C., et al. (2019). Astrocytic mechanisms involving kynurenic acid control Δ9-tetrahydrocannabinol-induced increases in glutamate release in brain reward-processing areas. *Molecular Neurobiology*, *56*(5), 3563–3575. https://doi.org/10.1007/s12035-018-1319-y.

Sengupta, T., Jaryal, A. K., & Mallick, H. N. (2016). Effects of NMDA and non-NMDA ionotropic glutamate receptors in the medial preoptic area on body temperature in awake rats. *Journal of Thermal Biology*, *61*, 1–7. https://doi.org/10.1016/j.jtherbio.2016.07.020.

Shang, Y., & Tang, Y. (2017). The central cannabinoid receptor type-2 (CB2) and chronic pain. *International Journal of Neuroscience, 127*(9), 812–823. https://doi.org/10.1080/00207454.2016.1257992.

Shibasaki, K., Ishizaki, Y., & Mandadi, S. (2013). Astrocytes express functional TRPV2 ion channels. *Biochemical and Biophysical Research Communications, 441*(2), 327–332. https://doi.org/10.1016/j.bbrc.2013.10.046.

Sierra, S., Luquin, N., Rico, A. J., Gómez-Bautista, V., Roda, E., Dopeso-Reyes, I. G., et al. (2015). Detection of cannabinoid receptors CB1 and CB2 within basal ganglia output neurons in macaques: changes following experimental parkinsonism. *Brain Structure and Function, 220*(5), 2721–2738. https://doi.org/10.1007/s00429-014-0823-8.

Solinas, M., Zangen, A., Thiriet, N., & Goldberg, S. R. (2004). β-Endorphin elevations in the ventral tegmental area regulate the discriminative effects of Δ-9-tetrahydrocannabinol. *European Journal of Neuroscience, 19*(12), 3183–3192. https://doi.org/10.1111/j.0953-816X.2004.03420.x.

Soria, G., Castañé, A., Berrendero, F., Ledent, C., Parmentier, M., Maldonado, R., et al. (2004). Adenosine A2A receptors are involved in physical dependence and place conditioning induced by THC. *European Journal of Neuroscience, 20*(8), 2203–2213. https://doi.org/10.1111/j.1460-9568.2004.03682.x.

Sousa, V. C., Assaife-Lopes, N., Ribeiro, J. A., Pratt, J. A., Brett, R. R., & Sebastião, A. M. (2011). Regulation of hippocampal cannabinoid CB1 receptor actions by adenosine A1 receptors and chronic caffeine administration: Implications for the effects of Δ9-tetrahydrocannabinol on spatial memory. *Neuropsychopharmacology, 36*(2), 472–487. https://doi.org/10.1038/npp.2010.179.

Spencer, S., Neuhofer, D., Chioma, V. C., Garcia-Keller, C., Schwartz, D. J., Allen, N., et al. (2018). A model of Δ9-tetrahydrocannabinol self-administration and reinstatement that alters synaptic plasticity in nucleus accumbens. *Biological Psychiatry, 84*(8), 601–610. https://doi.org/10.1016/j.biopsych.2018.04.016.

Spiller, K. J., Bi, G. H., He, Y., Galaj, E., Gardner, E. L., & Xi, Z. X. (2019). Cannabinoid CB(1) and CB(2) receptor mechanisms underlie cannabis reward and aversion in rats. *British Journal of Pharmacology, 176*(9), 1268–1281. https://doi.org/10.1111/bph.14625.

Spindle, T. R., Cone, E. J., Schlienz, N. J., Mitchell, J. M., Bigelow, G. E., Flegel, R., et al. (2018). Acute effects of smoked and vaporized cannabis in healthy adults who infrequently use cannabis: A crossover trial. *JAMA Network Open, 1*(7), e184841. https://doi.org/10.1001/jamanetworkopen.2018.4841. 30646391. PMCID: PMC6324384.

Stefano, G. B., Liu, Y., & Goligorsky, M. S. (1996). Cannabinoid receptors are coupled to nitric oxide release in invertebrate immunocytes, microglia, and human monocytes*. *Journal of Biological Chemistry, 271*(32), 19238–19242. https://doi.org/10.1074/jbc.271.32.19238.

Stella, N. (2010). Cannabinoid and cannabinoid-like receptors in microglia, astrocytes, and astrocytomas. *Glia, 58*(9), 1017–1030. https://doi.org/10.1002/glia.20983.

Stempel, A. V., Stumpf, A., Zhang, H.-Y., Özdoğan, T., Pannasch, U., Theis, A.-K., et al. (2016). Cannabinoid type 2 receptors mediate a cell type-specific plasticity in the hippocampus. *Neuron, 90*(4), 795–809. https://doi.org/10.1016/j.neuron.2016.03.034.

Sun, Y., Alexander, S. P. H., Garle, M. J., Gibson, C. L., Hewitt, K., Murphy, S. P., et al. (2007). Cannabinoid activation of PPAR alpha; a novel neuroprotective mechanism. *British Journal of Pharmacology, 152*(5), 734–743. https://doi.org/10.1038/sj.bjp.0707478.

Szabo, B., Siemes, S., & Wallmichrath, I. (2002). Short communication: Inhibition of GABAergic neurotransmission in the ventral tegmental area by cannabinoids. *European Journal of Neuroscience, 15*(12), 2057–2061. https://doi.org/10.1046/j.1460-9568.2002.02041.x.

Szkudlarek, H. J., Desai, S. J., Renard, J., Pereira, B., Norris, C., Jobson, C. E. L., et al. (2019). Δ-9-Tetrahydrocannabinol and Cannabidiol produce dissociable effects on prefrontal cortical executive function and regulation of affective behaviors. *Neuropsychopharmacology*, *44*(4), 817–825. https://doi.org/10.1038/s41386-018-0282-7.

Taffe, M. A., Creehan, K. M., & Vandewater, S. A. (2015). Cannabidiol fails to reverse hypothermia or locomotor suppression induced by Δ(9)-tetrahydrocannabinol in Sprague-Dawley rats. *British Journal of Pharmacology*, *172*(7), 1783–1791. https://doi.org/10.1111/bph.13024.

Taffe, M. A., Creehan, K. M., Vandewater, S. A., Kerr, T. M., & Cole, M. (2021). Effects of Δ^9-tetrahydrocannabinol (THC) vapor inhalation in Sprague-Dawley and Wistar rats. *Experimental and Clinical Psychopharmacology*, *29*(1), 1–13. https://doi.org/10.1037/pha0000373.

Takahashi, R. N., & Singer, G. (1979). Self-administration of Δ9-tetrahydrocannabinol by rats. *Pharmacology Biochemistry and Behavior*, *11*(6), 737–740. https://doi.org/10.1016/0091-3057(79)90274-0.

Takeda, S., Ikeda, E., Su, S., Harada, M., Okazaki, H., Yoshioka, Y., et al. (2014). Δ9-THC modulation of fatty acid 2-hydroxylase (FA2H) gene expression: Possible involvement of induced levels of PPARα in MDA-MB-231 breast cancer cells. *Toxicology*, *326*, 18–24. https://doi.org/10.1016/j.tox.2014.09.011.

Tanda, G., Munzar, P., & Goldberg, S. R. (2000). Self-administration behavior is maintained by the psychoactive ingredient of marijuana in squirrel monkeys. *Nature Neuroscience*, *3*(11), 1073–1074. https://doi.org/10.1038/80577.

Tanda, G., Pontieri, F. E., & Chiara, G. D. (1997). Cannabinoid and heroin activation of mesolimbic dopamine transmission by a common μ_1 opioid receptor mechanism. *Science*, *276*(5321), 2048. https://doi.org/10.1126/science.276.5321.2048.

Todd, S. M., & Arnold, J. C. (2016). Neural correlates of interactions between cannabidiol and Delta(9)-tetrahydrocannabinol in mice: implications for medical cannabis. *British Journal of Pharmacology*, *173*(1), 53–65. https://doi.org/10.1111/bph.13333.

Tseng, A. H., & Craft, R. M. (2004). CB1 receptor mediation of cannabinoid behavioral effects in male and female rats. *Psychopharmacology*, *172*(1), 25–30. https://doi.org/10.1007/s00213-003-1620-x.

Tsou, K., Mackie, K., Sañudo-Peña, M. C., & Walker, J. M. (1999). Cannabinoid CB1 receptors are localized primarily on cholecystokinin-containing GABAergic interneurons in the rat hippocampal formation. *Neuroscience*, *93*(3), 969–975. https://doi.org/10.1016/S0306-4522(99)00086-X.

Valjent, E., & Maldonado, R. (2000). A behavioural model to reveal place preference to Δ9-tetrahydrocannabinol in mice. *Psychopharmacology*, *147*(4), 436–438. https://doi.org/10.1007/s002130050013.

van der Stelt, M., & Di Marzo, V. (2003). The endocannabinoid system in the basal ganglia and in the mesolimbic reward system: implications for neurological and psychiatric disorders. *European Journal of Pharmacology*, *480*(1), 133–150. https://doi.org/10.1016/j.ejphar.2003.08.101.

Van Sickle, M. D., Duncan, M., Kingsley, P. J., Mouihate, A., Urbani, P., Mackie, K., et al. (2005). Identification and functional characterization of brainstem cannabinoid CB_2 receptors. *Science*, *310*(5746), 329–332. https://doi.org/10.1126/science.1115740.

Vann, R. E., Gamage, T. F., Warner, J. A., Marshall, E. M., Taylor, N. L., Martin, B. R., et al. (2008). Divergent effects of cannabidiol on the discriminative stimulus and place conditioning effects of Δ^9-tetrahydrocannabinol. *Drug and Alcohol Dependence*, *94*(1-3), 191–198. https://doi.org/10.1016/j.drugalcdep.2007.11.017.

Varvel, S. A., Bridgen, D. T., Tao, Q., Thomas, B. F., Martin, B. R., & Lichtman, A. H. (2005). Δ^9Tetrahydrocannbinol accounts for the antinociceptive, hypothermic, and cataleptic effects of marijuana in mice. *Journal of Pharmacology and Experimental Therapeutics, 314*(1), 329–337. https://doi.org/10.1124/jpet.104.080739.

Varvel, S. A., & Lichtman, A. H. (2002). Evaluation of CB_1 receptor knockout mice in the morris water maze. *Journal of Pharmacology and Experimental Therapeutics, 301*(3), 915–924. https://doi.org/10.1124/jpet.301.3.915.

Varvel, S. A., Wiley, J. L., Yang, R., Bridgen, D. T., Long, K., Lichtman, A. H., et al. (2006). Interactions between THC and cannabidiol in mouse models of cannabinoid activity. *Psychopharmacology, 186*(2), 226–234. https://doi.org/10.1007/s00213-006-0356-9.

Vickstrom, C. R., Liu, X., Liu, S., Hu, M.-M., Mu, L., Hu, Y., et al. (2021). Role of endocannabinoid signaling in a septohabenular pathway in the regulation of anxiety- and depressive-like behavior. *Molecular Psychiatry, 26*(7), 3178–3191. https://doi.org/10.1038/s41380-020-00905-1.

Vidal-Puig, A., Jimenez-Liñan, M., Lowell, B. B., Hamann, A., Hu, E., Spiegelman, B., et al. (1996). Regulation of PPAR gamma gene expression by nutrition and obesity in rodents. *The Journal of Clinical Investigation, 97*(11), 2553–2561. https://doi.org/10.1172/JCI118703.

Villapol, S. (2018). Roles of peroxisome proliferator-activated receptor gamma on brain and peripheral inflammation. *Cellular and Molecular Neurobiology, 38*(1), 121–132. https://doi.org/10.1007/s10571-017-0554-5.

Viñals, X., Moreno, E., Lanfumey, L., Cordomí, A., Pastor, A., de La Torre, R., et al. (2015). cognitive impairment induced by Delta9-tetrahydrocannabinol occurs through heteromers between cannabinoid CB1 and serotonin 5-HT2A receptors. *PLoS Biology, 13*(7), e1002194. https://doi.org/10.1371/journal.pbio.1002194.

Waksman, Y., Olson, J. M., Carlisle, S. J., & Cabral, G. A. (1999). The central cannabinoid receptor (CB1) mediates inhibition of nitric oxide production by rat microglial cells. *Journal of Pharmacology and Experimental Therapeutics, 288*(3), 1357–1366. Retrieved from https://jpet.aspetjournals.org/content/jpet/288/3/1357.full.pdf.

Wang, X. F., Galaj, E., Bi, G. H., Zhang, C., He, Y., Zhan, J., et al. (2020). Different receptor mechanisms underlying phytocannabinoid- versus synthetic cannabinoid-induced tetrad effects: Opposite roles of CB(1)/CB(2) versus GPR55 receptors. *British Journal of Pharmacology, 177*(8), 1865–1880. https://doi.org/10.1111/bph.14958.

Warden, A., Truitt, J., Merriman, M., Ponomareva, O., Jameson, K., Ferguson, L. B., et al. (2016). Localization of PPAR isotypes in the adult mouse and human brain. *Scientific Reports, 6*(1), 27618. https://doi.org/10.1038/srep27618.

Whiting, P. F., Wolff, R. F., Deshpande, S., Di Nisio, M., Duffy, S., Hernandez, A. V., et al. (2015). Cannabinoids for medical use: A systematic review and meta-analysis. *JAMA, 313*(24), 2456–2473. https://doi.org/10.1001/jama.2015.6358.

Wiebelhaus, J. M., Grim, T. W., Owens, R. A., Lazenka, M. F., Sim-Selley, L. J., Abdullah, R. A., et al. (2015). Δ^9-Tetrahydrocannabinol and endocannabinoid degradative enzyme inhibitors attenuate intracranial self-stimulation in mice. *Journal of Pharmacology and Experimental Therapeutics, 352*(2), 195–207. https://doi.org/10.1124/jpet.114.218677.

Wiley, J. L., & Martin, B. R. (2003). Cannabinoid pharmacological properties common to other centrally acting drugs. *European Journal of Pharmacology, 471*(3), 185–193. https://doi.org/10.1016/S0014-2999(03)01856-9.

World Health Organization. (2021). *Cannabis*. Alcohol, Drugs and Addictive Behaviors Unit.

Wu, C.-S., Chen, H., Sun, H., Zhu, J., Jew, C. P., Wager-Miller, J., et al. (2013). GPR55, a G-protein coupled receptor for lysophosphatidylinositol, plays a role in motor coordination. *PLoS One, 8*(4), e60314. https://doi.org/10.1371/journal.pone.0060314.

Xi, Z. X., Peng, X. Q., Li, X., Song, R., Zhang, H. Y., Liu, Q. R., et al. (2011). Brain cannabinoid CB_2 receptors modulate cocaine's actions in mice. *Nature Neuroscience*, *14*(9), 1160–1166. https://doi.org/10.1038/nn.2874.

Yu, X. H., Cao, C. Q., Martino, G., Puma, C., Morinville, A., St-Onge, S., et al. (2010). A peripherally restricted cannabinoid receptor agonist produces robust anti-nociceptive effects in rodent models of inflammatory and neuropathic pain. *Pain*, *151*(2), 337–344. https://doi.org/10.1016/j.pain.2010.07.019.

Zangen, A., Solinas, M., Ikemoto, S., Goldberg, S. R., & Wise, R. A. (2006). Two brain sites for cannabinoid reward. *The Journal of Neuroscience*, *26*(18), 4901–4907. https://doi.org/10.1523/jneurosci.3554-05.2006.

Zhang, H.-Y., Bi, G. H., Li, X., Li, J., Qu, H., Zhang, S. J., et al. (2015). Species differences in cannabinoid receptor 2 and receptor responses to cocaine self-administration in mice and rats. *Neuropsychopharmacology*, *40*(4), 1037–1051. https://doi.org/10.1038/npp.2014.297.

Zhang, H. Y., De Biase, L., Chandra, R., Shen, H., Liu, Q. R., Gardner, E., et al. (2021). Repeated cocaine administration upregulates CB2 receptor expression in striatal medium-spiny neurons that express dopamine D1 receptors in mice. *Acta Pharmacologica Sinica*. https://doi.org/10.1038/s41401-021-00712-6. 34316031.

Zhang, H.-Y., Gao, M., Liu, Q.-R., Bi, G.-H., Li, X., Yang, H.-J., et al. (2014). Cannabinoid CB_2 receptors modulate midbrain dopamine neuronal activity and dopamine-related behavior in mice. *Proceedings of the National Academy of Sciences*, *111*(46), E5007–E5015. https://doi.org/10.1073/pnas.1413210111.

Zhang, H.-Y., Gao, M., Shen, H., Bi, G.-H., Yang, H.-J., Liu, Q.-R., et al. (2017). Expression of functional cannabinoid CB2 receptor in VTA dopamine neurons in rats. *Addiction Biology*, *22*(3), 752–765. https://doi.org/10.1111/adb.12367.

Zhang, H.-Y., Shen, H., Gao, M., Ma, Z., Hempel, B. J., Bi, G.-H., et al. (2021). Cannabinoid CB2 receptors are expressed in glutamate neurons in the red nucleus and functionally modulate motor behavior in mice. *Neuropharmacology*, *189*, 108538. https://doi.org/10.1016/j.neuropharm.2021.108538.

Zhang, H. Y., Shen, H., Jordan, C. J., Liu, Q. R., Gardner, E. L., Bonci, A., et al. (2019). CB(2) receptor antibody signal specificity: correlations with the use of partial CB(2)-knockout mice and anti-rat CB(2) receptor antibodies. *Acta Pharmacologica Sinica*, *40*(3), 398–409. https://doi.org/10.1038/s41401-018-0037-3.

Zimmer, A., Valjent, E., König, M., Zimmer, A. M., Robledo, P., Hahn, H., et al. (2001). Absence of Δ-9-tetrahydrocannabinol dysphoric effects in dynorphin-deficient mice. *The Journal of Neuroscience*, *21*(23), 9499–9505. Retrieved from http://www.jneurosci.org/content/21/23/9499.abstract.

Zimmer, A., Zimmer, A. M., Hohmann, A. G., Herkenham, M., & Bonner, T. I. (1999). Increased mortality, hypoactivity, and hypoalgesia in cannabinoid CB1 receptor knockout mice. *Proceedings of the National Academy of Sciences*, *96*(10), 5780–5785. https://doi.org/10.1073/pnas.96.10.5780.

Zuardi, A. W., Shirakawa, I., Finkelfarb, E., & Karniol, I. G. (1982). Action of cannabidiol on the anxiety and other effects produced by delta 9-THC in normal subjects. *Psychopharmacology*, *76*(3), 245–250.

CHAPTER TEN

Potential therapeutic targets for the treatment of opioid abuse and pain

Norikazu Kiguchi[a,*] and Mei-Chuan Ko[b]

[a]Department of Physiological Sciences, School of Pharmaceutical Sciences, Wakayama Medical University, Wakayama, Japan
[b]Department of Physiology and Pharmacology, Wake Forest University School of Medicine, Winston-Salem, NC, United States
*Corresponding author: e-mail address: kiguchi@wakayama-med.ac.jp

Contents

1. Introduction 337
2. Opioid abuse 338
   2.1 Background of opioid abuse 338
   2.2 Treatment of opioid abuse 340
   2.3 G protein signaling-biased MOP receptor agonists 341
   2.4 Orexin-1 receptor antagonists 342
   2.5 NOP receptor agonists 343
   2.6 Emerging targets 345
3. Pain 346
   3.1 Background of pain 346
   3.2 Treatment of pain 347
   3.3 Treatment of pain by peripheral actions 348
4. Treatment of pain by spinal and supraspinal actions 353
   4.1 Cannabinoid receptor agonists 353
   4.2 NOP receptor agonists 355
5. Conclusions 357
Acknowledgments 358
Conflict of interest 358
References 358

Abstract

Although μ-opioid peptide (MOP) receptor agonists are effective analgesics available in clinical settings, their serious adverse effects put limits on their use. The marked increase in abuse and misuse of prescription opioids for pain relief and opioid overdose mortality in the past decade has seriously impacted society. Therefore, safe analgesics that produce potent analgesic effects without causing MOP receptor-related adverse effects are needed. This review highlights the potential therapeutic targets for the

Advances in Pharmacology, Volume 93
ISSN 1054-3589
https://doi.org/10.1016/bs.apha.2021.09.002

treatment of opioid abuse and pain based on available evidence generated through preclinical studies and clinical trials. To ameliorate the abuse-related effects of opioids, orexin-1 receptor antagonists and mixed nociceptin/MOP partial agonists have shown promising results in translational aspects of animal models. There are several promising non-opioid targets for selectively inhibiting pain-related responses, including nerve growth factor inhibitors, voltage-gated sodium channel inhibitors, and cannabinoid- and nociceptin-related ligands. We have also discussed several emerging and novel targets. The current medications for opioid abuse are opioid receptor-based ligands. Although neurobiological studies in rodents have discovered several non-opioid targets, there is a translational gap between rodents and primates. Given that the neuroanatomical aspects underlying opioid abuse and pain are different between rodents and primates, it is pivotal to investigate the functional profiles of these non-opioid compounds compared to those of clinically used drugs in non-human primate models before initiating clinical trials. More pharmacological studies of the functional efficacy, selectivity, and tolerability of these newly discovered compounds in non-human primates will accelerate the development of effective medications for opioid abuse and pain.

Abbreviations

CB cannabinoid
CB1R cannabinoid 1 receptor
CB2R cannabinoid 2 receptor
CBD cannabidiol
CNS central nervous system
DOP δ-opioid peptide
DORA dual orexin antagonist
DRG dorsal root ganglia
FDA Food and Drug Administration
GPCR G-protein coupled receptor
KOP κ-opioid peptide
MOP μ-opioid peptide
N/OFQ nociceptin/orphanin FQ
NAC nucleus accumbens
Na_v voltage-gated sodium channel
NGF nerve growth factor
NHP non-human primate
NK1 neurokinin-1
NOP nociceptin/orphanin FQ peptide
OA osteoarthritis
OUD opioid use disorder
OX1R orexin-1 receptor
OX2R orexin-2 receptor
PFC prefrontal cortex
SDH spinal dorsal horn
STING stimulator of interferon genes
TAAR1 trace amine-associated receptor 1

THC	Δ9-tetrahydrocannabinol
TrkA	tyrosine kinase A
TRPV1	transient receptor potential vanilloid 1
TTX	tetrodotoxin
VTA	ventral tegmental area

1. Introduction

Although nociceptive somatosensory systems, such as pain, are indispensable to detect abnormalities or disorders in organs and protect tissue damage, intractable pain associated with several chronic diseases should be effectively relieved. Pain is considered a burden that largely reduces quality of life and impairs productivity globally (Cohen, Vase, & Hooten, 2021; Collaborators et al., 2018). In the US, over 100 million adults experience chronic pain annually, and the annual total cost of pain, including direct costs, decreased wages, and lost productivity, largely eclipsed that of any other diseases such as heart diseases, cancer, and diabetes (Holmes, 2016). Thus, there is an unmet need to establish effective treatment strategies for intractable pain. People recognized different types of pain, such as burning and stabbing, and the opium poppy (*Papaver somniferum* L.) was used to relieve pain for thousands of years (Brook, Bennett, & Desai, 2017). In 1805, morphine was identified as the active pain-killing ingredient of the opium poppy. The discovery of morphine has had a huge impact that contributed to not only scientific knowledge but also human lives (Pain, 2016). Till date, this ingredient remains one of the most potent analgesics, and several of its derivatives or related compounds that act on μ-opioid peptide (MOP) receptors are widely used for the management of severe pain associated with serious diseases, such as cancer and myocardial infarction (Degenhardt et al., 2019; Kreek, Reed, & Butelman, 2019).

Opioid receptors were identified and cloned in the 1990s after several years of biochemical, physiological, and pharmacological research (Chen, Mestek, Liu, Hurley, & Yu, 1993; Evans, Keith, Morrison, Magendzo, & Edwards, 1992; Yasuda et al., 1993). Classical opioid receptors consist of three subtypes—MOP, δ-opioid peptide (DOP), and κ-opioid peptide (KOP) receptors. These receptors are widely distributed in the peripheral and central nervous system (CNS) and are particularly located in pain-processing regions, such as the dorsal root ganglia (DRG), spinal dorsal horn

(SDH), and brain in mammals (Corder, Castro, Bruchas, & Scherrer, 2018; Fields, 2004). Under physiological conditions, endogenous opioid peptides activate cognate opioid receptors to reduce pain and influence reward processing and mood through Gi-protein coupled receptor (GPCR) signaling. This in turn inhibits adenylate cyclase and voltage-gated calcium channels and activates inward potassium channels, resulting in a reduction in synaptic transmission (Darcq & Kieffer, 2018). Among the opioid receptors, the MOP receptor is known to be the sole receptor responsible for the analgesic effects of morphine. This observation is based on rodent studies that demonstrated that the deletion of the MOP receptor eliminates the analgesic effects of morphine (Matthes et al., 1996). The MOP receptor is also a key therapeutic target for clinically used opioids (such as oxycodone, fentanyl, methadone, buprenorphine), indicating that activation of the MOP receptor has substantial utility to relieve severe pain. However, MOP receptors also produce serious dose-limiting adverse effects such as abuse liability, respiratory depression, constipation, itching sensation, and physical dependence (Gunther et al., 2018). Although MOP receptor ligands are the strongest analgesics currently known to humans, these adverse effects often compromise therapeutic effects and cause serious problems, such as opioid use disorder (OUD).

Recently, an epidemic of opioid abuse and overdoses emerged in North America and a part of Europe. The marked increase in abuse and misuse of prescription opioids for pain relief and opioid overdose mortality in the past decade has had considerable impact on society (Dart et al., 2015; Degenhardt et al., 2014). Given that MOP receptor agonists are the only drugs that can relieve unbearable pain associated with cancer or some other medical conditions, it is pivotal to develop novel safe opioid analgesics that produce potent analgesic effects without causing MOP receptor-related adverse effects (Volkow & Collins, 2017). In this review, we have compiled evidence from preclinical and clinical studies to uncover the regulatory mechanisms of opioid abuse and analgesia and propose newly discovered targets as potential therapeutics for the treatment of opioid abuse and pain.

2. Opioid abuse

2.1 Background of opioid abuse

Opioid abuse is a brain disorder associated with behavioral, psychological, and neurochemical manifestations (Kreek et al., 2019). Although a breakthrough finding in the 1970s revealed the importance of dopamine systems, for several decades, key components of drug addiction have been considered responsible for dysregulation of dopaminergic neurotransmitter systems (Nutt, Lingford-Hughes, Erritzoe, & Stokes, 2015). Dopamine systems normally contribute to various brain functions. Further, dopamine neurons play an important role in attention and working memory and are necessary for regulating motivation, reward, and similar motor functions (Bromberg-Martin, Matsumoto, & Hikosaka, 2010). Moreover, dopamine is associated with the pathogenesis of a proportion of psychosis and involved in positive mood in humans (Cousins, Butts, & Young, 2009). Notably, the mesolimbic dopaminergic system, known as the reward system, originates from the ventral tegmental area (VTA) and projects into the corticolimbic regions, such as the nucleus accumbens (NAC) and the prefrontal cortex (PFC) (Kourrich, Calu, & Bonci, 2015). The majority of NAC neurons are medium spiny neurons that receive excitatory glutamatergic inputs from the PFC, thalamus, amygdala, and VTA; therefore, they are considered key reward-related neural circuits (Kourrich et al., 2015). Based on these data, drug addiction is hypothesized to be due to drugs that induce dopamine release and they are considered to have a risk of abuse. There is a significant causal link between dopamine levels and actions in the brain and addiction to psychostimulants (such as amphetamine and cocaine) (Bello et al., 2011; Sulzer, 2011). However, studies in rodents have demonstrated that blockade of dopamine receptors do not attenuate the rewarding effects of opioids (Fields & Margolis, 2015; Hnasko, Sotak, & Palmiter, 2005), and clinical trials could not support that this blockade was effective for the treatment of drug addiction in humans (Lingford-Hughes, Welch, Peters, Nutt, & British Association for Psychopharmacology, 2012; Rothman, 1994).

Preclinical animal studies have suggested that the opioid system largely contributes to reward and aversion and that dysregulation of opioid neurotransmission is crucial for drug abuse (Darcq & Kieffer, 2018). MOP receptors are widely distributed throughout the mesocorticolimbic circuitry in the brain (Corder et al., 2018). The prevailing disinhibition hypothesis proposes that activation of MOP receptors expressed by GABAergic interneurons in the VTA reduces local inhibition, subsequently resulting in the activation of dopamine neurons (Fields & Margolis, 2015; Morales & Margolis, 2017). However, as discussed above, such a hypothesis has not been confirmed as several brain regions that receive dopaminergic input, such as NAC, have abundant MOP receptors (Cui et al., 2014). Furthermore, dopamine-independent opioid reward based on MOP receptor-expressing neurons driving opioid reward outside the VTA has been demonstrated (Hnasko et al., 2005). MOP and KOP receptors oppositely regulate hedonic homeostasis, and MOP and KOP receptor agonists lead to euphoria and dysphoria, respectively. Unlike MOP receptors, KOP receptors in dopamine neurons of the VTA counteract MOP receptor-mediated activity in the NAC and PFC (Margolis et al., 2006) and disrupt behaviors. KOP receptors in the medium spiny neurons of the NAC regulate the input to the amygdala to negatively regulate motivational processes (Tejeda et al., 2017). Accumulating evidence suggests that nociceptin/orphanin FQ (N/OFQ) peptide (NOP) and its cognate receptor system, known as the fourth opioid receptor subtype, play unique roles in negatively regulating craving for abused drugs (Kiguchi, Ding, & Ko, 2020; Parker et al., 2019). Although evidence on the contribution of DOP receptors in opioid abuse is limited, four opioid receptor subtypes have been implicated in drug-dependent motivation underlying reward and abuse potential. Given that addiction is a complex mixture of behaviors and other neurological factors, there is no rationale to support that a single neurotransmitter (dopamine) could be associated with all aspects of addiction, suggesting that addiction can be considered a multiple-neurotransmitter disorder (Kreek et al., 2019; Nutt et al., 2015; Rasmussen, White, & Acri, 2019).

2.2 Treatment of opioid abuse

Currently there are three medications available for the treatment of OUD. These medications are methadone (a full MOP receptor agonist), buprenorphine (a low-efficacy partial MOP receptor agonist), and naltrexone (a MOP receptor antagonist). Each of these medications has its own unique pharmacological properties that require considerable knowledge and skills for appropriate prescribing (Kreek et al., 2019; Saxon, 2013; Schuckit, 2016). The appropriate use of these medications has also been limited by stigma, insufficient medical education, and inadequate resources (Kreek et al., 2019). Scientists have developed different strategies to address the opioid crisis. While reviewing the literature, we selected five approaches to update readers with recent findings. It should be noted that given the complex nature of opioid addiction, it is not realistic to expect a magic bullet to treat OUD. Successful treatment outcomes for patients with OUD require integration of both pharmacotherapy and psychosocial interventions

(Rasmussen et al., 2019; Volkow & Blanco, 2020). Here, we have focused on opioid-related compounds with improved side-effect profiles and those that could suppress the abuse liability of opioids.

2.3 G protein signaling-biased MOP receptor agonists

MOP receptor activation initiates two different signaling pathways—G protein signaling and β-arrestin recruitment (Whistler, Chuang, Chu, Jan, & von Zastrow, 1999; Zhang et al., 1998). Earlier studies using β-arrestin2 knockout mice have shown that the antinociceptive effect of morphine could be improved, that is, potentiation of morphine can be enhanced, tolerance to it can be slowly developed, and side effects such as respiratory depression and constipation due to its usage can be reduced (Bohn et al., 1999; Bohn, Gainetdinov, Lin, Lefkowitz, & Caron, 2000; Raehal, Walker, & Bohn, 2005). Therefore, a G protein signaling-biased ligand devoid of β-arrestin recruitment may exert enhanced analgesia with improved safety and tolerability (Luttrell, Maudsley, & Bohn, 2015; Schmid & Bohn, 2009; Violin, Crombie, Soergel, & Lark, 2014). Oliceridine (TRV130) was the first reported G protein-biased MOP receptor agonist (Chen et al., 2013). In rodents, oliceridine, a potent analgesic across several pain models, causes less respiratory depression and gastrointestinal dysfunction (DeWire et al., 2013). Although oliceridine has progressed to clinical trials and has been approved by the US Food and Drug Administration (FDA), its therapeutic window is not as wide as originally expected. Namely, an analgesic effect is seen and accompanied by respiratory depression (Soergel et al., 2014; Viscusi et al., 2016).

Recently, scientists have discovered a series of G protein signaling-biased MOP agonists as new chemical entities with different bias factors, i.e., the degree of separation measured in the G protein signaling and β-arrestin2 recruitment assays. Through computational docking of over 3 million molecules against the MOP receptor structure and further optimization, PZM21 was discovered as a G protein-biased MOP receptor agonist. This compound exerted antinociceptive effects without rewarding effects and respiratory depression in mice (Manglik et al., 2016). Studies have also shown that PZM21 produces morphine-like respiratory depression in mice (Hill et al., 2018) and oxycodone-like reinforcing effects in monkeys (Ding et al., 2020), indicating that there is no difference in the two major side effects of opioids (respiratory depression and abuse liability) between PZM21 and the other clinically used opioid analgesics.

SR-17018 was identified as a G protein-biased MOP agonist with the highest bias factor and minimal respiratory depression even at higher doses (Schmid et al., 2017). However, in another study, SR-17018, PZM21, and oliceridine displayed low intrinsic efficacy similar to that of buprenorphine in MOP receptor regulation, regardless of the downstream signaling pathways (Gillis et al., 2020). Given the correlation between the therapeutic windows and their intrinsic efficacies at the MOP receptor, it is reasonable to attribute the improved side-effect profile of G protein-biased MOP agonists to their low intrinsic efficacy (Azevedo Neto et al., 2020; Gillis et al., 2020). In particular, these G protein-biased MOP agonists with low intrinsic efficacy can function like buprenorphine, which explains their effectiveness in attenuating the abuse-related effects of opioids in animal models. Although substitution with SR-17018 in morphine-tolerant mice restored the antinociceptive effect of morphine in the hot plate test (Grim et al., 2020), additional studies are required to investigate the degree to which SR-17018 is different from buprenorphine in terms of its analgesic and adverse effects in different animal models. With regard to the retained abuse liability of G protein-biased MOP agonists (Ding et al., 2020; Zamarripa et al., 2018), it is difficult to ascertain how biased G protein signaling can substantially refine opioid therapeutics in response to the opioid crisis.

2.4 Orexin-1 receptor antagonists

Accumulated evidence on the orexin receptors has opened an exciting avenue for the treatment of drug abuse (Baimel et al., 2015; James, Mahler, Moorman, & Aston-Jones, 2017). Orexin neurons in the lateral hypothalamus project to several brain regions involved in reward and drug-seeking behavior (Harris, Wimmer, & Aston-Jones, 2005; Hopf, 2020). For example, the VTA has been demonstrated to be an important site of orexin signaling in drug abuse (James et al., 2017). Blockade of the orexin-1 receptor (OX1R) in the VTA attenuates the rewarding property of MOP receptor agonists (Zarepour, Fatahi, Sarihi, & Haghparast, 2014). Importantly, SB-334867, an OX1R antagonist, reduced heroin self-administration in rats (Smith & Aston-Jones, 2012). A recent study further demonstrated that SB-334867 decreased oxycodone self-administration, but the orexin-2 receptor (OX2R) antagonist TCSOX229 does not affect oxycodone self-administration in rats (Matzeu & Martin-Fardon, 2020). In addition, OX1R is critical for the expression of morphine withdrawal, and increased numbers of orexin-producing cells may play a role in maintaining opioid addiction (Georgescu et al., 2003; Sharf, Sarhan, & Dileone, 2008; Thannickal et al., 2018).

Using behavioral economics procedures, preclinical studies have also demonstrated that SB-334867 reduces motivation to consume highly abused opioid fentanyl and attenuates cue-induced reinstatement of fentanyl seeking (Fragale, Pantazis, James, & Aston-Jones, 2019). Considerable evidence supports that orexin-based therapies may represent an effective treatment strategy for addiction across a various drugs of abuse, including opioids, stimulants, alcohol, and nicotine (Fragale et al., 2021; Hopf, 2020). According to the available literature, OX1R antagonists are effective in inhibiting the motivation for drug rewards. In contrast, OX2R antagonists and dual orexin antagonists (DORAs) are useful for facilitating sleep (Fragale et al., 2021; Perrey & Zhang, 2020). Although ample evidence supports the therapeutic potential of OX1R antagonists in the treatment of opioid abuse in animal models, there is currently no FDA-approved OX1R antagonist. Nevertheless, a DORA, suvorexant, has been approved by the FDA for the treatment of insomnia. Several clinical trials have investigated the functional efficacy of suvorexant in patients with OUD and other substance use disorders (Fragale et al., 2021; James et al., 2020). Given that sleep impairment is often associated with OUD, it is worthwhile to wait for results of ongoing clinical trials of suvorexant. Further, preclinical studies rigorously comparing the functional efficacy and therapeutic window of OX1R antagonists and DORAs in the context of OUD-related endpoints will facilitate the future development of orexin-based ligands as a new treatment approach for OUD.

2.5 NOP receptor agonists

Recent research on the NOP receptor has opened another avenue as a potential medication for the dynamic epidemic of opioid abuse (Lin & Ko, 2013; Rasmussen et al., 2019; Toll, Bruchas, Calo, Cox, & Zaveri, 2016). Briefly, activation of the NOP receptor inhibits sensory processing, dopamine release, and neural transmission, which are considered viable targets for both pain and addiction (Kiguchi et al., 2020; Schroder, Lambert, Ko, & Koch, 2014; Toll et al., 2016). NOP agonists alone do not produce rewarding or aversive effects (Ko et al., 2009; Le Pen, Wichmann, Moreau, & Jenck, 2002). In an earlier study, the effects of opioids, measured by conditioned place preference, was blocked by selective NOP receptor agonists (Murphy, Lee, & Maidment, 1999). However, selective NOP receptor agonists did not display functional selectivity, that is, their sedative doses attenuated the reinforcing effects mediated by both opioids and food, measured by the self-administration assay (Podlesnik et al., 2011; Sukhtankar, Lagorio, & Ko, 2014). Given that opioid-induced rewarding and reinforcing effects are not fully mediated by dopamine signaling (Fields & Margolis, 2015; Nutt et al., 2015), selective NOP agonists may have mild-to-moderate efficacy in suppressing the abuse liability of opioids.

Clinical trials have documented that buprenorphine is an effective medication for OUD as it can reduce opioid craving and relapse risk (Kakko et al., 2019; Reimer, Vogelmann, Trümper, & Scherbaum, 2020). However, buprenorphine can produce moderate euphoric effects and physical dependency. It is also associated with an additional risk of diversion and misuse or abuse of medication (Johanson, Arfken, di Menza, & Schuster, 2012; Lavonas et al., 2014). Nonetheless, added naloxone in the commonly available formulations (e.g., suboxone) is expected to decrease abuse potential (Jones et al., 2017). Given that NOP receptor agonists synergistically enhance the antinociceptive effect of buprenorphine and partially inhibit MOP receptor-mediated reinforcing effects (Cremeans, Gruley, Kyle, & Ko, 2012; Ding et al., 2021), a ligand with mixed NOP/MOP receptor agonist activities may have a wider therapeutic window with fewer side effects (Kiguchi et al., 2020; Lin & Ko, 2013). This hypothesis is supported by the functional profile of BU08028, a buprenorphine analog, with additional NOP receptor binding affinity and efficacy, which shows improved analgesic potency and a lack of reinforcing effects and physical dependency (Ding et al., 2016). The promising therapeutic profile of mixed NOP/MOP partial agonists is not compound specific as this class of compounds in different chemical structures include safe analgesics without abuse potential and physical dependency in non-human primates (NHPs) (Ding et al., 2018; Kiguchi et al., 2019). More importantly, ligands with dual actions (such as partial MOP agonists and NOP agonists) can inhibit the reinforcing effects of oxycodone without affecting the reinforcing effects of food pellets in NHP self-administration models, possessing a functional selectivity for inhibiting opioid abuse-related effects (Ding et al., 2018). Although cebranopadol, a mixed NOP/MOP full agonist, has been developed as a safe analgesic (Calo & Lambert, 2018; Tzschentke, Linz, Koch, & Christoph, 2019), its moderate reinforcing strength may limit its use in a broader therapeutic context (Ding et al., 2021). Nonetheless, given the clinical utility of buprenorphine, its analogs with additional NOP receptor agonist activity and other "*centrally penetrant*" combined NOP/MOP partial agonists possess great potential for treating OUD. In particular, more preclinical studies should be undertaken to further investigate the functional efficacy of such ligands with different brain-penetrant degrees in the context of OUD-related endpoints in NHP models (Ding & Ko, 2021).

2.6 Emerging targets

After the discovery of trace amine-associated receptor 1 (TAAR1) and subsequent development of selective small-molecule TAAR1 agonists (Borowsky et al., 2001; Sotnikova, Caron, & Gainetdinov, 2009), there has been a growing interest in the therapeutic potential of this receptor (Tonelli & Cichero, 2020). TAAR1 agonists are known to reduce the firing rate of dopaminergic neurons (Revel et al., 2011) and have great potential as therapeutic targets for neuropsychiatric diseases and drug addiction (Liu & Li, 2018; Schwartz et al., 2018). Although TAAR1 agonists have been extensively demonstrated as a promising pharmacotherapy for psychostimulant addiction (Liu, Wu, & Li, 2020), little is known about whether these agonists can modulate the abuse-related effects of opioids. Importantly, a recent study demonstrated that RO5263397, a TAAR1 partial agonist, attenuates morphine intake and motivation to self-administer morphine and decreases cue- and drug-induced reinstatement of morphine-seeking behavior in rats (Liu et al., 2021). Selective inhibition of the reinforcing effects of morphine by RO5263397 without changing the antinociceptive effect of morphine warrants additional animal and human studies to develop an optimal treatment strategy to curb opioid abuse.

Ibogaine, an alkaloid extracted from plants from the family Apocynaceae such as *Tabernanthe iboga*, is classified as a hallucinogen owing to its psychedelic property (Iyer, Favela, Zhang, & Olson, 2021). Although human studies on the safety and efficacy of ibogaine are lacking, anecdotal reports and animal studies support that it can reduce opioid cravings and prevent relapse (Belgers et al., 2016). Ibogaine has been reported to cause acute motor impairment and cardiotoxicity in animals. However, additional studies are required to determine its risks and potential benefits. As ibogaine is a psychoplastogen that can promote functional and structural neural plasticity in addiction-related circuitry, chemists have concentrated on the function-oriented synthesis of analogs of iboga alkaloids (Iyer et al., 2021).

Importantly, tabernanthalog was discovered through a psychoplastogenic pharmacophore of ibogaine; it does not possess the toxicity and hallucinogenic effects of ibogaine (Cameron et al., 2021). Systemic administration of tabernanthalog reduced both heroin and sucrose self-administration, indicating that its inhibitory effect could be due to non-selective disruption of the operant response. Nonetheless, pretreatment with tabernanthalog prevented only cue-induced reinstatement of heroin and not sucrose-seeking behavior in rats (Cameron et al., 2021). These new findings encourage additional behavioral and neurochemical studies on tabernanthalog to determine its functional efficacy and selectivity across different animal models of OUD.

3. Pain

3.1 Background of pain

Primary sensory neurons transmit electrical impulses that encode specific sensory information to the CNS (the SDH and brainstem). Among heterogeneous sensory neurons, C- or Aδ-fibers are nociceptors that respond to noxious (such as thermal, mechanical, and chemical) stimuli that are essential for the recognition of pain, while Aβ-fibers play a role in sensing tactile information (Moehring, Halder, Seal, & Stucky, 2018; Peirs & Seal, 2016). For the detection and transmission of nociceptive information, specialized cation channels, such as transient receptor potential vanilloid 1 (TRPV1) and voltage-gated sodium channels (Na_vs), are necessary to amplify these signals for generation of action potential (Waxman & Zamponi, 2014). Subsequently, propagation of action potentials to the central terminals of sensory neurons leads to the release of neurotransmitters (such as glutamate and neuropeptides), which activate secondary CNS neurons by binding to postsynaptic cognate receptors. Primary sensory neurons input corresponding laminae in the SDH, which is the region for integration of peripheral input and descending supraspinal regulation. Most C- and Aδ-fibers form synapses in the superficial laminae (I and II), and Aβ-fibers project to deeper laminae (III–V) (Braz, Solorzano, Wang, & Basbaum, 2014; Moehring et al., 2018). The majority of SDH neurons consist of excitatory or inhibitory interneurons that locally modulate pain processing, while the other minor population is neurokinin-1 (NK1) receptor-expressing projection neurons located in laminae I (Peirs & Seal, 2016). Projection neurons convey pain information to several supraspinal areas such as the thalamus, parabrachial nucleus, amygdala, and cortex

(Todd, 2010). Recent studies have uncovered complicated pain-processing mechanisms at the peripheral and SDH levels, suggesting that these areas could be reasonable therapeutic targets for pain (Woolf, 2020).

Pain is classified into three types—nociceptive, neuropathic, and nociplastic according to its etiology, pathophysiology, anatomical presentation, intensity, and duration (Raja et al., 2020). Nociceptive pain is caused by the activation of nociceptors and is important for defensive behaviors under physiological conditions, while continued noxious stimuli lead to pathological nociceptive pain. For example, osteoarthritis (OA) causes intense joint pain based on hyperactivation of nociceptors (Basbaum, Bautista, Scherrer, & Julius, 2009). To deal with such pain, a pharmacotherapy directly targeting molecules expressed on nociceptors, for instance, TRPV1 and other cation channels, might be effective (Moran, McAlexander, Biro, & Szallasi, 2011). In the event of tissue injury and inflammation, alterations in nociceptor function cause hypersensitivity and spontaneous pain. Nevertheless, if the inflammation is acute and transient, non-steroidal anti-inflammatory drugs can effectively suppress inflammatory pain (Woolf, 2020). Neuropathic pain is elicited by lesions or disorders in the somatosensory nervous system and present allodynia (pain caused by innoxious stimuli) and hyperalgesia, which are exaggerated responses to noxious stimuli (Attal, Bouhassira, & Baron, 2018). Compared to inflammatory pain, neuropathic pain is normally intractable and long lasting because of structural and functional alterations occurring in the nervous system, at least in part, through neuro-immune mechanisms (Ji, Chamessian, & Zhang, 2016). Nociplastic pain is defined as pain occurring in the absence of noxious stimuli, inflammation, or damage to the nervous system (Fitzcharles et al., 2021). Thus, it is very challenging to appropriately control neuropathic and nociplastic pain because of their complicated mechanisms. To appropriately deal with different types of pain, the extent to which the component of pain is mechanistically linked needs to be determined.

3.2 Treatment of pain

Currently, there are a limited number of options that produce clinically meaningful analgesia, and efforts to develop novel effective analgesics are ongoing (Yekkirala, Roberson, Bean, & Woolf, 2017). Traditionally used analgesics, such as opioids, non-steroidal anti-inflammatory drugs, acetaminophen, and antiepileptics, were discovered first for their analgesic effects, after which the target molecules were identified. In contrast, serotonin-norepinephrine re-uptake inhibitors and gabapentinoids have been identified based on preclinical studies of pain-regulatory mechanisms (Woolf, 2020). Although it is necessary to use these drugs as front-line treatment, they do not sufficiently relieve some types of pain because of their dose-limiting adverse effects or diversity of pathophysiology (Attal & Bouhassira, 2015; Cohen et al., 2021). Given the complicated mechanisms of pain processing, it might be reasonable to discover novel analgesic targets based on preclinical studies. TRPV1, NK1 receptor, Na_Vs, and nerve growth factor (NGF) have been nominated as candidates for analgesics that block excessive input of somatosensory nociceptive information into the SDH. Despite numerous studies demonstrating that such molecules (i.e., TRPV1 and NK1 receptor) significantly contribute to several types of pain in rodents (Nilius & Szallasi, 2014; Steinhoff, von Mentzer, Geppetti, Pothoulakis, & Bunnett, 2014; Yekkirala et al., 2017), inhibitors for TRPV1 or NK1 receptor failed clinical human studies because of their lower efficacy than originally anticipated or unexpected adverse effects. These facts suggest that there are difficulties in developing novel analgesics that are safe and clinically effective. Hence, reliance on this approach alone may not be appropriate to identify clinically effective therapeutic targets. Human diseases and biological responses are not well simulated in rodents because of anatomical and functional gaps between rodents and humans (Balsters, Zerbi, Sallet, Wenderoth, & Mars, 2020; Seok et al., 2013; Warren et al., 2020). It is very important to conduct preclinical studies that replicate human pain conditions using multiple outcome measures and different species (Fig. 1).

3.3 Treatment of pain by peripheral actions

3.3.1 NGF inhibitors

Accumulating evidence suggests that neurotrophins, such as NGF and brain-derived neurotrophic factor, largely contribute to several types of pain through peripheral and central mechanisms (Ji, Xu, & Gao, 2014). NGF is the most characterized neurotrophin that activates nociceptive sensory neurons to convey pain signals from the periphery to the CNS, and its effects on pain processing have been well investigated (Denk, Bennett, & McMahon, 2017). Although NGF underlies the development of sensory neurons, it is also required to maintain the homeostasis of neurons and other tissues. NGF forms a ligand-receptor complex with the high-affinity receptor tyrosine kinase A (TrkA), and the complex is translocated to the nuclei of DRG

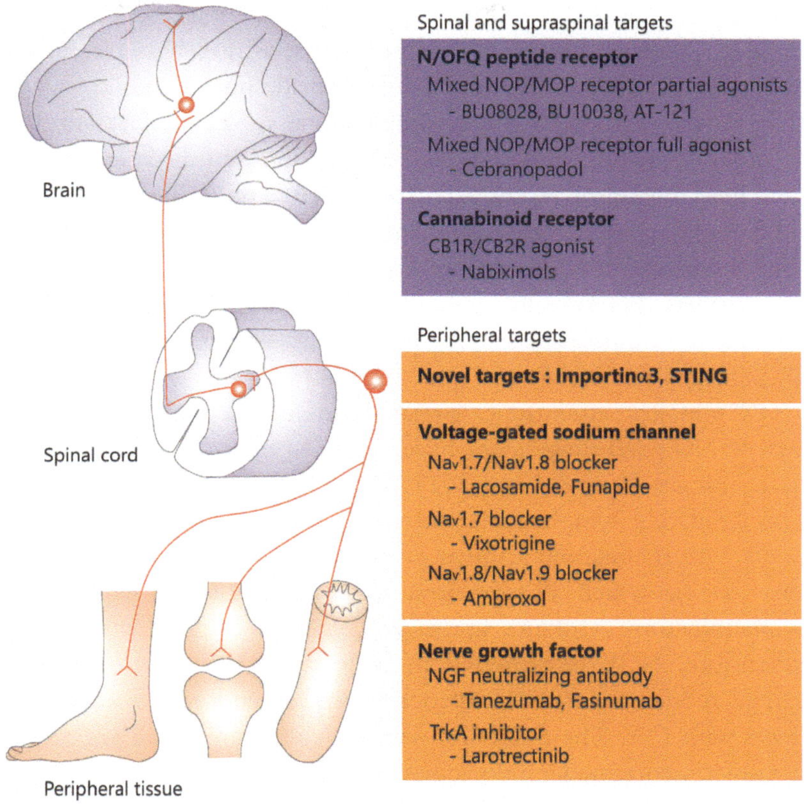

Fig. 1 Potential therapeutic targets for the treatment of pain. Primary sensory neurons transmit electrical impulses that encode specific sensory information to the spinal cord, subsequently projection neurons in the dorsal horn convey pain information to the brain. Given the complicated mechanisms of pain processing, it might be reasonable to discover novel analgesic targets based on preclinical studies. At the same time, it is also very important to conduct preclinical studies that replicate human pain conditions. CB1R; cannabinoid 1 receptor, CB2R; cannabinoid 2 receptor, MOP; μ- opioid peptide, Na_V; voltage-gated sodium channel, NGF; nerve growth factor, N/OFQ; nociceptin/orphanin FQ, NOP; nociceptin/orphanin FQ peptide, STING; stimulator of interferon genes, TrkA; tyrosine kinase A.

neurons. Subsequently, phosphorylation of the NGF-TrkA complex enhances gene transcription (Denk et al., 2017; Ehlers, Kaplan, Price, & Koliatsos, 1995). In response to nociceptive (such as thermal, mechanical, and chemical) stimuli, substance P and calcitonin gene-related peptide are upregulated by NGF-TrkA signaling. Although these neuropeptides are transported to the central terminals of sensory neurons, they can also be released from peripheral terminals to act as proinflammatory molecules in tissue (Wise, Seidel, & Lane, 2021). Moreover, NGF increases the excitability of DRG neurons when nociceptors, such as TRPV1, are activated, resulting in peripheral sensitization (Ji, Samad, Jin, Schmoll, & Woolf, 2002). Given that NGF is a multifunctional molecule that affects not only the C- and Aδ-fibers of DRG neurons but also the bone and other tissues, musculoskeletal diseases are closely related to NGF signaling among the different types of chronic pain (Lane & Corr, 2017). Notably, NGF plays an important role in bone metabolism and regeneration as documented in animal studies. Peripherally released NGF facilitates bone formation by increasing the number of osteoblasts in mice with bone fractures (Wise et al., 2021).

NGF inhibitors attenuate OA-related pain in mice, suggesting that inhibition of NGF signaling might have favorable effects on musculoskeletal pain in humans (Lane & Corr, 2017; Wise et al., 2021). NGF is expressed on accumulating lymphocytes and monocytes in the synovial fluid in patients with rheumatoid arthritis or OA (Barthel et al., 2009; Stoppiello et al., 2014), which is supported by findings that substance P and pro-inflammatory cytokines upregulate NGF in cultured synovial cells. Furthermore, NGF is expressed in bone-associated cells (such as subchondral mononuclear cells, osteoclasts, and chondrocytes) in tissues of patients with OA. The expression levels of NGF are associated with age and synovitis scores, suggesting a correlation between NGF and chronic pain caused by OA (Aso et al., 2019). Based on these findings, a number of small compounds and antibodies that inhibit NGF and TrkA functions have been tested in both preclinical and clinical studies. Larotrectinib, which inhibits TrkA, TrkB, and TrkC, has been approved for the treatment of solid tumors (Drilon et al., 2018). As the therapeutic potential of NGF antibodies has also been demonstrated in animal models of bone cancer pain, it is pivotal to further undertake clinical studies to assess the effectiveness of NGF inhibitors (Lucchesi et al., 2017). However, other small molecules, such as ASP7962, a TrkA antagonist, did not show the desired efficacy in patients with knee OA (Watt et al., 2019). Although, several monoclonal antibodies have been investigated, a majority of these molecules have not entered clinical trials because of lower efficacy or unexpected adverse effects, such as osteonecrosis. Tanezumab and fasinumab are currently being evaluated in clinical trials for OA and chronic low back pain with promising results for further consideration (Wise et al., 2021). Therefore, preclinical and clinical studies have supported the therapeutic potential of NGF-TrkA signaling for chronic pain associated with musculoskeletal diseases.

3.3.2 Na_v inhibitors

Among the different types of Na_vs that are expressed in humans, $Na_v1.7$, $Na_v1.8$, and $Na_v1.9$ are localized on DRG neurons and are crucial for peripheral signaling in nociceptive pain (Dib-Hajj, Yang, Black, & Waxman, 2013; Goodwin & McMahon, 2021). Na_vs consist of an ion-conducting pore-forming α subunit and one to two β subunits; their trafficking and gating properties are due to the α subunit. These Na_vs are divided into the tetrodotoxin (TTX)-sensitive subtype (Nav1.7) and the TTX-resistant subtype ($Na_v1.8$ and $Na_v1.9$). TTX-sensitive subtypes are activated more rapidly and show faster kinetics than TTX-resistant subtypes (Zeisel et al., 2018). Previous studies have indicated that mutations in the genes encoding these Na_vs are largely associated with sensitivity to pain in humans. This is because mutation leads to gain of function in $Na_v1.7$, which in turn activates $Na_v1.8$, which enhances pain (Bennett, Clark, Huang, Waxman, & Dib-Hajj, 2019). Furthermore, loss of function in $Na_v1.7$ results in loss of pain sensation due to different nociceptive stimuli without affecting other neurological functions (Cox et al., 2006; Goldberg et al., 2007). Although the mechanisms linking the loss of $Na_v1.7$ function and insensitivity to pain are not fully understood, it may be correlated to the fact that the majority of inactivating mutations of $Na_v1.7$ lead to a complete loss of channel function (Cox et al., 2006; McDermott et al., 2019). $Na_v1.8$ mutations have been identified in individuals with painful peripheral neuropathy (Faber et al., 2012), and a mutation causing a moderate loss of function in $Na_v1.8$ has been associated with reduced pain sensitivity (Duan et al., 2016). Based on preclinical studies in rodent models, $Na_v1.8$ contributes to neuropathic pain (Lai et al., 2002). Given that many preclinical and human studies have emphasized the potential role of $Na_v1.8$ in regulating pain at the peripheral level, it is essential to validate $Na_v1.8$ as a potential therapeutic target for pain (Alsaloum, Higerd, Effraim, & Waxman, 2020).

Moreover, locally administered non-selective Na_v blockers, such as lidocaine, suppress pain originating from different nociceptive stimuli. Funapide, an inhibitor of both $Na_v1.7$ and $Na_v1.8$, has been investigated for the treatment of inherited erythromelalgia, neuropathic pain, and post-herpetic neuralgia (Goldberg et al., 2012; Price et al., 2017). Although funapide showed promising results in clinical studies, multiple trials have failed to meet the endpoint (Alsaloum et al., 2020). Lacosamide, which is prescribed as an anticonvulsant inhibiting $Na_v1.7$ and $Na_v1.8$, has been tested in clinical studies for $Na_v1.7$-related small fiber neuropathy (de Greef et al., 2019), and currently available data suggest that this compound is effective in the treatment of painful neuropathy (Alsaloum et al., 2020). Moreover, various selective blockers of $Na_V1.7$ have also been tested in patients with chronic pain. For example, vixotrigine was tested for the treatment of lumbosacral radiculopathy and trigeminal neuralgia. The results of phase II trials suggest that vixotrigine has the potential to be an effective and safe treatment for small fiber neuropathy (Alsaloum et al., 2020). Ambroxol, a widely used mucoactive agent for bronchopulmonary diseases (Malerba & Ragnoli, 2008), inhibits TTX-resistant $Na_V1.8$ and $Na_V1.9$, rather than TTX-sensitive $Na_V1.7$, in DRG neurons (Weiser & Wilson, 2002). Ambroxol not only attenuates neuropathic pain, as seen in preclinical studies using various rodent models (Belkouch et al., 2014; Gaida, Klinder, Arndt, & Weiser, 2005), but also exerts analgesic effects at the peripheral level, as seen in clinical studies (Chenot, Weber, & Friede, 2014). In a recent phase III randomized controlled trial, ambroxol attenuated oropharyngeal pain (Sousa, Lakha, Brette, & Hitier, 2019). Nevertheless, the use of ambroxol for the treatment of neuropathic pain has only been supported by case reports, necessitating controlled clinical trials for neuropathic pain. Furthermore, other $Na_V1.8$ blockers, such as PF-0431082 and VX-150, manufactured by different pharmaceutical companies have also been tested in clinical trials. These new compounds, at least in part, demonstrate reasonable effects on several types of pain, and it is important to keep an eye on the results of the ongoing clinical studies.

3.3.3 Novel targets

More recently, newly discovered molecules regulating sensory processing have been identified in animal models of chronic pain. Importin α3, which is a key regulator of nucleocytoplasmic transport, induces nuclear import of c-Fos in DRG neurons (Marvaldi et al., 2020; Panayotis, Karpova, Kreutz, & Fainzilber, 2015). Importin α3 knockout or sensory neuron-specific knockdown attenuated responses to noxious stimuli and the maintenance phase of neuropathic pain in rodents (Marvaldi et al., 2020). Although c-Fos-related mechanisms underlie both peripheral and central levels of pain processing (Coggeshall, 2005), peripheral sensory neurons are targets of importin α3-dependent regulation of pain. Given that the expression patterns of both importin α3 and c-Fos are conserved between mice and humans (Ray et al., 2018), importin α3 might be a potential target for pain. Stimulator of interferon genes (STING) is an endoplasmic reticulum-bound DNA sensor that induces type I interferons and other cytokines that regulate immune responses (Hopfner & Hornung, 2020; Zhang et al., 1998). As STING is highly expressed in peripheral nociceptors, it was hypothesized that it may regulate nociception through interferon signaling. Although the loss of STING functions exhibited hypersensitivity to nociceptive stimuli and heightened nociceptor excitability, the intrathecal activation of STING exerted analgesic effects in mice with chemotherapy-induced peripheral neuropathy, nerve injury-induced neuropathic pain, and bone cancer pain (Donnelly et al., 2021). Importantly, the STING pathway exerts long-lasting analgesic effects in NHPs, and interferons directly suppress the excitability of nociceptors in mice and that of NHPs in humans through modulation of sodium and calcium channel function (Donnelly et al., 2021), indicating that STING can also be a novel peripheral target for chronic pain. Collectively, these results suggest that novel pain-regulatory molecules exhibiting different peripheral mechanisms are ideal candidates for the development of potent and non-opioid-based analgesics.

4. Treatment of pain by spinal and supraspinal actions

4.1 Cannabinoid receptor agonists

It has been traditionally known that cannabinoids (CBs), such as Δ9-tetrahydrocannabinol (THC) and cannabidiol (CBD), purified from *Cannabis sativa* have therapeutic effects against several neurological disorders (Friedman, French, & Maccarrone, 2019). Based on binding studies using radiolabeled THC, CB1 and CB2 receptors (CB1R and CB2R, respectively) have been identified as target receptors of naturally isolated CBs (Devane, Dysarz 3rd, Johnson, Melvin, & Howlett, 1988; Matsuda, Lolait, Brownstein, Young, & Bonner, 1990). Subsequently, the biochemical and physiological characteristics of endogenous ligands for CB1R and CB2R, which are anandamide and 2-arachidonoyl-glycerol, have been worked out (Devane et al., 1992; Sugiura et al., 1995). Similar to the opioid receptors, both CB1R and CB2R are GPCRs. Although CB1Rs are abundantly expressed in the brain, CB2Rs are highly expressed in the immune system and involved in several physiological functions (Cristino, Bisogno, & Di Marzo, 2020). As CB1Rs are located on presynaptic terminals of excitatory and inhibitory neurons, activation of CB1R signaling can inhibit voltage-gated calcium channels and vesicular release of neurotransmitters (such as GABA and glutamate) underlying regulation of mood, cognition, and perception in animals and humans (Bara, Ferland, Rompala,

Szutorisz, & Hurd, 2021; Cristino et al., 2020). In particular, accumulating evidence from studies using animal models suggests that CB1R agonists produce antinociception through the activation of CB1Rs at spinal or supraspinal levels (Donvito et al., 2018), indicating that CB1R agonists may be potential targets for centrally acting analgesics. Moreover, CB1Rs are also expressed on astrocytes that are not only involved in the regulation of synaptic plasticity in different brain areas and but also further located on progenitor stem cells and differentiate into neurons or astrocytes (Prenderville, Kelly, & Downer, 2015). Given that the patterns of CB1R activation and distribution may be altered in several CNS regions under pathological conditions (Cristino et al., 2020), CB1R may be considered a potential target for the treatment of neurological diseases. In contrast, CB2Rs are mainly expressed in CNS microglia in patients with multiple sclerosis and amyotrophic lateral sclerosis (Aymerich et al., 2018), and the activation of CB2Rs attenuates the expression of inflammatory cytokines associated with neurodegenerative disorders (Cassano et al., 2017). Thus, CB2Rs may have different functional properties and diverse therapeutic mechanisms than CB1Rs.

In view of the substantial anatomical and neurochemical overlap between opioid and CB systems (Le Foll, 2021; Rios, Gomes, & Devi, 2006), it was hypothesized that there is a therapeutic benefit of combining opioids and CBs for the treatment of pain. In this regard, a number of studies have demonstrated that non-analgesic doses of THC enhance opioid analgesia in rodents and NHPs (Babalonis & Walsh, 2020). The synergistic effects of opioid and CB combinations appeared to be rather selective for pain processing in animals, and the other unfavorable effects of CBs (such as hypothermia and hypoactivity) and opioids (such as respiratory depression) were not potentiated by such a combination (Welch, 2009). However, these findings have not been clearly confirmed in human studies. In fact, a combination of CBs and opioids demonstrated diverse results depending on the experimental setting in humans (Babalonis & Walsh, 2020). In addition, no substantial data are available to suggest that CBs are highly effective analgesics for different pain conditions, including chronic pain. However, considerable evidence suggests that the expression levels of CB1R and CB2R are altered not only in animal models but also in patients with multiple sclerosis and that the activation of CB1Rs and CB2Rs has a beneficial therapeutic effect (Baker et al., 2000; Cristino et al., 2020; Maresz et al., 2007). Nabiximols, a cannabis extract that includes THC and CBD, has shown promising results in clinical studies and has been approved in several countries for the treatment of neuropathic pain and spasticity in multiple sclerosis (Giacoppo, Bramanti, & Mazzon, 2017). Moreover, as the effects of nabiximols are based on neuroimmune regulation, treatment with nabiximols reduces circulating levels of inflammatory cytokines that usually enhance pathological pain (Orefice et al., 2016). Nabiximols are currently being investigated for the treatment of painful conditions associated with CNS disorders, such as stroke and glioblastoma (Marinelli et al., 2017). Since nabiximols have shown promising therapeutic effects in clinical studies for these diseases (Friedman et al., 2019), it is likely that CBs can also be useful for several types of neurological disorders.

4.2 NOP receptor agonists

As NOP receptors are located on the pain-processing pathways (the DRG, spinal cord, and brain), several studies have been conducted to understand the functional profiles of NOP receptors in regulating pain (Corder et al., 2018; Schroder et al., 2014). Similar to MOP receptors, presynaptic and postsynaptic NOP receptors can inhibit excitatory glutamatergic transmission via GPCR signaling in the SDH and brain (Winters, Christie, & Vaughan, 2019), indicating that NOP receptor activation may produce antinociception. In rodents, NOP receptor activation produces both dose- and pain modality-dependent bi-directional (pronociceptive or antinociceptive) effects at the spinal or supraspinal levels. (Schroder et al., 2014). Nevertheless, as peptidic and non-peptidic NOP receptor agonists suppress neuropathic pain in rodents (Kiguchi, Ding, Kishioka, & Ko, 2020; Toll et al., 2016), NOP receptor-related ligands may be effective for the treatment of neuropathic pain. In contrast, intrathecal, intracisternal, or systemic administration of NOP receptor agonists only produces antinociception in NHPs (Ding et al., 2015; Kiguchi & Ko, 2019; Ko et al., 2009). Notably, N/OFQ was found to be the most potent endogenous peptide among all opioid peptides, such as β-endorphin and enkephalins, for spinal analgesia in inflammatory pain conditions (Lee & Ko, 2015). Importantly, intrathecal administration of NOP receptor agonists produces potent antinociceptive effects without eliciting morphine-like adverse effects, such as itching, in NHPs (Kiguchi et al., 2020). Moreover, the combination of SCH221510, a NOP receptor agonist, and buprenorphine significantly enhanced the analgesic effect and did not cause adverse effects in NHPs (Cremeans et al., 2012). These results indicate the probability of synergistic analgesia by the co-activation of both NOP and MOP receptors in humans.

Given the preferable functional properties of the NOP receptor agonists, it has been hypothesized that mixed NOP/MOP receptor agonists may be safer opioid analgesics, without the undesirable adverse effects. Based on the understanding of the structure-activity relationship of NOP receptors, several candidates for novel ligands, acting on both NOP and MOP receptors with different affinities and partial agonist efficacies, have been investigated in preclinical studies (Kiguchi, Ding, Kishioka, & Ko, 2020; Zaveri & Meyer, 2019). In rodents, intrathecal administration of BU08028 (Khroyan et al., 2011) and SR16435 exerted antinociceptive and antiallodynic effects through the activation of NOP and MOP receptors (Sukhtankar, Zaveri, Husbands, & Ko, 2013). Recently, BU10038 was developed as a naltrexone-derived bifunctional NOP/MOP receptor agonist. Intrathecal BU10038 produced potent and long-lasting antinociceptive and antiallodynic effects compared to morphine in NHPs, and intrathecal BU10038 did not cause adverse effects, such as itching sensation, and tolerance. Unlike spinal analgesia, systemically administered NOP receptor agonists demonstrate integrated effects of peripheral, spinal, and supraspinal actions (Kiguchi et al., 2019). Systemic administration of BU08028 exerted morphine-comparable antinociceptive effects, but showed rewarding effects in rodents (Khroyan et al., 2011). However, it did not elicit reinforcing effects in NHPs (Ding et al., 2016), indicating that a translational gap exists with respect to the efficacy of mixed NOP/MOP receptor agonists between rodents and NHPs. A non-morphinan NOP/MOP receptor agonist, AT-121, produced potent antinociceptive and antiallodynic effects, which were almost 100-fold more potent than those of morphine, and was antagonized by either NOP or MOP receptor antagonist in NHPs (Ding et al., 2018). Moreover, the systemic administration of AT-121 lacks dose-limiting adverse effects such as abuse liability, itching sensation, respiratory depression, cardiovascular dysfunction, physical dependence, and opioid-induced hyperalgesia (Ding et al., 2018). Although these NOP/MOP receptor agonists have different binding profiles to NOP and MOP receptors (Kiguchi, Ding, Kishioka, & Ko, 2020), mixed NOP/MOP receptor partial agonists seem to have ideal functional profiles and, thus, may be developed as novel non-addictive and safe analgesics.

In rodents, cebranopadol has a half-life of 4.5 h and oral bioavailability of 13–23% and exerts dose-dependent antinociceptive effects via NOP and MOP receptor activation after systemic administration (Calo & Lambert, 2018; Linz et al., 2014). Notably, cebranopadol was >100-fold more potent and long-lasting than morphine-induced analgesia, producing potent anti-allodynic effects in different models of neuropathic pain; unlike morphine, it does not affect respiratory and motor functions at analgesic doses (Calo & Lambert, 2018; Linz et al., 2014). The beneficial effects of cebranopadol can be translated to NHPs as it produces potent antinociceptive and antihypersensitive effects compared to fentanyl after systemic or intrathecal administration with reduced side effects, such as a lack of respiratory depression and itching (Ding et al., 2021). Although cebranopadol caused reinforcing effects in the fixed-ratio schedule of self-administration, its reinforcing strength was lower than that of fentanyl (Ding et al., 2021). Given that MOP receptor activation mainly contributes to cebranopadol-induced antinociception in NHPs, it is necessary to consider the detectable reinforcing effects of cebranopadol for clinical use. In phase I and phase II clinical trials for analgesic indications, the pharmacokinetic properties of cebranopadol have been demonstrated in patients (Calo & Lambert, 2018; Kleideiter, Piana, Wang, Nemeth, & Gautrois, 2018). Although oral administration of cebranopadol produced drug-liking effects, they were less or shorter than those of the usual MOP receptor full agonist hydromorphone (Gohler et al., 2019). This observation was consistent with that of preclinical study on NHPs (Ding et al., 2021). In clinical trials, cebranopadol produced significant analgesic efficacy in patients with low back pain, cancer pain, or diabetic neuropathy, with fewer undesirable side effects such as miosis, respiratory depression, constipation, dizziness, and nausea (Christoph, Eerdekens, Kok, Volkers, & Freynhagen, 2017; Eerdekens et al., 2019; Kiguchi et al., 2020). Collectively, these findings support the concept of coactivation of NOP and MOP receptors for enhanced pain relief with reduced side effects.

5. Conclusions

This review highlights the recent progress in well-known targets and discusses exciting findings of emerging and novel targets for the treatment of opioid abuse and pain. Given that opioids are the most commonly prescribed analgesics for the treatment of moderate-to-severe pain, it is challenging to develop non-opioid analgesics that can replace opioids in clinical settings (Azzam, McDonald, & Lambert, 2019; Corbett, Henderson, McKnight, & Paterson, 2006). Nevertheless, biomedical science has evolved rapidly to discover innovative medications to treat opioid abuse and/or as safe, non-addictive interventions to manage pain (Rasmussen et al., 2019; Volkow & Collins, 2017; Woolf, 2020). There is a translational gap in the development of effective medications for opioid abuse and pain as behavioral and physiological responses to opioid-related ligands in rodents cannot be translated to primates (Ding & Ko, 2021; Kiguchi, Ding, & Ko, 2016). Rhesus macaques have genetic similarities to the human genome (Rhesus Macaque Genome et al., 2007) and this species plays a critical role in modeling human diseases and physiological responses that are not well simulated in rodents (Balsters et al., 2020; Seok et al., 2013; Warren et al., 2020). Although rodent studies have documented promising novel targets, few non-opioid targets have been validated in primates. To date, NHP studies have demonstrated that MOP receptor- or mixed opioid receptor subtype-based ligands are effective in alleviating opioid-induced adverse effects (Ding & Ko, 2021). Given the mounting evidence that neuroanatomical aspects of opioid and non-opioid receptors differ between rodents and primates (Bianchi et al., 2012; Hawkinson et al., 2007; Shiers et al., 2021; Yu et al., 2019), it is important to investigate the functional profiles of novel compounds extensively in NHP models before initiating expensive clinical trials. More pharmacological studies of the functional efficacy, selectivity, and tolerability of the novel compounds in NHP models will accelerate the development of effective medications for opioid abuse and pain to advance human medicine.

Acknowledgments

Funding was provided by the US National Institutes of Health, National Institute on Drug Abuse (DA053343, DA044450, and DA049580). The contents of this study are solely the responsibility of the authors and do not necessarily represent the official views of US federal agencies. We thank Editage for editing the manuscript.

Conflict of interest

N.K. and M.C.K. declare that there is no conflict of interest.

References

Alsaloum, M., Higerd, G. P., Effraim, P. R., & Waxman, S. G. (2020). Status of peripheral sodium channel blockers for non-addictive pain treatment. *Nature Reviews. Neurology*, *16*(12), 689–705. https://doi.org/10.1038/s41582-020-00415-2.

Aso, K., Shahtaheri, S. M., Hill, R., Wilson, D., McWilliams, D. F., & Walsh, D. A. (2019). Associations of symptomatic knee osteoarthritis with histopathologic features in subchondral bone. *Arthritis & Rhematology*, *71*(6), 916–924. https://doi.org/10.1002/art.40820.

Attal, N., & Bouhassira, D. (2015). Pharmacotherapy of neuropathic pain: which drugs, which treatment algorithms? *Pain*, *156*(Suppl 1), S104–S114. https://doi.org/10.1097/01.j.pain.0000460358.01998.15.

Attal, N., Bouhassira, D., & Baron, R. (2018). Diagnosis and assessment of neuropathic pain through questionnaires. *Lancet Neurology*, *17*(5), 456–466. https://doi.org/10.1016/S1474-4422(18)30071-1.

Aymerich, M. S., Aso, E., Abellanas, M. A., Tolon, R. M., Ramos, J. A., Ferrer, I., et al. (2018). Cannabinoid pharmacology/therapeutics in chronic degenerative disorders affecting the central nervous system. *Biochemical Pharmacology*, *157*, 67–84. https://doi.org/10.1016/j.bcp.2018.08.016.

Azevedo Neto, J., Costanzini, A., De Giorgio, R., Lambert, D. G., Ruzza, C., & Calò, G. (2020). Biased versus partial agonism in the search for safer opioid analgesics. *Molecules*, *25*(17), 3780. https://doi.org/10.3390/molecules25173870.

Azzam, A. A. H., McDonald, J., & Lambert, D. G. (2019). Hot topics in opioid pharmacology: Mixed and biased opioids. *British Journal of Anaesthesia*, *122*(6), e136–e145. https://doi.org/10.1016/j.bja.2019.03.006.

Babalonis, S., & Walsh, S. L. (2020). Therapeutic potential of opioid/cannabinoid combinations in humans: Review of the evidence. *European Neuropsychopharmacology*, *36*, 206–216. https://doi.org/10.1016/j.euroneuro.2020.03.002.

Baimel, C., Bartlett, S. E., Chiou, L. C., Lawrence, A. J., Muschamp, J. W., Patkar, O., et al. (2015). Orexin/hypocretin role in reward: Implications for opioid and other addictions. *British Journal of Pharmacology*, *172*(2), 334–348. https://doi.org/10.1111/bph.12639.

Baker, D., Pryce, G., Croxford, J. L., Brown, P., Pertwee, R. G., Huffman, J. W., et al. (2000). Cannabinoids control spasticity and tremor in a multiple sclerosis model. *Nature*, *404*(6773), 84–87. https://doi.org/10.1038/35003583.

Balsters, J. H., Zerbi, V., Sallet, J., Wenderoth, N., & Mars, R. B. (2020). Primate homologs of mouse cortico-striatal circuits. *eLife*, *9*. https://doi.org/10.7554/eLife.53680.

Bara, A., Ferland, J. N., Rompala, G., Szutorisz, H., & Hurd, Y. L. (2021). Cannabis and synaptic reprogramming of the developing brain. *Nature Reviews. Neuroscience*, *22*(7), 423–438. https://doi.org/10.1038/s41583-021-00465-5.

Barthel, C., Yeremenko, N., Jacobs, R., Schmidt, R. E., Bernateck, M., Zeidler, H., et al. (2009). Nerve growth factor and receptor expression in rheumatoid arthritis and spondyloarthritis. *Arthritis Research & Therapy*, *11*(3), R82. https://doi.org/10.1186/ar2716.

Basbaum, A. I., Bautista, D. M., Scherrer, G., & Julius, D. (2009). Cellular and molecular mechanisms of pain. *Cell*, *139*(2), 267–284. https://doi.org/10.1016/j.cell.2009.09.028.

Belgers, M., Leenaars, M., Homberg, J. R., Ritskes-Hoitinga, M., Schellekens, A. F., & Hooijmans, C. R. (2016). Ibogaine and addiction in the animal model, a systematic review and meta-analysis. *Translational Psychiatry*, *6*(5), e826. https://doi.org/10.1038/tp.2016.71.

Belkouch, M., Dansereau, M. A., Tetreault, P., Biet, M., Beaudet, N., Dumaine, R., et al. (2014). Functional up-regulation of Nav1.8 sodium channel in Abeta afferent fibers subjected to chronic peripheral inflammation. *Journal of Neuroinflammation*, *11*, 45. https://doi.org/10.1186/1742-2094-11-45.

Bello, E. P., Mateo, Y., Gelman, D. M., Noain, D., Shin, J. H., Low, M. J., et al. (2011). Cocaine supersensitivity and enhanced motivation for reward in mice lacking dopamine D2 autoreceptors. *Nature Neuroscience*, *14*(8), 1033–1038. https://doi.org/10.1038/nn.2862.

Bennett, D. L., Clark, A. J., Huang, J., Waxman, S. G., & Dib-Hajj, S. D. (2019). The role of voltage-gated sodium channels in pain signaling. *Physiological Reviews*, *99*(2), 1079–1151. https://doi.org/10.1152/physrev.00052.2017.

Bianchi, B. R., Zhang, X. F., Reilly, R. M., Kym, P. R., Yao, B. B., & Chen, J. (2012). Species comparison and pharmacological characterization of human, monkey, rat, and mouse TRPA1 channels. *The Journal of Pharmacology and Experimental Therapeutics*, *341*(2), 360–368. https://doi.org/10.1124/jpet.111.189902.

Bohn, L. M., Gainetdinov, R. R., Lin, F. T., Lefkowitz, R. J., & Caron, M. G. (2000). Mu-opioid receptor desensitization by beta-arrestin-2 determines morphine tolerance but not dependence. *Nature*, *408*(6813), 720–723. https://doi.org/10.1038/35047086.

Bohn, L. M., Lefkowitz, R. J., Gainetdinov, R. R., Peppel, K., Caron, M. G., & Lin, F. T. (1999). Enhanced morphine analgesia in mice lacking beta-arrestin 2. *Science*, *286*(5449), 2495–2498.

Borowsky, B., Adham, N., Jones, K. A., Raddatz, R., Artymyshyn, R., Ogozalek, K. L., et al. (2001). Trace amines: identification of a family of mammalian G protein-coupled receptors. *Proceedings of the National Academy of Sciences of the United States of America*, *98*(16), 8966–8971. https://doi.org/10.1073/pnas.151105198.

Braz, J., Solorzano, C., Wang, X., & Basbaum, A. I. (2014). Transmitting pain and itch messages: a contemporary view of the spinal cord circuits that generate gate control. *Neuron*, *82*(3), 522–536. https://doi.org/10.1016/j.neuron.2014.01.018.

Bromberg-Martin, E. S., Matsumoto, M., & Hikosaka, O. (2010). Dopamine in motivational control: rewarding, aversive, and alerting. *Neuron*, *68*(5), 815–834. https://doi.org/10.1016/j.neuron.2010.11.022.

Brook, K., Bennett, J., & Desai, S. P. (2017). The chemical history of morphine: An 8000-year journey, from resin to de-novo synthesis. *Journal of Anesthesia History*, *3*(2), 50–55. https://doi.org/10.1016/j.janh.2017.02.001.

Calo, G., & Lambert, D. G. (2018). Nociceptin/orphanin FQ receptor ligands and translational challenges: focus on cebranopadol as an innovative analgesic. *British Journal of Anaesthesia*, *121*(5), 1105–1114. https://doi.org/10.1016/j.bja.2018.06.024.

Cameron, L. P., Tombari, R. J., Lu, J., Pell, A. J., Hurley, Z. Q., Ehinger, Y., et al. (2021). A non-hallucinogenic psychedelic analogue with therapeutic potential. *Nature*, *589*(7842), 474–479. https://doi.org/10.1038/s41586-020-3008-z.

Cassano, T., Calcagnini, S., Pace, L., De Marco, F., Romano, A., & Gaetani, S. (2017). Cannabinoid receptor 2 signaling in neurodegenerative disorders: From pathogenesis to a promising therapeutic target. *Frontiers in Neuroscience*, *11*, 30. https://doi.org/10.3389/fnins.2017.00030.

Chen, Y., Mestek, A., Liu, J., Hurley, J. A., & Yu, L. (1993). Molecular cloning and functional expression of a mu-opioid receptor from rat brain. *Molecular Pharmacology*, *44*(1), 8–12. Retrieved from https://www.ncbi.nlm.nih.gov/pubmed/8393525.

Chen, X. T., Pitis, P., Liu, G., Yuan, C., Gotchev, D., Cowan, C. L., et al. (2013). Structure-activity relationships and discovery of a G protein biased mu opioid receptor ligand, [(3-methoxythiophen-2-yl)methyl]({2-[(9R)-9-(pyridin-2-yl)-6-oxaspiro-[4.5]decan- 9-yl]ethyl})amine (TRV130), for the treatment of acute severe pain. *Journal of Medicinal Chemistry*, *56*(20), 8019–8031. https://doi.org/10.1021/jm4010829.

Chenot, J. F., Weber, P., & Friede, T. (2014). Efficacy of Ambroxol lozenges for pharyngitis: A meta-analysis. *BMC Family Practice*, *15*, 45. https://doi.org/10.1186/1471-2296-15-45.

Christoph, A., Eerdekens, M. H., Kok, M., Volkers, G., & Freynhagen, R. (2017). Cebranopadol, a novel first-in-class analgesic drug candidate: First experience in patients with chronic low back pain in a randomized clinical trial. *Pain*, *158*(9), 1813–1824. https://doi.org/10.1097/j.pain.0000000000000986.

Coggeshall, R. E. (2005). Fos, nociception and the dorsal horn. *Progress in Neurobiology*, 77(5), 299–352. https://doi.org/10.1016/j.pneurobio.2005.11.002.

Cohen, S. P., Vase, L., & Hooten, W. M. (2021). Chronic pain: An update on burden, best practices, and new advances. *Lancet*, *397*(10289), 2082–2097. https://doi.org/10.1016/S0140-6736(21)00393-7.

Collaborators, U. S. B. o. D, Mokdad, A. H., Ballestros, K., Echko, M., Glenn, S., Olsen, H. E., et al. (2018). The State of US Health, 1990-2016: Burden of diseases, injuries, and risk factors among US states. *JAMA*, *319*(14), 1444–1472. https://doi.org/10.1001/jama.2018.0158.

Corbett, A. D., Henderson, G., McKnight, A. T., & Paterson, S. J. (2006). 75 years of opioid research: The exciting but vain quest for the Holy Grail. *British Journal of Pharmacology, 147*(Suppl 1), S153–S162. https://doi.org/10.1038/sj.bjp.0706435.

Corder, G., Castro, D. C., Bruchas, M. R., & Scherrer, G. (2018). Endogenous and exogenous opioids in pain. *Annual Review of Neuroscience, 41*, 453–473. https://doi.org/10.1146/annurev-neuro-080317-061522.

Cousins, D. A., Butts, K., & Young, A. H. (2009). The role of dopamine in bipolar disorder. *Bipolar Disorders, 11*(8), 787–806. https://doi.org/10.1111/j.1399-5618.2009.00760.x.

Cox, J. J., Reimann, F., Nicholas, A. K., Thornton, G., Roberts, E., Springell, K., et al. (2006). An SCN9A channelopathy causes congenital inability to experience pain. *Nature, 444*(7121), 894–898. https://doi.org/10.1038/nature05413.

Cremeans, C. M., Gruley, E., Kyle, D. J., & Ko, M. C. (2012). Roles of mu-opioid receptors and nociceptin/orphanin FQ peptide receptors in buprenorphine-induced physiological responses in primates. *The Journal of Pharmacology and Experimental Therapeutics, 343*(1), 72–81. https://doi.org/10.1124/jpet.112.194308.

Cristino, L., Bisogno, T., & Di Marzo, V. (2020). Cannabinoids and the expanded endocannabinoid system in neurological disorders. *Nature Reviews. Neurology, 16*(1), 9–29. https://doi.org/10.1038/s41582-019-0284-z.

Cui, Y., Ostlund, S. B., James, A. S., Park, C. S., Ge, W., Roberts, K. W., et al. (2014). Targeted expression of mu-opioid receptors in a subset of striatal direct-pathway neurons restores opiate reward. *Nature Neuroscience, 17*(2), 254–261. https://doi.org/10.1038/nn.3622.

Darcq, E., & Kieffer, B. L. (2018). Opioid receptors: drivers to addiction? *Nature Reviews. Neuroscience, 19*(8), 499–514. https://doi.org/10.1038/s41583-018-0028-x.

Dart, R. C., Surratt, H. L., Cicero, T. J., Parrino, M. W., Severtson, S. G., Bucher-Bartelson, B., et al. (2015). Trends in opioid analgesic abuse and mortality in the United States. *The New England Journal of Medicine, 372*(3), 241–248. https://doi.org/10.1056/NEJMsa1406143.

de Greef, B. T. A., Hoeijmakers, J. G. J., Geerts, M., Oakes, M., Church, T. J. E., Waxman, S. G., et al. (2019). Lacosamide in patients with Nav1.7 mutations-related small fibre neuropathy: A randomized controlled trial. *Brain, 142*(2), 263–275. https://doi.org/10.1093/brain/awy329.

Degenhardt, L., Charlson, F., Mathers, B., Hall, W. D., Flaxman, A. D., Johns, N., et al. (2014). The global epidemiology and burden of opioid dependence: results from the global burden of disease 2010 study. *Addiction, 109*(8), 1320–1333. https://doi.org/10.1111/add.12551.

Degenhardt, L., Grebely, J., Stone, J., Hickman, M., Vickerman, P., Marshall, B. D. L., et al. (2019). Global patterns of opioid use and dependence: harms to populations, interventions, and future action. *Lancet, 394*(10208), 1560–1579. https://doi.org/10.1016/S0140-6736(19)32229-9.

Denk, F., Bennett, D. L., & McMahon, S. B. (2017). Nerve growth factor and pain mechanisms. *Annual Review of Neuroscience, 40*, 307–325. https://doi.org/10.1146/annurev-neuro-072116-031121.

Devane, W. A., Dysarz, F. A., 3rd, Johnson, M. R., Melvin, L. S., & Howlett, A. C. (1988). Determination and characterization of a cannabinoid receptor in rat brain. *Molecular Pharmacology, 34*(5), 605–613. Retrieved from https://www.ncbi.nlm.nih.gov/pubmed/2848184.

Devane, W. A., Hanus, L., Breuer, A., Pertwee, R. G., Stevenson, L. A., Griffin, G., et al. (1992). Isolation and structure of a brain constituent that binds to the cannabinoid receptor. *Science, 258*(5090), 1946–1949. https://doi.org/10.1126/science.1470919.

DeWire, S. M., Yamashita, D. S., Rominger, D. H., Liu, G., Cowan, C. L., Graczyk, T. M., et al. (2013). A G protein-biased ligand at the mu-opioid receptor is potently analgesic with reduced gastrointestinal and respiratory dysfunction compared with morphine. *The Journal of Pharmacology and Experimental Therapeutics, 344*(3), 708–717. https://doi.org/10.1124/jpet.112.201616.

Dib-Hajj, S. D., Yang, Y., Black, J. A., & Waxman, S. G. (2013). The Na(V)1.7 sodium channel: from molecule to man. *Nature Reviews. Neuroscience, 14*(1), 49–62. https://doi.org/10.1038/nrn3404.

Ding, H., Czoty, P. W., Kiguchi, N., Cami-Kobeci, G., Sukhtankar, D. D., Nader, M. A., et al. (2016). A novel orvinol analog, BU08028, as a safe opioid analgesic without abuse liability in primates. *Proceedings of the National Academy of Sciences of the United States of America, 113*(37), E5511–E5518. https://doi.org/10.1073/pnas.1605295113.

Ding, H., Hayashida, K., Suto, T., Sukhtankar, D. D., Kimura, M., Mendenhall, V., et al. (2015). Supraspinal actions of nociceptin/orphanin FQ, morphine and substance P in regulating pain and itch in non-human primates. *British Journal of Pharmacology, 172*(13), 3302–3312. https://doi.org/10.1111/bph.13124.

Ding, H., Kiguchi, N., Perrey, D. A., Nguyen, T., Czoty, P. W., Hsu, F. C., et al. (2020). Antinociceptive, reinforcing, and pruritic effects of the G-protein signalling-biased mu opioid receptor agonist PZM21 in non-human primates. *British Journal of Anaesthesia, 125*(4), 596–604. https://doi.org/10.1016/j.bja.2020.06.057.

Ding, H., Kiguchi, N., Yasuda, D., Daga, P. R., Polgar, W. E., Lu, J. J., et al. (2018). A bifunctional nociceptin and mu opioid receptor agonist is analgesic without opioid side effects in nonhuman primates. *Science Translational Medicine, 10*(456), eaar3483. https://doi.org/10.1126/scitranslmed.aar3483.

Ding, H., & Ko, M. C. (2021). Translational value of non-human primates in opioid research. *Experimental Neurology, 338*, 113602. https://doi.org/10.1016/j.expneurol.2021.113602.

Ding, H., Trapella, C., Kiguchi, N., Hsu, F. C., Calo, G., & Ko, M. C. (2021). Functional profile of systemic and intrathecal cebranopadol in nonhuman primates. *Anesthesiology, 135*(3), 482–493. https://doi.org/10.1097/ALN.0000000000003848.

Donnelly, C. R., Jiang, C., Andriessen, A. S., Wang, K., Wang, Z., Ding, H., et al. (2021). STING controls nociception via type I interferon signalling in sensory neurons. *Nature, 591*(7849), 275–280. https://doi.org/10.1038/s41586-020-03151-1.

Donvito, G., Nass, S. R., Wilkerson, J. L., Curry, Z. A., Schurman, L. D., Kinsey, S. G., et al. (2018). The endogenous cannabinoid system: A budding source of targets for treating inflammatory and neuropathic pain. *Neuropsychopharmacology, 43*(1), 52–79. https://doi.org/10.1038/npp.2017.204.

Drilon, A., Laetsch, T. W., Kummar, S., DuBois, S. G., Lassen, U. N., Demetri, G. D., et al. (2018). Efficacy of Larotrectinib in TRK fusion-positive cancers in adults and children. *The New England Journal of Medicine, 378*(8), 731–739. https://doi.org/10.1056/NEJMoa1714448.

Duan, G., Han, C., Wang, Q., Guo, S., Zhang, Y., Ying, Y., et al. (2016). A SCN10A SNP biases human pain sensitivity. *Molecular Pain, 12*. https://doi.org/10.1177/1744806916666083.

Eerdekens, M. H., Kapanadze, S., Koch, E. D., Kralidis, G., Volkers, G., Ahmedzai, S. H., et al. (2019). Cancer-related chronic pain: Investigation of the novel analgesic drug candidate cebranopadol in a randomized, double-blind, noninferiority trial. *European Journal of Pain, 23*(3), 577–588. https://doi.org/10.1002/ejp.1331.

Ehlers, M. D., Kaplan, D. R., Price, D. L., & Koliatsos, V. E. (1995). NGF-stimulated retrograde transport of trkA in the mammalian nervous system. *The Journal of Cell Biology, 130*(1), 149–156. https://doi.org/10.1083/jcb.130.1.149.

Evans, C. J., Keith, D. E., Jr., Morrison, H., Magendzo, K., & Edwards, R. H. (1992). Cloning of a delta opioid receptor by functional expression. *Science, 258*(5090), 1952–1955. https://doi.org/10.1126/science.1335167.

Faber, C. G., Lauria, G., Merkies, I. S., Cheng, X., Han, C., Ahn, H. S., et al. (2012). Gain-of-function Nav1.8 mutations in painful neuropathy. *Proceedings of the National Academy of Sciences of the United States of America*, *109*(47), 19444–19449. https://doi.org/10.1073/pnas.1216080109.

Fields, H. (2004). State-dependent opioid control of pain. *Nature Reviews. Neuroscience*, *5*(7), 565–575. https://doi.org/10.1038/nrn1431.

Fields, H. L., & Margolis, E. B. (2015). Understanding opioid reward. *Trends in Neurosciences*, *38*(4), 217–225. https://doi.org/10.1016/j.tins.2015.01.002.

Fitzcharles, M. A., Cohen, S. P., Clauw, D. J., Littlejohn, G., Usui, C., & Hauser, W. (2021). Nociplastic pain: Towards an understanding of prevalent pain conditions. *Lancet*, *397*(10289), 2098–2110. https://doi.org/10.1016/S0140-6736(21)00392-5.

Fragale, J. E., James, M. H., Avila, J. A., Spaeth, A. M., Aurora, R. N., Langleben, D., et al. (2021). The insomnia-addiction positive feedback loop: Role of the orexin system. *Frontiers of Neurology and Neuroscience*, *45*, 117–127. https://doi.org/10.1159/000514965.

Fragale, J. E., Pantazis, C. B., James, M. H., & Aston-Jones, G. (2019). The role of orexin-1 receptor signaling in demand for the opioid fentanyl. *Neuropsychopharmacology*, *44*(10), 1690–1697. https://doi.org/10.1038/s41386-019-0420-x.

Friedman, D., French, J. A., & Maccarrone, M. (2019). Safety, efficacy, and mechanisms of action of cannabinoids in neurological disorders. *Lancet Neurology*, *18*(5), 504–512. https://doi.org/10.1016/S1474-4422(19)30032-8.

Gaida, W., Klinder, K., Arndt, K., & Weiser, T. (2005). Ambroxol, a Nav1.8-preferring Na(+) channel blocker, effectively suppresses pain symptoms in animal models of chronic, neuropathic and inflammatory pain. *Neuropharmacology*, *49*(8), 1220–1227. https://doi.org/10.1016/j.neuropharm.2005.08.004.

Georgescu, D., Zachariou, V., Barrot, M., Mieda, M., Willie, J. T., Eisch, A. J., et al. (2003). Involvement of the lateral hypothalamic peptide orexin in morphine dependence and withdrawal. *The Journal of Neuroscience*, *23*(8), 3106–3111.

Giacoppo, S., Bramanti, P., & Mazzon, E. (2017). Sativex in the management of multiple sclerosis-related spasticity: An overview of the last decade of clinical evaluation. *Multiple Sclerosis and Related Disorders*, *17*, 22–31. https://doi.org/10.1016/j.msard.2017.06.015.

Gillis, A., Gondin, A. B., Kliewer, A., Sanchez, J., Lim, H. D., Alamein, C., et al. (2020). Low intrinsic efficacy for G protein activation can explain the improved side effect profiles of new opioid agonists. *Science Signaling*, *13*(625), eaaz3140. https://doi.org/10.1126/scisignal.aaz3140.

Gillis, A., Kliewer, A., Kelly, E., Henderson, G., Christie, M. J., Schulz, S., et al. (2020). Critical assessment of G protein-biased agonism at the μ-opioid receptor. *Trends in Pharmacological Sciences*, *41*(12), 947–959. https://doi.org/10.1016/j.tips.2020.09.009.

Gohler, K., Sokolowska, M., Schoedel, K. A., Nemeth, R., Kleideiter, E., Szeto, I., et al. (2019). Assessment of the abuse potential of cebranopadol in nondependent recreational opioid users: A phase 1 randomized controlled study. *Journal of Clinical Psychopharmacology*, *39*(1), 46–56. https://doi.org/10.1097/JCP.0000000000000995.

Goldberg, Y. P., MacFarlane, J., MacDonald, M. L., Thompson, J., Dube, M. P., Mattice, M., et al. (2007). Loss-of-function mutations in the Nav1.7 gene underlie congenital indifference to pain in multiple human populations. *Clinical Genetics*, *71*(4), 311–319. https://doi.org/10.1111/j.1399-0004.2007.00790.x.

Goldberg, Y. P., Price, N., Namdari, R., Cohen, C. J., Lamers, M. H., Winters, C., et al. (2012). Treatment of Na(v)1.7-mediated pain in inherited erythromelalgia using a novel sodium channel blocker. *Pain*, *153*(1), 80–85. https://doi.org/10.1016/j.pain.2011.09.008.

Goodwin, G., & McMahon, S. B. (2021). The physiological function of different voltage-gated sodium channels in pain. *Nature Reviews. Neuroscience*, *22*(5), 263–274. https://doi.org/10.1038/s41583-021-00444-w.

Grim, T. W., Schmid, C. L., Stahl, E. L., Pantouli, F., Ho, J. H., Acevedo-Canabal, A., et al. (2020). A G protein signaling-biased agonist at the μ-opioid receptor reverses morphine tolerance while preventing morphine withdrawal. *Neuropsychopharmacology*, *45*(2), 416–425. https://doi.org/10.1038/s41386-019-0491-8.

Gunther, T., Dasgupta, P., Mann, A., Miess, E., Kliewer, A., Fritzwanker, S., et al. (2018). Targeting multiple opioid receptors - improved analgesics with reduced side effects? *British Journal of Pharmacology*, *175*(14), 2857–2868. https://doi.org/10.1111/bph.13809.

Harris, G. C., Wimmer, M., & Aston-Jones, G. (2005). A role for lateral hypothalamic orexin neurons in reward seeking. *Nature*, *437*(7058), 556–559. https://doi.org/10.1038/nature04071.

Hawkinson, J. E., Szoke, B. G., Garofalo, A. W., Hom, D. S., Zhang, H., Dreyer, M., et al. (2007). Pharmacological, pharmacokinetic, and primate analgesic efficacy profile of the novel bradykinin B1 Receptor antagonist ELN441958. *The Journal of Pharmacology and Experimental Therapeutics*, *322*(2), 619–630. https://doi.org/10.1124/jpet.107.120352.

Hill, R., Disney, A., Conibear, A., Sutcliffe, K., Dewey, W., Husbands, S., et al. (2018). The novel mu-opioid receptor agonist PZM21 depresses respiration and induces tolerance to antinociception. *British Journal of Pharmacology*, *175*(13), 2653–2661. https://doi.org/10.1111/bph.14224.

Hnasko, T. S., Sotak, B. N., & Palmiter, R. D. (2005). Morphine reward in dopamine-deficient mice. *Nature*, *438*(7069), 854–857. https://doi.org/10.1038/nature04172.

Holmes, D. (2016). The pain drain. *Nature*, *535*(7611), S2–S3. https://doi.org/10.1038/535S2a.

Hopf, F. W. (2020). Recent perspectives on orexin/hypocretin promotion of addiction-related behaviors. *Neuropharmacology*, *168*, 108013. https://doi.org/10.1016/j.neuropharm.2020.108013.

Hopfner, K. P., & Hornung, V. (2020). Molecular mechanisms and cellular functions of cGAS-STING signalling. *Nature Reviews. Molecular Cell Biology*, *21*(9), 501–521. https://doi.org/10.1038/s41580-020-0244-x.

Iyer, R. N., Favela, D., Zhang, G., & Olson, D. E. (2021). The iboga enigma: the chemistry and neuropharmacology of iboga alkaloids and related analogs. *Natural Product Reports*, *38*(2), 307–329. https://doi.org/10.1039/d0np00033g.

James, M. H., Fragale, J. E., Aurora, R. N., Cooperman, N. A., Langleben, D. D., & Aston-Jones, G. (2020). Repurposing the dual orexin receptor antagonist suvorexant for the treatment of opioid use disorder: why sleep on this any longer? *Neuropsychopharmacology*, *45*(5), 717–719. https://doi.org/10.1038/s41386-020-0619-x.

James, M. H., Mahler, S. V., Moorman, D. E., & Aston-Jones, G. (2017). A decade of orexin/hypocretin and addiction: Where are we now? *Current Topics in Behavioral Neurosciences*, *33*, 247–281. https://doi.org/10.1007/7854_2016_57.

Ji, R. R., Chamessian, A., & Zhang, Y. Q. (2016). Pain regulation by non-neuronal cells and inflammation. *Science*, *354*(6312), 572–577. https://doi.org/10.1126/science.aaf8924.

Ji, R. R., Samad, T. A., Jin, S. X., Schmoll, R., & Woolf, C. J. (2002). p38 MAPK activation by NGF in primary sensory neurons after inflammation increases TRPV1 levels and maintains heat hyperalgesia. *Neuron*, *36*(1), 57–68. https://doi.org/10.1016/s0896-6273(02)00908-x.

Ji, R. R., Xu, Z. Z., & Gao, Y. J. (2014). Emerging targets in neuroinflammation-driven chronic pain. *Nature Reviews. Drug Discovery*, *13*(7), 533–548. https://doi.org/10.1038/nrd4334.

Johanson, C. E., Arfken, C. L., di Menza, S., & Schuster, C. R. (2012). Diversion and abuse of buprenorphine: Findings from national surveys of treatment patients and physicians. *Drug and Alcohol Dependence*, *120*(1-3), 190–195. https://doi.org/10.1016/j.drugalcdep.2011.07.019.

Jones, J. D., Manubay, J. M., Mogali, S., Metz, V. E., Madera, G., Martinez, S., et al. (2017). Abuse liability of intravenous buprenorphine vs. buprenorphine/naloxone: Importance of absolute naloxone amount. *Drug and Alcohol Dependence*, *179*, 362–369. https://doi.org/10.1016/j.drugalcdep.2017.06.033.

Kakko, J., Alho, H., Baldacchino, A., Molina, R., Nava, F. A., & Shaya, G. (2019). Craving in opioid use disorder: From neurobiology to clinical practice. *Frontiers in Psychiatry*, *10*, 592. https://doi.org/10.3389/fpsyt.2019.00592.

Khroyan, T. V., Polgar, W. E., Cami-Kobeci, G., Husbands, S. M., Zaveri, N. T., & Toll, L. (2011). The first universal opioid ligand, (2S)-2-[(5R,6R,7R,14S)-N-cyclopropylmethyl-4,5-epoxy-6,14-ethano-3-hydroxy-6-meth oxymorphinan-7-yl]-3,3-dimethylpentan-2-ol (BU08028): characterization of the in vitro profile and in vivo behavioral effects in mouse models of acute pain and cocaine-induced reward. *The Journal of Pharmacology and Experimental Therapeutics*, *336*(3), 952–961. https://doi.org/10.1124/jpet.110.175620.

Kiguchi, N., Ding, H., Cami-Kobeci, G., Sukhtankar, D. D., Czoty, P. W., DeLoid, H. B., et al. (2019). BU10038 as a safe opioid analgesic with fewer side-effects after systemic and intrathecal administration in primates. *British Journal of Anaesthesia*, *122*(6), e146–e156. https://doi.org/10.1016/j.bja.2018.10.065.

Kiguchi, N., Ding, H., Kishioka, S., & Ko, M. C. (2020). Nociceptin/Orphanin FQ Peptide Receptor-Related Ligands as Novel Analgesics. *Current Topics in Medicinal Chemistry*, *20*(31), 2878–2888. https://doi.org/10.2174/1568026620666200508082615.

Kiguchi, N., Ding, H., & Ko, M. C. (2016). Central N/OFQ-NOP receptor system in pain modulation. *Advances in Pharmacology*, *75*, 217–243. https://doi.org/10.1016/bs.apha.2015.10.001.

Kiguchi, N., Ding, H., & Ko, M. C. (2020). Therapeutic potentials of NOP and MOP receptor coactivation for the treatment of pain and opioid abuse. *Journal of Neuroscience Research*. https://doi.org/10.1002/jnr.24624.

Kiguchi, N., & Ko, M. C. (2019). Effects of NOP-related ligands in nonhuman primates. *Handbook of Experimental Pharmacology*, *254*, 323–343. https://doi.org/10.1007/164_2019_211.

Kleideiter, E., Piana, C., Wang, S., Nemeth, R., & Gautrois, M. (2018). Clinical pharmacokinetic characteristics of cebranopadol, a novel first-in-class analgesic. *Clinical Pharmacokinetics*, *57*(1), 31–50. https://doi.org/10.1007/s40262-017-0545-1.

Ko, M. C., Woods, J. H., Fantegrossi, W. E., Galuska, C. M., Wichmann, J., & Prinssen, E. P. (2009). Behavioral effects of a synthetic agonist selective for nociceptin/orphanin FQ peptide receptors in monkeys. *Neuropsychopharmacology*, *34*(9), 2088–2096. https://doi.org/10.1038/npp.2009.33.

Kourrich, S., Calu, D. J., & Bonci, A. (2015). Intrinsic plasticity: An emerging player in addiction. *Nature Reviews. Neuroscience*, *16*(3), 173–184. https://doi.org/10.1038/nrn3877.

Kreek, M. J., Reed, B., & Butelman, E. R. (2019). Current status of opioid addiction treatment and related preclinical research. *Science Advances*, *5*(10), eaax9140. https://doi.org/10.1126/sciadv.aax9140.

Lai, J., Gold, M. S., Kim, C. S., Bian, D., Ossipov, M. H., Hunter, J. C., et al. (2002). Inhibition of neuropathic pain by decreased expression of the tetrodotoxin-resistant sodium channel, NaV1.8. *Pain*, *95*(1-2), 143–152. https://doi.org/10.1016/s0304-3959(01)00391-8.

Lane, N. E., & Corr, M. (2017). Osteoarthritis in 2016: Anti-NGF treatments for pain—Two steps forward, one step back? *Nature Reviews Rheumatology*, *13*(2), 76–78. https://doi.org/10.1038/nrrheum.2016.224.

Lavonas, E. J., Severtson, S. G., Martinez, E. M., Bucher-Bartelson, B., Le Lait, M. C., Green, J. L., et al. (2014). Abuse and diversion of buprenorphine sublingual tablets and film. *Journal of Substance Abuse Treatment*, *47*(1), 27–34. https://doi.org/10.1016/j.jsat.2014.02.003.

Le Foll, B. (2021). Opioid-sparing effects of cannabinoids: Myth or reality? *Progress in Neuro-Psychopharmacology & Biological Psychiatry*, *106*, 110065. https://doi.org/10.1016/j.pnpbp.2020.110065.

Le Pen, G., Wichmann, J., Moreau, J. L., & Jenck, F. (2002). The orphanin receptor agonist RO 64-6198 does not induce place conditioning in rats. *Neuroreport*, *13*(4), 451–454. https://doi.org/10.1097/00001756-200203250-00018.

Lee, H., & Ko, M. C. (2015). Distinct functions of opioid-related peptides and gastrin-releasing peptide in regulating itch and pain in the spinal cord of primates. *Scientific Reports*, *5*, 11676. https://doi.org/10.1038/srep11676.

Lin, A. P., & Ko, M. C. (2013). The therapeutic potential of nociceptin/orphanin FQ receptor agonists as analgesics without abuse liability. *ACS Chemical Neuroscience*, *4*(2), 214–224. https://doi.org/10.1021/cn300124f.

Lingford-Hughes, A. R., Welch, S., Peters, L., Nutt, D. J., & British Association for Psychopharmacology, E. R. G. (2012). BAP updated guidelines: evidence-based guidelines for the pharmacological management of substance abuse, harmful use, addiction and comorbidity: recommendations from BAP. *Journal of Psychopharmacology*, *26*(7), 899–952. https://doi.org/10.1177/0269881112444324.

Linz, K., Christoph, T., Tzschentke, T. M., Koch, T., Schiene, K., Gautrois, M., et al. (2014). Cebranopadol: a novel potent analgesic nociceptin/orphanin FQ peptide and opioid receptor agonist. *The Journal of Pharmacology and Experimental Therapeutics*, *349*(3), 535–548. https://doi.org/10.1124/jpet.114.213694.

Liu, J. F., & Li, J. X. (2018). TAAR1 in addiction: Looking beyond the tip of the iceberg. *Frontiers in Pharmacology*, *9*, 279. https://doi.org/10.3389/fphar.2018.00279.

Liu, J., Seaman, R., Jr., Johnson, B., Wu, R., Vu, J., Tian, J., et al. (2021). Activation of trace amine-associated receptor 1 selectively attenuates the reinforcing effects of morphine. *British Journal of Pharmacology*, *178*(4), 933–945. https://doi.org/10.1111/bph.15335.

Liu, J., Wu, R., & Li, J. X. (2020). TAAR1 and psychostimulant addiction. *Cellular and Molecular Neurobiology*, *40*(2), 229–238. https://doi.org/10.1007/s10571-020-00792-8.

Lucchesi, M., Lanzetta, G., Antonuzzo, A., Rozzi, A., Sardi, I., Favre, C., et al. (2017). Developing drugs in cancer-related bone pain. *Critical Reviews in Oncology/Hematology*, *119*, 66–74. https://doi.org/10.1016/j.critrevonc.2017.08.005.

Luttrell, L. M., Maudsley, S., & Bohn, L. M. (2015). Fulfilling the promise of "biased" G protein-coupled receptor agonism. *Molecular Pharmacology*, *88*(3), 579–588. https://doi.org/10.1124/mol.115.099630.

Malerba, M., & Ragnoli, B. (2008). Ambroxol in the 21st century: Pharmacological and clinical update. *Expert Opinion on Drug Metabolism & Toxicology*, *4*(8), 1119–1129. https://doi.org/10.1517/17425255.4.8.1119.

Manglik, A., Lin, H., Aryal, D. K., McCorvy, J. D., Dengler, D., Corder, G., et al. (2016). Structure-based discovery of opioid analgesics with reduced side effects. *Nature*, *537*(7619), 185–190. https://doi.org/10.1038/nature19112.

Maresz, K., Pryce, G., Ponomarev, E. D., Marsicano, G., Croxford, J. L., Shriver, L. P., et al. (2007). Direct suppression of CNS autoimmune inflammation via the cannabinoid receptor CB1 on neurons and CB2 on autoreactive T cells. *Nature Medicine*, *13*(4), 492–497. https://doi.org/10.1038/nm1561.

Margolis, E. B., Lock, H., Chefer, V. I., Shippenberg, T. S., Hjelmstad, G. O., & Fields, H. L. (2006). Kappa opioids selectively control dopaminergic neurons projecting to the prefrontal cortex. *Proceedings of the National Academy of Sciences of the United States of America*, *103*(8), 2938–2942. https://doi.org/10.1073/pnas.0511159103.

Marinelli, L., Balestrino, M., Mori, L., Puce, L., Rosa, G. M., Giorello, L., et al. (2017). A randomised controlled cross-over double-blind pilot study protocol on THC:CBD oromucosal spray efficacy as an add-on therapy for post-stroke spasticity. *BMJ Open*, 7(9), e016843. https://doi.org/10.1136/bmjopen-2017-016843.

Marvaldi, L., Panayotis, N., Alber, S., Dagan, S. Y., Okladnikov, N., Koppel, I., et al. (2020). Importin alpha3 regulates chronic pain pathways in peripheral sensory neurons. *Science*, *369*(6505), 842–846. https://doi.org/10.1126/science.aaz5875.

Matsuda, L. A., Lolait, S. J., Brownstein, M. J., Young, A. C., & Bonner, T. I. (1990). Structure of a cannabinoid receptor and functional expression of the cloned cDNA. *Nature*, *346*(6284), 561–564. https://doi.org/10.1038/346561a0.

Matthes, H. W., Maldonado, R., Simonin, F., Valverde, O., Slowe, S., Kitchen, I., et al. (1996). Loss of morphine-induced analgesia, reward effect and withdrawal symptoms in mice lacking the mu-opioid-receptor gene. *Nature*, *383*(6603), 819–823. https://doi.org/10.1038/383819a0.

Matzeu, A., & Martin-Fardon, R. (2020). Targeting the orexin system for prescription opioid use disorder: Orexin-1 receptor blockade prevents oxycodone taking and seeking in rats. *Neuropharmacology*, *164*, 107906. https://doi.org/10.1016/j.neuropharm.2019.107906.

McDermott, L. A., Weir, G. A., Themistocleous, A. C., Segerdahl, A. R., Blesneac, I., Baskozos, G., et al. (2019). Defining the functional role of NaV1.7 in human nociception. *Neuron*, *101*(5), 905–919. e908 https://doi.org/10.1016/j.neuron.2019.01.047.

Moehring, F., Halder, P., Seal, R. P., & Stucky, C. L. (2018). Uncovering the cells and circuits of touch in normal and pathological settings. *Neuron*, *100*(2), 349–360. https://doi.org/10.1016/j.neuron.2018.10.019.

Morales, M., & Margolis, E. B. (2017). Ventral tegmental area: cellular heterogeneity, connectivity and behaviour. *Nature Reviews. Neuroscience*, *18*(2), 73–85. https://doi.org/10.1038/nrn.2016.165.

Moran, M. M., McAlexander, M. A., Biro, T., & Szallasi, A. (2011). Transient receptor potential channels as therapeutic targets. *Nature Reviews. Drug Discovery*, *10*(8), 601–620. https://doi.org/10.1038/nrd3456.

Murphy, N. P., Lee, Y., & Maidment, N. T. (1999). Orphanin FQ/nociceptin blocks acquisition of morphine place preference. *Brain Research*, *832*(1-2), 168–170.

Nilius, B., & Szallasi, A. (2014). Transient receptor potential channels as drug targets: From the science of basic research to the art of medicine. *Pharmacological Reviews*, *66*(3), 676–814. https://doi.org/10.1124/pr.113.008268.

Nutt, D. J., Lingford-Hughes, A., Erritzoe, D., & Stokes, P. R. (2015). The dopamine theory of addiction: 40 years of highs and lows. *Nature Reviews. Neuroscience*, *16*(5), 305–312. https://doi.org/10.1038/nrn3939.

Orefice, N. S., Alhouayek, M., Carotenuto, A., Montella, S., Barbato, F., Comelli, A., et al. (2016). Oral palmitoylethanolamide treatment is associated with reduced cutaneous adverse effects of interferon-beta1a and circulating proinflammatory cytokines in relapsing-remitting multiple sclerosis. *Neurotherapeutics*, *13*(2), 428–438. https://doi.org/10.1007/s13311-016-0420-z.

Pain, S. (2016). Painful progress. *Nature*, *535*(7611), S18–S19. https://doi.org/10.1038/535S18a.

Panayotis, N., Karpova, A., Kreutz, M. R., & Fainzilber, M. (2015). Macromolecular transport in synapse to nucleus communication. *Trends in Neurosciences*, *38*(2), 108–116. https://doi.org/10.1016/j.tins.2014.12.001.

Parker, K. E., Pedersen, C. E., Gomez, A. M., Spangler, S. M., Walicki, M. C., Feng, S. Y., et al. (2019). A paranigral VTA nociceptin circuit that constrains motivation for reward. *Cell*, *178*(3), 653–671. e619. https://doi.org/10.1016/j.cell.2019.06.034.

Peirs, C., & Seal, R. P. (2016). Neural circuits for pain: Recent advances and current views. *Science*, *354*(6312), 578–584. https://doi.org/10.1126/science.aaf8933.

Perrey, D. A., & Zhang, Y. (2020). Therapeutics development for addiction: Orexin-1 receptor antagonists. *Brain Research*, *1731*, 145922. https://doi.org/10.1016/j.brainres.2018.08.025.

Podlesnik, C. A., Ko, M. C., Winger, G., Wichmann, J., Prinssen, E. P., & Woods, J. H. (2011). The effects of nociceptin/orphanin FQ receptor agonist Ro 64-6198 and diazepam on antinociception and remifentanil self-administration in rhesus monkeys. *Psychopharmacology*, *213*(1), 53–60. https://doi.org/10.1007/s00213-010-2012-7.

Prenderville, J. A., Kelly, A. M., & Downer, E. J. (2015). The role of cannabinoids in adult neurogenesis. *British Journal of Pharmacology*, *172*(16), 3950–3963. https://doi.org/10.1111/bph.13186.

Price, N., Namdari, R., Neville, J., Proctor, K. J., Kaber, S., Vest, J., et al. (2017). Safety and efficacy of a topical sodium channel inhibitor (TV-45070) in patients with postherpetic neuralgia (PHN): A randomized, controlled, proof-of-concept, crossover study, with a subgroup analysis of the Nav1.7 R1150W genotype. *The Clinical Journal of Pain*, *33*(4), 310–318. https://doi.org/10.1097/AJP.0000000000000408.

Raehal, K. M., Walker, J. K., & Bohn, L. M. (2005). Morphine side effects in beta-arrestin 2 knockout mice. *The Journal of Pharmacology and Experimental Therapeutics*, *314*(3), 1195–1201. https://doi.org/10.1124/jpet.105.087254.

Raja, S. N., Carr, D. B., Cohen, M., Finnerup, N. B., Flor, H., Gibson, S., et al. (2020). The revised International Association for the Study of Pain definition of pain: concepts, challenges, and compromises. *Pain*, *161*(9), 1976–1982. https://doi.org/10.1097/j.pain.0000000000001939.

Rasmussen, K., White, D. A., & Acri, J. B. (2019). NIDA's medication development priorities in response to the opioid crisis: ten most wanted. *Neuropsychopharmacology*, *44*(4), 657–659. https://doi.org/10.1038/s41386-018-0292-5.

Ray, P., Torck, A., Quigley, L., Wangzhou, A., Neiman, M., Rao, C., et al. (2018). Comparative transcriptome profiling of the human and mouse dorsal root ganglia: an RNA-seq-based resource for pain and sensory neuroscience research. *Pain*, *159*(7), 1325–1345. https://doi.org/10.1097/j.pain.0000000000001217.

Reimer, J., Vogelmann, T., Trümper, D., & Scherbaum, N. (2020). Impact of buprenorphine dosage on the occurrence of relapses in patients with opioid dependence. *European Addiction Research*, *26*(2), 77–84. https://doi.org/10.1159/000505294.

Revel, F. G., Moreau, J. L., Gainetdinov, R. R., Bradaia, A., Sotnikova, T. D., Mory, R., et al. (2011). TAAR1 activation modulates monoaminergic neurotransmission, preventing hyperdopaminergic and hypoglutamatergic activity. *Proceedings of the National Academy of Sciences of the United States of America*, *108*(20), 8485–8490. https://doi.org/10.1073/pnas.1103029108.

Rhesus Macaque Genome, S., Analysis, C., Gibbs, R. A., Rogers, J., Katze, M. G., Bumgarner, R., et al. (2007). Evolutionary and biomedical insights from the rhesus macaque genome. *Science*, *316*(5822), 222–234. https://doi.org/10.1126/science.1139247.

Rios, C., Gomes, I., & Devi, L. A. (2006). Mu opioid and CB1 cannabinoid receptor interactions: reciprocal inhibition of receptor signaling and neuritogenesis. *British Journal of Pharmacology*, *148*(4), 387–395. https://doi.org/10.1038/sj.bjp.0706757.

Rothman, R. B. (1994). A review of the effects of dopaminergic agents in humans: Implications for medication development. *NIDA Research Monograph*, *145*, 67–87. Retrieved from https://www.ncbi.nlm.nih.gov/pubmed/8742808.

Saxon, A. J. (2013). Treatment of opioid dependence. In *Research and Development of Opioid-Related Ligands* (pp. 61–102). American Chemical Society Publications.

Schmid, C. L., & Bohn, L. M. (2009). Physiological and pharmacological implications of beta-arrestin regulation. *Pharmacology & Therapeutics*, *121*(3), 285–293. https://doi.org/10.1016/j.pharmthera.2008.11.005.

Schmid, C. L., Kennedy, N. M., Ross, N. C., Lovell, K. M., Yue, Z., Morgenweck, J., et al. (2017). Bias factor and therapeutic window correlate to predict safer opioid analgesics. *Cell*, *171*(5), 1165–1175. e1113 https://doi.org/10.1016/j.cell.2017.10.035.

Schroder, W., Lambert, D. G., Ko, M. C., & Koch, T. (2014). Functional plasticity of the N/OFQ-NOP receptor system determines analgesic properties of NOP receptor agonists. *British Journal of Pharmacology*, *171*(16), 3777–3800. https://doi.org/10.1111/bph.12744.

Schuckit, M. A. (2016). Treatment of opioid-use disorders. *The New England Journal of Medicine*, *375*(4), 357–368. https://doi.org/10.1056/NEJMra1604339.

Schwartz, M. D., Canales, J. J., Zucchi, R., Espinoza, S., Sukhanov, I., & Gainetdinov, R. R. (2018). Trace amine-associated receptor 1: A multimodal therapeutic target for neuropsychiatric diseases. *Expert Opinion on Therapeutic Targets*, *22*(6), 513–526. https://doi.org/10.1080/14728222.2018.1480723.

Seok, J., Warren, H. S., Cuenca, A. G., Mindrinos, M. N., Baker, H. V., Xu, W., et al. (2013). Genomic responses in mouse models poorly mimic human inflammatory diseases. *Proceedings of the National Academy of Sciences of the United States of America*, *110*(9), 3507–3512. https://doi.org/10.1073/pnas.1222878110.

Sharf, R., Sarhan, M., & Dileone, R. J. (2008). Orexin mediates the expression of precipitated morphine withdrawal and concurrent activation of the nucleus accumbens shell. *Biological Psychiatry*, *64*(3), 175–183. https://doi.org/10.1016/j.biopsych.2008.03.006.

Shiers, S. I., Sankaranarayanan, I., Jeevakumar, V., Cervantes, A., Reese, J. C., & Price, T. J. (2021). Convergence of peptidergic and non-peptidergic protein markers in the human dorsal root ganglion and spinal dorsal horn. *Journal of Comparative Neurology*, *529*(10), 2771–2788. https://doi.org/10.1002/cne.25122.

Smith, R. J., & Aston-Jones, G. (2012). Orexin/hypocretin 1 receptor antagonist reduces heroin self-administration and cue-induced heroin seeking. *The European Journal of Neuroscience*, *35*(5), 798–804. https://doi.org/10.1111/j.1460-9568.2012.08013.x.

Soergel, D. G., Subach, R. A., Burnham, N., Lark, M. W., James, I. E., Sadler, B. M., et al. (2014). Biased agonism of the mu-opioid receptor by TRV130 increases analgesia and reduces on-target adverse effects versus morphine: A randomized, double-blind, placebo-controlled, crossover study in healthy volunteers. *Pain*, *155*(9), 1829–1835. https://doi.org/10.1016/j.pain.2014.06.011.

Sotnikova, T. D., Caron, M. G., & Gainetdinov, R. R. (2009). Trace amine-associated receptors as emerging therapeutic targets. *Molecular Pharmacology*, *76*(2), 229–235. https://doi.org/10.1124/mol.109.055970.

Sousa, R., Lakha, D. R., Brette, S., & Hitier, S. (2019). A randomized, double-blind, placebo-controlled study to assess the efficacy and safety of ambroxol hard-boiled lozenges in patients with acute pharyngitis. *Pulm Ther*, *5*(2), 201–211. https://doi.org/10.1007/s41030-019-00100-w.

Steinhoff, M. S., von Mentzer, B., Geppetti, P., Pothoulakis, C., & Bunnett, N. W. (2014). Tachykinins and their receptors: Contributions to physiological control and the mechanisms of disease. *Physiological Reviews*, *94*(1), 265–301. https://doi.org/10.1152/physrev.00031.2013.

Stoppiello, L. A., Mapp, P. I., Wilson, D., Hill, R., Scammell, B. E., & Walsh, D. A. (2014). Structural associations of symptomatic knee osteoarthritis. *Arthritis & Rhematology*, *66*(11), 3018–3027. https://doi.org/10.1002/art.38778.

Sugiura, T., Kondo, S., Sukagawa, A., Nakane, S., Shinoda, A., Itoh, K., et al. (1995). 2-Arachidonoylglycerol: a possible endogenous cannabinoid receptor ligand in brain. *Biochemical and Biophysical Research Communications*, *215*(1), 89–97. https://doi.org/10.1006/bbrc.1995.2437.

Sukhtankar, D. D., Lagorio, C. H., & Ko, M. C. (2014). Effects of the NOP agonist SCH221510 on producing and attenuating reinforcing effects as measured by drug self-administration in rats. *European Journal of Pharmacology*, *745*, 182–189. https://doi.org/10.1016/j.ejphar.2014.10.029.

Sukhtankar, D. D., Zaveri, N. T., Husbands, S. M., & Ko, M. C. (2013). Effects of spinally administered bifunctional nociceptin/orphanin FQ peptide receptor/mu-opioid receptor ligands in mouse models of neuropathic and inflammatory pain. *The Journal of Pharmacology and Experimental Therapeutics*, *346*(1), 11–22. https://doi.org/10.1124/jpet.113.203984.

Sulzer, D. (2011). How addictive drugs disrupt presynaptic dopamine neurotransmission. *Neuron*, *69*(4), 628–649. https://doi.org/10.1016/j.neuron.2011.02.010.

Tejeda, H. A., Wu, J., Kornspun, A. R., Pignatelli, M., Kashtelyan, V., Krashes, M. J., et al. (2017). Pathway- and cell-specific kappa-opioid receptor modulation of excitation-inhibition balance differentially gates D1 and D2 accumbens neuron activity. *Neuron*, *93*(1), 147–163. https://doi.org/10.1016/j.neuron.2016.12.005.

Thannickal, T. C., John, J., Shan, L., Swaab, D. F., Wu, M. F., Ramanathan, L., et al. (2018). Opiates increase the number of hypocretin-producing cells in human and mouse brain and reverse cataplexy in a mouse model of narcolepsy. *Science Translational Medicine*, *10*(447). https://doi.org/10.1126/scitranslmed.aao4953.

Todd, A. J. (2010). Neuronal circuitry for pain processing in the dorsal horn. *Nature Reviews. Neuroscience*, *11*(12), 823–836. https://doi.org/10.1038/nrn2947.

Toll, L., Bruchas, M. R., Calo, G., Cox, B. M., & Zaveri, N. T. (2016). Nociceptin/orphanin FQ receptor structure, signaling, ligands, functions, and interactions with opioid systems. *Pharmacological Reviews*, *68*(2), 419–457. https://doi.org/10.1124/pr.114.009209.

Tonelli, M., & Cichero, E. (2020). Trace amine associated receptor 1 (TAAR1) modulators: a patent review (2010-present). *Expert Opinion on Therapeutic Patents*, *30*(2), 137–145. https://doi.org/10.1080/13543776.2020.1708900.

Tzschentke, T. M., Linz, K., Koch, T., & Christoph, T. (2019). Cebranopadol: A novel first-in-class potent analgesic acting via NOP and opioid receptors. *Handbook of Experimental Pharmacology*, *254*, 367–398. https://doi.org/10.1007/164_2019_206.

Violin, J. D., Crombie, A. L., Soergel, D. G., & Lark, M. W. (2014). Biased ligands at G-protein-coupled receptors: promise and progress. *Trends in Pharmacological Sciences*, *35*(7), 308–316. https://doi.org/10.1016/j.tips.2014.04.007.

Viscusi, E. R., Webster, L., Kuss, M., Daniels, S., Bolognese, J. A., Zuckerman, S., et al. (2016). A randomized, phase 2 study investigating TRV130, a biased ligand of the mu-opioid receptor, for the intravenous treatment of acute pain. *Pain*, *157*(1), 264–272. https://doi.org/10.1097/j.pain.0000000000000363.

Volkow, N. D., & Blanco, C. (2020). The changing opioid crisis: Development, challenges and opportunities. *Molecular Psychiatry*, *26*(1), 218–233. https://doi.org/10.1038/s41380-41020-40661-41384.

Volkow, N. D., & Collins, F. S. (2017). The role of science in addressing the opioid crisis. *The New England Journal of Medicine*, *377*(4), 391–394. https://doi.org/10.1056/NEJMsr1706626.

Warren, W. C., Harris, R. A., Haukness, M., Fiddes, I. T., Murali, S. C., Fernandes, J., et al. (2020). Sequence diversity analyses of an improved rhesus macaque genome enhance its biomedical utility. *Science*, *370*(6523). https://doi.org/10.1126/science.abc6617.

Watt, F. E., Blauwet, M. B., Fakhoury, A., Jacobs, H., Smulders, R., & Lane, N. E. (2019). Tropomyosin-related kinase A (TrkA) inhibition for the treatment of painful knee osteoarthritis: results from a randomized controlled phase 2a trial. *Osteoarthritis and Cartilage*, *27*(11), 1590–1598. https://doi.org/10.1016/j.joca.2019.05.029.

Waxman, S. G., & Zamponi, G. W. (2014). Regulating excitability of peripheral afferents: Emerging ion channel targets. *Nature Neuroscience*, *17*(2), 153–163. https://doi.org/10.1038/nn.3602.

Weiser, T., & Wilson, N. (2002). Inhibition of tetrodotoxin (TTX)-resistant and TTX-sensitive neuronal Na(+) channels by the secretolytic ambroxol. *Molecular Pharmacology*, *62*(3), 433–438. https://doi.org/10.1124/mol.62.3.433.

Welch, S. P. (2009). Interaction of the cannabinoid and opioid systems in the modulation of nociception. *International Review of Psychiatry*, *21*(2), 143–151. https://doi.org/10.1080/09540260902782794.

Whistler, J. L., Chuang, H. H., Chu, P., Jan, L. Y., & von Zastrow, M. (1999). Functional dissociation of mu opioid receptor signaling and endocytosis: implications for the biology of opiate tolerance and addiction. *Neuron*, *23*(4), 737–746.

Winters, B. L., Christie, M. J., & Vaughan, C. W. (2019). Electrophysiological Actions of N/OFQ. *Handbook of Experimental Pharmacology*, *254*, 91–130. https://doi.org/10.1007/164_2019_205.

Wise, B. L., Seidel, M. F., & Lane, N. E. (2021). The evolution of nerve growth factor inhibition in clinical medicine. *Nature Reviews Rheumatology*, *17*(1), 34–46. https://doi.org/10.1038/s41584-020-00528-4.

Woolf, C. J. (2020). Capturing novel non-opioid pain targets. *Biological Psychiatry*, *87*(1), 74–81. https://doi.org/10.1016/j.biopsych.2019.06.017.

Yasuda, K., Raynor, K., Kong, H., Breder, C. D., Takeda, J., Reisine, T., et al. (1993). Cloning and functional comparison of kappa and delta opioid receptors from mouse brain. *Proceedings of the National Academy of Sciences of the United States of America*, *90*(14), 6736–6740. https://doi.org/10.1073/pnas.90.14.6736.

Yekkirala, A. S., Roberson, D. P., Bean, B. P., & Woolf, C. J. (2017). Breaking barriers to novel analgesic drug development. *Nature Reviews. Drug Discovery*, *16*(8), 545–564. https://doi.org/10.1038/nrd.2017.87.

Yu, H., Zhao, T., Liu, S., Wu, Q., Johnson, O., Wu, Z., et al. (2019). MRGPRX4 is a bile acid receptor for human cholestatic itch. *eLife*, *8*, e48431. https://doi.org/10.7554/eLife.48431.

Zamarripa, C., Edwards, S. R., Qureshi, H. N., Yi, J. N., Blough, B. E., & Freeman, K. B. (2018). The G-protein biased mu-opioid agonist, TRV130, produces reinforcing and antinociceptive effects that are comparable to oxycodone in rats. *Drug and Alcohol Dependence*, *192*, 158–162. https://doi.org/10.1016/j.drugalcdep.2018.08.002.

Zarepour, L., Fatahi, Z., Sarihi, A., & Haghparast, A. (2014). Blockade of orexin-1 receptors in the ventral tegmental area could attenuate the lateral hypothalamic stimulation-induced potentiation of rewarding properties of morphine. *Neuropeptides*, *48*(3), 179–185. https://doi.org/10.1016/j.npep.2014.04.003.

Zaveri, N. T., & Meyer, M. E. (2019). NOP-targeted nonpeptide ligands. *Handbook of Experimental Pharmacology*, *254*, 37–67. https://doi.org/10.1007/164_2019_213.

Zeisel, A., Hochgerner, H., Lonnerberg, P., Johnsson, A., Memic, F., van der Zwan, J., et al. (2018). Molecular architecture of the mouse nervous system. *Cell*, *174*(4), 999–1014. e1022 https://doi.org/10.1016/j.cell.2018.06.021.

Zhang, J., Ferguson, S. S., Barak, L. S., Bodduluri, S. R., Laporte, S. A., Law, P. Y., et al. (1998). Role for G protein-coupled receptor kinase in agonist-specific regulation of mu-opioid receptor responsiveness. *Proceedings of the National Academy of Sciences of the United States of America*, *95*(12), 7157–7162.

CHAPTER ELEVEN

Trace amine-associated receptor 1 and drug abuse

Ruyan Wu[a,b], Jianfeng Liu[c], and Jun-Xu Li[b,*]

[a]Medical College of Yangzhou University, Yangzhou, China
[b]Department of Pharmacology and Toxicology, University at Buffalo, Buffalo, NY, United States
[c]Department of Psychological and Brain Sciences, College of Liberal Arts, Texas A&M University, College Station, TX, United States
[*]Corresponding author: e-mail address: junxuli@buffalo.edu

Contents

1. Introduction 375
2. The implication of TAAR1 in the brain 376
3. Neural mechanisms of TAAR1 in drug addiction 378
   3.1 Dopaminergic system 378
   3.2 Cellular signaling 385
   3.3 Neuroanatomic sites of TAAR1 actions 386
4. TAAR1 and psychostimulants 386
   4.1 Amphetamines 386
   4.2 Cocaine 388
   4.3 Nicotine 389
5. TAAR1 and opioids 390
   5.1 Morphine 390
6. TAAR1 and alcohol 392
7. Current challenges 392
   7.1 TAAR1 and other drugs of abuse 392
   7.2 TAAR1 agonists and antagonists 393
   7.3 Clinical studies of TAAR1 agonists 394
8. Conclusion 394
Acknowledgments 395
Conflict of interest 395
References 395

Abstract

Trace amine-associated receptor 1 (TAAR1) is the best characterized receptor selectively activated by trace amines. It is broadly expressed in the monoaminergic system in the brain including ventral tegmental area (VTA), nucleus accumbens (NAc), dorsal raphe (DR) and substantial nigra (SN). Extensive studies have suggested that TAAR1 plays an important role in the modulation of monoaminergic system, especially dopamine (DA) transmission which may underlie the mechanisms by which TAAR1 interventions affect drug abuse-like behaviors. TAAR1 activation inhibits the rewarding and

Advances in Pharmacology, Volume 93
ISSN 1054-3589
https://doi.org/10.1016/bs.apha.2021.10.005

reinforcing effects of drugs from different classes including psychostimulants, opioid and alcohol as well as drug-induced increase in DA accumulation. The mechanisms of TAAR1's function in mediating drug abuse-like behaviors are not clear. However, it is hypothesized that TAAR1 interaction with DA transporter (DAT) and dopamine D2 receptor (D2) and the subsequent modulation of cellular cascades may contribute to the effects of TAAR1 in regulating drug abuse. Further studies are needed to investigate the role of TAAR1 in other drugs of abuse-related behaviors and its safety and efficacy for prolonged medications. Together, TAAR1 inhibits drug-induced DA transmission and drug abuse-related behaviors. Therefore, TAAR1 may be a promising therapeutic target for the treatment of drug addiction.

Abbreviations

3-MT	3-methoxytyramine
BRET	bioluminescence resonance energy transfer
CFA	Complete Freund's adjuvant
CPA	conditioned place aversion
CPP	conditioned place preference
CTA	conditioned taste aversion
DA	dopamine
DAT	dopamine transporter
DR	dorsal raphe
GPCR	G-protein coupled receptors
ICSS	intracranial self-stimulation
IUPHAR	International Union of Pharmacology
LA	long-access
LC	locus coeruleus
LLA	locomotor-like activity
LORR	loss of righting reflex
MDMA, ecstasy	3,4-methylenedioxymethamphetamine
METH	methamphetamine
NAc	nucleus accumbens
NE	norepinephrine
OCT	p-octopamine
PEA	β-phenylethylamine
PNSS	positive and negative symptom scale
POHA	para-hydroxyamphetamine
ShA	short-access
SN	substantial nigra
TAAR1	Trace amine-associated receptor 1
TAAR1-KO	TAAR1 knockout
TAAR1-OE	TAAR1 overexpression
TAs	trace-amine receptors
TBC	two-bottle choice
TRP	tryptamine
TYR	p-tyramine
VTA	ventral tegmental area
WT	wide-type

1. Introduction

The research and interest in trace amines, which include β-phenylethylamine (PEA), p-tyramine (TYR), tryptamine (TRP), and p-octopamine (OCT), dates back to almost 50 years ago (Boulton, 1974, 1980; Sandler et al., 1980). Trace amines (TA) represent a group of endogenous amines which express at levels that are at least 100-fold lower than those of classic monoamine transmitters such as dopamine (DA), serotonin and norepinephrine (NE) (Berry, 2004; Grandy, 2007). Although trace amines share the most obvious structural similarity with the well-established classic amines (Fig. 1) and are implicated to exert physiological effects in the brain (Berry, 2007; Burchett & Hicks, 2006), their functions remained largely unknown for decades due to the lack of specific receptors (Miller, 2011). Fortunately, in 2001, a new family of G-protein coupled receptors (GPCR), termed Trace-Amine Receptors (TAs), were cloned by two independent groups (Borowsky et al., 2001; Bunzow et al., 2001) where two members of this family (TA_1 and TA_2) were reported to be selectively activated by trace amines.

Four years later, a new TA receptor nomenclature was suggested to be changed to Trace Amine-Associated Receptor (TAAR) since only TA_1 and TA_2 can be activated by trace amines (Lindemann & Hoener, 2005). Thus, TA_1 was renamed as TAAR1 (Lindemann & Hoener, 2005). However, it

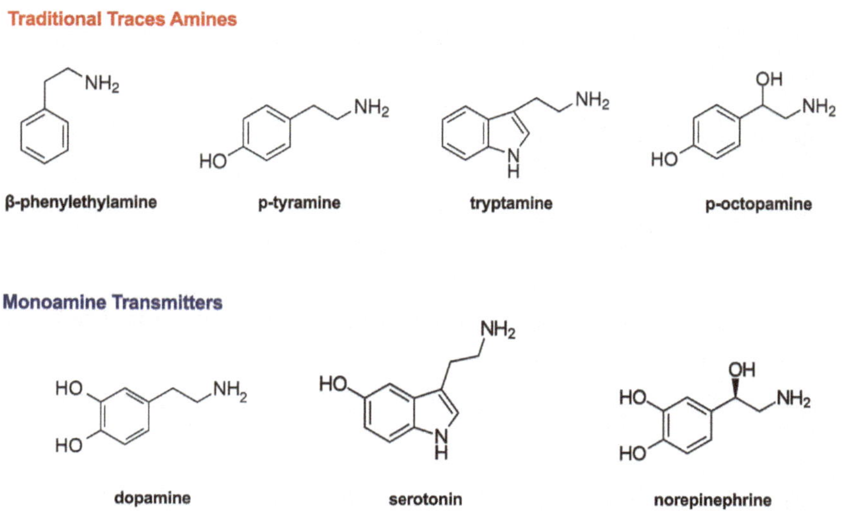

Fig. 1 Structures of representative trace amines and classic monoamine transmitters.

was later suggested by the International Union of Pharmacology (IUPHAR) that the name of receptor remained TA_1 in 2009 (Maguire et al., 2009). While the IUPHAR's suggestion is based on the tradition that receptor be named for their endogenous ligands (Gainetdinov, Hoener, & Berry, 2018), it presents an uncomfortable condition in this field since almost all recent studies refer to this receptor as TAAR1 (Lam, Espinoza, Gerasimov, Gainetdinov, & Salahpour, 2015). Therefore, we will also be using the TAAR1 in this review for simplicity and consistency.

2. The implication of TAAR1 in the brain

Because TAAR4 (previous TA_2) is actually a pseudogene in humans (Liu, Kusumi, Ulpian, Tallerico, & Seeman, 1998; Maguire et al., 2009), most of the subsequent research interest focused on TAAR1. The human, rat and mouse TAAR1 coupled to a $G\alpha_s$ class G-protein and increased cAMP accumulation (Borowsky et al., 2001; Bunzow et al., 2001; Hartmann, Sherriff, & Kent, 1995). While all TAARs (except for TAAR1) are expressed in the olfactory epithelium and shown to potentially function as a group of olfactory receptors (Dewan, Pacifico, Zhan, Rinberg, & Bozza, 2013; Liberles & Buck, 2006; Zhang, Pacifico, Cawley, Feinstein, & Bozza, 2013), TAAR1 mRNA was reported in several brain regions including amygdala, hippocampus, dorsal root ganglia and cerebellum (Borowsky et al., 2001). The expression of TAAR1 was also found in spinal cord and periphery where its role in regulating immune functions was overlooked, mainly because the TAAR1 presence was further shown in several key monoaminergic brain regions including ventral tegmental area (VTA), locus coeruleus (LC), dorsal raphe (DR), substantial nigra (SN), hypothalamus, striatum and frontal cortex (Di Cara et al., 2011; Lindemann et al., 2008; Revel et al., 2011; Xie et al., 2007). In addition, the gene for TAAR1 in humans is mapped to chromosome 6q23.2, a putative susceptibility locus for schizophrenia and mood disorders (Lindemann et al., 2005; Lindemann & Hoener, 2005). These studies strongly suggest that TAAR1 is involved in the modulation of monoaminergic system and therefore participate in the regulation of neuropsychiatric disorders like schizophrenia, depression, Parkinson's disease, bipolar disorder and drug addiction.

The potential role of TAAR1 in modulation monoaminergic transmission was further suggested by studies of genetic animal models. From 2007 to 2011, three separate groups generated TAAR1 knockout

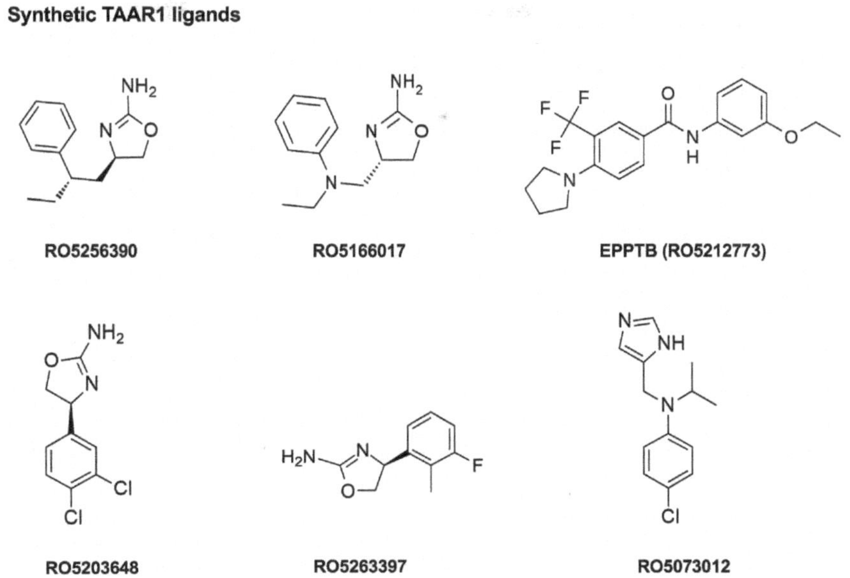

Fig. 2 Structures of synthetic TAAR1 ligands (full agonists: RO5256390, RO5166017; antagonist: EPPTB; partial agonists: RO5203648, RO5263397, RO5273012).

animals (Di Cara et al., 2011; Lindemann et al., 2008; Wolinsky et al., 2007). It is shown that TAAR1-KO mice have no differences in sensor and motor functions like motor coordination and spontaneous locomotor activity, however, they demonstrate an impairment of sensorimotor gating function, which might be a phenotype related to schizophrenia (Wolinsky et al., 2007). They also have increased sensitivity to the behavioral and neurochemical responses to amphetamine and higher proportion of high affinity D2 receptors in the striatum (Lindemann et al., 2008; Wolinsky et al., 2007). Moreover, knockout of TAAR1 induces a remarkable increase in the spontaneous firing rate of VTA dopaminergic neurons and DR serotonergic neurons which might be due to TAAR1's role in tonic activation of inwardly rectifying potassium ion channels in these neurons in order to reduce basal firing rate (Bradaia et al., 2009; Lindemann et al., 2008; Revel et al., 2011). In addition to TAAR1-KO animals, a transgenic TAAR1 overexpression model (TAAR1-OE) was generated in 2012 (Revel et al., 2012). Mice overexpressing TAAR1 show hyposensitivity to amphetamine which is the opposite of TAAR1-KO animals (Revel, Meyer, et al., 2012). However, they also show the similar augmented spontaneous firing rate in VTA dopaminergic neurons and DR serotonergic neurons as TAAR1-KO mice (Revel, Meyer, et al., 2012). This finding is difficult to interpret since in these animals, TAAR1 was overexpressed in the brain regions which do not normally express TAAR1 (Lam et al., 2015). Nevertheless, these studies further supported the role of TAAR1 in mediating dopaminergic, glutamatergic and serotonergic system and led to the excitement of exploring TAAR1 in different neuropsychiatric disorders.

Considering the fact that endogenous ligands of TAAR1 have effects through targets other than TAAR1 itself (Burchett & Hicks, 2006; Ledonne et al., 2010; Panas et al., 2010), however, the lack of highly selective ligands challenged the examinations whether modulations of TAAR1 could be potential therapeutic strategies to improve these neuropsychiatric disorders. Fortunately, the development of highly potent and selective full (RO5166017, RO5263390) (Revel et al., 2011, 2013) and partial (RO5203648, RO5263397) (Revel et al., 2012, 2013) agonists and first antagonist (EPPTB) (Bradaia et al., 2009) contributed substantially to the identification of TAAR1 biological functions (Fig. 2). Among all the neuropsychiatric disorders that TAAR1 is involved in, drug addiction is best characterized. In this review, we will focus on the role of TAAR1 in regulating drug addiction and its underlying mechanisms. We will be discussing the effects of TAAR1 modulation in addiction to different drug classes, including psychostimulants (amphetamines/cocaine/nicotine), opioid (morphine) and alcohol with the studies of selective and characterized TAAR1 ligands and transgenetic animal models (Table 1).

3. Neural mechanisms of TAAR1 in drug addiction

3.1 Dopaminergic system

The inhibitory effect of TAAR1 was thought to be at least partially through regulations of dopaminergic system (Fig. 3). It is reported that methamphetamine (METH) interacts with TAAR1 and subsequently inhibits DA uptake, enhance DA efflux and induces DAT internalization, and these effects are dependent on TAAR1 (Xie & Miller, 2009). For example, METH-induced inhibition of DA uptake was observed in TAAR1 and DAT co-transfected cells and WT mouse and monkey striatal synaptosomes but not in DAT-only transfected cells or in striatal synaptosomes of TAAR1-KO mice (Xie & Miller, 2009). TAAR1 activation was enhanced by co-expression of monoamine transporters and this effect could be blocked by monoamine transporter antagonists (Xie et al., 2007; Xie & Miller, 2007). Furthermore, DA activation of TAAR1 induced C-FOS-luciferase expression only in the presence of DAT (Xie et al., 2007).

Table 1 Modulations of TAAR1 activity on addiction-related behaviors of drugs.

Drug	TAAR1 modulation	Species	Behavior	Effect	Reference
Amphetamine	TAAR1 knockout	Mouse	Locomotor activity	Enhanced	Wolinsky et al. (2007)
	TAAR1 overexpression	Mouse	Locomotor activity	Reduced	Revel, Meyer, et al. (2012)
	TAAR1 partial agonist RO5073012	Mouse	Locomotor activity	Enhanced	
	TAAR1 knockout	Mouse	Locomotor activity	Enhanced	Achat-Mendes, Lynch, Sullivan, Vallender, and Miller (2012)
	TAAR1 knockout	Mouse	Locomotor activity	Enhanced	Sukhanov et al. (2016)
		Mouse	Priming-induced reinstatement of amphetamine-induced CPP	Enhanced	
METH	TAAR1 knockout	Mouse	Locomotor activity	Enhanced	Achat-Mendes et al. (2012)
	TAAR1 knockout	Mouse	METH-induced CPP	Enhanced	
	Non-functional allele of *Taar1*	Mouse	METH intake	Enhanced	Harkness, Shi, Janowsky, and Phillips (2015)
		Mouse	METH-induced CTA and hypothermia	Reduced	
	TAAR1 polymorphism	Human	METH craving	Enhanced	Loftis et al. (2019)
	TAAR1 partial agonist RO5263397	Rat	Expression of METH induced-behavioral sensitization	Reduced	Jing, Zhang, and Li (2014)
			METH self-administration	Reduced	
			Cue- and drug-induced reinstatement of METH-seeking	Reduced	
	TAAR1 partial agonist RO5203648	Rat	METH-stimulated hyperactivity	Reduced	Cotter et al. (20150
			Development of METH sensitization	Reduced	
			METH self-administration	Reduced	

Continued

Table 1 Modulations of TAAR1 activity on addiction-related behaviors of drugs.—cont'd

Drug	TAAR1 modulation	Species	Behavior	Effect	Reference
	TAAR1 partial agonist RO5263397	Rat	Break-point for METH	Reduced	Pei, Asif-Malik, Hoener, and Canales (2017)
			Drug-primed reinstatement of METH-seeking	Reduced	
	TAAR1 partial agonist RO5263397	Rat	METH-induced premature response	Reduced	Xue, Siemian, Johnson, Zhang, and Li (2018)
Cocaine	TAAR1 partial agonist RO5203648	Rat and mouse	Cocaine-induced hyperlocomotion	Reduced	Revel, Moreau, et al. (2012)
		Rat	Cocaine taking	Reduced	
	TAAR1 partial agonist RO5203648 and full agonist RO5256390	Rat	Cocaine-seeking	Reduced	Pei et al. (2014)
	TAAR1 partial agonist RO5203648	Rat	Drug-primed reinstatement of cocaine-seeking	Reduced	
	TAAR1 partial agonist RO5263397	Rat	Expression of cocaine-induced behavioral sensitization	Reduced	Thorn, Zhang, Zhang, and Li (2014)
			Development of cocaine-induced behavioral sensitization	No effect	
			Cocaine CPP	Reduced	
			Cue- and drug-induced reinstatement	Reduced	
			Elasticity of cocaine demand curve	Reduced	
	TAAR1 partial agonist RO5203648 and full agonist RO5256390	Rat	Cocaine dose-response curve	Reduced	Pei, Mortas, Hoener, and Canales (2015)
	TAAR1 full agonist RO5256390	Rat	ICSS threshold	Reduced	

Table 1 Modulations of TAAR1 activity on addiction-related behaviors of drugs.—cont'd

Drug	TAAR1 modulation	Species	Behavior	Effect	Reference
	TAAR1 partial agonist RO5263397	Rat	Induction of CPP induced behavioral sensitization	Reduced	Thorn, Zhang, et al. (2014)
	TAAR1 full agonist RO5166017	Rat	Expression of cocaine CPP	Reduced	Liu, Thorn, Zhang, and Li (2016)
	TAAR1 full agonist RO5166017 (intra-VTA, PrL)	Rat	Cue- and drug-induced reinstatement	Reduced	Liu, Siemian, Seaman Jr., Zhang, and Li (2017)
	TAAR1 full agonist RO5166017 (intra-NAc core)	Rat	Cue-induced reinstatement	Reduced	
	TAAR1 full agonist RO5166017 (intra-NAc shell)	Rat	Drug-induced reinstatement	Reduced	
	TAAR1 full agonist RO5256390 and partial agonist RO5263397	Mice	Cocaine-induced hyperactivity	Reduced	Revel et al. (2013)
	TAAR1 full agonist RO5166017	Mice	Cocaine-induced hyperactivity	Reduced	Revel et al. (2011)
	TAAR1 partial agonist RO5263397	Rat	Cocaine intake, tolerance, binge intake	Reduced	Liu et al. (2020)
			Cue- and drug-induced reinstatement	Reduced	
			Yohimbine-induced reinstatement	Reduced	
Nicotine	TAAR1 partial agonist RO5263397	Rat	Nicotine-induced hyperlocomotion	Reduced	Sukhanov, Dorofeikova, Dolgorukova, Dorotenko, and Gainetdinov (2018)

Continued

Table 1 Modulations of TAAR1 activity on addiction-related behaviors of drugs.—cont'd

Drug	TAAR1 modulation	Species	Behavior	Effect	Reference
			Development and expression of nicotine sensitization	Reduced	
	TAAR1 knockout	Mice	Nicotine-induced hyperlocomotion	No effect	
	TAAR1 partial agonist RO5263397	Rat	Expression and development of nicotine sensitization	Reduced	Liu et al. (2018)
			Discriminative effects of nicotine	Reduced	
			Nicotine demand curve	Reduced	
			Nicotine-induced hypothermia	No effect	
	TAAR1 full agonist RO5166017 (systemic and intra-NAc)	Rat	Reinstatement of nicotine-seeking	Reduced	
	TAAR1 knockout	Rat	Nicotine-seeking	Enhanced	
Morphine	TAAR1 knockout	Mouse	Morphine-induced CPP	No effects	Achat-Mendes et al. (2012)
	TAAR1 partial agonist RO5263397	Mouse	Expression of morphine-induced sensitization	Reduced	Liu et al. (2021)
		Rat	Morphine intake, progressive ratio test	Reduced	
		Rat	Cue- and drug-induced reinstatement of morphine-seeking	Reduced	
		Mouse/rat	morphine CPP	No effect	
		Mouse	Naltrexone-induced jumping and CPA	No effect	
		Mouse	Hot water tail immersion test	No effect	
		Rat	CFA-induced inflammatory test	No effect	

Table 1 Modulations of TAAR1 activity on addiction-related behaviors of drugs.—cont'd

Drug	TAAR1 modulation	Species	Behavior	Effect	Reference
Alcohol	TAAR1 knockout	Mouse	Preference for and consumption of ethanol	Enhanced	Lynch et al. (2013)
			Sedative-like effects of acute ethanol	Enhanced	
			Locomotor activity induced by acute ethanol	Reduced	
	TAAR1 partial agonist RO5263397	Mouse	Expression and development of ethanol-induced sensitization	Reduced	Wu et al. (2020)
	TAAR1 knockout	Mouse	Ethanol-induced sensitization	No effect	

TAAR1, trace amine-associated receptor 1; METH, methamphetamine; CPP, conditioned place preference; CTA, conditioned taste aversion; ICSS, intracranial self-stimulation; CPA, conditioned place aversion,

Recent study also showed that amphetamines mediates the trafficking of both DA and glutamate transporters by increasing the activation of small GTPase RhoA and of protein kinase A (Underhill et al., 2014; Underhill, Colt, & Amara, 2020; Wheeler et al., 2015) and this regulation is dependent on the direct activation of TAAR1 by its coupling to two G proteins G_{13} and Gs α-subunits (Underhill et al., 2021). Moreover, although intracellular entry through DAT may not be prerequisite for METH-induced activation of TAAR1 signaling, DAT serves as an important avenue for the access to the cytoplasm. Therefore, octopamine, which is a potent agonist of TAAR1 and a poor substrate for DAT, did not activate RhoA in the cells (Underhill et al., 2021). However, Yue et al. showed that RO5203648 blocked cocaine-induced DA overflow in the nucleus accumbens without altering DA half-life, suggesting that partial activation of TAAR1 by RO5203648 attenuated DA overflow by mechanisms other interaction with DAT (Pei et al., 2014). Consistently, RO5166017 did not affect the half-life of DA in the NAc and striatum (Leo et al., 2014) and decreased the hyperlocomotion in DAT-KO mice (Revel et al., 2011), suggesting that the inhibitory effect of TAAR1 in drug addiction might be independent of DAT.

Bradaia et al. found that antagonism of TAAR1 by acute application of EPPTB increased the potency of DA at D2 auto-receptor in dopaminergic

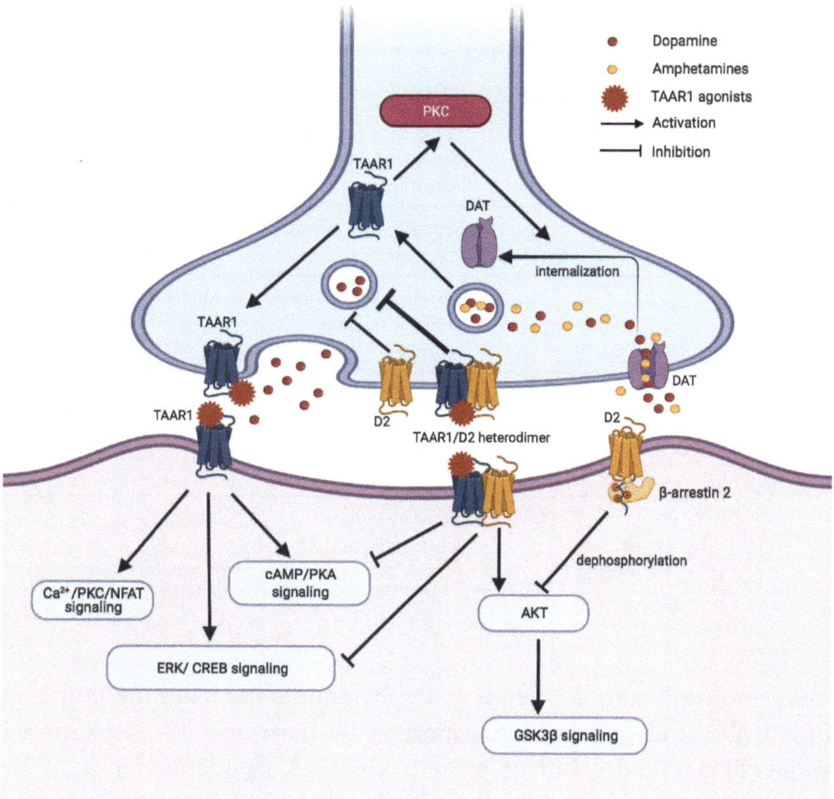

Fig. 3 Schematic representation of the functional interaction of TAAR1 with dopaminergic system. It is hypothesized that in the pre-synaptic membrane, DATs might serve as conduits for the entry of dopamine and amphetamines into the membrane which then induces activation of intracellular TAAR1. This TAAR1 activation promotes PKC-mediated internalization of DAT, which results in increased dopamine efflux. TAAR1 activation might also trigger trafficking of TAAR1 into the plasma membrane and potentiate D2-mediated inhibition of dopamine transmission. In the post-synaptic membrane, TAAR1 activation signals through cAMP/PKA and ERK/CREB which can be inhibited by the activation of TAAR1/D2 heterodimers. TAAR1/D2 heterodimers activation might also reverse the inhibition of β-arrestin 2/AKT/GSK3β pathway induced by D2 activation. TAAR1 can also signals through Ca^{2+}/PKC/NFAT pathway. TAAR1, trace amine-associated receptor 1; D2, dopamine D2 receptors; PKA, protein kinase A; PKC, protein kinase C; ERK1/2, extracellular signal-regulated protein kinases 1 and 2; AKT, protein kinase B; GSK3β, glycogen synthase kinase 3β; CREB, cAMP response element binding protein; NFAT, nuclear factor of activated T-cells.

neurons (Bradaia et al., 2009). Espinoa et al. further explored the interaction between TAAR1 and D2 using a bioluminescence resonance energy transfer (BRET) biosensor for cAMP (Espinoza et al., 2011). They discovered that TAAR1 agonist PEA induced increase of cAMP was enhanced by

D2 receptor antagonists (haloperidol, raclopride, and amisulpride) (Espinoza et al., 2011). Furthermore, TAAR1 and D2 receptor were able to form heterodimers when co-expressed in HEK 293 cells, and this effect was disrupted by D2 receptor antagonist haloperidol (Espinoza et al., 2011). However, haloperidol induced c-Fos activation in the striatum and catalepsy were significantly attenuated in TAAR1-KO mice (Espinoza et al., 2011). In addition, RO5256390 blockade of cocaine-induced DA release in slices of NAc was blocked by the antagonism of D2 receptor (Asif-Malik, Hoener, & Canales, 2017). Taken together, these data suggest that the interactions of TAAR1 and D2 receptor might underlie the functions of TAAR1 in modulations of monoaminergic system.

3.2 Cellular signaling

Consistent studies have suggested that the TAAR1 expression is probably intracellular. It was challenging to study TAAR1 initially because of the lack of expression at the plasma membrane *in vitro* as observed in microscopy images (Miller, 2011). Thus, many earlier studies of TAAR1 pharmacology required modifications to the receptor so as to increase its membrane expression (Bunzow et al., 2001; Lindemann & Hoener, 2005; Reese, Bunzow, Arttamangkul, Sonders, & Grandy, 2007; Wainscott et al., 2007). Moreover, it is shown that rhesus monkey TAAR1 interacts with monoamine transporters and thus provide an access by which TAAR1 ligands can enter the cytoplasm and bind to TAAR1. A more recent study suggested that trace amines action is dependent on intracellular uptake by pentamidine-sensitive Na(+)-independent membrane transporters but not monoamine transporters (Gozal et al., 2014). Furthermore, since traces amine have delayed onset in locomotor-like activity (LLA) in rat neonatal spinal cord compared with serotonin (Gozal et al., 2014), it supports the hypothesis that TAAR1 locates in intracellular compartments and its activation requires intracellular transportation.

TAAR1 couples to Gαs protein and increases the accumulation of cAMP upon activation. Moreover, it is speculated that TAAR1 may also signal directly or indirectly through β-arrestin 2/Akt/GSK3 pathway. The β-arrestin 2 knock-out mice showed similar hypoactivity in response to amphetamine as TAAR1-OE mice (Revel, Meyer, et al., 2012). However, in the striatum of TAAR1-KO mice, an overexpression of D2 receptors was observed, paralleled with a selective inhibition of AKT/GSK3 signaling pathway (Espinoza et al., 2015). While the interaction of TAAR1 with D2 receptor reduced the β-arrestin 2 recruitment to D2 receptor, cAMP signaling of TAAR1 was reduced in the presence of D2 receptor (Harmeier et al., 2015). These findings suggest that β-arrestin 2/Akt/GSK3 signaling may be an important pathway for TAAR1 function and the activation of TAAR1/D2 receptor heterodimers negatively regulates this signaling. In addition, TAAR1 activation by 3-methoxytyramine (3-MT) significantly increased the phosphorylation of ERK and CREB in mouse striatum while in TAAR1-KO mice, the responses caused by 3-MT was significantly attenuated (Sotnikova et al., 2010). In contrast, upon the interaction with D2 receptor, activation of TAAR1 leads to a reduction in phosphorylation of ERK and CREB (Harmeier et al., 2015), suggesting the involvement of ERK/CREB signaling in TAAR1's functions. Moreover, TAAR1 activation was shown to increase the phosphorylation of PKC and PKA in HEK293 transfected cells (Panas et al., 2012).

3.3 Neuroanatomic sites of TAAR1 actions

TAAR1 is expressed in a wide range of brain regions especially in the dopaminergic system, however, studies using systemic manipulations of TAAR1 cannot answer the question that which brain regions are crucial for TAAR1's function. By using local microinfusions into different brain regions including PFC, NAc, VTA, Amygdala and SN, our group identified that TAAR1 in specific brain regions of reward system plays distinct role in drug addiction (Liu et al., 2017). For example, microinfusion of RO5166017 into the VTA and prelimbic area of medial PFC attenuated both cue- and drug-induced reinstatement of cocaine-seeking. Moreover, RO5266017 within the NAc core and shell were key to cue- and drug-induced seeking behavior, respectively (Liu et al., 2017). However, RO5166017 in brain regions like SN, Amygdala and infralimbic PFC may not participate in cocaine relapse-like behaviors (Liu et al., 2017).

4. TAAR1 and psychostimulants

4.1 Amphetamines

When first cloned in 2001, TAAR1 was shown to be activated potently by amphetamine and its analogues like METH, para-hydroxyamphetamine (POHA) and 3,4-Methylenedioxymethamphetamine (MDMA, ecstasy) (Borowsky et al., 2001; Bunzow et al., 2001). As we know that trace amines are TAAR1 agonists, they show high level of structural and physiological similarities with amphetamine. Therefore, β-PEA has been described as endogenous "amphetamine" (Borison, Mosnaim, & Sabelli, 1975; Janssen, Leysen, Megens, & Awouters, 1999). It was further characterized by Grandy lab and others that both S-(+)- and R-(−) isomers of METH were full agonists at mouse and human-rat chimera TAAR1 while were partial agonists at rat TAAR1 (Lewin, Miller, & Gilmour, 2011; Reese et al., 2007), and TAAR1 had a stereoselective binding site for compounds in the amphetamine class *in vitro* (Simmler, Buchy, Chaboz, Hoener, & Liechti, 2016).

The findings from *in vitro* studies suggest that TAAR1 may play a role in the effects of psychostimulants *in vivo*. In fact, enhanced behavioral and neurochemical responses of amphetamine were observed in mice lacking the TAAR1 gene (TAAR1-KO) compared with their wide-type (WT) littermates (Wolinsky et al., 2007). On the contrary, TAAR1-OE mice showed hyposensitivity to the psychostimulant effects of amphetamine (Revel, Meyer, et al., 2012). These studies suggest that TAAR1 may be implicated in the rewarding effects of psychostimulants. By measuring locomotor activity and conditioned place preference (CPP), it was shown that *d*-amphetamine and METH produced higher levels of locomotion in TAAR1-KO mice (Achat-Mendes et al., 2012; Sukhanov et al., 2016). Moreover, TAAR1-KO mice acquired METH-induced CPP earlier and retained CPP longer than WT mice (Achat-Mendes et al., 2012). This finding was later supported by the study which showed that TAAR1-KO mice consumed more METH and demonstrated less sensitivity to METH-induced hypothermia and conditioned taste aversion (CTA) (Harkness et al., 2015; Miner, Elmore, Baumann, Phillips, & Janowsky, 2017), implicating an inhibitory role of TAAR1 in the effects of amphetamines. Most recently, it is shown that *TAAR1* gene variants contribute to the increased METH intake (Reed et al., 2017; Reed et al., 2021; Stafford et al., 2019) which is consistent with a report that the V288V polymorphism in *TAAR1* gene increases drug craving in individuals with METH dependence (Loftis et al., 2019).

With the utilization of TAAR1 selective agonists, the role of TAAR1 in amphetamines stimulant effects was further clarified. In 2014, Jing et al. first examined the TAAR1 partial agonist RO5263397 in addiction-related behaviors of METH (Jing et al., 2014). They found that RO5263397 dose-dependently reduced the expression METH-induced behavioral sensitization. Using the self-administration model, a gold standard animal model for drug addiction research, they further reported that RO5263397 decreased the cue- and drug-induced reinstatement of METH-seeking behavior (Jing et al., 2014). Meanwhile, RO5263397 also reduced the break-point for METH self-administration, a behavioral model of motivation (Pei et al., 2017). Similarly, another partial agonist RO5203648 showed consistent inhibitory effects demonstrated by the decreased METH-induced hyperactivity, sensitization and self-administration (Cotter et al., 2015). Importantly, both agonists showed no effect on operant responding maintained by sucrose (Cotter et al., 2015; Jing et al., 2014) and were not self-administered when tested as a METH's substitute, indicating no abuse potential (Cotter et al., 2015; Pei et al., 2017). Moreover, neurochemical data showed that RO5203648 and RO5263397 inhibited METH-induced increase of extracellular DA levels in the NAc and in the slices of the NAc, respectively (Cotter et al., 2015; Pei et al., 2017), which might contribute to its inhibitory effects in METH addiction-related behaviors. In regards to METH-induced impulsivity, an important trait related to drug addiction, RO5263397 was also able to attenuate acute but not chronic METH-induced premature responses (Xue et al., 2018). The increased impulsivity caused by discontinuation of METH treatment was reduced by RO5263397 as well (Xue et al., 2018). Consistently, while TAAR1-KO mice showed perseverative and impulsive phenotype, activation of TAAR1 by RO5166017 and RO5203648 reduced premature impulsive responses observed in the fixed-interval conditioning schedule in WT mice (Espinoza et al., 2015).

4.2 Cocaine

Cocaine is an DA modulator as it is known to increase DA accumulation in the NAc resulted from blockade of DA reuptake through interaction with DA transporter (DAT) (Greco & Garris, 2003). While cocaine is not an agonist of TAAR1, recent studies support a critical role of TAAR1 in mediating DA transmission. For example, TAAR1-KO mice showed increased spontaneous firing rate of dopaminergic neurons in the VTA and higher expression of high-affinity D2 receptors in the striatum (Lindemann et al., 2008). Furthermore, similar to TAAR1 endogenous agonist p-tyramine, the pharmacologically selective full agonist RO5166017 inhibited the firing frequency of dopaminergic neurons in brain slice of WT but not TAAR1-KO mice, which can be blocked by TAAR1 selective antagonist EPPTB (Revel et al., 2011). TAAR1 agonists RO5166017, RO5256390, RO5263397, and RO5203648 were able to attenuate cocaine-induced hyperlocomotion and drug-taking behaviors (Revel et al., 2011, 2013; Revel, Moreau, et al., 2012). The inhibitory role of TAAR1 in the regulation of dopaminergic system strongly suggest that

TAAR1 could be a potential therapeutic target for the treatment of cocaine addiction.

In light of this, more studies have tested the effect of TAAR1 activation in abuse-related effects of cocaine. Canales lab examined the effects partial and full activation of TAAR1 on cocaine-taking, cocaine-induced lowering in intracranial self-stimulation (ICSS) and relapse-like behaviors (Pei et al., 2014, 2015). They found that both RO5256390 and RO5203648 suppressed the reinforcing and rewarding effects of cocaine as evidenced by a downward shift in the cocaine dose-response curve and the prevention of cocaine-induced changes in ICSS (Pei et al., 2015). The inhibitory role of TAAR1 was further supported by the findings that RO5256390 and RO5203648 attenuated cocaine-seeking both in withdrawal and extinction-reinstatement paradigms (Pei et al., 2014). Meanwhile, our lab showed consistent findings. RO5263397 and RO5166017 blocked the induction and expression of cocaine-induced behavioral sensitization and CPP and suppressed the dose-effect response of cocaine, respectively (Liu et al., 2016; Thorn, Jing, et al., 2014; Thorn, Zhang, et al., 2014). Moreover, RO5263397 decreased the cue- and drug-induced reinstatement of cocaine-seeking while suppressed the motivation of cocaine in behavioral economic analysis (Thorn, Jing, et al., 2014). Recently, our group further characterized the role of TAAR1 in compulsive cocaine use using an extended access self-administration model (Liu et al., 2020). Here, RO5263397 reduced cocaine intake in this model without developing tolerance and decreased cue- and stress-induced relapse-like behaviors after prolonged abstinence (Liu et al., 2020), further strengthening the importance of TAAR1 in cocaine addiction.

4.3 Nicotine

Nicotine produces stimulant effects by binding to the nicotinic acetylcholine receptors within the mesocorticolimbic system to modulate DA transmission (Subramaniyan & Dani, 2015). In fact, nicotine increases the firing rate and phasic bursts in the dopaminergic neurons in the VTA and its projecting areas, resulting in enhanced DA release (Stoker & Markou, 2013; Zhang, Doyon, Clark, Phillips, & Dani, 2009). As TAAR1 mediates central dopaminergic system, recent studies have begun to illustrate whether TAAR1 played a role in nicotine addiction-like behavior. It was shown that RO5263397 attenuated the acute reinforcing effect of nicotine as evidenced by decreased nicotine-induced hyperactivity (Sukhanov et al., 2018). Moreover, RO5263397 prevented the development of nicotine-induced sensitization and reduced the hyperactivity in nicotine-sensitized rats (Sukhanov et al., 2018). A more comprehensive study from our lab further examined the ability of TAAR1 in mediating nicotine addiction-like behavior (Liu et al., 2018). Consistent with previous study, we showed that TAAR1 activation by RO5263397 reduced the expression and development of nicotine-induced sensitization (Liu et al., 2018). TAAR1 activation attenuated the discriminative effects of nicotine, nicotine intake and shifted the demand curve for nicotine downward (Liu et al., 2018). For relapse-like behaviors, we found that TAAR1 activation suppressed the cue- and drug-induced reinstatement of nicotine-seeking behavior while knockout of TAAR1 further enhanced this effect (Liu et al., 2018). Moreover, TAAR1 activation reduced nicotine-induced c-Fos expression and DA release in the NAc, which might contribute to the inhibitory effects of TAAR1 in nicotine addiction (Liu et al., 2018). Meanwhile, local activation of TAAR1 in the NAc reduced the nicotine-seeking behavior, suggesting that the NAc is important for TAAR1's effects in the reinstatement of nicotine-seeking (Liu et al., 2018).

While nicotine has a modest reinforcing effect compared with other psychostimulants (Mansvelder, Keath, & McGehee, 2002; Nestler, 2005), the pronounced withdrawal symptoms after drug discontinuation contribute substantially to the development of nicotine addiction (Epping-Jordan, Watkins, Koob, & Markou, 1998; Hughes, Higgins, & Bickel, 1994; Koob & Bloom, 1988). However, the involvement of TAAR1 in the negative reinforcement of drug addiction has not been studied. Using the short-access (ShA, 1h) and long-access (LA, 21h) self-administration models, we have found that rats in the LA group showed more robust withdrawal symptoms than those from ShA group, evidenced by increased anxiety-like behavior, hyperalgesia and augmented withdrawal signs induced by drug abstinence (Wu et al., 2021). Importantly, RO5263397 was able to attenuate those withdrawal-related effects in rats, suggesting a role in mediating withdrawal-related effects of nicotine (Wu et al., 2021). However, the neural mechanisms through which TAAR1 mediates nicotine's withdrawal effects remain unclear, which is currently under investigation.

5. TAAR1 and opioids

5.1 Morphine

Studies of the role of TAAR1 in morphine addiction are limited. It was previously showed by Achat-Mendes et al. that both TAAR1-KO and

WT mice developed the same preference for morphine in CPP paradigm (Achat-Mendes et al., 2012). Moreover, there was no difference between TAAR1-KO and WT mice in the extinction and reinstatement of morphine-induced CPP (Achat-Mendes et al., 2012), suggesting that endogenous TAAR1 is not important for morphine-induced CPP. However, although TAAR1-KO animals had similar infusions in nicotine self-administration as their WT counterparts, TAAR1 agonist was able to reduce the nicotine intake in WT rats (Liu et al., 2018). Thus, the result that TAAR1-KO mice had similar morphine CPP may not rule out the possibility that TAAR1 is involved in other morphine addiction-like behaviors.

This hypothesis was recently tested by our group using a battery of behavioral assays including morphine-induced behavioral sensitization, morphine self-administration, morphine-induced CPP and two different pain models (Liu et al., 2021). In this study, RO5263397 decreased the expression of morphine-induced behavioral sensitization in WT but not TAAR1-KO mice (Liu et al., 2021). RO5263397 in the doses that did not affect food-maintained response shifted the dose-effect curve of morphine self-administration downward and reduced the breakpoint in a progressive ratio test (Liu et al., 2021). RO5263397 also attenuated the relapse-like behaviors of morphine as it decreased the cue- and drug-induced reinstatement of morphine-seeking behavior (Liu et al., 2021). Importantly, RO5263397 alone did not affect the locomotor activity and reinstate morphine-seeking behavior (Liu et al., 2021). Interestingly, RO5263397 had no effect on morphine-induced CPP both in mice and rats (Liu et al., 2021), which is consistent with previous study. This finding suggests that TAAR1 may not participate in the mechanisms underlying morphine CPP (Liu et al., 2021). Nonetheless, these studies suggest that TAAR1 inhibits the reinforcing and rewarding effects of morphine.

Similar to nicotine addiction, morphine addiction is also marked with a robust withdrawal effect after drug discontinuation. However, RO5263397 did not alter naltrexone-induced jumping behaviors and the expression of naltrexone-precipitated conditioned place aversion (CPA) in morphine-dependent mice (Liu et al., 2021), suggesting that activation of TAAR1 by RO5263397 did not affect the negative effects of morphine in mice. Considering that TAAR1 attenuated the withdrawal effects of nicotine but not morphine, it seems that the mechanisms underlying negative reinforcement may differ from different drug classes. As morphine is a powerful analgesic, it is worth testing whether TAAR1 activation could affect the analgesic effect of morphine. Using two different pain models (acute thermal pain and chronic inflammatory pain), RO5263397 was shown not to affect tail withdrawal in the hot water tail immersion test and withdrawal threshold in the Complete Freund's adjuvant (CFA)-induced inflammation test (Liu et al., 2021). Taken together, activation of TAAR1 did not change the antinociceptive effect of morphine, which suggests that TAAR1 activation might be an efficient therapeutic strategy for patients with comorbidity of drug addiction and pain.

6. TAAR1 and alcohol

It was shown that TAAR1-KO mice displayed significantly higher preference and intake for ethanol in two-bottle choice (TBC) test compared with WT mice (Lynch et al., 2013). However, this effect was not observed in TBC with sucrose, suggesting the specificity to the drug (Lynch et al., 2013). TAAR1-KO mice also had enhanced sedative-like effects of ethanol shown by severer motor impairment in loss of righting reflex (LORR) test (Lynch et al., 2013). Moreover, they also showed less ethanol induced locomotor stimulating effects, demonstrating less reinforcing effect of ethanol in the lack of TAAR1 (Lynch et al., 2013). Meanwhile, TAAR1-KO mice had similar blood ethanol level with WT mice, suggesting that these effects were not due to the differences in clearance rates between these two groups (Lynch et al., 2013). A more recent study tested the effect of TAAR1 activation in ethanol-induced behavioral sensitization (Wu et al., 2020). RO5263397 significantly decreased the expression and development of ethanol-induced behavioral sensitization both in female and male WT mice (Wu et al., 2020). Furthermore, while TAAR1-KO mice developed comparable levels of sensitization, RO5263397 had no effect in this behavior in TAAR1-KO mice (Wu et al., 2020). These results suggest that TAAR1 is involved in addiction-like behaviors and TAAR1 agonist may be useful to treat alcohol-related disorders.

7. Current challenges

7.1 TAAR1 and other drugs of abuse

So far, we have discussed the essential roles of TAAR1 in modulations of addiction-like behaviors of several drugs of abuse including amphetamines, cocaine, nicotine, morphine and alcohol. It is clear that TAAR1 activation negatively mediates the rewarding and reinforcing effects of most of the studied drugs of abuse, of which its role in modulation of dopaminergic system contributes substantially to the effects observed. Pharmacological studies also suggest that highly potent and selective TAAR1 agonists might be useful for the treatment of drug addiction.

However, although the accumulating evidence form the past several decades provide us with much knowledge about the function of TAAR1 and its role in drug addiction, there are still blanks to be filled in the near future. For example, there are limited studies focused on the role of TAAR1 in opioids except for the only two studies of morphine (Achat-Mendes et al., 2012; Liu et al., 2021). We have demonstrated that TAAR1 activation inhibits the reinforcing effects of morphine while sparing its analgesic effects (Liu et al., 2021). Thus, it will be interesting to test if this effect can be generalized to other opioids with higher potency, like fentanyl or remifentanil. The results from these studies could greatly help to curb the current opioid epidemic. Moreover, few studies have examined the effect of TAAR1 activation using ethanol self-administration or CPP model which could otherwise be useful to measure the effects of TAAR1 in mediating the rewarding effects, motivation and relapse-like behaviors of ethanol. Such studies could add valuable information for the potential of TAAR1 agonists to treat alcohol addiction.

7.2 TAAR1 agonists and antagonists

The studies of TAAR1 agonists suggest that these compounds showed good pharmacokinetic properties and efficacy in regulating addiction of many drugs of abuse. Intriguingly, TAAR1 partial agonists RO5263397 and RO5203648 increased the firing rate of dopaminergic neurons in the brain slices (Revel et al., 2013; Revel, Moreau, et al., 2012), the effect similar to what was seen in the TAAR1 antagonist EPPTB (Bradaia et al., 2009). However, one of the pharmacological properties of partial agonists is that they can act as an agonist or antagonist dependent on endogenous intrinsic activity of the receptor (Lam et al., 2015). Moreover, it is suggested that TAAR1 is tonically active or constitutively activated to downregulate DA neuron firing frequency (Lindemann et al., 2008). Therefore, it is possible that TAAR1 partial agonists have "inhibiting effects" *in vitro*. Nevertheless, the above *in vivo* behavioral studies showed that the partial agonists act in a similar fashion as TAAR1 full agonists like RO5166017 and RO5256390 (Liu et al., 2020; Revel et al., 2011, 2013). Based on these data, TAAR1 agonists may serve as promising therapeutic targets for the treatment of drug addiction. As the treatment of drug addiction requires repeated and long-term medications, it is important to determine whether repeated TAAR1 activation could cause tolerance or toxicity. These preclinical studies will provide crucial data to support future clinical developments.

Thus far, EPPTB is the only TAAR1 antagonist that has been identified. It is a highly potent mouse TAAR1-selective antagonist that prevents the reduction of firing rate of dopaminergic neurons induced by TYR *in vitro* (Bradaia et al., 2009). EPPTB could also increase the firing rate of DA neurons in the brain slices from WT but not TAAR1-KO mice (Bradaia et al., 2009), ruling out off-target effects. However, EPPTB is mostly inactive at rat and human TAAR1s (Berry, Gainetdinov, Hoener, & Shahid, 2017) and even in mice, the pharmacokinetic properties prevent the *in vivo* use of EPPTB (Bradaia et al., 2009). Therefore, the development of new TAAR1 antagonists with more favorable pharmacological profiles could boost the progress in elucidating TAAR1's function. Moreover, TAAR1 antagonists may also have therapeutic potentials for the treatment of hypodopaminergic diseases, such as Parkinson's disease (Alvarsson et al., 2015).

7.3 Clinical studies of TAAR1 agonists

With the promising preclinical data of the role of TAAR1 in mediating neuropsychiatric disorders, several clinical trials for TAAR1 agonists have been initiated for the treatment of mental disorders. RG7351, a partial agonist on TAAR1, is currently under phase I clinical trial by Hoffmann–La Roche for the treatment of depression. In a 4-week randomized, controlled clinical trial, SEP-363856, a compound that act on TAAR1 and 5-HT1A other than dopamine D2 receptors, significantly alleviated the severe psychotic symptoms in patients with schizophrenia as evidenced by remarkable reduction in the Positive and Negative Symptom scale (PNSS) (Koblan et al., 2020). Certainly, longer and larger trials are needed to confirm the effects of SEP-363856 in schizophrenia, but it represents an important step forward to develop novel treatments for mental disorders. Although there remains a long way ahead, it might be promising to test their efficacy for the treatment of drug addiction as well in the future.

8. Conclusion

TAAR1 negatively regulates addiction to different drug classes including psychostimulants, opioid and alcohol. The extensive inhibitory effect of TAAR1 agonists on drug addiction suggests that TAAR1 agonists might serve as potential and effective pharmacological therapeutics for the treatment of drug addiction. The mechanism underlying TAAR1's function in drug addiction mainly involves modulation of dopaminergic system. Emerging evidence suggests that the interaction of TAAR1 with DAT and D2 receptors contribute substantially to the regulation of DA transmission. Together with the subsequent downstream cellular signaling including β-arrestin 2/Akt/GSK3 pathway, ERK/CREB pathway and PKA/PKC activation, TAAR1 induced-neurobiological alterations underlie the overall behavioral output. However, more studies are needed to further understand the role of TAAR1 in addiction to other drugs of abuse and examine the potency and efficacy of novel pharmacotherapy for drug addiction based on TAAR1.

Acknowledgments

This work was supported by the National Institutes of Health National Institute on Drug Abuse (Grant number R01DA047967 to J-X.L.). The content is solely the responsibility of the authors and does not necessarily represent the official views of the National Institutes of Health.

Conflict of interest

The authors declare no conflicts of interest.

References

Achat-Mendes, C., Lynch, L. J., Sullivan, K. A., Vallender, E. J., & Miller, G. M. (2012). Augmentation of methamphetamine-induced behaviors in transgenic mice lacking the trace amine-associated receptor 1. *Pharmacology, Biochemistry, and Behavior, 101*(2), 201–207. https://doi.org/10.1016/j.pbb.2011.10.025.

Alvarsson, A., Zhang, X., Stan, T. L., Schintu, N., Kadkhodaei, B., Millan, M. J., et al. (2015). Modulation by trace amine-associated receptor 1 of experimental parkinsonism, L-DOPA responsivity, and glutamatergic neurotransmission. *The Journal of Neuroscience, 35*(41), 14057–14069. https://doi.org/10.1523/JNEUROSCI.1312-15.2015.

Asif-Malik, A., Hoener, M. C., & Canales, J. J. (2017). Interaction between the trace amine-associated receptor 1 and the dopamine D2 receptor controls Cocaine's neurochemical actions. *Scientific Reports*, 7(1), 13901. https://doi.org/10.1038/s41598-017-14472-z.

Berry, M. D. (2004). Mammalian central nervous system trace amines. Pharmacologic amphetamines, physiologic neuromodulators. *Journal of Neurochemistry, 90*(2), 257–271. https://doi.org/10.1111/j.1471-4159.2004.02501.x.

Berry, M. D. (2007). The potential of trace amines and their receptors for treating neurological and psychiatric diseases. *Reviews on Recent Clinical Trials, 2*(1), 3–19. https://doi.org/10.2174/157488707779318107.

Berry, M. D., Gainetdinov, R. R., Hoener, M. C., & Shahid, M. (2017). Pharmacology of human trace amine-associated receptors: Therapeutic opportunities and challenges. *Pharmacology & Therapeutics, 180*, 161–180. https://doi.org/10.1016/j.pharmthera.2017.07.002.

Borison, R. L., Mosnaim, A. D., & Sabelli, H. C. (1975). Brain 2-phenylethylamine as a major mediator for the central actions of amphetamine and methylphenidate. *Life Sciences, 17*(8), 1331–1343. https://doi.org/10.1016/0024-3205(75)90147-2.

Borowsky, B., Adham, N., Jones, K. A., Raddatz, R., Artymyshyn, R., Ogozalek, K. L., et al. (2001). Trace amines: Identification of a family of mammalian G protein-coupled receptors. *Proceedings of the National Academy of Sciences of the United States of America*, *98*(16), 8966–8971. https://doi.org/10.1073/pnas.151105198.

Boulton, A. A. (1974). Letter: Amines and theories in psychiatry. *Lancet*, *2*(7871), 52–53. https://doi.org/10.1016/s0140-6736(74)91390-7.

Boulton, A. A. (1980). Trace amines and mental disorders. *The Canadian Journal of Neurological Sciences*, 7(3), 261–263. https://doi.org/10.1017/s0317167100023313.

Bradaia, A., Trube, G., Stalder, H., Norcross, R. D., Ozmen, L., Wettstein, J. G., et al. (2009). The selective antagonist EPPTB reveals TAAR1-mediated regulatory mechanisms in dopaminergic neurons of the mesolimbic system. *Proceedings of the National Academy of Sciences of the United States of America*, *106*(47), 20081–20086. https://doi.org/10.1073/pnas.0906522106.

Bunzow, J. R., Sonders, M. S., Arttamangkul, S., Harrison, L. M., Zhang, G., Quigley, D. I., et al. (2001). Amphetamine, 3,4-methylenedioxymethamphetamine, lysergic acid diethylamide, and metabolites of the catecholamine neurotransmitters are agonists of a rat trace amine receptor. *Molecular Pharmacology*, *60*(6), 1181–1188. https://doi.org/10.1124/mol.60.6.1181.

Burchett, S. A., & Hicks, T. P. (2006). The mysterious trace amines: Protean neuromodulators of synaptic transmission in mammalian brain. *Progress in Neurobiology*, *79*(5–6), 223–246. https://doi.org/10.1016/j.pneurobio.2006.07.003.

Cotter, R., Pei, Y., Mus, L., Harmeier, A., Gainetdinov, R. R., Hoener, M. C., et al. (2015). The trace amine-associated receptor 1 modulates methamphetamine's neurochemical and behavioral effects. *Frontiers in Neuroscience*, *9*, 39. https://doi.org/10.3389/fnins.2015.00039.

Dewan, A., Pacifico, R., Zhan, R., Rinberg, D., & Bozza, T. (2013). Non-redundant coding of aversive odours in the main olfactory pathway. *Nature*, *497*(7450), 486–489. https://doi.org/10.1038/nature12114.

Di Cara, B., Maggio, R., Aloisi, G., Rivet, J. M., Lundius, E. G., Yoshitake, T., et al. (2011). Genetic deletion of trace amine 1 receptors reveals their role in auto-inhibiting the actions of ecstasy (MDMA). *The Journal of Neuroscience*, *31*(47), 16928–16940. https://doi.org/10.1523/JNEUROSCI.2502-11.2011.

Epping-Jordan, M. P., Watkins, S. S., Koob, G. F., & Markou, A. (1998). Dramatic decreases in brain reward function during nicotine withdrawal. *Nature*, *393*(6680), 76–79. https://doi.org/10.1038/30001.

Espinoza, S., Ghisi, V., Emanuele, M., Leo, D., Sukhanov, I., Sotnikova, T. D., et al. (2015). Postsynaptic D2 dopamine receptor supersensitivity in the striatum of mice lacking TAAR1. *Neuropharmacology*, *93*, 308–313. https://doi.org/10.1016/j.neuropharm.2015.02.010.

Espinoza, S., Lignani, G., Caffino, L., Maggi, S., Sukhanov, I., Leo, D., et al. (2015). TAAR1 modulates cortical glutamate NMDA receptor function. *Neuropsychopharmacology*, *40*(9), 2217–2227. https://doi.org/10.1038/npp.2015.65.

Espinoza, S., Salahpour, A., Masri, B., Sotnikova, T. D., Messa, M., Barak, L. S., et al. (2011). Functional interaction between trace amine-associated receptor 1 and dopamine D2 receptor. *Molecular Pharmacology*, *80*(3), 416–425. https://doi.org/10.1124/mol.111.073304.

Gainetdinov, R. R., Hoener, M. C., & Berry, M. D. (2018). Trace amines and their receptors. *Pharmacological Reviews*, *70*(3), 549–620. https://doi.org/10.1124/pr.117.015305.

Gozal, E. A., O'Neill, B. E., Sawchuk, M. A., Zhu, H., Halder, M., Chou, C. C., et al. (2014). Anatomical and functional evidence for trace amines as unique modulators of locomotor function in the mammalian spinal cord. *Frontiers in Neural Circuits*, *8*, 134. https://doi.org/10.3389/fncir.2014.00134.

Grandy, D. K. (2007). Trace amine-associated receptor 1-family archetype or iconoclast? *Pharmacology & Therapeutics*, *116*(3), 355–390. https://doi.org/10.1016/j.pharmthera.2007.06.007.

Greco, P. G., & Garris, P. A. (2003). In vivo interaction of cocaine with the dopamine transporter as measured by voltammetry. *European Journal of Pharmacology*, *479*(1–3), 117–125. https://doi.org/10.1016/j.ejphar.2003.08.062.

Harkness, J. H., Shi, X., Janowsky, A., & Phillips, T. J. (2015). Trace amine-associated receptor 1 regulation of methamphetamine intake and related traits. *Neuropsychopharmacology*, *40*(9), 2175–2184. https://doi.org/10.1038/npp.2015.61.

Harmeier, A., Obermueller, S., Meyer, C. A., Revel, F. G., Buchy, D., Chaboz, S., et al. (2015). Trace amine-associated receptor 1 activation silences GSK3beta signaling of TAAR1 and D2R heteromers. *European Neuropsychopharmacology*, *25*(11), 2049–2061. https://doi.org/10.1016/j.euroneuro.2015.08.011.

Hartmann, P., Sherriff, J., & Kent, J. (1995). Maternal nutrition and the regulation of milk synthesis. *The Proceedings of the Nutrition Society*, *54*(2), 379–389. https://doi.org/10.1079/pns19950007.

Hughes, J. R., Higgins, S. T., & Bickel, W. K. (1994). Nicotine withdrawal versus other drug withdrawal syndromes: Similarities and dissimilarities. *Addiction*, *89*(11), 1461–1470. https://doi.org/10.1111/j.1360-0443.1994.tb03744.x.

Janssen, P. A., Leysen, J. E., Megens, A. A., & Awouters, F. H. (1999). Does phenylethylamine act as an endogenous amphetamine in some patients? *The International Journal of Neuropsychopharmacology*, *2*(3), 229–240. https://doi.org/10.1017/S1461145799001522.

Jing, L., Zhang, Y., & Li, J. X. (2014). Effects of the trace amine associated receptor 1 agonist RO5263397 on abuse-related behavioral indices of methamphetamine in rats. *The International Journal of Neuropsychopharmacology*, *18*(4). https://doi.org/10.1093/ijnp/pyu060.

Koblan, K. S., Kent, J., Hopkins, S. C., Krystal, J. H., Cheng, H., Goldman, R., et al. (2020). A non-D2-receptor-binding drug for the treatment of schizophrenia. *The New England Journal of Medicine*, *382*(16), 1497–1506. https://doi.org/10.1056/NEJMoa1911772.

Koob, G. F., & Bloom, F. E. (1988). Cellular and molecular mechanisms of drug dependence. *Science*, *242*(4879), 715–723. https://doi.org/10.1126/science.2903550.

Lam, V. M., Espinoza, S., Gerasimov, A. S., Gainetdinov, R. R., & Salahpour, A. (2015). In-vivo pharmacology of trace-amine associated receptor 1. *European Journal of Pharmacology*, *763*(Pt. B), 136–142. https://doi.org/10.1016/j.ejphar.2015.06.026.

Ledonne, A., Federici, M., Giustizieri, M., Pessia, M., Imbrici, P., Millan, M. J., et al. (2010). Trace amines depress D(2)-autoreceptor-mediated responses on midbrain dopaminergic cells. *British Journal of Pharmacology*, *160*(6), 1509–1520. https://doi.org/10.1111/j.1476-5381.2010.00792.x.

Leo, D., Mus, L., Espinoza, S., Hoener, M. C., Sotnikova, T. D., & Gainetdinov, R. R. (2014). Taar1-mediated modulation of presynaptic dopaminergic neurotransmission: Role of D2 dopamine autoreceptors. *Neuropharmacology*, *81*, 283–291. https://doi.org/10.1016/j.neuropharm.2014.02.007.

Lewin, A. H., Miller, G. M., & Gilmour, B. (2011). Trace amine-associated receptor 1 is a stereoselective binding site for compounds in the amphetamine class. *Bioorganic & Medicinal Chemistry*, *19*(23), 7044–7048. https://doi.org/10.1016/j.bmc.2011.10.007.

Liberles, S. D., & Buck, L. B. (2006). A second class of chemosensory receptors in the olfactory epithelium. *Nature*, *442*(7103), 645–650. https://doi.org/10.1038/nature05066.

Lindemann, L., Ebeling, M., Kratochwil, N. A., Bunzow, J. R., Grandy, D. K., & Hoener, M. C. (2005). Trace amine-associated receptors form structurally and functionally distinct subfamilies of novel G protein-coupled receptors. *Genomics*, *85*(3), 372–385. https://doi.org/10.1016/j.ygeno.2004.11.010.

Lindemann, L., & Hoener, M. C. (2005). A renaissance in trace amines inspired by a novel GPCR family. *Trends in Pharmacological Sciences*, *26*(5), 274–281. https://doi.org/10.1016/j.tips.2005.03.007.

Lindemann, L., Meyer, C. A., Jeanneau, K., Bradaia, A., Ozmen, L., Bluethmann, H., et al. (2008). Trace amine-associated receptor 1 modulates dopaminergic activity. *The Journal of Pharmacology and Experimental Therapeutics*, *324*(3), 948–956. https://doi.org/10.1124/jpet.107.132647.

Liu, J., Johnson, B., Wu, R., Seaman, R., Jr., Vu, J., Zhu, Q., et al. (2020). TAAR1 agonists attenuate extended-access cocaine self-administration and yohimbine-induced reinstatement of cocaine-seeking. *British Journal of Pharmacology*, *177*(15), 3403–3414. https://doi.org/10.1111/bph.15061.

Liu, I. S., Kusumi, I., Ulpian, C., Tallerico, T., & Seeman, P. (1998). A serotonin-4 receptor-like pseudogene in humans. *Brain Research. Molecular Brain Research*, *53*(1–2), 98–103. https://doi.org/10.1016/s0169-328x(97)00283-0.

Liu, J., Seaman, R., Jr., Johnson, B., Wu, R., Vu, J., Tian, J., et al. (2021). Activation of trace amine-associated receptor 1 selectively attenuates the reinforcing effects of morphine. *British Journal of Pharmacology*, *178*(4), 933–945. https://doi.org/10.1111/bph.15335.

Liu, J. F., Seaman, R., Jr., Siemian, J. N., Bhimani, R., Johnson, B., Zhang, Y., et al. (2018). Role of trace amine-associated receptor 1 in nicotine's behavioral and neurochemical effects. *Neuropsychopharmacology*, *43*(12), 2435–2444. https://doi.org/10.1038/s41386-018-0017-9.

Liu, J. F., Siemian, J. N., Seaman, R., Jr., Zhang, Y., & Li, J. X. (2017). Role of TAAR1 within the subregions of the mesocorticolimbic dopaminergic system in cocaine-seeking behavior. *The Journal of Neuroscience*, *37*(4), 882–892. https://doi.org/10.1523/JNEUROSCI.2006-16.2016.

Liu, J. F., Thorn, D. A., Zhang, Y., & Li, J. X. (2016). Effects of trace amine-associated receptor 1 agonists on the expression, reconsolidation, and extinction of cocaine reward memory. *The International Journal of Neuropsychopharmacology*, *19*(7). https://doi.org/10.1093/ijnp/pyw009.

Loftis, J. M., Lasarev, M., Shi, X., Lapidus, J., Janowsky, A., Hoffman, W. F., et al. (2019). Trace amine-associated receptor gene polymorphism increases drug craving in individuals with methamphetamine dependence. *PLoS One*, *14*(10), e0220270. https://doi.org/10.1371/journal.pone.0220270.

Lynch, L. J., Sullivan, K. A., Vallender, E. J., Rowlett, J. K., Platt, D. M., & Miller, G. M. (2013). Trace amine associated receptor 1 modulates behavioral effects of ethanol. *Substance Abuse*, *7*, 117–126. https://doi.org/10.4137/SART.S12110.

Maguire, J. J., Parker, W. A., Foord, S. M., Bonner, T. I., Neubig, R. R., & Davenport, A. P. (2009). International Union of Pharmacology. LXXII. Recommendations for trace amine receptor nomenclature. *Pharmacological Reviews*, *61*(1), 1–8. https://doi.org/10.1124/pr.109.001107.

Mansvelder, H. D., Keath, J. R., & McGehee, D. S. (2002). Synaptic mechanisms underlie nicotine-induced excitability of brain reward areas. *Neuron*, *33*(6), 905–919. https://doi.org/10.1016/s0896-6273(02)00625-6.

Miller, G. M. (2011). The emerging role of trace amine-associated receptor 1 in the functional regulation of monoamine transporters and dopaminergic activity. *Journal of Neurochemistry*, *116*(2), 164–176. https://doi.org/10.1111/j.1471-4159.2010.07109.x.

Miner, N. B., Elmore, J. S., Baumann, M. H., Phillips, T. J., & Janowsky, A. (2017). Trace amine-associated receptor 1 regulation of methamphetamine-induced neurotoxicity. *Neurotoxicology*, *63*, 57–69. https://doi.org/10.1016/j.neuro.2017.09.006.

Nestler, E. J. (2005). Is there a common molecular pathway for addiction? *Nature Neuroscience*, *8*(11), 1445–1449. https://doi.org/10.1038/nn1578.

Panas, H. N., Lynch, L. J., Vallender, E. J., Xie, Z., Chen, G. L., Lynn, S. K., et al. (2010). Normal thermoregulatory responses to 3-iodothyronamine, trace amines and amphetamine-like psychostimulants in trace amine associated receptor 1 knockout mice. *Journal of Neuroscience Research*, *88*(9), 1962–1969. https://doi.org/10.1002/jnr.22367.

Panas, M. W., Xie, Z., Panas, H. N., Hoener, M. C., Vallender, E. J., & Miller, G. M. (2012). Trace amine associated receptor 1 signaling in activated lymphocytes. *Journal of Neuroimmune Pharmacology*, 7(4), 866–876. https://doi.org/10.1007/s11481-011-9321-4.

Pei, Y., Asif-Malik, A., Hoener, M., & Canales, J. J. (2017). A partial trace amine-associated receptor 1 agonist exhibits properties consistent with a methamphetamine substitution treatment. *Addiction Biology*, *22*(5), 1246–1256. https://doi.org/10.1111/adb.12410.

Pei, Y., Lee, J., Leo, D., Gainetdinov, R. R., Hoener, M. C., & Canales, J. J. (2014). Activation of the trace amine-associated receptor 1 prevents relapse to cocaine seeking. *Neuropsychopharmacology*, *39*(10), 2299–2308. https://doi.org/10.1038/npp.2014.88.

Pei, Y., Mortas, P., Hoener, M. C., & Canales, J. J. (2015). Selective activation of the trace amine-associated receptor 1 decreases cocaine's reinforcing efficacy and prevents cocaine-induced changes in brain reward thresholds. *Progress in Neuro-Psychopharmacology & Biological Psychiatry*, *63*, 70–75. https://doi.org/10.1016/j.pnpbp.2015.05.014.

Reed, C., Baba, H., Zhu, Z., Erk, J., Mootz, J. R., Varra, N. M., et al. (2017). A spontaneous mutation in Taar1 impacts methamphetamine-related traits exclusively in DBA/2 mice from a single vendor. *Frontiers in Pharmacology*, *8*, 993. https://doi.org/10.3389/fphar.2017.00993.

Reed, C., Stafford, A. M., Mootz, J. R. K., Baba, H., Erk, J., & Phillips, T. J. (2021). A breeding strategy to identify modifiers of high genetic risk for methamphetamine intake. *Genes, Brain, and Behavior*, *20*(2), e12667. https://doi.org/10.1111/gbb.12667.

Reese, E. A., Bunzow, J. R., Arttamangkul, S., Sonders, M. S., & Grandy, D. K. (2007). Trace amine-associated receptor 1 displays species-dependent stereoselectivity for isomers of methamphetamine, amphetamine, and para-hydroxyamphetamine. *The Journal of Pharmacology and Experimental Therapeutics*, *321*(1), 178–186. https://doi.org/10.1124/jpet.106.115402.

Revel, F. G., Meyer, C. A., Bradaia, A., Jeanneau, K., Calcagno, E., Andre, C. B., et al. (2012). Brain-specific overexpression of trace amine-associated receptor 1 alters monoaminergic neurotransmission and decreases sensitivity to amphetamine. *Neuropsychopharmacology*, *37*(12), 2580–2592. https://doi.org/10.1038/npp.2012.109.

Revel, F. G., Moreau, J. L., Gainetdinov, R. R., Bradaia, A., Sotnikova, T. D., Mory, R., et al. (2011). TAAR1 activation modulates monoaminergic neurotransmission, preventing hyperdopaminergic and hypoglutamatergic activity. *Proceedings of the National Academy of Sciences of the United States of America*, *108*(20), 8485–8490. https://doi.org/10.1073/pnas.1103029108.

Revel, F. G., Moreau, J. L., Gainetdinov, R. R., Ferragud, A., Velazquez-Sanchez, C., Sotnikova, T. D., et al. (2012). Trace amine-associated receptor 1 partial agonism reveals novel paradigm for neuropsychiatric therapeutics. *Biological Psychiatry*, *72*(11), 934–942. https://doi.org/10.1016/j.biopsych.2012.05.014.

Revel, F. G., Moreau, J. L., Pouzet, B., Mory, R., Bradaia, A., Buchy, D., et al. (2013). A new perspective for schizophrenia: TAAR1 agonists reveal antipsychotic- and antidepressant-like activity, improve cognition and control body weight. *Molecular Psychiatry*, *18*(5), 543–556. https://doi.org/10.1038/mp.2012.57.

Sandler, M., Ruthven, C. R., Goodwin, B. L., Reynolds, G. P., Rao, V. A., & Coppen, A. (1980). Trace amine deficit in depressive illness: The phenylalanine connexion. *Acta Psychiatrica Scandinavica. Supplementum*, *280*, 29–39. Retrieved from https://www.ncbi.nlm.nih.gov/pubmed/6773301.

Simmler, L. D., Buchy, D., Chaboz, S., Hoener, M. C., & Liechti, M. E. (2016). In vitro characterization of psychoactive substances at rat, mouse, and human trace amine-associated receptor 1. *The Journal of Pharmacology and Experimental Therapeutics*, *357*(1), 134–144. https://doi.org/10.1124/jpet.115.229765.

Sotnikova, T. D., Beaulieu, J. M., Espinoza, S., Masri, B., Zhang, X., Salahpour, A., et al. (2010). The dopamine metabolite 3-methoxytyramine is a neuromodulator. *PLoS One*, *5*(10), e13452. https://doi.org/10.1371/journal.pone.0013452.

Stafford, A. M., Reed, C., Baba, H., Walter, N. A., Mootz, J. R., Williams, R. W., et al. (2019). Taar1 gene variants have a causal role in methamphetamine intake and response and interact with Oprm1. *eLife*, *8*. https://doi.org/10.7554/eLife.46472.

Stoker, A. K., & Markou, A. (2013). Unraveling the neurobiology of nicotine dependence using genetically engineered mice. *Current Opinion in Neurobiology*, *23*(4), 493–499. https://doi.org/10.1016/j.conb.2013.02.013.

Subramaniyan, M., & Dani, J. A. (2015). Dopaminergic and cholinergic learning mechanisms in nicotine addiction. *Annals of the New York Academy of Sciences*, *1349*, 46–63. https://doi.org/10.1111/nyas.12871.

Sukhanov, I., Caffino, L., Efimova, E. V., Espinoza, S., Sotnikova, T. D., Cervo, L., et al. (2016). Increased context-dependent conditioning to amphetamine in mice lacking TAAR1. *Pharmacological Research*, *103*, 206–214. https://doi.org/10.1016/j.phrs.2015.11.002.

Sukhanov, I., Dorofeikova, M., Dolgorukova, A., Dorotenko, A., & Gainetdinov, R. R. (2018). Trace amine-associated receptor 1 modulates the locomotor and sensitization effects of nicotine. *Frontiers in Pharmacology*, *9*, 329. https://doi.org/10.3389/fphar.2018.00329.

Thorn, D. A., Jing, L., Qiu, Y., Gancarz-Kausch, A. M., Galuska, C. M., Dietz, D. M., et al. (2014). Effects of the trace amine-associated receptor 1 agonist RO5263397 on abuse-related effects of cocaine in rats. *Neuropsychopharmacology*, *39*(10), 2309–2316. https://doi.org/10.1038/npp.2014.91.

Thorn, D. A., Zhang, C., Zhang, Y., & Li, J. X. (2014). The trace amine associated receptor 1 agonist RO5263397 attenuates the induction of cocaine behavioral sensitization in rats. *Neuroscience Letters*, *566*, 67–71. https://doi.org/10.1016/j.neulet.2014.02.024.

Underhill, S. M., Colt, M. S., & Amara, S. G. (2020). Amphetamine stimulates endocytosis of the norepinephrine and neuronal glutamate transporters in cultured locus coeruleus neurons. *Neurochemical Research*, *45*(6), 1410–1419. https://doi.org/10.1007/s11064-019-02939-6.

Underhill, S. M., Hullihen, P. D., Chen, J., Fenollar-Ferrer, C., Rizzo, M. A., Ingram, S. L., et al. (2021). Amphetamines signal through intracellular TAAR1 receptors coupled to Galpha13 and GalphaS in discrete subcellular domains. *Molecular Psychiatry*, *26*(4), 1208–1223. https://doi.org/10.1038/s41380-019-0469-2.

Underhill, S. M., Wheeler, D. S., Li, M., Watts, S. D., Ingram, S. L., & Amara, S. G. (2014). Amphetamine modulates excitatory neurotransmission through endocytosis of the glutamate transporter EAAT3 in dopamine neurons. *Neuron*, *83*(2), 404–416. https://doi.org/10.1016/j.neuron.2014.05.043.

Wainscott, D. B., Little, S. P., Yin, T., Tu, Y., Rocco, V. P., He, J. X., et al. (2007). Pharmacologic characterization of the cloned human trace amine-associated receptor1 (TAAR1) and evidence for species differences with the rat TAAR1. *The Journal of Pharmacology and Experimental Therapeutics*, *320*(1), 475–485. https://doi.org/10.1124/jpet.106.112532.

Wheeler, D. S., Underhill, S. M., Stolz, D. B., Murdoch, G. H., Thiels, E., Romero, G., et al. (2015). Amphetamine activates Rho GTPase signaling to mediate dopamine transporter internalization and acute behavioral effects of amphetamine. *Proceedings of the National Academy of Sciences of the United States of America*, *112*(51), E7138–E7147. https://doi.org/10.1073/pnas.1511670112.

Wolinsky, T. D., Swanson, C. J., Smith, K. E., Zhong, H., Borowsky, B., Seeman, P., et al. (2007). The trace amine 1 receptor knockout mouse: An animal model with relevance to schizophrenia. *Genes, Brain, and Behavior*, *6*(7), 628–639. https://doi.org/10.1111/j.1601-183X.2006.00292.x.

Wu, R, Liu, J, Johnson, B, Huang, Y, Zhang, Y, & Li, JX. (2021). Activation of trace amine-associated receptor 1 attenuates nicotine withdrawal-related effects. *Addiction Biology*, *25*, e13075.

Wu, R., Liu, J., Wang, K., Huang, Y., Zhang, Y., & Li, J. X. (2020). Effects of a trace amine-associated receptor 1 agonist RO 5263397 on ethanol-induced behavioral sensitization. *Behavioural Brain Research*, *390*, 112641. https://doi.org/10.1016/j.bbr.2020.112641.

Xie, Z., & Miller, G. M. (2007). Trace amine-associated receptor 1 is a modulator of the dopamine transporter. *The Journal of Pharmacology and Experimental Therapeutics*, *321*(1), 128–136. https://doi.org/10.1124/jpet.106.117382.

Xie, Z., & Miller, G. M. (2009). A receptor mechanism for methamphetamine action in dopamine transporter regulation in brain. *The Journal of Pharmacology and Experimental Therapeutics*, *330*(1), 316–325. https://doi.org/10.1124/jpet.109.153775.

Xie, Z., Westmoreland, S. V., Bahn, M. E., Chen, G. L., Yang, H., Vallender, E. J., et al. (2007). Rhesus monkey trace amine-associated receptor 1 signaling: Enhancement by monoamine transporters and attenuation by the D2 autoreceptor in vitro. *The Journal of Pharmacology and Experimental Therapeutics*, *321*(1), 116–127. https://doi.org/10.1124/jpet.106.116863.

Xue, Z., Siemian, J. N., Johnson, B. N., Zhang, Y., & Li, J. X. (2018). Methamphetamine-induced impulsivity during chronic methamphetamine treatment in rats: Effects of the TAAR 1 agonist RO5263397. *Neuropharmacology*, *129*, 36–46. https://doi.org/10.1016/j.neuropharm.2017.11.012.

Zhang, L., Doyon, W. M., Clark, J. J., Phillips, P. E., & Dani, J. A. (2009). Controls of tonic and phasic dopamine transmission in the dorsal and ventral striatum. *Molecular Pharmacology*, *76*(2), 396–404. https://doi.org/10.1124/mol.109.056317.

Zhang, J., Pacifico, R., Cawley, D., Feinstein, P., & Bozza, T. (2013). Ultrasensitive detection of amines by a trace amine-associated receptor. *The Journal of Neuroscience*, *33*(7), 3228–3239. https://doi.org/10.1523/JNEUROSCI.4299-12.2013.

CHAPTER TWELVE

Substance abuse and neurotransmission

Sarah Davis and Jun Zhu*
Department of Drug Discovery and Biomedical Sciences, College of Pharmacy, University of South Carolina, Columbia, SC, United States
*Corresponding author: e-mail address: zhuj@cop.sc.edu

Contents

1. Introduction 404
2. Cocaine 406
   2.1 Cocaine targets of neurotransmission 406
   2.2 Cocaine-induced long-lasting changes in neurotransmission 407
3. Methamphetamine 409
   3.1 Methamphetamine targets of neurotransmission 409
   3.2 Therapeutic strategies for methamphetamine abuse 410
4. Amphetamine 411
   4.1 Amphetamine targets of neurotransmission 411
5. Opioids 412
   5.1 Opioid targets of neurotransmission 413
   5.2 Fentanyl 413
   5.3 Heroin 415
   5.4 Pharmacotherapies for opioid abuse 416
6. Alcohol 417
   6.1 Alcohol-mediated effects on neurotransmission 417
   6.2 Pharmacotherapies for alcohol use disorder 418
7. Nicotine 419
   7.1 Nicotine targets of neurotransmission 419
8. Drugs of abuse and HIV-1 421
9. Considerations regarding COVID-19 423
10. Conclusion 423
Acknowledgments 424
Conflict of interest 424
References 424

Abstract

The number of people who suffer from a substance abuse disorder has continued to rise over the last decade; particularly, the number of drug-related overdose deaths has sharply increased during the COVID-19 pandemic. Converging lines of clinical observations, supported by imaging and neuropsychological performance testing, have

Advances in Pharmacology, Volume 93
ISSN 1054-3589
https://doi.org/10.1016/bs.apha.2021.10.007

demonstrated that substance abuse-induced dysregulation of neurotransmissions in the brain is critical for development and expression of the addictive properties of abused substances. Recent scientific advances have allowed for better understanding of the neurobiological processes that mediates drugs of abuse and addiction. This chapter presents the past classic concepts and the recent advances in our knowledge about how cocaine, amphetamines, opioids, alcohol, and nicotine alter multiple neurotransmitter systems, which contribute to the behaviors associated with each drug. Additionally, we discuss the interactive effects of HIV-1 or COVID-19 and substance abuse on neurotransmission and neurobiological pathways. Finally, we introduce therapeutic strategies for development of pharmacotherapies for substance abuse disorders.

Abbreviations

5-HT	serotonin
AMPAR	α-amino-3-hydroxy-5-methyl-4-isoxazolepropionic acid receptors
AMPH	amphetamine
DA	dopamine
DAT	dopamine transporter
GABA	γ-aminobutyric acid
GLU	glutamate
M-,K-,D-, OR	μ-, κ-, δ- receptors
METH	methamphetamine
MSN	medium spiny neuron
NAc	nucleus accumbens
nAChRs	nicotinic acetylcholine receptors
NE	norepinephrine
NET	norepinephrine transporter
NMDAR	*N*-methyl-D-aspartic acid receptors
ROS	reactive oxygen species
SERT	serotonin transporter
Tat	transactivator of transcription
VMAT-2	vesicular monoamine transporter 2
VTA	ventral tegmental area
σ1R	σ1-receptor

1. Introduction

Substance abuse presents a significant and growing health crisis in the United States. The provisional data for the center for disease control (CDC) indicates a drastic increase of the number of overdose related deaths during the COVID-19 pandemic (Ahmad, Rossen, & Sutton, 2021). Furthermore, during the COVID-19 pandemic there has been an increase in the self-reported use of substances of abuse, particularly due to the increase in stressors imposed by the pandemic (Czeisler et al., 2021). The number of overdose-related deaths has continued to increase over the last 5 years, and from November 2019 through November 2020 there was a record high of 90,722 reported deaths. Importantly, a recent study found that the medical cost associated with substance abuse in 2017 was approximately $13.2 billion (Peterson, Li, Xu, Mikosz, & Luo, 2021). Understanding how these drugs of abuse impact neurotransmission is critical for addressing this health crisis. For this chapter, we review recent advances in knowledge made in understanding how commonly abused substances, including cocaine, amphetamines, fentanyl, heroin, alcohol, and nicotine, impact neurotransmission on a molecular level. We discuss the direct effects of these substances on their molecular targets, which lead to dysregulation of neuro-signaling, and their indirect (downstream) effects on neuro-signaling with the hope of highlighting potential targets for therapeutic intervention. While progression from substance abuse to addiction is a critical area of interest, the development from of substance abuse to substance addiction has been discussed, and is not the primary focus for this chapter (Uhl, Koob, & Cable, 2019; Wise & Koob, 2014). This chapter will focus on the general neurochemical effects elicited by these abused substances and how they impact behavior outcomes.

Changes in neurotransmission due to abused substances will be discussed in the context of relevant neurocircuitry pathways. For instance, abused substances either directly or indirectly, alter dopaminergic transmission in the mesocorticolimbic pathway, leading to the development and expression of drug dependence. There is a debate regarding the specific direction of dopaminergic tone (increased or decreased) which is critical for developing addiction (Samaha, Khoo, Ferrario, & Robinson, 2021). Regardless, alterations in DA neurotransmission within the mesolimbic pathway are critical for mediating substance induced behaviors. The mesolimbic pathway includes dopaminergic projections from the ventral tegmental area (VTA) to the Nucleus Accumbens (NAc) (Volkow, Wang, Fowler, & Tomasi, 2012). The glutamatergic projections from the NAc to the prefrontal cortex (PFC) make up the mesocortical pathway, which is key factor for memory formation and is implicated in the long-lasting effects of drug use (Feltenstein, See, & Fuchs, 2021). Synaptic plasticity (strength of synaptic transmission) in response to acute drug use mediates the long-lasting molecular changes which store drug experience and promote relapse (Zhang & Bramham, 2020). Synaptic plasticity and dysregulation of dopaminergic transmission are central to drug induced adaptations in neurotransmission signaling.

However, other neurotransmitter signaling systems are also affected, including serotonin (5-HT), norepinephrine (NE), γ-aminobutyric acid (GABA), and acetylcholine (ACh). Furthermore, the endogenous opioid system, which has direct influence on dopaminergic signaling, is also associated with susceptibility to substance abuse disorders (Butelman, Yuferov, & Kreek, 2012). These signaling systems are the most prominent direct molecular targets and downstream mediators associated with neuroadaptations in response to abused drugs.

2. Cocaine

2.1 Cocaine targets of neurotransmission

Cocaine abuse is a highly prevalent health crisis in the United States. In 2014, there was an estimated 900,000 adults nationwide living with cocaine use disorder (CUD), while in 2018 there were 19 million users worldwide (Lipari & Van Horn, 2017; United Nations Office on Drugs and Crime (UNODC), 2020). The primary driver of cocaine-induced dysregulation of neurotransmission has been attributed to the direct inhibition of the dopamine transporter (DAT) by cocaine, leading to increased extracellular DA levels (Rocha et al., 1998). Cocaine interacts with the dopamine (DA) uptake site on DATs with an inhibitory concentration in the micromolar range. However, many higher affinity DAT inhibitors do not share the behavioral response of cocaine, suggesting that cocaine may interact with DAT through alternative binding sties. A recent computational modeling study has revealed that cocaine binds to a novel high-affinity second binding site allosterically (Xu & Chen, 2020). Indeed, a recent study found that cocaine at nanomolar levels can elicit neural autophagic degradation of DAT *in vitro* and *in vivo*, suggesting a potential mechanism for how cocaine increases extracellular levels of DA despite having a weak affinity for DAT (Harraz et al., 2021). DAT function and availability are regulated by its endocytic trafficking and dynamic conformational changes (Fagan, Kearney, & Melikian, 2020). Cocaine promotes the outward-facing conformation of DAT, which was associated with reduced oligomerization of DAT and subsequently reduced endocytosis of the transporter (Sorkina et al., 2021). Thus, in the context of cocaine-mediated endocytosis of DAT, there is a need for improved tools to fully understand how cocaine regulates DAT trafficking.

In addition to DAT, cocaine has been found to directly interact with the norepinephrine (NE) transporter (NET), serotonin (5-HT) transporter (SERT), and the σ1-receptor (σ1R) (Blakely, De Felice, & Hartzell, 1994; Ravna, Sylte, & Dahl, 2003). Increased NE released from the Locus

Coeruleus (LC) as a result of cocaine inhibition of NET is thought to drive the α1b-adrenoceptor (α -AR)-mediated increases in glutamate (GLU) transmission from the medial prefrontal cortex (mPFC), which is critical for cocaine reinstatement (Zhu et al., 2017). Cocaine induces an increase in extracellular 5-HT through inhibition of SERT, which then activates 5-HT1B receptors on D2R MSNs, consequently inhibiting GABA transmission on the GABAergic neurons in the ventral palladium (Matsui & Alvarez, 2018). Cocaine-induced alteration of serotoninergic signaling has been implicated as a key mediating factor for cocaine-induced reinforcement. Lastly, σ1R is primarily an endoplasmic reticulum protein, however, it has several roles including regulation of Ca^{2+} dynamics as well as regulation of Na^{+}, K^{+}, and Cl^{-} channels (Maurice & Su, 2009). Recent advances suggest that σ1R interacts with DA molecular targets. This includes increasing D2R function, as well as interacting directly with DAT to promote occupation of its outward-facing conformation, subsequently promoting cocaine binding (Beggiato et al., 2017; Hong et al., 2017).

2.2 Cocaine-induced long-lasting changes in neurotransmission

A prominent neuroadaptation driven by cocaine is the development of silent synapses, which are considered as key aspects of cocaine memories related to reinforcement and relapse. The cocaine-generated silent synapses are immature glutamatergic synapses characterized by a decreased ratio of the glutamatergic ionotropic receptors, α-amino-3-hydroxy-5-methyl-4-isoxazolepropionic acid (AMPA) to *N*-methyl-D-aspartic acid receptors (NMDARs) (Dong, Taylor, Wolf, & Shaham, 2017). The cocaine-generated silent synapses are unsilenced and become matured by replacing GLUN2B subunits with GLUN2A subunits in NMDARs (Smaga, Sanak, & Filip, 2019). How cocaine induces the changes in NMDAR stoichiometry is still unclear, however, activation of D1 receptors modulating NMDAR-mediated GLU signaling presents a potential mechanism. Glutamatergic inputs from the paraventricular nucleus of the thalamus (PVT) to the NAc medium spiny neurons (MSNs) are essential in formation of the silent synapses and cocaine-related memories. These particular silent synapses are important for acquisition of cocaine self-administration but not for incubation of cocaine craving (Neumann et al., 2016). Therefore, the long-lasting incubation of cocaine is dependent on specific neurocircuitry pathways in order to store cocaine experience necessary for cocaine reinstatement. A study found that infralimbic and prelimbic medial prefrontal cortex (mPFC) inputs to the NAc also undergo silent-synapse formation in response to cocaine. These projections undergo different unsilencing mechanisms, and more importantly, unsilencing the infralimbic to NAc projection potentiated relapse, whereas unsilencing of the mPFC to NAc inhibited cocaine craving (Ma et al., 2014). Thus, targeting the functional states of cocaine-generated silent synapses can disrupt cocaine memories and reduce cocaine-mediated behavior.

Cocaine-induced adaptive changes in neurotransmission are mediated through functional expression of D1 or D2 receptors on NAc MSNs (Zinsmaier, Dong, & Huang, 2021). Cocaine-induced silent synapses are formed at D1R MSNs and are unsilenced by recruiting AMPARs to increase AMPAR/NMDAR (Graziane et al., 2016). These NAc MSNs also differ in that D1R contain the opioid neuropeptide dynorphin (Dyn) and the D2R, enkephalin (Enk). Cocaine increases Enk levels, likely through activation of D1R and NMDAR-mediated pathways. Increased Enk can further modulate dopaminergic and glutamatergic signaling through various opioid receptor interactions, even influencing AMPA trafficking (Mongi-Bragato, Avalos, Guzmán, Bollati, & Cancela, 2018). This evidence supports that long-lasting neuroadaptation in response to cocaine occurs in MSNs through both silent synapses and the endogenous opioid system.

Traditionally, it was believed that cocaine-induced inhibition of DAT is primarily responsible for cocaine-driven behavior (Rocha et al., 1998). However, research since has implicated multiple neuronal pathways in contributing to cocaine-driven behavior. Therefore, alternatives to targeting DAT have been developed as therapeutic approaches to treatment of CUD, including D3 receptor antagonists, 5-HT receptor agonists, and *N*-acetylcysteine (NIDA, 2020). To date, there are no FDA approved pharmacotherapies for treatment of CUD based on the following potential reasons: (1) There are molecular interactions between the treatment and therapeutic target outside of key neurocircuitry pathways creating off target effects; (2) Treatments only target one neurotransmitter system, which are insufficient to completely abolish drug-induced behaviors; and (3) CUD patients may take more than one substance as many drug users co-abuse psychostimulants, thereby complicating their state of dysregulated neurotransmission. For example, the orexin neuropeptide system presents a shared target in co-abused cocaine and alcohol and thus a possible avenue for therapeutic development (James, Fragale, O'Connor, Zimmer, & Aston-Jones, 2021). Understanding the effects of co-abused substance drugs on neurotransmissions and neuronal pathways will be beneficial for developing therapeutic strategies for treatment of co-abused substances.

3. Methamphetamine

3.1 Methamphetamine targets of neurotransmission

In 2017, an estimated 964,000 people had a methamphetamine (METH) use disorder in the United States (Chomchai & Chomchai, 2015; NIDA, 2019). Our earliest understanding of METH-induced dysregulation of neurotransmission involves alterations in dopaminergic signaling through inhibition of DATs (Fleckenstein, Metzger, Wilkins, Gibb, & Hanson, 1997). Further, the vesicular monoamine transporter (VMAT-2), the primary transporter in vesicle membrane responsible for reuptake of monoamines into presynaptic vesicles for storage, was implicated in driving METH-induced dysregulation of DA and behavior (Fukushima et al., 2007; Fumagalli et al., 1999). This led to our current model for METH induced dysregulation of neurotransmission in which METH inhibits reuptake of DA via the VMAT-2 thereby increasing cytosolic DA which then reverse transports through DAT and increases extracellular DA until all stored DA is depleted (Nickell, Siripurapu, Vartak, Crooks, & Dwoskin, 2014). There is evidence that supports the effects of METH on DA homeostasis are driven not only temporally but also bidirectionally by the concentration of METH (Branch & Beckstead, 2012). Additionally, METH exerts its neurotoxic effect on DA metabolism by directly inhibiting monoamine oxidase (MAO) (Mantle, Tipton, & Garrett, 1976) which leads to autoxidation of DA and generation of ROS and subsequent neurodegeneration (Meiser, Weindl, & Hiller, 2013). It has been postulated that ROS formed by drugs of abuse can regulate protein function through s-glutathionylation (GSH) modification at cysteine residues (Womersley & Uys, 2016). A recent study found indirect evidence supporting a possible mechanism in which ROS formed in response to METH promoted GSH modification of VMAT-2 to inhibit VMAT-2 function (Hedges et al., 2018). Lastly, METH interacts directly with σ1R, and recent evidence supports σ1R mediates METH effects on DA through direct interactions with DAT (Sambo et al., 2017). These findings highlight recent advances regarding METH-induced alterations of neurotransmission specific to the dopaminergic system.

In addition to the dopaminergic system, other signaling systems, including GLU, NE, and 5-HT neurotransmission, are also implicated by METH use (Ferrucci, Giorgi, Bartalucci, Busceti, & Fornai, 2013; Nordahl, Salo, & Leamon, 2003; Szumlinski et al., 2017). One possible mechanism underlying METH-induced increases in GLU transmission involves the vesicular glutamate transporter (VGLUT2), as heterozygous deletion of VGLUT2 reduced locomotor response to METH and attenuated METH-induced increases in DA and GLU (Shen, Chen, Marino, McDevitt, & Xi, 2021). Moreover, the metabotropic GLU receptor, mGlu5, mediates METH effects on DA dynamics and behavior. Negative allosteric modulators of mGlu5 attenuated METH effects on striatal DA and METH-conditioned place preference (Petzold, Szumlinski, & London, 2021). On the other hand, METH also increases NE levels via inhibition of both NET and presynaptic α-adrenergic receptors (α-ARs) (Ferrucci et al., 2019). Although METH is a potent inhibitor of NET ($K_I = 110\,nM$) compared to SERT ($K_I = 31.74\,\mu M$), persistent reductions in SERT expression are observed in METH abusers (Han & Gu, 2006; Sekine et al., 2006). Further, homozygous deletion of SERT in its knock-out mouse model shows a reduction of METH-induced locomotor activity and an increase in 5-HT levels (Igari et al., 2015). A recent meta-analysis identified that functional variants of brain derived neurotrophic factor (BDNF) and fatty acid amide hydrolase (FAAH) are significantly associated with METH abuse disorder (Guerin et al., 2021). This finding is relevant to neurotransmission, as a recent study found that BDNF plays a role mediating METH effects on serotonergic cells (Sepulveda, Manning, Gogos, Hale, & van den Buuse, 2021). These studies highlight the role of nondopaminergic systems in mediating METH abuse.

3.2 Therapeutic strategies for methamphetamine abuse

Given that METH dysregulates dopaminergic transmission by targeting DAT and VMAT2, the novel compound GZ-793A was developed, which targets both DAT and VMAT-2. GZ-793A inhibits METH-induced DA release and reduces METH-induced self-administration and reinstatement of drug seeking (Alvers et al., 2012; Beckmann et al., 2012; Horton, Nickell, Zheng, Crooks, & Dwoskin, 2013). Additionally, a new study identified that NBI-98782, a metabolite of the VMAT-2 inhibitor valbenazine, attenuated AMPH-induced DA and NE efflux and reduced AMPH-induced locomotor activity in mice (Huang et al., 2020). Targeting VMAT-2 and DAT for reducing METH-induced dysregulation of DA system presents a potential therapeutic strategy for treatment of METH abuse.

Pharmacotherapies have been tested in the clinical setting for treatment of METH dependence. A recent systematic literature review reported that stimulant agonists such as dexamphetamine and methylphenidate may show promise; however, evaluating the efficacy of pharmacotherapies is complicated, as most METH users have co-morbidities (e.g., other drugs of abuse, depression or anxiety). Therefore, further investigation in larger sample sizes is necessary (Siefried, Acheson, Lintzeris, & Ezard, 2020). A promising clinical trial showed that a combined regiment of the antidepressant bupropion and the opioid-receptor antagonist naltrexone improved patient outcomes (% of negative-urine samples over 5–6, and 11–12 weeks) compared to placebo (13.6% vs 2.5%) (Trivedi et al., 2021). While this regiment was indeed effective and supports the use of combined pharmacotherapies for treatment, overall response was low. Future work aimed at combined pharmacotherapies which target multiple METH interactions will likely be key to developing highly effective treatment of METH dependence.

4. Amphetamine

4.1 Amphetamine targets of neurotransmission

Amphetamine (AMPH) is a structural analog of METH and is used as a prescription treatment for attention deficit hyperactive disorder (ADHD). Although METH is easier to access recreationally, the two drugs share molecular mechanisms and behavioral outcomes and are therefore often used interchangeably (Chou, Huang, & Jiann, 2015). Here, we highlight the similarities and differences between AMPH and METH impacts on behavior and neurotransmission.

Both AMPH and METH have the same mechanism underlying dysregulation of DA neurotransmission through inhibition of VMAT-2 and DAT (Carboni et al., 2001; Jones, Gainetdinov, Wightman, & Caron, 1998; Takahashi et al., 1997). Additionally, both AMPH and METH share the same nondopaminergic targets including MAOs, catechol-O-methyltransferase (COMT), SERT, and NET (Sulzer, Sonders, Poulsen, & Galli, 2005). As with METH, AMPH has a concentration dependent effect on mediating extracellular DA levels (Felmer, Janson, Summers, & Wallace, 2019; Siciliano, Calipari, Ferris, & Jones, 2014). However, METH is five times more effective than AMPH at releasing DA via efflux through DAT and inhibiting DA clearance through DAT (Goodwin et al., 2009). Homozygous deletion of DAT in mice prevented AMPH-induced locomotor activity, indicating DAT as a critical component for AMPH-induced behavior (Giros, Jaber, Jones, Wightman, & Caron, 1996). AMPH increases extracellular DA through reverse transport via DAT therefore understanding the specific mechanism for AMPH-mediated DA efflux has been a key area of interest (Kahlig et al., 2005). Early evidence indicated roles for both intracellular Ca^{2+} and physical association with protein kinase Cβ (PKCβ) in mediating DA efflux through DAT (Johnson, Guptaroy, Lund, Shamban, & Gnegy, 2005). In agreement with this, phosphorylation of DAT by AMPHs specifically (not cocaine) by PKCβ was crucial for promoting AMPH-induced DA efflux though DAT (Foster et al., 2012). Evidence supports that other proteins and molecules including syntaxin 1A, G protein βγ (Gβγ) subunits, and phosphatidylinositol (4,5)-bisphosphate (PIP_2) help to facilitate AMPH-induced DA efflux through DAT (Belovich et al., 2021; Binda et al., 2008; Mauna et al., 2019). Further, recent evidence has also identified the organic cation transporter 3 (OCT3), which non-selectively transports monoamines, as another transporter protein which undergoes AMPH-induced DA efflux (Mayer et al., 2018). Understanding the molecular mechanism for AMPH-induced DA efflux through DAT may identify novel therapeutic targets for alleviating AMPH-induced behavior (Sitte & Freissmuth, 2015).

AMPH also dysregulates non-dopaminergic forms of neurotransmission. AMPH-induced conditioned place preference and locomotor activity are dependent on functional expression of NET (Mannangatti, Ramamoorthy, & Jayanthi, 2018). Pharmacological evidence supports that AMPH-stimulated NE release may contribute to AMPH-induced behavior (Rothman et al., 2001). In addition to NE, AMPH also increases GLU transmission. Increased GLU levels may be a result of endocytosis of the GLU transporter. AMPH-induced endocytosis of EAAT3 is mediated by the trace amine-associated receptor, TAAR1 (Underhill, Colt, & Amara, 2020; Wolf, Xue, Li, & Wavak, 2000). In addition to EAAT3, the major GLU transporter GLT-1 also mediates AMPH-induced behavior. AMPH-induced locomotor activity was reduced in conditional GLT-1 KO mice (Fischer et al., 2018). Another study found that AMPH did not induce changes in GLT-1 expression in the mPFC or NAc. However, this study found that β-lactam antibiotic ceftriaxone, which restores GLT-1 expression, reduced AMPH-induced drug seeking and cue-induced reinstatement of drug seeking behavior (Garcia, Arndt, & Cain, 2019). AMPH-induced dysregulation of non-dopaminergic neurotransmission is an important area of research which warrants further exploration.

5. Opioids

Persistent pain affects nearly 100 million adults in the United States, with an economic cost between $560 and $635 billion annually (Gaskin & Richard, 2012). The overuse of opioids prescribed for pain has led to the prevalence of opioid use disorder (OUD), and in recent years, is linked to the increased use of cheaper illicit opioids such as heroin and fentanyl (Stoicea et al., 2019), which accounted for 66.4% of all overdose deaths in 2016 (Seth, Scholl, Rudd, & Bacon, 2018). Development of pharmacotherapies are not only critical for treatment of ongoing OUD, but non addictive opioid alternatives as pharmacotherapy for pain management is crucial in mitigating the development of OUD. For the purposes of this review, we will focus on ongoing developments related to the molecular mechanism of illicit opioids of abuse.

5.1 Opioid targets of neurotransmission

Opioids include a class of drugs used for treatment of pain that act at opioid receptors including μ-(MOR), κ-(KOR), and δ-(DOR) receptors (Sun, Chen, Chen, & Pan, 2019; Wang, 2019). Differential localization of opioid receptors throughout the CNS have been characterized and attributed to the receptor-specific effects of mediating analgesia (inability to feel pain), dysphoria (unease), and other autonomic functions, and is detailed further in review (Valentino & Volkow, 2018). Additionally, how interactions between the opioid morphine and addiction related pathways has been extensively discussed in a recent review (Kupnicka et al., 2020). For the purposes of this chapter, we will focus on fentanyl and heroin effects on neurotransmission.

5.2 Fentanyl

Fentanyl is typically used for treatment of patients with severe pain; however, the illicit use of fentanyl has increased over the past several years (Hedegaard, Miniño, & Warner, 2018). Recent evidence shows an increase in the incidence of fentanyl-related overdose deaths (Davis & Behm, 2020). Fentanyl is a powerful synthetic opioid analgesic that is similar to morphine but has high lipophilicity and is 100 times more potent as a high affinity agonist for MOR compared to other opioid receptors (DOR, KOR) (Maguire et al., 1992). Recently, the binding mode of fentanyl to MOR has been characterized (Vo, Mahinthichaichan, Shen, & Ellis, 2021). Fentanyl acts as a biased agonist of MOR to promote a unique signaling cascade through activation of MOR, which favors downstream signaling through β-arrestin-2 over G-protein signaling (Comer & Cahill, 2019). Neurochemical effects of fentanyl include dysregulation of DA, GLU, and GABA transmission. Fentanyl increases DA in the NAc through activation of MOR and DOR (Yoshida et al., 1999). Interestingly, a recent study found that treatment with a growth hormone secretagogue receptor (GHS-R1A) antagonist reduced fentanyl-induced increases in DA in the NAc and reduced fentanyl-conditioned place preference in rats (Sustkova-Fiserova et al., 2020). The mechanism by which GHS-R1A mediates fentanyl effects on neurotransmission is still under investigation. Fentanyl also dysregulates GLU and GABA transmission, as has been previously observed in the peripheral nervous system (Fu, Tsen, Lee, Lui, & Chan, 1997; Griffioen et al., 2004). A recent study found that fentanyl increased GABA release and decreased GLU release in the anterior hypothalamus of rats (Pourzitaki et al., 2018). How fentanyl reduces GLU release is not fully understood, however, endogenous opioids have been shown to act in a retrograde manner to inhibit excitatory transmission thereby presenting a possible mechanism for this phenomenon (Iremonger & Bains, 2009).

The MOR antagonist naloxone is the primary treatment for opioid overdose (Baumann, Kopajtic, & Madras, 2018). Converging lines of evidence have found that repeated administration of naloxone is needed in fentanyl-related overdoses, in part due to the short half-life (30–90 min) of naloxone (Faul et al., 2017; Somerville et al., 2017). However, it is not entirely clear why multiple doses of naloxone are needed. There is evidence that respiratory complications arise during fentanyl-related overdoses specifically (Fairbairn, Coffin, & Walley, 2017). These respiratory complications, referred to as "wooden chest syndrome," cause muscle rigidity which occurs quickly (within 2 min) (Pergolizzi, Webster, Vortsman, Ann LeQuang, & Raffa, 2021). Early evidence regarding the pharmaceutical action of fentanyl suggested the role of NE and cholinergic systems in mediating fentanyl off target effects (Atcheson, Rowbotham, & Lambert, 1993). This is of interest, as recent evidence suggests a possible role for these systems in mediating fentanyl-related respiratory and cardiovascular failure (Torralva & Janowsky, 2019). Further research to improve the treatment of fentanyl-related overdoses is warranted (Comer, Pravetoni, Coop, Baumann, & Cunningham, 2021; Pergolizzi et al., 2021; Volkow, 2021). Improving the efficacy of treatment administered will likely improve the survival outcome of those experiencing a fentanyl-related overdose. This would be particularly beneficial in rural areas, where emergency response times are longer (Faul et al., 2017), and bystander intervention is necessary to swiftly treat the patient (Somerville et al., 2017). In addition to naloxone, targeting the effects of fentanyl on NE and cholinergic systems presents one possible approach for improving therapeutic treatment of fentanyl-related overdoses.

Lastly, recent *in vitro* evidence supports possible interaction between fentanyl and several non-MOR targets involved in neurotransmission. Fentanyl binds 5-HT receptors (5-HT_{1A} and 5-HT_{2A}), acting as an agonist at 5-HT_{1A}, and produces efflux of 5-HT (Baldo & Rose, 2020). Furthermore, a recent pharmacological study was done to identify potential non-MOR molecular targets for fentanyl. This study found *in vitro* evidence which supports several possible non-MOR interactions for fentanyl. This includes binding of fentanyl to NE receptors (α_1-ADr), weak inhibition of uptake through at DAT, SERT, and NET, partial antagonist action at DA receptors (D4.4), and inhibition of uptake through VMAT-2 (Torralva et al., 2020). Future *in vivo* work is necessary to validate these molecules as molecular targets for fentanyl and to determine whether these interactions contribute to fentanyl-induced behaviors.

5.3 Heroin

Heroin use in the United States has continued to increase since 2000 and in 2015 the societal cost of heroin use disorder was an estimated $51.2 billion (Jiang, Lee, Lee, & Pickard, 2017). Heroin is a prodrug form of morphine that is readily metabolized into 6-monoacetylmorphine (6-MAM) and morphine (Rook, Huitema, van den Brink, van Ree, & Beijnen, 2006; Sawynok, 1986). Heroin acts as a highly addictive analgesic drug through interaction with MORs (Wang et al., 2016). The long-standing hypothesis of opioid reward is that opioid activation of MORs in GABAergic interneurons in the VTA disinhibits dopaminergic neurons thereby increasing DA in the reward pathway (Corre et al., 2018). However, this model has been repeatedly challenged. Early evidence found that MORs are expressed throughout the VTA and heroin is self-administered in the absence of DA terminals (Pettit, Ettenberg, Bloom, & Koob, 1984). A recent study found that conditional KO mice lacking MOR in the striatum had no locomotor response and reduced motivation to heroin; however, heroin-conditioned place preference remained intact (Charbogne et al., 2017). Further, another study found that inhibition and activation of MORs in the substantia nigra had a greater impact on reducing, and reinstating (respectively) drug seeking behavior in response to heroin compared to GABAergic VTA neurons (Galaj et al., 2020). This evidence supports a role for MORs in regions besides the VTA for promoting heroin-induced behaviors.

Although the relationship between MORs and the reward pathway is not fully elucidated, there is evidence which indicates heroin use is associated with dysregulation of dopaminergic and serotonergic function. For instance, DAT expression is increased in early heroin addicted rat models and decreased availability of DAT was observed in heroin users using

PET scan imaging (Li, Xia, Li, Yin, & Liang, 2017; Xu et al., 2017). As well, genetic variants of DA receptors (Lachowicz et al., 2020; Zhan et al., 2018) as well as serotonergic molecules, appear to correlate with heroin dependence (Cao, LaRocque, & Li, 2013; Yin et al., 2016). However, whether heroin alters dopaminergic and serotonergic function remains controversial. Single photon emission computed tomography (SPECT) showed no difference in DAT and SERT levels between healthy individuals and heroin users (Cosgrove et al., 2010). Therefore, more work is needed to discern the impact of heroin on DA and 5-HT signaling.

Glutamatergic function is associated with heroin relapse (Knackstedt & Kalivas, 2009). GLU release in the NAc core of rats is necessary for heroin seeking, which can be blocked by inhibition of AMPA receptors (LaLumiere & Kalivas, 2008). As previously discussed in the cocaine section, generation of silent synapses are thought to be key to storing cocaine experience, and unsilencing these synapses is key for reinstatement of drug seeking behavior. Cocaine forms silent synapses on D1R-MSNs by increasing NMDARs containing the GLUN2B subunit whereas morphine preferentially forms silent synapses on D2R-MSNs by insertion of AMPARs. Unsilencing of synapses for cocaine involves strengthening of D1R by insertion of AMPARs, whereas morphine involves removal of AMPARs on D2R-MSNS. Although the mechanism for unsilencing synapses differs between morphine and cocaine, both drugs lead to an increase in D1R/D2R-MSN synapses (Hearing, Graziane, Dong, & Thomas, 2018). Heroin also impacts astrocytic function (Reynolds, Mahajan, Sykes, & Nair, 2006), thereby mediating heroin's effects on GLU levels, as astrocytes are important for mediating for the glutamate-glutamine cycle. Heroin induces dynamic changes in expression of the GLU transporter GLT-1 in NAc astrocytes, and the role of plasticity in specific astrocytic populations in mediating heroin-seeking behavior is an ongoing area of research (Kruyer & Kalivas, 2021). Molecules involved in GLU function may yield possible therapeutic targets for treatment of heroin-induced relapse.

5.4 Pharmacotherapies for opioid abuse

Three types of FDA approved treatments are available for OUD: buprenorphine, a partial MOR agonist and KOR antagonist; naltrexone, an opioid receptor antagonist; and methadone, an MOR agonist (Helm, Trescot, Colson, Sehgal, & Silverman, 2008). Despite this, financial and regulation barriers remain and have prevented universal accessibility to these treatments (Meyer, 2020; Sharma et al., 2017). Furthermore, because buprenorphine and methadone act as agonists there is the potential for development of withdrawal symptoms, therefore these drugs are often prescribed below the minimal dosage required to be effective (Volkow, Jones, Einstein, & Wargo, 2019). While these drugs focus on treatment of OUD, another MOR high affinity antagonist, naloxone, is the primary treatment for opioid overdose (Chou et al., 2017; Wang, Frankfurt, & Burns, 2008). There is indeed evidence of the benefits of naloxone in the reversal of opioid overdose, however, similar to that of treatments for OUD, the barriers are in place regarding naloxone access which need to be addressed (Behar, Bagnulo, & Coffin, 2018; Smart, Pardo, & Davis, 2021).

6. Alcohol

6.1 Alcohol-mediated effects on neurotransmission

According to the National Institute on Alcohol Abuse and Alcoholism (NIAAA) there were 14.1 million adults and 414,000 adolescents who had an alcohol use disorder (AUD) in 2019 (NIAAA, 2021). Alcohol differs from the previously discussed drugs of abuse in that to date, there is no consensus that alcohol (ethanol) has a specific molecular target for which it binds and mediates dysregulation of neurotransmission. Evidence that supports potential direct molecular targets of ethanol is detailed in review, with possible direct targets including alcohol dehydrogenase (ADH), nicotinic acetylcholine receptors (nAChR), glycine receptors (GlyR), GABA receptors, NMDARs, Ca^{2+}-activated K^{+} (BK channels), G-protein-coupled inwardly rectifying K^{+} channels (GIRK,), and indirect targets primarily consisting of downstream signaling factors, genetic regulators, and σ1Rs (Abrahao, Salinas, & Lovinger, 2017; Quadir, Cottone, & Sabino, 2019).

Glutamate transmission is differentially affected across the CNS in response to acute and chronic alcohol use. Molecular targets in the glutamatergic system, including ionotropic and metabotropic receptors, may present potential therapeutic targets for treatment of AUD (Burnett, Chandler, & Trantham-Davidson, 2016; Joffe, Centanni, Jaramillo, Winder, & Conn, 2018; Johnson & Lovinger, 2020). Antagonism of the metabotropic GLU receptor, mGluR5, prevented alcohol induced relapse in rats (Adams, Short, & Lawrence, 2010). Recent advances using positron emission tomography (PET) imaging have identified a link between mGluR5 availability (specifically cortical and mesolimbic) and long-term relapse in patients who abuse alcohol (Ceccarini et al., 2020; Joo et al., 2021). Additionally, acute alcohol use inhibits the ionotropic GLU receptor NMDAR while chronic alcohol use upregulates NMDAR function. Changes in NMDAR function are important as downstream signaling pathways activated by NMDARs influence synaptic plasticity and alcohol related behaviors (Morisot & Ron, 2017). Lastly, dysregulation of glutamatergic transmission is a key area of interest regarding co-abuse of cocaine and alcohol. Alcohol and cocaine individually increase GLU levels in the NAc through downregulating expression of the GLU transporter, GLT-1 (Fischer, Houston, & Rebec, 2013; Gass & Olive, 2008; Sari & Sreemantula, 2012), however, the effects of cocaine and alcohol effects on GLT-1 expression are nonadditive (Hammad, Althobaiti, Das, & Sari, 2017; Stennett, Padovan-Hernandez, & Knackstedt, 2020). Understanding the role of glutamatergic molecules in mediating alcohol and alcohol/cocaine abuse is of interest for future investigation.

An important polysubstance abuse cohort to consider is those who abuse alcohol and nicotine. People who smoke are 10 times more likely to abuse alcohol, and conversely an estimated 70–80% of alcoholics smoke (Cross, Lotfipour, & Leslie, 2017). Indeed, alcohol and nicotine share molecular mechanisms for acquiring self-administration (Li, Volkow, Baler, & Egli, 2007) and the mechanisms for nicotine specifically are discussed in the next section. Alcohol exploits the dopaminergic reward system by increasing DA in the NAc to drive alcohol seeking behavior, however, polymorphisms of DA molecular targets are not highly associated with AUD (Bhaskar & Kumar, 2014; Ma & Zhu, 2014). Instead, alcohol effects on dopaminergic reward pathways are mediated by interactions with nicotinic receptors (nAChRs) (Miller & Kamens, 2020). Activation of nAChRs activates DA release by increasing firing of dopaminergic neurons in the VTA, which is regulated by different nAChR subunit compositions (Mameli-Engvall et al., 2006). How nAChRs modulate alcohol and nicotine induced behaviors, respectively, is detailed in review (Miller & Kamens, 2020; Wittenberg, Wolfman, De Biasi, & Dani, 2020). Future work should consider nAChRs as a highly probably mediator underlying polysubstance abuse of alcohol and nicotine and as a potential therapeutic target for alleviating co-morbid abuse of alcohol and nicotine.

6.2 Pharmacotherapies for alcohol use disorder

Current FDA-approved medications for treating AUD include naltrexone (general opioid receptor antagonist), disulfiram (acetaldehyde dehydrogenase inhibitor), and acamprosate (NMDA receptor antagonist, positive allosteric $GABA_A$ modulator) (Castrén, Mäkelä, & Alho, 2019). Naltrexone is significantly effective in reducing alcohol relapse to heavy drinking, however, the degree of its effectiveness is minimal (Kranzler & Soyka, 2018; Palpacuer et al., 2018). A current approach for treatment of AUD is the development of selective KOR antagonists (Banks, 2020). Activation of KOR by the endogenous opioid peptide dynorphin (Dyn) inhibits dopaminergic firing. Acute and chronic alcohol use increases Dyn released from the D1R NAc MSNs, leading to upregulation of KOR function. How KOR function mediates alcohol-induced behavior varies based on the model used (Karkhanis & Al-Hasani, 2020; Karkhanis, Holleran, & Jones, 2017). Further research is needed to understand how KOR mediates alcohol induced behaviors for the development of KOR based therapeutic treatment of AUD.

7. Nicotine

7.1 Nicotine targets of neurotransmission

Nicotine, through activation of neuronal nicotinic acetylcholine receptors (nAChRs) in the brain (Dani, Jenson, Broussard, & De Biasi, 2011), triggers the release of several neurotransmitters including DA, acetylcholine (ACh), Glu, 5-HT, and epinephrine (Schmidt, Rupprecht, & Addy, 2019). Repeated nicotine exposure in smokers causes a number of neuroadaptations, including persistent desensitization of the predominant $\alpha4\beta2$ nAChRs (Bertrand & Terry, 2018; Feduccia, Chatterjee, & Bartlett, 2012; Zoli, Pucci, Vilella, & Gotti, 2018), strengthening glutamatergic synapses onto dopaminergic neurons (Mao, Gallagher, & McGehee, 2011; Saal, Dong, Bonci, & Malenka, 2003), altering midbrain GABAergic circuitry (Grilli et al., 2012) and upregulating D2 DA receptors in the NAc (Novak, Seeman, & Le Foll, 2010). These neuroadaptations have a great impact on diverse neurotransmissions in the mesocorticolimbic pathway, which contribute to the pathophysiology of smoking behavior and nicotine addiction. Similar to all drugs of abuse, nicotine activates $\beta2$-containing nAChRs expressed on dopaminergic neurons (Mameli-Engvall et al., 2006) and possible $\alpha7$ nAChRs expressed on glutamatergic afferents (Mansvelder & McGehee, 2000) in the VTA and subsequently results in DA release in the NAc (Di Chiara, 2000; Laviolette & van der Kooy, 2004). Dopaminergic transmission has been strongly implicated in the reinforcing and withdrawal effects of nicotine, evidenced by (1) alteration of DA transmission within the mesolimbic reward system by systemic administration of nicotine and during nicotine withdrawal (Di Chiara, 2000; Natividad, Tejeda, Torres, & O'Dell, 2010) and (2) reducing the reinforcing effects of nicotine by blocking DA receptors (Diaz et al., 2000; Liu et al., 2010). Furthermore, bupropion and varenicline that are clinically used for treatment of nicotine dependence are associated with targeting dopaminergic neurotransmission (Ericson, Löf, Stomberg, & Söderpalm, 2009; Paterson, 2009; Prochaska & Benowitz, 2016). Considering that glutamatergic transmission plays a crucial rule in the reinforcing effects of nicotine, there is growing interest in glutamate-based therapeutic strategies (Liechti & Markou, 2008). The underlying mechanism is that following administration of nicotine, activation of GLU receptors on dopaminergic neurons in the VTA by released GLU increases firing of VTA dopaminergic neurons, leading to DA release in the NAc and nicotine reward (Grillner & Svensson, 2000). Several animal studies show that nicotine-induced DA release can be reduced by administering GLU receptor antagonists (Fu, Matta, Gao, Brower, & Sharp, 2000) and GLU receptors are decreased during nicotine withdrawal (Dravolina et al., 2007; Mansvelder & McGehee, 2000). These findings suggest that therapeutic targeting glutamatergic transmission could be beneficial to smoking-cessation.

The activity of the VTA dopaminergic transmission is regulated by local GABA-releasing neurons and GLU-releasing neurons (Morales & Margolis, 2017). GABAergic transmission displays an inhibitory effect on the activation of mesolimbic dopaminergic neurons, which reduces nicotine reward and reinforcement. Acute nicotine exposure increases GABA release from the VTA GABAergic neurons, whereas chronic nicotine exposure decreases the nicotine-induced GABA release by desensitizing β2-containing nAChRs, leading to reduced inhibition of VTA dopaminergic neurons and enhanced DA release in the NAc (Mansvelder, Keath, & McGehee, 2002). The effect of GABAergic activity on nicotine reward and reinforcement is evidenced by systemic administration of $GABA_B$ receptor agonists (Fattore et al., 2009; Franklin et al., 2009; Vlachou et al., 2011). Given that DA is a precursor of NE, the stress-induced nicotine-seeking during withdrawal is mediated by NE transmission (Mantsch, Baker, Funk, Lê, & Shaham, 2016), evidenced by the stress-induced reinstatement of nicotine seeking which can be attenuated by activation of α2 adrenergic receptors (Zislis, Desai, Prado, Shah, & Bruijnzeel, 2007). In addition, recent studies show that 5-HT receptors are involved in nicotine seeking (Fletcher et al., 2012; Schmidt et al., 2019). In addition to these traditional neurotransmitters, emerging evidence shows that many neuropeptide systems such as KOR

(Shippenberg, Zapata, & Chefer, 2007), hypocretin and corticotropin-releasing factor are related to stress-induced nicotine reinforcement and reinstatement (Bruijnzeel, 2017). These findings may provide novel preventive strategies for smoking cessation.

8. Drugs of abuse and HIV-1

HIV-1-associated neurocognitive disorders (HAND) are highly prevalent in the era of efficacious combination antiretroviral therapies (cART), with a greater number of HIV-infected persons living longer (Heaton et al., 2010, 2011). Drugs of abuse, such as METH and cocaine have been shown to increase the incidence of HAND, exacerbate its severity, and enhance viral replication (Nath, Maragos, Avison, Schmitt, & Berger, 2001; Soontornniyomkij et al., 2016). Perturbation of dopaminergic neurotransmission has been demonstrated as a mediating factor in HAND in concurrent drug abusers (Berger & Arendt, 2000; Gaskill et al., 2009; Gaskill, Miller, Gamble-George, Yano, & Khoshbouei, 2017; Purohit, Rapaka, & Shurtleff, 2011). HIV-1 viral proteins are associated with the persistence of HIV-related neuropathology and subsequent neurocognitive impairments observed in HAND (Brack-Werner, 1999; Frankel & Young, 1998; Gaskill et al., 2009; Johnston et al., 2001; Power et al., 1998). Persistent viral replication and expression of HIV-1 viral proteins within the CNS can accelerate damage in the mesocorticolimbic DA system (Berger & Arendt, 2000; Koutsilieri, Sopper, Scheller, ter Meulen, & Riederer, 2002; Nath, Jankovic, & Pettigrew, 1987) and to the brain pathways controlling motivation (Berridge, 2007; Everitt & Robbins, 2005; Wise & Bozarth, 1987). Therapy-naïve HIV patients display increased levels of DA and decreased DA turnover in the early stages of HIV infection (Scheller et al., 2010) which may initiate compensatory mechanisms eventually resulting in decreased DA levels (Kumar et al., 2009; Kumar, Ownby, Waldrop-Valverde, Fernandez, & Kumar, 2011; Sardar, Czudek, & Reynolds, 1996) and dopaminergic neuron damage (Chang et al., 2008; Wang et al., 2004) in the advanced stages of HIV infection. Importantly, the HIV-induced elevated DA level in CNS of HIV-infected patients can stimulate viral replication in human macrophages within DA-rich brain regions (Gaskill, Calderon, Coley, & Berman, 2013; Gaskill et al., 2009; Gaskill, Yano, Kalpana, Javitch, & Berman, 2014), which has been implicated in the pathophysiology of HAND (Li, Li, Steiner, & Nath, 2009).

Among the HIV viral proteins, the transactivator of transcription (Tat) protein plays a crucial role in viral replication in the early stage of HIV infection and the pathophysiological effects on development of HAND (King, Eugenin, Buckner, & Berman, 2006; Rappaport et al., 1999), as Tat protein has been detected in dopaminergic-rich brain areas (Del Valle et al., 2000; Hudson et al., 2000; Lamers et al., 2010) and in the sera (Westendorp et al., 1995; Xiao et al., 2000) of HIV-1 infected patients (Johnson et al., 2013). Our published work has demonstrated that Tat protein induces dysregulation of dopaminergic neurotransmission by inhibiting DA transport through DAT in cells expressing human DAT (Midde et al., 2013, 2015; Quizon et al., 2016), multiple HIV-1 viral protein transgenic rat model (Zhu et al., 2016), and HIV-1 Tat transgenic mouse model (Strauss et al., 2020). Notably, studying single Tat protein would allow us to identify protein targets for Tat binding and develop therapeutic approaches to prevent Tat-mediated neurological damages. Moreover, studying single Tat protein will provide insight into fully understanding the consequence of combined neurological effects of the viral proteins on the CNS. Recent studies show that other viral proteins, such as gp120 and Nef, can also influence DAT activity (Acharjee et al., 2014; Hu, Sheng, & Rock, 2013). On the other hand, clinical observations have demonstrated that DAT activity is dramatically reduced in HIV-infected patients, which is exacerbated in cocaine abusers (Chang et al., 2008; Wang et al., 2004). Interplay of Tat and cocaine augments synaptic DA release by inhibiting DAT activity (Ferris, Frederick-Duus, Fadel, Mactutus, & Booze, 2009; Zhu, Mactutus, Wallace, & Booze, 2009), which may be consistent with animal study that the transgenic expression of Tat in the mouse brain potentiates cocaine reward (Paris et al., 2014). The underlying mechanism of the Tat-induced inhibition of DAT-mediated DA reuptake is through Tat binding to allosteric binding site(s) on DAT, not by interacting with the DA uptake site (Yuan et al., 2015; Zhu et al., 2009; Zhu, Ananthan, Mactutus, & Booze, 2011). Furthermore, given that DAT-mediated DA transport process is dynamically regulated by three typical conformational states: Outward-open → Outward-occluded → Inward-open, cocaine and Tat protein prefer the outward-open state that causes inhibition of DA uptake (Yuan, Huang, Zhu, & Zhan, 2016). This mechanism has been validated by a novel DAT allosteric modulator which attenuates Tat-induced inhibition of DAT-mediated DA transport (Sun et al., 2017). Thus, developing allosteric modulators that decrease the affinity and maximal binding potential of Tat could be a viable approach for reversing Tat-induced dysregulation of the DA system.

9. Considerations regarding COVID-19

The topic of long-term COVID-19 effects on neuropsychiatric symptoms is an emerging field of great interest. While there is evidence of depression and neuroinflammation due to COVID-19, it has been reported that there is potential interplay between severe acute respiratory syndrome coronavirus 2 (SARS-CoV-2) infection and neurotransmission, such as dopaminergic and serotoninergic systems (Attademo & Bernardini, 2021; Boldrini, Canoll, & Klein, 2021). This is due to the discovery that angiotensin 1 converting enzyme 2 (ACE2), a host receptor for SARS-CoV-2, is co-expressed with dopa decarboxylase (DDC), a major enzyme in the DA and 5-HT synthesis pathways (Nataf, 2020). Furthermore, a new study reports that dopaminergic neurons derived from human pluripotent stem cells are susceptible to SARS-CoV-2 infection (Chen et al., 2021). Dysregulation of dopaminergic and serotonergic systems is critical for the development of substance abuse disorders. As described in the previous section, HIV-1 induces neuropathological changes in dopaminergic signaling which increases susceptibility to development of substance abuse disorders. Based on emerging evidence and our published work from comorbidity of HIV-1 and substance abuse, we hypothesize that COVID-19 infection may induce neuropathological changes which impact neurotransmission, such as dysregulation of dopaminergic and serotonergic systems, which may greatly impact susceptibility to development of substance abuse disorders as well as neurocognitive impairments. We anticipate that the long-term impact of COVID-19 on neurotransmission will be an important area of interest requiring further research.

10. Conclusion

In this chapter, we discuss recent advances made in understanding how commonly abused substances, including cocaine, amphetamines, opioids, alcohol, and nicotine, impact neurotransmission on a molecular level. Every abused substance covered in this chapter impacts more than one neurotransmitter system, and each system plays a role in mediating certain elements of drug induced behaviors. For instance, GLU signaling generally underlies reinstatement of drug seeking, whereas dopaminergic signaling is key for acute self-administration. Abused substances induce dysregulation of neurotransmission in key neurocircuitry pathways, which act together in concert to invoke a range of drug taking behaviors. Future work is needed to understand the impact of co-abused substances on neurotransmission. Molecular factors which mediate dysregulation of neurotransmission for more than one substance of abuse should be investigated as possible therapeutic targets for polysubstance abuse cohorts (e.g., nAChRs for alcohol/ nicotine users). Translational research which integrates basic sciences and clinical observations on the neurobiological processes induced by these substances will aid in the development of effective therapeutic strategies for treatment of substance abuse disorders.

Acknowledgments

This work was supported by National Institutes of Health National Institute on Drug Abuse (R01DA035714 and R01DA047924). The authors acknowledge Dr. Ana Jimenez Torres and Katherine Porter for their help in editing the chapter.

Conflict of interest

The authors have no conflicts of interest to declare.

References

Abrahao, K. P., Salinas, A. G., & Lovinger, D. M. (2017). Alcohol and the brain: Neuronal molecular targets, synapses, and circuits. *Neuron, 96*(6), 1223–1238. https://doi.org/https://doi.org/10.1016/j.neuron.2017.10.032.

Acharjee, S., Branton, W. G., Vivithanaporn, P., Maingat, F., Paul, A. M., Dickie, P., et al. (2014). HIV-1 Nef expression in microglia disrupts dopaminergic and immune functions with associated mania-like behaviors. *Brain, Behavior, and Immunity, 40*, 74–84. https://doi.org/https://doi.org/10.1016/j.bbi.2014.02.016.

Adams, C. L., Short, J. L., & Lawrence, A. J. (2010). Cue-conditioned alcohol seeking in rats following abstinence: Involvement of metabotropic glutamate 5 receptors. *British Journal of Pharmacology, 159*(3), 534–542. https://doi.org/https://doi.org/10.1111/j.1476-5381.2009.00562.x.

Ahmad, F. B., Rossen, L. M., & Sutton, P. (2021). *Provisional drug overdose death counts*. Retrieved June 13, 2021, from https://www.cdc.gov/nchs/nvss/vsrr/drug-overdose-data.htm.

Alvers, K. M., Beckmann, J. S., Zheng, G., Crooks, P. A., Dwoskin, L. P., & Bardo, M. T. (2012). The effect of VMAT2 inhibitor GZ-793A on the reinstatement of methamphetamine-seeking in rats. *Psychopharmacology, 224*(2), 255–262. https://doi.org/https://doi.org/10.1007/s00213-012-2748-3.

Atcheson, R., Rowbotham, D. J., & Lambert, D. G. (1993). Fentanyl inhibits the uptake of [3H]noradrenaline in cultured neuronal cells. *British Journal of Anaesthesia, 71*(4), 540–543. https://doi.org/https://doi.org/10.1093/bja/71.4.540.

Attademo, L., & Bernardini, F. (2021). Are dopamine and serotonin involved in COVID-19 pathophysiology? *The European Journal of Psychiatry, 35*(1), 62–63. https://doi.org/https://doi.org/10.1016/j.ejpsy.2020.10.004.

Baldo, B. A., & Rose, M. A. (2020). The anaesthetist, opioid analgesic drugs, and serotonin toxicity: A mechanistic and clinical review. *British Journal of Anaesthesia, 124*(1), 44–62. https://doi.org/https://doi.org/10.1016/j.bja.2019.08.010.

Banks, M. L. (2020). The rise and fall of kappa-opioid receptors in drug abuse research. *Handbook of Experimental Pharmacology*, *258*, 147–165. https://doi.org/https://doi.org/10.1007/164_2019_268.

Baumann, M. H., Kopajtic, T. A., & Madras, B. K. (2018). Pharmacological research as a key component in mitigating the opioid overdose crisis. *Trends in Pharmacological Sciences*, *39*(12), 995–998. https://doi.org/https://doi.org/10.1016/j.tips.2018.09.006.

Beckmann, J. S., Denehy, E. D., Zheng, G., Crooks, P. A., Dwoskin, L. P., & Bardo, M. T. (2012). The effect of a novel VMAT2 inhibitor, GZ-793A, on methamphetamine reward in rats. *Psychopharmacology*, *220*(2), 395–403. https://doi.org/https://doi.org/10.1007/s00213-011-2488-9.

Beggiato, S., Borelli, A. C., Borroto-Escuela, D., Corbucci, I., Tomasini, M. C., Marti, M., et al. (2017). Cocaine modulates allosteric D2-σ1 receptor-receptor interactions on dopamine and glutamate nerve terminals from rat striatum. *Cellular Signalling*, *40*, 116–124. https://doi.org/https://doi.org/10.1016/j.cellsig.2017.09.007.

Behar, E., Bagnulo, R., & Coffin, P. O. (2018). Acceptability and feasibility of naloxone prescribing in primary care settings: A systematic review. *Preventive Medicine*, *114*, 79–87. https://doi.org/https://doi.org/10.1016/j.ypmed.2018.06.005.

Belovich, A. N., Aguilar, J. I., Mabry, S. J., Cheng, M. H., Zanella, D., Hamilton, P. J., et al. (2021). A network of phosphatidylinositol (4,5)-bisphosphate (PIP2) binding sites on the dopamine transporter regulates amphetamine behavior in drosophila melanogaster. *Molecular Psychiatry*, *26*(8), 4417–4430. https://doi.org/10.1038/s41380-019-0620-0. Epub December 3, 2019.

Berger, J. R., & Arendt, G. (2000). HIV dementia: The role of the basal ganglia and dopaminergic systems. *Journal of Psychopharmacology*, *14*(3), 214–221. https://doi.org/https://doi.org/10.1177/026988110001400304.

Berridge, K. C. (2007). The debate over dopamine's role in reward: The case for incentive salience. *Psychopharmacology*, *191*(3), 391–431. https://doi.org/https://doi.org/10.1007/s00213-006-0578-x.

Bertrand, D., & Terry, A. V. (2018). The wonderland of neuronal nicotinic acetylcholine receptors. *Biochemical Pharmacology*, *151*, 214–225. https://doi.org/https://doi.org/10.1016/j.bcp.2017.12.008.

Bhaskar, L. V. K. S., & Kumar, S. A. (2014). Polymorphisms in genes encoding dopamine signalling pathway and risk of alcohol dependence: A systematic review. *Acta Neuropsychiatrica*, *26*(2), 69–80. https://doi.org/https://doi.org/10.1017/neu.2013.27.

Binda, F., Dipace, C., Bowton, E., Robertson, S. D., Lute, B. J., Fog, J. U., et al. (2008). Syntaxin 1A interaction with the dopamine transporter promotes amphetamine-induced dopamine efflux. *Molecular Pharmacology*, *74*(4), 1101–1108. https://doi.org/https://doi.org/10.1124/mol.108.048447.

Blakely, R. D., De Felice, L. J., & Hartzell, H. C. (1994). Molecular physiology of norepinephrine and serotonin transporters. *Journal of Experimental Biology*, *196*, 263–281. https://doi.org/https://doi.org/10.1242/jeb.196.1.263.

Boldrini, M., Canoll, P. D., & Klein, R. S. (2021). How COVID-19 affects the brain. *JAMA Psychiatry*, *78*(6), 682–683. https://doi.org/https://doi.org/10.1001/jamapsychiatry.2021.0500.

Brack-Werner, R. (1999). Astrocytes: HIV cellular reservoirs and important participants in neuropathogenesis. *AIDS*, *13*(1), 1–22. https://doi.org/https://doi.org/10.1097/00002030-199901140-00003.

Branch, S. Y., & Beckstead, M. J. (2012). Methamphetamine produces bidirectional, concentration-dependent effects on dopamine neuron excitability and dopamine-mediated synaptic currents. *Journal of Neurophysiology*, *108*(3), 802–809. https://doi.org/https://doi.org/10.1152/jn.00094.2012.

Bruijnzeel, A. W. (2017). Neuropeptide systems and new treatments for nicotine addiction. *Psychopharmacology, 234*(9–10), 1419–1437. https://doi.org/https://doi.org/10.1007/s00213-016-4513-5.

Burnett, E. J., Chandler, L. J., & Trantham-Davidson, H. (2016). Glutamatergic plasticity and alcohol dependence-induced alterations in reward, affect and cognition. *Progress in Neuro-Psychopharmacology & Biological Psychiatry, 65*, 309–320. https://doi.org/https://doi.org/10.1016/j.pnpbp.2015.08.012.

Butelman, E. R., Yuferov, V., & Kreek, M. J. (2012). κ-Opioid receptor/dynorphin system: Genetic and pharmacotherapeutic implications for addiction. *Trends in Neurosciences, 35*(10), 587–596. https://doi.org/https://doi.org/10.1016/j.tins.2012.05.005.

Cao, J., LaRocque, E., & Li, D. (2013). Associations of the 5-hydroxytryptamine (serotonin) receptor 1B gene (HTR1B) with alcohol, cocaine, and heroin abuse. *American Journal of Medical Genetics. Part B, Neuropsychiatric Genetics, 162B*(2), 169–176. https://doi.org/https://doi.org/10.1002/ajmg.b.32128.

Carboni, E., Spielewoy, C., Vacca, C., Nosten-Bertrand, M., Giros, B., & Di Chiara, G. (2001). Cocaine and amphetamine increase extracellular dopamine in the nucleus accumbens of mice lacking the dopamine transporter gene. *The Journal of Neuroscience, 21*(9). RC141: 1–4. https://doi.org/https://doi.org/10.1523/JNEUROSCI.21-09-j0001.2001.

Castrén, S., Mäkelä, N., & Alho, H. (2019). Selecting an appropriate alcohol pharmacotherapy: Review of recent findings. *Current Opinion in Psychiatry, 32*(4), 266–274. https://doi.org/https://doi.org/10.1097/YCO.0000000000000512.

Ceccarini, J., Leurquin-Sterk, G., Crunelle, C. L., de Laat, B., Bormans, G., Peuskens, H., et al. (2020). Recovery of decreased metabotropic glutamate receptor 5 availability in abstinent alcohol-dependent patients. *Journal of Nuclear Medicine, 61*(2), 256–262. https://doi.org/https://doi.org/10.2967/jnumed.119.228825.

Chang, L., Wang, G.-J., Volkow, N. D., Ernst, T., Telang, F., Logan, J., et al. (2008). Decreased brain dopamine transporters are related to cognitive deficits in HIV patients with or without cocaine abuse. *NeuroImage, 42*(2), 869–878. https://doi.org/https://doi.org/10.1016/j.neuroimage.2008.05.011.

Charbogne, P., Gardon, O., Martín-García, E., Keyworth, H. L., Matsui, A., Mechling, A. E., et al. (2017). Mu opioid receptors in gamma-aminobutyric Acidergic forebrain neurons moderate motivation for heroin and palatable food. *Biological Psychiatry, 81*(9), 778–788. https://doi.org/https://doi.org/10.1016/j.biopsych.2016.12.022.

Chen, S., Han, Y., Yang, L., Kim, T., Nair, M., Harschnitz, O., et al. (2021). SARS-CoV-2 infection causes dopaminergic neuron senescence. *Research Square*. https://doi.org/10.21203/rs.3.rs-513461/v1.

Chomchai, C., & Chomchai, S. (2015). Global patterns of methamphetamine use. *Current Opinion in Psychiatry, 28*(4), 269–274. https://doi.org/https://doi.org/10.1097/YCO.0000000000000168.

Chou, N.-H., Huang, Y.-J., & Jiann, B.-P. (2015). The impact of illicit use of amphetamine on male sexual functions. *The Journal of Sexual Medicine, 12*(8), 1694–1702. https://doi.org/https://doi.org/10.1111/jsm.12926.

Chou, R., Korthuis, P. T., McCarty, D., Coffin, P. O., Griffin, J. C., Davis-O'Reilly, C., et al. (2017). Management of Suspected Opioid Overdose with Naloxone in out-of--hospital settings: A systematic review. *Annals of Internal Medicine, 167*(12), 867–875. https://doi.org/https://doi.org/10.7326/M17-2224.

Comer, S. D., & Cahill, C. M. (2019). Fentanyl: Receptor pharmacology, abuse potential, and implications for treatment. *Neuroscience and Biobehavioral Reviews, 106*, 49–57. https://doi.org/https://doi.org/10.1016/j.neubiorev.2018.12.005.

Comer, S. D., Pravetoni, M., Coop, A., Baumann, M. H., & Cunningham, C. W. (2021). Potential unintended consequences of class-wide drug scheduling based on chemical structure: A cautionary tale for fentanyl-related compounds. *Drug and Alcohol Dependence, 221*, 108530. https://doi.org/https://doi.org/10.1016/j.drugalcdep.2021.108530.

Corre, J., van Zessen, R., Loureiro, M., Patriarchi, T., Tian, L., Pascoli, V., et al. (2018). Dopamine neurons projecting to medial shell of the nucleus accumbens drive heroin reinforcement. *eLife*, 7, e39945. https://doi.org/10.7554/eLife.39945.

Cosgrove, K. P., Tellez-Jacques, K., Pittman, B., Petrakis, I., Baldwin, R. M., Tamagnan, G., et al. (2010). Dopamine and serotonin transporter availability in chronic heroin users: A [^{123}I]β-CIT SPECT imaging study. *Psychiatry Research*, *184*(3), 192–195. https://doi.org/https://doi.org/10.1016/j.pscychresns.2010.08.001.

Cross, S. J., Lotfipour, S., & Leslie, F. M. (2017). Mechanisms and genetic factors underlying co-use of nicotine and alcohol or other drugs of abuse. *The American Journal of Drug and Alcohol Abuse*, *43*(2), 171–185. https://doi.org/https://doi.org/10.1080/00952990.2016.1209512.

Czeisler, M.É., Drane, A., Winnay, S. S., Capodilupo, E. R., Czeisler, C. A., Rajaratnam, S. M., et al. (2021). Mental health, substance use, and suicidal ideation among unpaid caregivers in the United States during the COVID-19 pandemic: Relationships to age, race/ethnicity, employment, and caregiver intensity. *SSRN Electronic Journal*, *295*, 1259–1268. https://doi.org/10.1016/j.jad.2021.08.130.

Dani, J. A., Jenson, D., Broussard, J. I., & De Biasi, M. (2011). Neurophysiology of nicotine addiction. *Journal of Addiction Research & Therapy*, *S1*(1). https://doi.org/10.4172/2155-6105.S1-001.

Davis, M. P., & Behm, B. (2020). Reasons to avoid fentanyl. *Annals of Palliative Medicine*, *9*(2), 611–624. https://doi.org/10.21037/apm.2020.01.12.

Del Valle, L., Croul, S., Morgello, S., Amini, S., Rappaport, J., & Khalili, K. (2000). Detection of HIV-1 tat and JCV capsid protein, VP1, in AIDS brain with progressive multifocal leukoencephalopathy. *Journal of Neurovirology*, *6*(3), 221–228.

Di Chiara, G. (2000). Role of dopamine in the behavioural actions of nicotine related to addiction. *European Journal of Pharmacology*, *393*(1–3), 295–314. https://doi.org/https://doi.org/10.1016/s0014-2999(00)00122-9.

Diaz, J., Pilon, C., Le Foll, B., Gros, C., Triller, A., Schwartz, J. C., et al. (2000). Dopamine D3 receptors expressed by all mesencephalic dopamine neurons. *The Journal of Neuroscience*, *20*(23), 8677–8684.

Dong, Y., Taylor, J. R., Wolf, M. E., & Shaham, Y. (2017). Circuit and synaptic plasticity mechanisms of drug relapse. *The Journal of Neuroscience*, *37*(45), 10867–10876. https://doi.org/https://doi.org/10.1523/JNEUROSCI.1821-17.2017.

Dravolina, O. A., Zakharova, E. S., Shekunova, E. V., Zvartau, E. E., Danysz, W., & Bespalov, A. Y. (2007). mGlu1 receptor blockade attenuates cue- and nicotine-induced reinstatement of extinguished nicotine self-administration behavior in rats. *Neuropharmacology*, *52*(2), 263–269. https://doi.org/https://doi.org/10.1016/j.neuropharm.2006.07.023.

Ericson, M., Löf, E., Stomberg, R., & Söderpalm, B. (2009). The smoking cessation medication varenicline attenuates alcohol and nicotine interactions in the rat mesolimbic dopamine system. *The Journal of Pharmacology and Experimental Therapeutics*, *329*(1), 225–230. https://doi.org/https://doi.org/10.1124/jpet.108.147058.

Everitt, B. J., & Robbins, T. W. (2005). Neural systems of reinforcement for drug addiction: From actions to habits to compulsion. *Nature Neuroscience*, *8*(11), 1481–1489. https://doi.org/https://doi.org/10.1038/nn1579.

Fagan, R. R., Kearney, P. J., & Melikian, H. E. (2020). In situ regulated dopamine transporter trafficking: there's no place like home. *Neurochemical Research*, *45*(6), 1335–1343. https://doi.org/https://doi.org/10.1007/s11064-020-03001-6.

Fairbairn, N., Coffin, P. O., & Walley, A. Y. (2017). Naloxone for heroin, prescription opioid, and illicitly made fentanyl overdoses: Challenges and innovations responding to a dynamic epidemic. *The International Journal on Drug Policy*, *46*, 172–179. https://doi.org/https://doi.org/10.1016/j.drugpo.2017.06.005.

Fattore, L., Spano, M. S., Cossu, G., Scherma, M., Fratta, W., & Fadda, P. (2009). Baclofen prevents drug-induced reinstatement of extinguished nicotine-seeking behaviour and nicotine place preference in rodents. *European Neuropsychopharmacology*, *19*(7), 487–498. https://doi.org/https://doi.org/10.1016/j.euroneuro.2009.01.007.

Faul, M., Lurie, P., Kinsman, J. M., Dailey, M. W., Crabaugh, C., & Sasser, S. M. (2017). Multiple naloxone administrations among emergency medical service providers is increasing. *Prehospital Emergency Care*, *21*(4), 411–419. https://doi.org/https://doi.org/10.1080/10903127.2017.1315203.

Feduccia, A. A., Chatterjee, S., & Bartlett, S. E. (2012). Neuronal nicotinic acetylcholine receptors: Neuroplastic changes underlying alcohol and nicotine addictions. *Frontiers in Molecular Neuroscience*, *5*, 83. https://doi.org/https://doi.org/10.3389/fnmol.2012.00083.

Felmer, A. C., Janson, M. T., Summers, K. E., & Wallace, L. J. (2019). Extracellular dopamine kinetic parameters consistent with amphetamine effects. *Synapse*, *73*(12), e22129. https://doi.org/https://doi.org/10.1002/syn.22129.

Feltenstein, M. W., See, R. E., & Fuchs, R. A. (2021). Neural substrates and circuits of drug addiction. *Cold Spring Harbor Perspectives in Medicine*, *11*(4). https://doi.org/https://doi.org/10.1101/cshperspect.a039628.

Ferris, M. J., Frederick-Duus, D., Fadel, J., Mactutus, C. F., & Booze, R. M. (2009). In vivo microdialysis in awake, freely moving rats demonstrates HIV-1 tat-induced alterations in dopamine transmission. *Synapse*, *63*(3), 181–185. https://doi.org/https://doi.org/10.1002/syn.20594.

Ferrucci, M., Giorgi, F. S., Bartalucci, A., Busceti, C. L., & Fornai, F. (2013). The effects of locus coeruleus and norepinephrine in methamphetamine toxicity. *Current Neuropharmacology*, *11*(1), 80–94. https://doi.org/https://doi.org/10.2174/157015913804999522.

Ferrucci, M., Limanaqi, F., Ryskalin, L., Biagioni, F., Busceti, C. L., & Fornai, F. (2019). The effects of amphetamine and methamphetamine on the release of norepinephrine, dopamine and acetylcholine from the brainstem reticular formation. *Frontiers in Neuroanatomy*, *13*, 48. https://doi.org/https://doi.org/10.3389/fnana.2019.00048.

Fischer, K. D., Houston, A. C. W., Desai, R. I., Doyle, M. R., Bergman, J., Mian, M., et al. (2018). Behavioral phenotyping and dopamine dynamics in mice with conditional deletion of the glutamate transporter GLT-1 in neurons: Resistance to the acute locomotor effects of amphetamine. *Psychopharmacology*, *235*(5), 1371–1387. https://doi.org/https://doi.org/10.1007/s00213-018-4848-1.

Fischer, K. D., Houston, A. C. W., & Rebec, G. V. (2013). Role of the major glutamate transporter GLT1 in nucleus accumbens core versus shell in cue-induced cocaine-seeking behavior. *The Journal of Neuroscience*, *33*(22), 9319–9327. https://doi.org/https://doi.org/10.1523/JNEUROSCI.3278-12.2013.

Fleckenstein, A. E., Metzger, R. R., Wilkins, D. G., Gibb, J. W., & Hanson, G. R. (1997). Rapid and reversible effects of methamphetamine on dopamine transporters. *The Journal of Pharmacology and Experimental Therapeutics*, *282*(2), 834–838.

Fletcher, P. J., Rizos, Z., Noble, K., Soko, A. D., Silenieks, L. B., Lê, A. D., et al. (2012). Effects of the 5-HT2C receptor agonist Ro60-0175 and the 5-HT2A receptor antagonist M100907 on nicotine self-administration and reinstatement. *Neuropharmacology*, *62*(7), 2288–2298. https://doi.org/https://doi.org/10.1016/j.neuropharm.2012.01.023.

Foster, J. D., Yang, J.-W., Moritz, A. E., Challasivakanaka, S., Smith, M. A., Holy, M., et al. (2012). Dopamine transporter phosphorylation site threonine 53 regulates substrate reuptake and amphetamine-stimulated efflux. *The Journal of Biological Chemistry*, *287*(35), 29702–29712. https://doi.org/https://doi.org/10.1074/jbc.M112.367706.

Frankel, A. D., & Young, J. A. (1998). HIV-1: Fifteen proteins and an RNA. *Annual Review of Biochemistry*, *67*, 1–25. https://doi.org/https://doi.org/10.1146/annurev.biochem.67.1.1.

Franklin, T. R., Harper, D., Kampman, K., Kildea-McCrea, S., Jens, W., Lynch, K. G., et al. (2009). The GABA B agonist baclofen reduces cigarette consumption in a preliminary double-blind placebo-controlled smoking reduction study. *Drug and Alcohol Dependence, 103*(1–2), 30–36. https://doi.org/https://doi.org/10.1016/j.drugalcdep.2009.02.014.

Fu, Y., Matta, S. G., Gao, W., Brower, V. G., & Sharp, B. M. (2000). Systemic nicotine stimulates dopamine release in nucleus accumbens: Re-evaluation of the role of N-methyl-D-aspartate receptors in the ventral tegmental area. *The Journal of Pharmacology and Experimental Therapeutics, 294*(2), 458–465.

Fu, M. J., Tsen, L. Y., Lee, T. Y., Lui, P. W., & Chan, S. H. (1997). Involvement of cerulospinal glutamatergic neurotransmission in fentanyl-induced muscular rigidity in the rat. *Anesthesiology, 87*(6), 1450–1459. https://doi.org/https://doi.org/10.1097/00000542-199712000-00024.

Fukushima, S., Shen, H., Hata, H., Ohara, A., Ohmi, K., Ikeda, K., et al. (2007). Methamphetamine-induced locomotor activity and sensitization in dopamine transporter and vesicular monoamine transporter 2 double mutant mice. *Psychopharmacology, 193*(1), 55–62. https://doi.org/https://doi.org/10.1007/s00213-007-0749-4.

Fumagalli, F., Gainetdinov, R. R., Wang, Y. M., Valenzano, K. J., Miller, G. W., & Caron, M. G. (1999). Increased methamphetamine neurotoxicity in heterozygous vesicular monoamine transporter 2 knock-out mice. *The Journal of Neuroscience, 19*(7), 2424–2431.

Galaj, E., Han, X., Shen, H., Jordan, C. J., He, Y., Humburg, B., et al. (2020). Dissecting the role of GABA neurons in the VTA versus SNr in opioid reward. *The Journal of Neuroscience, 40*(46), 8853–8869. https://doi.org/https://doi.org/10.1523/JNEUROSCI.0988-20.2020.

Garcia, E. J., Arndt, D. L., & Cain, M. E. (2019). Dynamic interactions of ceftriaxone and environmental variables suppress amphetamine seeking. *Brain Research, 1712*, 63–72. https://doi.org/https://doi.org/10.1016/j.brainres.2019.01.044.

Gaskill, P. J., Calderon, T. M., Coley, J. S., & Berman, J. W. (2013). Drug induced increases in CNS dopamine alter monocyte, macrophage and T cell functions: Implications for HAND. *Journal of Neuroimmune Pharmacology, 8*(3), 621–642. https://doi.org/https://doi.org/10.1007/s11481-013-9443-y.

Gaskill, P. J., Calderon, T. M., Luers, A. J., Eugenin, E. A., Javitch, J. A., & Berman, J. W. (2009). Human immunodeficiency virus (HIV) infection of human macrophages is increased by dopamine: A bridge between HIV-associated neurologic disorders and drug abuse. *The American Journal of Pathology, 175*(3), 1148–1159. https://doi.org/https://doi.org/10.2353/ajpath.2009.081067.

Gaskill, P. J., Miller, D. R., Gamble-George, J., Yano, H., & Khoshbouei, H. (2017). HIV, tat and dopamine transmission. *Neurobiology of Disease, 105*, 51–73. https://doi.org/https://doi.org/10.1016/j.nbd.2017.04.015.

Gaskill, P. J., Yano, H. H., Kalpana, G. V., Javitch, J. A., & Berman, J. W. (2014). Dopamine receptor activation increases HIV entry into primary human macrophages. *PLoS One, 9*(9), e108232. https://doi.org/https://doi.org/10.1371/journal.pone.0108232.

Gaskin, D. J., & Richard, P. (2012). The economic costs of pain in the United States. *The Journal of Pain, 13*(8), 715–724. https://doi.org/https://doi.org/10.1016/j.jpain.2012.03.009.

Gass, J. T., & Olive, M. F. (2008). Glutamatergic substrates of drug addiction and alcoholism. *Biochemical Pharmacology, 75*(1), 218–265. https://doi.org/https://doi.org/10.1016/j.bcp.2007.06.039.

Giros, B., Jaber, M., Jones, S. R., Wightman, R. M., & Caron, M. G. (1996). Hyperlocomotion and indifference to cocaine and amphetamine in mice lacking the dopamine transporter. *Nature, 379*(6566), 606–612. https://doi.org/https://doi.org/10.1038/379606a0.

Goodwin, J. S., Larson, G. A., Swant, J., Sen, N., Javitch, J. A., Zahniser, N. R., et al. (2009). Amphetamine and methamphetamine differentially affect dopamine transporters in vitro and in vivo. *The Journal of Biological Chemistry*, *284*(5), 2978–2989. https://doi.org/https://doi.org/10.1074/jbc.M805298200.

Graziane, N. M., Sun, S., Wright, W. J., Jang, D., Liu, Z., Huang, Y. H., et al. (2016). Opposing mechanisms mediate morphine- and cocaine-induced generation of silent synapses. *Nature Neuroscience*, *19*(7), 915–925. https://doi.org/https://doi.org/10.1038/nn.4313.

Griffioen, K. J. S., Venkatesan, P., Huang, Z.-G., Wang, X., Bouairi, E., Evans, C., et al. (2004). Fentanyl inhibits GABAergic neurotransmission to cardiac vagal neurons in the nucleus ambiguus. *Brain Research*, *1007*(1–2), 109–115. https://doi.org/https://doi.org/10.1016/j.brainres.2004.02.010.

Grilli, M., Summa, M., Salamone, A., Olivero, G., Zappettini, S., Di Prisco, S., et al. (2012). In vitro exposure to nicotine induces endocytosis of presynaptic AMPA receptors modulating dopamine release in rat nucleus accumbens nerve terminals. *Neuropharmacology*, *63*(5), 916–926. https://doi.org/https://doi.org/10.1016/j.neuropharm.2012.06.049.

Grillner, P., & Svensson, T. H. (2000). Nicotine-induced excitation of midbrain dopamine neurons in vitro involves ionotropic glutamate receptor activation. *Synapse*, *38*(1), 1–9. https://doi.org/10.1002/1098-2396(200010)38:1 < 1::AID-SYN1 > 3.0.CO;2-A.

Guerin, A. A., Nestler, E. J., Berk, M., Lawrence, A. J., Rossell, S. L., & Kim, J. H. (2021). Genetics of methamphetamine use disorder: A systematic review and meta-analyses of gene association studies. *Neuroscience and Biobehavioral Reviews*, *120*, 48–74. https://doi.org/https://doi.org/10.1016/j.neubiorev.2020.11.001.

Hammad, A. M., Althobaiti, Y. S., Das, S. C., & Sari, Y. (2017). Effects of repeated cocaine exposure and withdrawal on voluntary ethanol drinking, and the expression of glial glutamate transporters in mesocorticolimbic system of P rats. *Molecular and Cellular Neurosciences*, *82*, 58–65. https://doi.org/https://doi.org/10.1016/j.mcn.2017.04.008.

Han, D. D., & Gu, H. H. (2006). Comparison of the monoamine transporters from human and mouse in their sensitivities to psychostimulant drugs. *BMC Pharmacology*, *6*, 6. https://doi.org/https://doi.org/10.1186/1471-2210-6-6.

Harraz, M. M., Guha, P., Kang, I. G., Semenza, E. R., Malla, A. P., Song, Y. J., et al. (2021). Cocaine-induced locomotor stimulation involves autophagic degradation of the dopamine transporter. *Molecular Psychiatry*, *26*(2), 370–382. https://doi.org/https://doi.org/10.1038/s41380-020-00978-y.

Hearing, M., Graziane, N., Dong, Y., & Thomas, M. J. (2018). Opioid and psychostimulant plasticity: Targeting overlap in nucleus accumbens glutamate signaling. *Trends in Pharmacological Sciences*, *39*(3), 276–294. https://doi.org/https://doi.org/10.1016/j.tips.2017.12.004.

Heaton, R. K., Clifford, D. B., Franklin, D. R., Woods, S. P., Ake, C., Vaida, F., et al. (2010). HIV-associated neurocognitive disorders persist in the era of potent antiretroviral therapy: CHARTER study. *Neurology*, *75*(23), 2087–2096. https://doi.org/https://doi.org/10.1212/WNL.0b013e318200d727.

Heaton, R. K., Franklin, D. R., Ellis, R. J., McCutchan, J. A., Letendre, S. L., Leblanc, S., et al. (2011). HIV-associated neurocognitive disorders before and during the era of combination antiretroviral therapy: Differences in rates, nature, and predictors. *Journal of Neurovirology*, *17*(1), 3–16. https://doi.org/https://doi.org/10.1007/s13365-010-0006-1.

Hedegaard, H., Miniño, A. M., & Warner, M. (2018). Drug overdose deaths in the United States, 1999-2017. *NCHS Data Brief*, *329*, 1–8.

Hedges, D. M., Obray, J. D., Yorgason, J. T., Jang, E. Y., Weerasekara, V. K., Uys, J. D., et al. (2018). Methamphetamine induces dopamine release in the nucleus Accumbens through a sigma receptor-mediated pathway. *Neuropsychopharmacology*, *43*(6), 1405–1414. https://doi.org/https://doi.org/10.1038/npp.2017.291.

Helm, S., Trescot, A. M., Colson, J., Sehgal, N., & Silverman, S. (2008). Opioid antagonists, partial agonists, and agonists/antagonists: The role of office-based detoxification. *Pain Physician, 11*(2), 225–235.

Hong, W. C., Yano, H., Hiranita, T., Chin, F. T., McCurdy, C. R., Su, T.-P., et al. (2017). The sigma-1 receptor modulates dopamine transporter conformation and cocaine binding and may thereby potentiate cocaine self-administration in rats. *The Journal of Biological Chemistry, 292*(27), 11250–11261. https://doi.org/https://doi.org/10.1074/jbc.M116.774075.

Horton, D. B., Nickell, J. R., Zheng, G., Crooks, P. A., & Dwoskin, L. P. (2013). GZ-793A, a lobelane analog, interacts with the vesicular monoamine transporter-2 to inhibit the effect of methamphetamine. *Journal of Neurochemistry, 127*(2), 177–186. https://doi.org/https://doi.org/10.1111/jnc.12371.

Hu, S., Sheng, W. S., & Rock, R. B. (2013). CB2 receptor agonists protect human dopaminergic neurons against damage from HIV-1 gp120. *PLoS One, 8*(10), e77577. https://doi.org/https://doi.org/10.1371/journal.pone.0077577.

Huang, M., He, W., Rajagopal, L., Kudwa, A., Grigoriadis, D. E., & Meltzer, H. Y. (2020). Effects of NBI-98782, a selective vesicular monoamine transporter 2 (VMAT2) inhibitor, on neurotransmitter efflux and phencyclidine-induced locomotor activity: Relevance to tardive dyskinesia and antipsychotic action. *Pharmacology, Biochemistry, and Behavior, 190*, 172872. https://doi.org/https://doi.org/10.1016/j.pbb.2020.172872.

Hudson, L., Liu, J., Nath, A., Jones, M., Raghavan, R., Narayan, O., et al. (2000). Detection of the human immunodeficiency virus regulatory protein tat in CNS tissues. *Journal of Neurovirology, 6*(2), 145–155.

Igari, M., Shen, H.-W., Hagino, Y., Fukushima, S., Kasahara, Y., Lesch, K.-P., et al. (2015). Attenuated methamphetamine-induced locomotor sensitization in serotonin transporter knockout mice is restored by serotonin 1B receptor antagonist treatment. *Behavioural Pharmacology, 26*(1–2), 167–179. https://doi.org/https://doi.org/10.1097/FBP.0000000000000120.

Iremonger, K. J., & Bains, J. S. (2009). Retrograde opioid signaling regulates glutamatergic transmission in the hypothalamus. *The Journal of Neuroscience, 29*(22), 7349–7358. https://doi.org/https://doi.org/10.1523/JNEUROSCI.0381-09.2009.

James, M. H., Fragale, J. E., O'Connor, S. L., Zimmer, B. A., & Aston-Jones, G. (2021). The orexin (hypocretin) neuropeptide system is a target for novel therapeutics to treat cocaine use disorder with alcohol coabuse. *Neuropharmacology, 183*, 108359. https://doi.org/https://doi.org/10.1016/j.neuropharm.2020.108359.

Jiang, R., Lee, I., Lee, T. A., & Pickard, A. S. (2017). The societal cost of heroin use disorder in the United States. *PLoS One, 12*(5), e0177323. https://doi.org/https://doi.org/10.1371/journal.pone.0177323.

Joffe, M. E., Centanni, S. W., Jaramillo, A. A., Winder, D. G., & Conn, P. J. (2018). Metabotropic glutamate receptors in alcohol use disorder: Physiology, plasticity, and promising pharmacotherapies. *ACS Chemical Neuroscience, 9*(9), 2188–2204. https://doi.org/https://doi.org/10.1021/acschemneuro.8b00200.

Johnson, L. A., Guptaroy, B., Lund, D., Shamban, S., & Gnegy, M. E. (2005). Regulation of amphetamine-stimulated dopamine efflux by protein kinase C beta. *The Journal of Biological Chemistry, 280*(12), 10914–10919. https://doi.org/https://doi.org/10.1074/jbc.M413887200.

Johnson, K. A., & Lovinger, D. M. (2020). Allosteric modulation of metabotropic glutamate receptors in alcohol use disorder: Insights from preclinical investigations. *Advances in Pharmacology, 88*, 193–232. https://doi.org/https://doi.org/10.1016/bs.apha.2020.02.002.

Johnson, T. P., Patel, K., Johnson, K. R., Maric, D., Calabresi, P. A., Hasbun, R., et al. (2013). Induction of IL-17 and nonclassical T-cell activation by HIV-tat protein. *Proceedings of the National Academy of Sciences of the United States of America, 110*(33), 13588–13593. https://doi.org/https://doi.org/10.1073/pnas.1308673110.

Johnston, J. B., Zhang, K., Silva, C., Shalinsky, D. R., Conant, K., Ni, W., et al. (2001). HIV-1 tat neurotoxicity is prevented by matrix metalloproteinase inhibitors. *Annals of Neurology*, *49*(2), 230–241. https://doi.org/10.1002/1531-8249(20010201)49:2<230::aid-ana43>3.0.co;2-o.

Jones, S. R., Gainetdinov, R. R., Wightman, R. M., & Caron, M. G. (1998). Mechanisms of amphetamine action revealed in mice lacking the dopamine transporter. *The Journal of Neuroscience*, *18*(6), 1979–1986. https://doi.org/https://doi.org/10.1523/JNEUROSCI.18-06-01979.1998.

Joo, Y.-H., Kim, J.-H., Kim, H.-K., Son, Y.-D., Cumming, P., & Kim, J.-H. (2021). Functional analysis of brain imaging suggests changes in the availability of mGluR5 and altered connectivity in the cerebral cortex of long-term abstaining males with alcohol dependence: A preliminary study. *Life (Basel, Switzerland)*, *11*(6). https://doi.org/10.3390/life11060506.

Kahlig, K. M., Binda, F., Khoshbouei, H., Blakely, R. D., McMahon, D. G., Javitch, J. A., et al. (2005). Amphetamine induces dopamine efflux through a dopamine transporter channel. *Proceedings of the National Academy of Sciences of the United States of America*, *102*(9), 3495–3500. https://doi.org/https://doi.org/10.1073/pnas.0407737102.

Karkhanis, A. N., & Al-Hasani, R. (2020). Dynorphin and its role in alcohol use disorder. *Brain Research*, *1735*, 146742. https://doi.org/https://doi.org/10.1016/j.brainres.2020.146742.

Karkhanis, A., Holleran, K. M., & Jones, S. R. (2017). Dynorphin/kappa opioid receptor signaling in preclinical models of alcohol, drug, and food addiction. *International Review of Neurobiology*, *136*, 53–88. https://doi.org/https://doi.org/10.1016/bs.irn.2017.08.001.

King, J. E., Eugenin, E. A., Buckner, C. M., & Berman, J. W. (2006). HIV tat and neurotoxicity. *Microbes and Infection*, *8*(5), 1347–1357. https://doi.org/https://doi.org/10.1016/j.micinf.2005.11.014.

Knackstedt, L. A., & Kalivas, P. W. (2009). Glutamate and reinstatement. *Current Opinion in Pharmacology*, *9*(1), 59–64. https://doi.org/https://doi.org/10.1016/j.coph.2008.12.003.

Koutsilieri, E., Sopper, S., Scheller, C., ter Meulen, V., & Riederer, P. (2002). Involvement of dopamine in the progression of AIDS dementia complex. *Journal of Neural Transmission*, *109*(3), 399–410. https://doi.org/https://doi.org/10.1007/s007020200032.

Kranzler, H. R., & Soyka, M. (2018). Diagnosis and pharmacotherapy of alcohol use disorder: A review. *The Journal of the American Medical Association*, *320*(8), 815–824. https://doi.org/https://doi.org/10.1001/jama.2018.11406.

Kruyer, A., & Kalivas, P. W. (2021). Astrocytes as cellular mediators of cue reactivity in addiction. *Current Opinion in Pharmacology*, *56*, 1–6. https://doi.org/https://doi.org/10.1016/j.coph.2020.07.009.

Kumar, A. M., Fernandez, J. B., Singer, E. J., Commins, D., Waldrop-Valverde, D., Ownby, R. L., et al. (2009). Human immunodeficiency virus type 1 in the central nervous system leads to decreased dopamine in different regions of postmortem human brains. *Journal of Neurovirology*, *15*(3), 257–274. https://doi.org/https://doi.org/10.1080/13550280902973952.

Kumar, A. M., Ownby, R. L., Waldrop-Valverde, D., Fernandez, B., & Kumar, M. (2011). Human immunodeficiency virus infection in the CNS and decreased dopamine availability: Relationship with neuropsychological performance. *Journal of Neurovirology*, *17*(1), 26–40. https://doi.org/https://doi.org/10.1007/s13365-010-0003-4.

Kupnicka, P., Kojder, K., Metryka, E., Kapczuk, P., Jeżewski, D., Gutowska, I., et al. (2020). Morphine-element interactions: The influence of selected chemical elements on neural pathways associated with addiction. *Journal of Trace Elements in Medicine and Biology*, *60*, 126495. https://doi.org/https://doi.org/10.1016/j.jtemb.2020.126495.

Lachowicz, M., Chmielowiec, J., Chmielowiec, K., Suchanecka, A., Masiak, J., Michałowska-Sawczyn, M., et al. (2020). Significant association of *DRD2* and *ANKK1* genes with rural heroin dependence and relapse in men. *Annals of Agricultural and Environmental Medicine: AAEM, 27*(2), 269–273. https://doi.org/10.26444/aaem/119940.

LaLumiere, R. T., & Kalivas, P. W. (2008). Glutamate release in the nucleus accumbens core is necessary for heroin seeking. *The Journal of Neuroscience, 28*(12), 3170–3177. https://doi.org/https://doi.org/10.1523/JNEUROSCI.5129-07.2008.

Lamers, S. L., Salemi, M., Galligan, D. C., Morris, A., Gray, R., Fogel, G., et al. (2010). Human immunodeficiency virus-1 evolutionary patterns associated with pathogenic processes in the brain. *Journal of Neurovirology, 16*(3), 230–241. https://doi.org/https://doi.org/10.3109/13550281003735709.

Laviolette, S. R., & van der Kooy, D. (2004). The neurobiology of nicotine addiction: Bridging the gap from molecules to behaviour. *Nature Reviews. Neuroscience, 5*(1), 55–65. https://doi.org/https://doi.org/10.1038/nrn1298.

Li, W., Li, G., Steiner, J., & Nath, A. (2009). Role of tat protein in HIV neuropathogenesis. *Neurotoxicity Research, 16*(3), 205–220. https://doi.org/https://doi.org/10.1007/s12640-009-9047-8.

Li, T.-K., Volkow, N. D., Baler, R. D., & Egli, M. (2007). The biological bases of nicotine and alcohol co-addiction. *Biological Psychiatry, 61*(1), 1–3. https://doi.org/https://doi.org/10.1016/j.biopsych.2006.11.004.

Li, Y., Xia, B., Li, R., Yin, D., & Liang, W. (2017). Changes in expression of dopamine, its receptor, and transporter in nucleus Accumbens of heroin-addicted rats with brain-derived neurotrophic factor (BDNF) overexpression. *Medical Science Monitor, 23*, 2805–2815. https://doi.org/10.12659/msm.904670.

Liechti, M. E., & Markou, A. (2008). Role of the glutamatergic system in nicotine dependence. *CNS Drugs, 22*(9), 705–724. https://doi.org/https://doi.org/10.2165/00023210-200822090-00001.

Lipari, R. N., & Van Horn, S. L. (2017). Trends in substance use disorders among adults aged 18 or older. In *The CBHSQ report*. Rockville (MD): Substance Abuse and Mental Health Services Administration (US).

Liu, X., Jernigen, C., Gharib, M., Booth, S., Caggiula, A. R., & Sved, A. F. (2010). Effects of dopamine antagonists on drug cue-induced reinstatement of nicotine-seeking behavior in rats. *Behavioural Pharmacology, 21*(2), 153–160. https://doi.org/https://doi.org/10.1097/FBP.0b013e328337be95.

Ma, Y.-Y., Lee, B. R., Wang, X., Guo, C., Liu, L., Cui, R., et al. (2014). Bidirectional modulation of incubation of cocaine craving by silent synapse-based remodeling of prefrontal cortex to accumbens projections. *Neuron, 83*(6), 1453–1467. https://doi.org/https://doi.org/10.1016/j.neuron.2014.08.023.

Ma, H., & Zhu, G. (2014). The dopamine system and alcohol dependence. *Shanghai Archives of Psychiatry, 26*(2), 61–68. https://doi.org/https://doi.org/10.3969/j.issn.1002-0829.2014.02.002.

Maguire, P., Tsai, N., Kamal, J., Cometta-Morini, C., Upton, C., & Loew, G. (1992). Pharmacological profiles of fentanyl analogs at mu, delta and kappa opiate receptors. *European Journal of Pharmacology, 213*(2), 219–225. https://doi.org/https://doi.org/10.1016/0014-2999(92)90685-w.

Mameli-Engvall, M., Evrard, A., Pons, S., Maskos, U., Svensson, T. H., Changeux, J.-P., et al. (2006). Hierarchical control of dopamine neuron-firing patterns by nicotinic receptors. *Neuron, 50*(6), 911–921. https://doi.org/https://doi.org/10.1016/j.neuron.2006.05.007.

Mannangatti, P., Ramamoorthy, S., & Jayanthi, L. D. (2018). Interference of norepinephrine transporter trafficking motif attenuates amphetamine-induced locomotor hyperactivity and conditioned place preference. *Neuropharmacology, 128*, 132–141. https://doi.org/https://doi.org/10.1016/j.neuropharm.2017.10.005.

Mansvelder, H. D., Keath, J. R., & McGehee, D. S. (2002). Synaptic mechanisms underlie nicotine-induced excitability of brain reward areas. *Neuron*, *33*(6), 905–919. https://doi.org/https://doi.org/10.1016/s0896-6273(02)00625-6.

Mansvelder, H. D., & McGehee, D. S. (2000). Long-term potentiation of excitatory inputs to brain reward areas by nicotine. *Neuron*, *27*(2), 349–357. https://doi.org/https://doi.org/10.1016/s0896-6273(00)00042-8.

Mantle, T. J., Tipton, K. F., & Garrett, N. J. (1976). Inhibition of monoamine oxidase by amphetamine and related compounds. *Biochemical Pharmacology*, *25*(18), 2073–2077. https://doi.org/https://doi.org/10.1016/0006-2952(76)90432-9.

Mantsch, J. R., Baker, D. A., Funk, D., Lê, A. D., & Shaham, Y. (2016). Stress-induced reinstatement of drug seeking: 20 years of Progress. *Neuropsychopharmacology*, *41*(1), 335–356. https://doi.org/https://doi.org/10.1038/npp.2015.142.

Mao, D., Gallagher, K., & McGehee, D. S. (2011). Nicotine potentiation of excitatory inputs to ventral tegmental area dopamine neurons. *The Journal of Neuroscience*, *31*(18), 6710–6720. https://doi.org/https://doi.org/10.1523/JNEUROSCI.5671-10.2011.

Matsui, A., & Alvarez, V. A. (2018). Cocaine inhibition of synaptic transmission in the ventral pallidum is pathway-specific and mediated by serotonin. *Cell Reports*, *23*(13), 3852–3863. https://doi.org/https://doi.org/10.1016/j.celrep.2018.05.076.

Mauna, J. C., Harris, S. S., Pino, J. A., Edwards, C. M., DeChellis-Marks, M. R., Bassi, C. D., et al. (2019). G protein βγ subunits play a critical role in the actions of amphetamine. *Translational Psychiatry*, *9*(1), 81. https://doi.org/https://doi.org/10.1038/s41398-019-0387-8.

Maurice, T., & Su, T.-P. (2009). The pharmacology of sigma-1 receptors. *Pharmacology & Therapeutics*, *124*(2), 195–206. https://doi.org/https://doi.org/10.1016/j.pharmthera.2009.07.001.

Mayer, F. P., Schmid, D., Owens, W. A., Gould, G. G., Apuschkin, M., Kudlacek, O., et al. (2018). An unsuspected role for organic cation transporter 3 in the actions of amphetamine. *Neuropsychopharmacology*, *43*(12), 2408–2417. https://doi.org/https://doi.org/10.1038/s41386-018-0053-5.

Meiser, J., Weindl, D., & Hiller, K. (2013). Complexity of dopamine metabolism. *Cell Communication and Signaling: CCS*, *11*(1), 34. https://doi.org/https://doi.org/10.1186/1478-811X-11-34.

Meyer, R. E. (2020). Pharmacotherapy of substance use disorders. *Journal of Clinical Psychopharmacology*, *40*(4), 330–333. https://doi.org/https://doi.org/10.1097/JCP.0000000000001218.

Midde, N. M., Huang, X., Gomez, A. M., Booze, R. M., Zhan, C.-G., & Zhu, J. (2013). Mutation of tyrosine 470 of human dopamine transporter is critical for HIV-1 tat-induced inhibition of dopamine transport and transporter conformational transitions. *Journal of Neuroimmune Pharmacology*, *8*(4), 975–987. https://doi.org/https://doi.org/10.1007/s11481-013-9464-6.

Midde, N. M., Yuan, Y., Quizon, P. M., Sun, W.-L., Huang, X., Zhan, C.-G., et al. (2015). Mutations at tyrosine 88, lysine 92 and tyrosine 470 of human dopamine transporter result in an attenuation of HIV-1 tat-induced inhibition of dopamine transport. *Journal of Neuroimmune Pharmacology*, *10*(1), 122–135. https://doi.org/https://doi.org/10.1007/s11481-015-9583-3.

Miller, C. N., & Kamens, H. M. (2020). The role of nicotinic acetylcholine receptors in alcohol-related behaviors. *Brain Research Bulletin*, *163*, 135–142. https://doi.org/https://doi.org/10.1016/j.brainresbull.2020.07.017.

Mongi-Bragato, B., Avalos, M. P., Guzmán, A. S., Bollati, F. A., & Cancela, L. M. (2018). Enkephalin as a pivotal player in neuroadaptations related to psychostimulant addiction. *Frontiers in Psychiatry*, *9*, 222. https://doi.org/https://doi.org/10.3389/fpsyt.2018.00222.

Morales, M., & Margolis, E. B. (2017). Ventral tegmental area: Cellular heterogeneity, connectivity and behaviour. *Nature Reviews. Neuroscience*, *18*(2), 73–85. https://doi.org/https://doi.org/10.1038/nrn.2016.165.

Morisot, N., & Ron, D. (2017). Alcohol-dependent molecular adaptations of the NMDA receptor system. *Genes, Brain, and Behavior*, *16*(1), 139–148. https://doi.org/https://doi.org/10.1111/gbb.12363.

Nataf, S. (2020). An alteration of the dopamine synthetic pathway is possibly involved in the pathophysiology of COVID-19. *Journal of Medical Virology*, *92*(10), 1743–1744. https://doi.org/https://doi.org/10.1002/jmv.25826.

Nath, A., Jankovic, J., & Pettigrew, L. C. (1987). Movement disorders and AIDS. *Neurology*, *37*(1), 37–41. https://doi.org/https://doi.org/10.1212/wnl.37.1.37.

Nath, A., Maragos, W. F., Avison, M. J., Schmitt, F. A., & Berger, J. R. (2001). Acceleration of HIV dementia with methamphetamine and cocaine. *Journal of Neurovirology*, 7(1), 66–71. https://doi.org/https://doi.org/10.1080/135502801300069737.

Natividad, L. A., Tejeda, H. A., Torres, O. V., & O'Dell, L. E. (2010). Nicotine withdrawal produces a decrease in extracellular levels of dopamine in the nucleus accumbens that is lower in adolescent versus adult male rats. *Synapse*, *64*(2), 136–145. https://doi.org/https://doi.org/10.1002/syn.20713.

Neumann, P. A., Wang, Y., Yan, Y., Wang, Y., Ishikawa, M., Cui, R., et al. (2016). Cocaine-induced synaptic alterations in thalamus to nucleus Accumbens projection. *Neuropsychopharmacology*, *41*(9), 2399–2410. https://doi.org/https://doi.org/10.1038/npp.2016.52.

NIAAA. (2021). *Understanding Alcohol Use Disorder*. NIAAA.

Nickell, J. R., Siripurapu, K. B., Vartak, A., Crooks, P. A., & Dwoskin, L. P. (2014). The vesicular monoamine transporter-2: An important pharmacological target for the discovery of novel therapeutics to treat methamphetamine abuse. *Advances in Pharmacology*, *69*, 71–106. https://doi.org/https://doi.org/10.1016/B978-0-12-420118-7.00002-0.

NIDA. (2019). *Methamphetamine drug facts*. NIDA.

NIDA. (2020). *How is cocaine addiction treated?*. NIDA.

Nordahl, T. E., Salo, R., & Leamon, M. (2003). Neuropsychological effects of chronic methamphetamine use on neurotransmitters and cognition: A review. *The Journal of Neuropsychiatry and Clinical Neurosciences*, *15*(3), 317–325. https://doi.org/https://doi.org/10.1176/jnp.15.3.317.

Novak, G., Seeman, P., & Le Foll, B. (2010). Exposure to nicotine produces an increase in dopamine D2(high) receptors: A possible mechanism for dopamine hypersensitivity. *The International Journal of Neuroscience*, *120*(11), 691–697. https://doi.org/https://doi.org/10.3109/00207454.2010.513462.

Palpacuer, C., Duprez, R., Huneau, A., Locher, C., Boussageon, R., Laviolle, B., et al. (2018). Pharmacologically controlled drinking in the treatment of alcohol dependence or alcohol use disorders: A systematic review with direct and network meta-analyses on nalmefene, naltrexone, acamprosate, baclofen and topiramate. *Addiction*, *113*(2), 220–237. https://doi.org/https://doi.org/10.1111/add.13974.

Paris, J. J., Carey, A. N., Shay, C. F., Gomes, S. M., He, J. J., & McLaughlin, J. P. (2014). Effects of conditional central expression of HIV-1 tat protein to potentiate cocaine-mediated psychostimulation and reward among male mice. *Neuropsychopharmacology*, *39*(2), 380–388. https://doi.org/https://doi.org/10.1038/npp.2013.201.

Paterson, N. E. (2009). Behavioural and pharmacological mechanisms of bupropion's anti-smoking effects: Recent preclinical and clinical insights. *European Journal of Pharmacology*, *603*(1–3), 1–11. https://doi.org/https://doi.org/10.1016/j.ejphar.2008.12.009.

Pergolizzi, J. V., Webster, L. R., Vortsman, E., Ann LeQuang, J., & Raffa, R. B. (2021). Wooden chest syndrome: The atypical pharmacology of fentanyl overdose. *Journal of Clinical Pharmacy and Therapeutics*. https://doi.org/10.1111/jcpt.13484.

Peterson, C., Li, M., Xu, L., Mikosz, C. A., & Luo, F. (2021). Assessment of annual cost of substance use disorder in US hospitals. *JAMA Network Open*, *4*(3), e210242. https://doi.org/https://doi.org/10.1001/jamanetworkopen.2021.0242.

Pettit, H. O., Ettenberg, A., Bloom, F. E., & Koob, G. F. (1984). Destruction of dopamine in the nucleus accumbens selectively attenuates cocaine but not heroin self-administration in rats. *Psychopharmacology*, *84*(2), 167–173. https://doi.org/https://doi.org/10.1007/BF00427441.

Petzold, J., Szumlinski, K. K., & London, E. D. (2021). Targeting mGlu5 for methamphetamine use disorder. *Pharmacology & Therapeutics*, *224*, 107831. https://doi.org/https://doi.org/10.1016/j.pharmthera.2021.107831.

Pourzitaki, C., Tsaousi, G., Papazisis, G., Kyrgidis, A., Zacharis, C., Kritis, A., et al. (2018). Fentanyl and naloxone effects on glutamate and GABA release rates from anterior hypothalamus in freely moving rats. *European Journal of Pharmacology*, *834*, 169–175. https://doi.org/https://doi.org/10.1016/j.ejphar.2018.07.029.

Power, C., McArthur, J. C., Nath, A., Wehrly, K., Mayne, M., Nishio, J., et al. (1998). Neuronal death induced by brain-derived human immunodeficiency virus type 1 envelope genes differs between demented and nondemented AIDS patients. *Journal of Virology*, *72*(11), 9045–9053. https://doi.org/https://doi.org/10.1128/JVI.72.11.9045-9053.1998.

Prochaska, J. J., & Benowitz, N. L. (2016). The past, present, and future of nicotine addiction therapy. *Annual Review of Medicine*, *67*, 467–486. https://doi.org/https://doi.org/10.1146/annurev-med-111314-033712.

Purohit, V., Rapaka, R., & Shurtleff, D. (2011). Drugs of abuse, dopamine, and HIV-associated neurocognitive disorders/HIV-associated dementia. *Molecular Neurobiology*, *44*(1), 102–110. https://doi.org/https://doi.org/10.1007/s12035-011-8195-z.

Quadir, S. G., Cottone, P., & Sabino, V. (2019). Role of sigma receptors in alcohol addiction. *Frontiers in Pharmacology*, *10*, 687. https://doi.org/https://doi.org/10.3389/fphar.2019.00687.

Quizon, P. M., Sun, W.-L., Yuan, Y., Midde, N. M., Zhan, C.-G., & Zhu, J. (2016). Molecular mechanism: The human dopamine transporter histidine 547 regulates basal and HIV-1 tat protein-inhibited dopamine transport. *Scientific Reports*, *6*, 39048. https://doi.org/https://doi.org/10.1038/srep39048.

Rappaport, J., Joseph, J., Croul, S., Alexander, G., Del Valle, L., Amini, S., et al. (1999). Molecular pathway involved in HIV-1-induced CNS pathology: Role of viral regulatory protein, tat. *Journal of Leukocyte Biology*, *65*(4), 458–465. https://doi.org/https://doi.org/10.1002/jlb.65.4.458.

Ravna, A. W., Sylte, I., & Dahl, S. G. (2003). Molecular mechanism of citalopram and cocaine interactions with neurotransmitter transporters. *The Journal of Pharmacology and Experimental Therapeutics*, *307*(1), 34–41. https://doi.org/https://doi.org/10.1124/jpet.103.054593.

Reynolds, J. L., Mahajan, S. D., Sykes, D., & Nair, M. P. N. (2006). Heroin-induces differential protein expression by Normal human astrocytes (NHA). *American Journal of Infectious Diseases*, *2*(2), 49–57. https://doi.org/https://doi.org/10.3844/ajidsp.2006.49.57.

Rocha, B. A., Fumagalli, F., Gainetdinov, R. R., Jones, S. R., Ator, R., Giros, B., et al. (1998). Cocaine self-administration in dopamine-transporter knockout mice. *Nature Neuroscience*, *1*(2), 132–137. https://doi.org/https://doi.org/10.1038/381.

Rook, E. J., Huitema, A. D. R., van den Brink, W., van Ree, J. M., & Beijnen, J. H. (2006). Pharmacokinetics and pharmacokinetic variability of heroin and its metabolites: Review of the literature. *Current Clinical Pharmacology*, *1*(1), 109–118. https://doi.org/https://doi.org/10.2174/157488406775268219.

Rothman, R. B., Baumann, M. H., Dersch, C. M., Romero, D. V., Rice, K. C., Carroll, F. I., et al. (2001). Amphetamine-type central nervous system stimulants release norepinephrine more potently than they release dopamine and serotonin. *Synapse*, *39*(1), 32–41. https://doi.org/10.1002/1098-2396(20010101)39:1<32::AID-SYN5>3.0.CO;2-3.
Saal, D., Dong, Y., Bonci, A., & Malenka, R. C. (2003). Drugs of abuse and stress trigger a common synaptic adaptation in dopamine neurons. *Neuron*, *37*(4), 577–582. https://doi.org/https://doi.org/10.1016/s0896-6273(03)00021-7.
Samaha, A.-N., Khoo, S. Y.-S., Ferrario, C. R., & Robinson, T. E. (2021). Dopamine "ups and downs" in addiction revisited. *Trends in Neurosciences*, *44*(7), 516–526. https://doi.org/https://doi.org/10.1016/j.tins.2021.03.003.
Sambo, D. O., Lin, M., Owens, A., Lebowitz, J. J., Richardson, B., Jagnarine, D. A., et al. (2017). The sigma-1 receptor modulates methamphetamine dysregulation of dopamine neurotransmission. *Nature Communications*, *8*(1), 2228. https://doi.org/https://doi.org/10.1038/s41467-017-02087-x.
Sardar, A. M., Czudek, C., & Reynolds, G. P. (1996). Dopamine deficits in the brain: The neurochemical basis of parkinsonian symptoms in AIDS. *Neuroreport*, 7(4), 910–912. https://doi.org/https://doi.org/10.1097/00001756-199603220-00015.
Sari, Y., & Sreemantula, S. N. (2012). Neuroimmunophilin GPI-1046 reduces ethanol consumption in part through activation of GLT1 in alcohol-preferring rats. *Neuroscience*, *227*, 327–335. https://doi.org/https://doi.org/10.1016/j.neuroscience.2012.10.007.
Sawynok, J. (1986). The therapeutic use of heroin: A review of the pharmacological literature. *Canadian Journal of Physiology and Pharmacology*, *64*(1), 1–6. https://doi.org/https://doi.org/10.1139/y86-001.
Scheller, C., Arendt, G., Nolting, T., Antke, C., Sopper, S., Maschke, M., et al. (2010). Increased dopaminergic neurotransmission in therapy-naïve asymptomatic HIV patients is not associated with adaptive changes at the dopaminergic synapses. *Journal of Neural Transmission*, *117*(6), 699–705. https://doi.org/https://doi.org/10.1007/s00702-010-0415-6.
Schmidt, H. D., Rupprecht, L. E., & Addy, N. A. (2019). Neurobiological and neurophysiological mechanisms underlying nicotine seeking and smoking relapse. *Molecular Neuropsychiatry*, *4*(4), 169–189. https://doi.org/https://doi.org/10.1159/000494799.
Sekine, Y., Ouchi, Y., Takei, N., Yoshikawa, E., Nakamura, K., Futatsubashi, M., et al. (2006). Brain serotonin transporter density and aggression in abstinent methamphetamine abusers. *Archives of General Psychiatry*, *63*(1), 90–100. https://doi.org/https://doi.org/10.1001/archpsyc.63.1.90.
Sepulveda, M., Manning, E. E., Gogos, A., Hale, M., & van den Buuse, M. (2021). Long-term effects of young-adult methamphetamine on dorsal raphe serotonin systems in mice: Role of brain-derived neurotrophic factor. *Brain Research*, *1762*, 147428. https://doi.org/https://doi.org/10.1016/j.brainres.2021.147428.
Seth, P., Scholl, L., Rudd, R. A., & Bacon, S. (2018). Overdose deaths involving opioids, cocaine, and psychostimulants - United States, 2015-2016. *MMWR. Morbidity and Mortality Weekly Report*, *67*(12), 349–358. https://doi.org/10.15585/mmwr.mm6712a1.
Sharma, A., Kelly, S. M., Mitchell, S. G., Gryczynski, J., O'Grady, K. E., & Schwartz, R. P. (2017). Update on barriers to pharmacotherapy for opioid use disorders. *Current Psychiatry Reports*, *19*(6), 35. https://doi.org/https://doi.org/10.1007/s11920-017-0783-9.
Shen, H., Chen, K., Marino, R. A. M., McDevitt, R. A., & Xi, Z.-X. (2021). Deletion of VGLUT2 in midbrain dopamine neurons attenuates dopamine and glutamate responses to methamphetamine in mice. *Pharmacology, Biochemistry, and Behavior*, *202*, 173104. https://doi.org/https://doi.org/10.1016/j.pbb.2021.173104.
Shippenberg, T. S., Zapata, A., & Chefer, V. I. (2007). Dynorphin and the pathophysiology of drug addiction. *Pharmacology & Therapeutics*, *116*(2), 306–321. https://doi.org/https://doi.org/10.1016/j.pharmthera.2007.06.011.

Siciliano, C. A., Calipari, E. S., Ferris, M. J., & Jones, S. R. (2014). Biphasic mechanisms of amphetamine action at the dopamine terminal. *The Journal of Neuroscience*, *34*(16), 5575–5582. https://doi.org/https://doi.org/10.1523/JNEUROSCI.4050-13.2014.

Siefried, K. J., Acheson, L. S., Lintzeris, N., & Ezard, N. (2020). Pharmacological treatment of methamphetamine/amphetamine dependence: A systematic review. *CNS Drugs*, *34*(4), 337–365. https://doi.org/https://doi.org/10.1007/s40263-020-00711-x.

Sitte, H. H., & Freissmuth, M. (2015). Amphetamines, new psychoactive drugs and the monoamine transporter cycle. *Trends in Pharmacological Sciences*, *36*(1), 41–50. https://doi.org/https://doi.org/10.1016/j.tips.2014.11.006.

Smaga, I., Sanak, M., & Filip, M. (2019). Cocaine-induced changes in the expression of NMDA receptor subunits. *Current Neuropharmacology*, *17*(11), 1039–1055. https://doi.org/https://doi.org/10.2174/1570159X17666190617101726.

Smart, R., Pardo, B., & Davis, C. S. (2021). Systematic review of the emerging literature on the effectiveness of naloxone access laws in the United States. *Addiction*, *116*(1), 6–17. https://doi.org/https://doi.org/10.1111/add.15163.

Somerville, N. J., O'Donnell, J., Gladden, R. M., Zibbell, J. E., Green, T. C., Younkin, M., et al. (2017). Characteristics of fentanyl overdose - Massachusetts, 2014-2016. *MMWR. Morbidity and Mortality Weekly Report*, *66*(14), 382–386. https://doi.org/10.15585/mmwr.mm6614a2.

Soontornniyomkij, V., Kesby, J. P., Morgan, E. E., Bischoff-Grethe, A., Minassian, A., Brown, G. G., et al. (2016). Effects of HIV and methamphetamine on brain and behavior: Evidence from human studies and animal models. *Journal of Neuroimmune Pharmacology*, *11*(3), 495–510. https://doi.org/https://doi.org/10.1007/s11481-016-9699-0.

Sorkina, T., Cheng, M. H., Bagalkot, T. R., Wallace, C., Watkins, S. C., Bahar, I., et al. (2021). Direct coupling of oligomerization and oligomerization-driven endocytosis of the dopamine transporter to its conformational mechanics and activity. *The Journal of Biological Chemistry*, *100430*. https://doi.org/https://doi.org/10.1016/j.jbc.2021.100430.

Stennett, B. A., Padovan-Hernandez, Y., & Knackstedt, L. A. (2020). Sequential cocaine-alcohol self-administration produces adaptations in rat nucleus accumbens core glutamate homeostasis that are distinct from those produced by cocaine self-administration alone. *Neuropsychopharmacology*, *45*(3), 441–450. https://doi.org/https://doi.org/10.1038/s41386-019-0452-2.

Stoicea, N., Costa, A., Periel, L., Uribe, A., Weaver, T., & Bergese, S. D. (2019). Current perspectives on the opioid crisis in the US healthcare system: A comprehensive literature review. *Medicine*, *98*(20), e15425. https://doi.org/https://doi.org/10.1097/MD.0000000000015425.

Strauss, M., O'Donovan, B., Ma, Y., Xiao, Z., Lin, S., Bardo, M. T., et al. (2020). [3H]dopamine uptake through the dopamine and norepinephrine transporters is decreased in the prefrontal cortex of transgenic mice expressing HIV-1 Transactivator of transcription protein. *The Journal of Pharmacology and Experimental Therapeutics*, *374*(2), 241–251. https://doi.org/https://doi.org/10.1124/jpet.120.266023.

Sulzer, D., Sonders, M. S., Poulsen, N. W., & Galli, A. (2005). Mechanisms of neurotransmitter release by amphetamines: A review. *Progress in Neurobiology*, *75*(6), 406–433. https://doi.org/https://doi.org/10.1016/j.pneurobio.2005.04.003.

Sun, J., Chen, S.-R., Chen, H., & Pan, H.-L. (2019). μ-Opioid receptors in primary sensory neurons are essential for opioid analgesic effect on acute and inflammatory pain and opioid-induced hyperalgesia. *The Journal of Physiology*, *597*(6), 1661–1675. https://doi.org/https://doi.org/10.1113/JP277428.

Sun, W.-L., Quizon, P. M., Yuan, Y., Zhang, W., Ananthan, S., Zhan, C.-G., et al. (2017). Allosteric modulatory effects of SRI-20041 and SRI-30827 on cocaine and HIV-1 tat protein binding to human dopamine transporter. *Scientific Reports*, 7(1), 3694. https://doi.org/https://doi.org/10.1038/s41598-017-03771-0.

Sustkova-Fiserova, M., Puskina, N., Havlickova, T., Lapka, M., Syslova, K., Pohorala, V., et al. (2020). Ghrelin receptor antagonism of fentanyl-induced conditioned place preference, intravenous self-administration, and dopamine release in the nucleus accumbens in rats. *Addiction Biology*, *25*(6), e12845. https://doi.org/https://doi.org/10.1111/adb.12845.

Szumlinski, K. K., Lominac, K. D., Campbell, R. R., Cohen, M., Fultz, E. K., Brown, C. N., et al. (2017). Methamphetamine addiction vulnerability: The glutamate, the bad, and the ugly. *Biological Psychiatry*, *81*(11), 959–970. https://doi.org/https://doi.org/10.1016/j.biopsych.2016.10.005.

Takahashi, N., Miner, L. L., Sora, I., Ujike, H., Revay, R. S., Kostic, V., et al. (1997). VMAT2 knockout mice: Heterozygotes display reduced amphetamine-conditioned reward, enhanced amphetamine locomotion, and enhanced MPTP toxicity. *Proceedings of the National Academy of Sciences of the United States of America*, *94*(18), 9938–9943. https://doi.org/https://doi.org/10.1073/pnas.94.18.9938.

Torralva, R., Eshleman, A. J., Swanson, T. L., Schmachtenberg, J. L., Schutzer, W. E., Bloom, S. H., et al. (2020). Fentanyl but not morphine interacts with nonopioid recombinant human neurotransmitter receptors and transporters. *The Journal of Pharmacology and Experimental Therapeutics*, *374*(3), 376–391. https://doi.org/https://doi.org/10.1124/jpet.120.265561.

Torralva, R., & Janowsky, A. (2019). Noradrenergic mechanisms in fentanyl-mediated rapid death explain failure of naloxone in the opioid crisis. *The Journal of Pharmacology and Experimental Therapeutics*, *371*(2), 453–475. https://doi.org/https://doi.org/10.1124/jpet.119.258566.

Trivedi, M. H., Walker, R., Ling, W., Dela Cruz, A., Sharma, G., Carmody, T., et al. (2021). Bupropion and naltrexone in methamphetamine use disorder. *The New England Journal of Medicine*, *384*(2), 140–153. https://doi.org/https://doi.org/10.1056/NEJMoa2020214.

Uhl, G. R., Koob, G. F., & Cable, J. (2019). The neurobiology of addiction. *Annals of the New York Academy of Sciences*, *1451*(1), 5–28. https://doi.org/https://doi.org/10.1111/nyas.13989.

Underhill, S. M., Colt, M. S., & Amara, S. G. (2020). Amphetamine stimulates endocytosis of the norepinephrine and neuronal glutamate transporters in cultured locus coeruleus neurons. *Neurochemical Research*, *45*(6), 1410–1419. https://doi.org/https://doi.org/10.1007/s11064-019-02939-6.

United Nations Office on Drugs and Crime (UNODC). (2020). *World drug report 2020: Booklet 2 - drug use and health consequences*. (United Nations).

Valentino, R. J., & Volkow, N. D. (2018). Untangling the complexity of opioid receptor function. *Neuropsychopharmacology*, *43*(13), 2514–2520. https://doi.org/https://doi.org/10.1038/s41386-018-0225-3.

Vlachou, S., Guery, S., Froestl, W., Banerjee, D., Benedict, J., Finn, M. G., et al. (2011). Repeated administration of the GABAB receptor positive modulator BHF177 decreased nicotine self-administration, and acute administration decreased cue-induced reinstatement of nicotine seeking in rats. *Psychopharmacology*, *215*(1), 117–128. https://doi.org/https://doi.org/10.1007/s00213-010-2119-x.

Vo, Q. N., Mahinthichaichan, P., Shen, J., & Ellis, C. R. (2021). How μ-opioid receptor recognizes fentanyl. *Nature Communications*, *12*(1), 984. https://doi.org/https://doi.org/10.1038/s41467-021-21262-9.

Volkow, N. D. (2021). The epidemic of fentanyl misuse and overdoses: Challenges and strategies. *World Psychiatry: Official Journal of the World Psychiatric Association (WPA)*, *20*(2), 195–196. https://doi.org/https://doi.org/10.1002/wps.20846.

Volkow, N. D., Jones, E. B., Einstein, E. B., & Wargo, E. M. (2019). Prevention and treatment of opioid misuse and addiction: A review. *JAMA Psychiatry*, *76*(2), 208–216. https://doi.org/https://doi.org/10.1001/jamapsychiatry.2018.3126.

Volkow, N. D., Wang, G.-J., Fowler, J. S., & Tomasi, D. (2012). Addiction circuitry in the human brain. *Annual Review of Pharmacology and Toxicology*, *52*, 321–336. https://doi.org/https://doi.org/10.1146/annurev-pharmtox-010611-134625.

Wang, S. (2019). Historical review: Opiate addiction and opioid receptors. *Cell Transplantation*, *28*(3), 233–238. https://doi.org/https://doi.org/10.1177/0963689718811060.

Wang, X.-F., Barbier, E., Chiu, Y.-T., He, Y., Zhan, J., Bi, G.-H., et al. (2016). T394A mutation at the μ opioid receptor blocks opioid tolerance and increases vulnerability to heroin self-administration in mice. *The Journal of Neuroscience*, *36*(40), 10392–10403. https://doi.org/https://doi.org/10.1523/JNEUROSCI.0603-16.2016.

Wang, G.-J., Chang, L., Volkow, N. D., Telang, F., Logan, J., Ernst, T., et al. (2004). Decreased brain dopaminergic transporters in HIV-associated dementia patients. *Brain: A Journal of Neurology*, *127*(Pt 11), 2452–2458. https://doi.org/https://doi.org/10.1093/brain/awh269.

Wang, H.-Y., Frankfurt, M., & Burns, L. H. (2008). High-affinity naloxone binding to filamin a prevents mu opioid receptor-Gs coupling underlying opioid tolerance and dependence. *PLoS One*, *3*(2), e1554. https://doi.org/https://doi.org/10.1371/journal.pone.0001554.

Westendorp, M. O., Frank, R., Ochsenbauer, C., Stricker, K., Dhein, J., Walczak, H., et al. (1995). Sensitization of T cells to CD95-mediated apoptosis by HIV-1 tat and gp120. *Nature*, *375*(6531), 497–500. https://doi.org/https://doi.org/10.1038/375497a0.

Wise, R. A., & Bozarth, M. A. (1987). A psychomotor stimulant theory of addiction. *Psychological Review*, *94*(4), 469–492. https://doi.org/https://doi.org/10.1037/0033-295X.94.4.469.

Wise, R. A., & Koob, G. F. (2014). The development and maintenance of drug addiction. *Neuropsychopharmacology*, *39*(2), 254–262. https://doi.org/https://doi.org/10.1038/npp.2013.261.

Wittenberg, R. E., Wolfman, S. L., De Biasi, M., & Dani, J. A. (2020). Nicotinic acetylcholine receptors and nicotine addiction: A brief introduction. *Neuropharmacology*, *177*, 108256. https://doi.org/https://doi.org/10.1016/j.neuropharm.2020.108256.

Wolf, M. E., Xue, C. J., Li, Y., & Wavak, D. (2000). Amphetamine increases glutamate efflux in the rat ventral tegmental area by a mechanism involving glutamate transporters and reactive oxygen species. *Journal of Neurochemistry*, *75*(4), 1634–1644. https://doi.org/https://doi.org/10.1046/j.1471-4159.2000.0751634.x.

Womersley, J. S., & Uys, J. D. (2016). S-Glutathionylation and redox protein signaling in drug addiction. *Progress in Molecular Biology and Translational Science*, *137*, 87–121. https://doi.org/https://doi.org/10.1016/bs.pmbts.2015.10.001.

Xiao, H., Neuveut, C., Tiffany, H. L., Benkirane, M., Rich, E. A., Murphy, P. M., et al. (2000). Selective CXCR4 antagonism by tat: Implications for in vivo expansion of coreceptor use by HIV-1. *Proceedings of the National Academy of Sciences of the United States of America*, *97*(21), 11466–11471. https://doi.org/https://doi.org/10.1073/pnas.97.21.11466.

Xu, L., & Chen, L. Y. (2020). Identification of a new allosteric binding site for cocaine in dopamine transporter. *Journal of Chemical Information and Modeling*, *60*(8), 3958–3968. https://doi.org/https://doi.org/10.1021/acs.jcim.0c00346.

Xu, S., Liu, Y., Li, Y., Deng, Y., Yuan, J., Lv, R., et al. (2017). Availability of dopamine transporters in heroin-dependent subjects: A 18F-FECNT PET imaging study. *Psychiatry Research: Neuroimaging*, *263*, 121–126. https://doi.org/https://doi.org/10.1016/j.pscychresns.2017.03.011.

Yin, F., Ji, Y., Zhang, J., Guo, H., Huang, X., Lai, J., et al. (2016). Polymorphisms in the 5-hydroxytryptamine receptor 3B gene are associated with heroin dependence in the Chinese Han population. *Neuroscience Letters*, *635*, 123–129. https://doi.org/https://doi.org/10.1016/j.neulet.2016.10.033.

Yoshida, Y., Koide, S., Hirose, N., Takada, K., Tomiyama, K., Koshikawa, N., et al. (1999). Fentanyl increases dopamine release in rat nucleus accumbens: Involvement of mesolimbic mu- and delta-2-opioid receptors. *Neuroscience*, *92*(4), 1357–1365. https://doi.org/https://doi.org/10.1016/s0306-4522(99)00046-9.

Yuan, Y., Huang, X., Midde, N. M., Quizon, P. M., Sun, W.-L., Zhu, J., et al. (2015). Molecular mechanism of HIV-1 tat interacting with human dopamine transporter. *ACS Chemical Neuroscience*, *6*(4), 658–665. https://doi.org/https://doi.org/10.1021/acschemneuro.5b00001.

Yuan, Y., Huang, X., Zhu, J., & Zhan, C.-G. (2016). Computational modeling of human dopamine transporter structures, mechanism and its interaction with HIV-1 transactivator of transcription. *Future Medicinal Chemistry*, *8*(17), 2077–2089. https://doi.org/https://doi.org/10.4155/fmc-2016-0138.

Zhan, J., Jordan, C. J., Bi, G.-H., He, X.-H., Gardner, E. L., Wang, Y.-L., et al. (2018). Genetic deletion of the dopamine D3 receptor increases vulnerability to heroin in mice. *Neuropharmacology*, *141*, 11–20. https://doi.org/https://doi.org/10.1016/j.neuropharm.2018.08.016.

Zhang, H., & Bramham, C. R. (2020). Bidirectional dysregulation of AMPA receptor-mediated synaptic transmission and plasticity in brain disorders. *Frontiers in Synaptic Neuroscience*, *12*, 26. https://doi.org/https://doi.org/10.3389/fnsyn.2020.00026.

Zhu, J., Ananthan, S., Mactutus, C. F., & Booze, R. M. (2011). Recombinant human immunodeficiency virus-1 transactivator of transcription1-86 allosterically modulates dopamine transporter activity. *Synapse*, *65*(11), 1251–1254. https://doi.org/https://doi.org/10.1002/syn.20949.

Zhu, J., Mactutus, C. F., Wallace, D. R., & Booze, R. M. (2009). HIV-1 tat protein-induced rapid and reversible decrease in [3H]dopamine uptake: Dissociation of [3H]dopamine uptake and [3H]2beta-carbomethoxy-3-beta-(4-fluorophenyl)tropane (WIN 35,428) binding in rat striatal synaptosomes. *The Journal of Pharmacology and Experimental Therapeutics*, *329*(3), 1071–1083. https://doi.org/https://doi.org/10.1124/jpet.108.150144.

Zhu, F., Wu, Q., Li, J., Grycel, K., Liu, B., Sun, X., et al. (2017). A single dose of cocaine potentiates glutamatergic synaptic transmission onto locus coeruleus neurons. *Cell Calcium*, *67*, 11–20. https://doi.org/https://doi.org/10.1016/j.ceca.2017.07.007.

Zhu, J., Yuan, Y., Midde, N. M., Gomez, A. M., Sun, W.-L., Quizon, P. M., et al. (2016). HIV-1 transgenic rats display an increase in [(3)H]dopamine uptake in the prefrontal cortex and striatum. *Journal of Neurovirology*, *22*(3), 282–292. https://doi.org/https://doi.org/10.1007/s13365-015-0391-6.

Zinsmaier, A. K., Dong, Y., & Huang, Y. H. (2021). Cocaine-induced projection-specific and cell type-specific adaptations in the nucleus accumbens. *Molecular Psychiatry*. https://doi.org/10.1038/s41380-021-01112-2.

Zislis, G., Desai, T. V., Prado, M., Shah, H. P., & Bruijnzeel, A. W. (2007). Effects of the CRF receptor antagonist D-Phe CRF(12-41) and the alpha2-adrenergic receptor agonist clonidine on stress-induced reinstatement of nicotine-seeking behavior in rats. *Neuropharmacology*, *53*(8), 958–966. https://doi.org/https://doi.org/10.1016/j.neuropharm.2007.09.007.

Zoli, M., Pucci, S., Vilella, A., & Gotti, C. (2018). Neuronal and extraneuronal nicotinic acetylcholine receptors. *Current Neuropharmacology*, *16*(4), 338–349. https://doi.org/https://doi.org/10.2174/1570159X15666170912110450.

Kolibri 360 GmbH
Ferdinand-Jühlke-Straße 7
99095 Erfurt, Deutschland
produktsicherheit@kolibri360.de